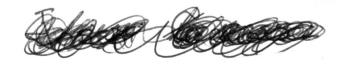

THE PRINCIPLES AND PRACTICE OF

ADDICTIONS IN PSYCHIATRY

NORMAN S. MILLER, M.D.
Associate Professor of Psychiatry and Neurology
Chief of Division of Addiction Programs
Departments of Psychiatry and Neurology
University of Illinois at Chicago
Chicago, Illinois

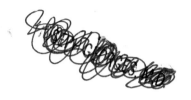

THE PRINCIPLES AND PRACTICE OF
ADDICTIONS IN PSYCHIATRY

W.B. SAUNDERS COMPANY
A Division of Harcourt Brace & Company
Philadelphia • London • Toronto • Montreal • Sydney • Tokyo

W.B. SAUNDERS COMPANY
A Division of Harcourt Brace & Company

The Curtis Center
Independence Square West
Philadelphia, Pennsylvania 19106

Library of Congress Cataloging-in-Publication Data

The principles and practice of addictions in psychiatry / [edited] by Norman S.
Miller.

p.   cm.

ISBN 0–7216–5211–5

1. Dual diagnosis.   2. Substance abuse.   I. Miller, Norman S.
   [DNLM: 1. Behavior, Addictive—psychology.   2. Behavior, Addictive—
   diagnosis.   3. Behavior, Addictive—therapy.   4. Mental Disorders.
   WM 176 P957 1997]

RC564.68.P75   1997   616.86—dc20

DNLM/DLC   95–20662

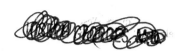

To those who wish to treat addicted patients without threat of judgment and fear of stigma.

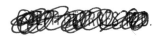

CONTRIBUTORS

Susan Adams, M.A.
Project Coordinator, Program for Mental Health Services Research on Women and Gender, Department of Psychiatry, University of Illinois, Chicago, Illinois
The Course of Alcoholism in Men and Women

John P. Allen, Ph.D., M.P.A.
Chief, Treatment Research Branch, National Institute of Alcohol Abuse and Alcoholism, Rockville, Maryland
Experimental Pharmacological Agents to Reduce Alcohol, Cocaine, and Opiate Use

Jacqueline M. Amato, M.D.
Psychiatry Resident, University of Illinois, Chicago, Illinois
Treatment of Addiction in Adolescent Populations

Robert M. Anthenelli, M.D.
Assistant Professor of Psychiatry, University of California, San Diego, School of Medicine, La Jolla, California; Director, Dual Diagnosis Treatment Program, San Diego Veterans Affairs Medical Center, San Diego, California
A Basic Clinical Approach to Diagnosis in Patients with Comorbid Psychiatric and Substance Use Disorders

Frank J. Ayd, Jr., M.D.
Clinical Professor of Psychiatry, West Virginia University, Charleston Division, Charleston, West Virginia; Emeritus Director of Education and Research, Taylor Manor Hospital, Ellicott City, Maryland; Editor, International Drug Therapy Newsletter, Baltimore, Maryland
Psychopharmacotherapy for the Addicted Borderline or Antisocial Patient

Dennis Beedle, M.D.
Assistant Professor, Department of Psychiatry, University of Illinois College of Medicine, Chicago, Illinois
Differential Diagnosis of Substance Abuse and Dependence

Laura J. Bierut, M.D.
Instructor, Washington University School of Medicine, Department of Psychiatry, St. Louis, Missouri
Familial and Genetic Studies of Comorbidity of Addictive and Psychiatric Disorders

Sheila B. Blume, M.D., C.A.C.
Clinical Professor of Psychiatry, State University of New York at Stony Brook, School of Medicine, Stony Brook, New York; Medical Director, Alcoholism, Chemical Dependency, and Compulsive Gambling Programs, South Oaks Hospital, Amityville, New York
Pathological Gambling

Remi J. Cadoret, M.D.
Professor of Psychiatry, Department of Psychiatry, University of Iowa School of Medicine, Iowa City, Iowa
Genetic Factors in Human Drug Abuse and Addiction

Zack Zdenek Cernovsky, Ph.D., C. Psych.
Assistant Professor, Faculty of Medicine, University of Western Ontario, London, Ontario, Canada; Director of Research and Program Evaluation, Addiction Rehabilitation Unit, St. Thomas Psychiatric Hospital, St. Thomas, Ontario, Canada
Implementing a Dual-Diagnosis Program and Treatment Outcome

John N. Chappel, M.D.
Professor of Psychiatry, School of Medicine, University of Nevada, Reno, Nevada; Medical Director Addictions Programs, West Hills Hospital, Reno, Nevada
Addiction Psychiatry and Long-Term Recovery in 12-Step Programs; Spirituality and Addiction Psychiatry

Ondrej Chudoba, M.D.
Assistant Professor of Psychiatry, University of Illinois at Chicago, Department of Psychiatry, Chicago, Illinois; Staff Physician, Veterans Affairs West Side Medical Center, Chicago, Illinois
Consultation/Liaison: An Intervention in Drug and Alcohol Addiction

Gregory B. Collins, M.D.
Assistant Professor, Ohio State University College of Medicine, Columbus, Ohio; Section Head, Alcohol and Drug Recovery Center, Department of Psychiatry, The Cleveland Clinic Foundation, Cleveland, Ohio
Inpatient and Outpatient Treatment of Alcoholism—Essential Features; Emerging Concepts of Alcoholism Treatment: Challenges and Controversies

Wilson M. Compton, III, M.D.
Assistant Professor of Psychiatry, Washington University School of Medicine, St. Louis, Missouri
The Medical Basis of Addictive Disorders

Amin N. Daghestani, M.D.
Professor of Psychiatry, Loyola University Medical Center, Maywood, Illinois; Director of Graduate Education in Psychiatry, Loyola University Medical Center, Maywood, Illinois
Forensic and Ethical Issues in Addiction Psychiatry

John M. Davis, M.D.
Gilman Professor of Psychiatry and Research Professor of Medicine, University of Illinois at Chicago, Chicago, Illinois; Director of Research, Illinois State Psychiatric Institute, Chicago, Illinois
Neurochemical Findings in Alcoholism and Drug Addiction and Psychiatric Comorbidity; Psychopharmacotherapy for the Addicted Borderline or Antisocial Patient; Psychopharmacotherapy for the Dually Diagnosed: Novel Approaches

Eric Devor, Ph.D.
Assistant Professor, Department of Psychiatry, University of Iowa College of Medicine, Iowa City, Iowa
Genetic Factors in Human Drug Abuse and Addiction

Stephen H. Dinwiddie, M.D.
Assistant Professor of Psychiatry, Washington University School of Medicine, Department of Psychiatry, St. Louis, Missouri; Attending Staff, Barnes Hospital, St. Louis, Missouri
Genetics of Alcoholism; Familial and Genetic Studies of Comorbidity of Addictive and Psychiatric Disorders

Robert E. Drake, M.D., Ph.D.
Professor of Psychiatry and Community and Family Medicine, Dartmouth Medical School, Lebanon, New Hampshire; Director, New Hampshire–Dartmouth Psychiatric Research Center, Concord, New Hampshire
Treatment of Comorbid Disorders with a Case Manager Approach

Robert L. DuPont, M.D.
Clinical Professor of Psychiatry, Georgetown University School of Medicine-Medical Center, Washington, D.C.
Psychotherapy in Addictive Disorders

Michael S. Easton, M.D.
Assistant Professor, Rush Medical College of Rush University, Chicago, Illinois; Director, Rush Chemical Dependency Program; Medical Director, Alcoholism Research Program, Rush Presbyterian–St. Luke's Medical Center, Chicago, Illinois
Treatment Outcomes for Addictive Disorders in Psychiatric Settings

Jan Fawcett, M.D.
Professor and Chairman, Department of Psychiatry, Rush Medical College of Rush University, Rush Presbyterian–St. Luke's Medical Center, Chicago, Illinois
Treatment Outcomes for Addictive Disorders in Psychiatric Settings

James Fine, M.D.
Addictive Disease Hospital, Brooklyn, New York
Epidemiology of Comorbidity in Addiction Psychiatry

Joseph A. Flaherty, M.D.
Professor and Deputy Head, Department of Psychiatry, University of
Illinois at Chicago, Chicago, Illinois
*The Course of Alcoholism in Men and Women; Managed Care for Psychiatric and
Addictive Disorders*

Marc Galanter, M.D.
Professor of Psychiatry, New York University, New York, New York;
Director, Division of Alcoholism and Drug Abuse, New York University
Medical Center, New York, New York
Network Therapy: A Practical Approach to the Office Treatment of Addiction

David R. Gastfriend, M.D.
Assistant Professor, Harvard Medical School, Boston, Massachusetts; Chief,
Addiction Services, Department of Psychiatry, Massachusetts General
Hospital, Boston, Massachusetts
Pharmacological Treatments for Psychiatric Symptoms in Addiction Populations

Mark S. Gold, M.D.
Professor, University of Florida Brain Institute, Departments of
Neuroscience, Psychiatry, Community Health and Family Medicine,
College of Medicine, Gainesville, Florida
*The Neurobiology of Addictive Disorders: The Role of Dopamine, Endorphin, and
Serotonin; Eating Disorders and Addictions: Behavioral and Neurobiological
Similarities*

David L. Goldberg, M.D.
Department of Psychiatry, University of Illinois at Chicago, Chicago,
Illinois
Treatment of Adolescent Addiction and Behavior Disorders

R. Jeffrey Goldsmith, M.D.
Associate Professor of Clinical Psychiatry, Department of Psychiatry,
College of Medicine, University of Cincinnati, Cincinnati, Ohio; Staff
Psychiatrist, Director of Addiction Medicine Fellowship, Cincinnati
Veterans Affairs Medical Center, Cincinnati, Ohio
*The Integrated Psychology for Addiction Psychiatry; The Elements of
Contemporary Treatment*

David A. Gorelick, M.D., Ph.D.
Chief, Treatment Branch, National Institute on Drug Abuse, Baltimore,
Maryland
*Experimental Pharmacological Agents to Reduce Alcohol, Cocaine, and Opiate
Use*

Samuel B. Guze, M.D.
Professor of Psychiatry and Head, Department of Psychiatry, Washington
University School of Medicine, St. Louis, Missouri
The Medical Basis of Addictive Disorders

Norman G. Hoffmann, Ph.D.
Hoffmann Health Care Institute, Minneapolis, Minnesota
Abstinence-Based Treatment and Depression

Richard R. Irons, M.D.
Associate Program Director, Alcohol and Drug Abuse Program, The
Menninger Clinic, Topeka, Kansas
Addictive Sexual Disorders

Carl Isenhart, Psy.D.
Assistant Professor, Department of Psychiatry, University of Minnesota
School of Medicine, Minneapolis, Minnesota; Administrative Coordinator,
Addictive Disorders Section, Department of Veterans Affairs Medical
Center, Minneapolis, Minnesota
New and Experimental Psychosocial Therapies in Alcoholism and Addiction

Philip G. Janicak, M.D.
Professor of Psychiatry, University of Illinois at Chicago, Chicago, Illinois;
Medical Director, Psychiatric Institute, University of Illinois at Chicago,
Chicago, Illinois
*Psychopharmacotherapy for the Addicted Borderline or Antisocial Patient;
Psychopharmacotherapy for the Dually Diagnosed: Novel Approaches*

Sajiv John, M.D.
Resident, Department of Psychiatry, The University of Chicago Hospitals,
Chicago, Illinois
Anxiety Disorders and Addictions

Steven M. Juergens, M.D.
Assistant Clinical Professor of Psychiatry, University of Washington,
Seattle, Washington; Medical Director, Virginia Mason Outpatient
Chemical Dependency Program, Virginia Mason Medical Center, Seattle,
Washington
Benzodiazepines, Other Sedative, Hypnotic, and Anxiolytic Drugs, and Addiction

Yifrah Kaminer, M.D.
Associate Professor of Psychiatry, Department of Psychiatry, University of
Connecticut Health Center, Farmington, Connecticut; Faculty at the
Alcohol Research Center, University of Connecticut Health Center,
Farmington, Connecticut
Pharmacotherapy for Adolescents with Psychoactive Substance Use Disorders

Kathleen Kim, M.D.
Visiting Associate Professor, Department of Psychiatry, University of
Illinois at Chicago, Chicago, Illinois; Associate Director of Clinical Services,
Department of Psychiatry, University of Illinois at Chicago, Chicago,
Illinois
*The Course of Alcoholism in Men and Women; Managed Care for Psychiatric and
Addictive Disorders*

Debra L. Klamen, M.D.
Director, Undergraduate Medical Education in Psychiatry, Department of
Psychiatry, University of Illinois, Chicago, Illinois
Abstinence-Based Treatment and Depression

Lial Kofoed, M.D., M.S.

Professor, Department of Psychiatry, University of South Dakota School of
Medicine, Sioux Falls, South Dakota; Chief of Psychiatry, Royal C. Johnson
Veterans Affairs Medical Center, Sioux Falls, South Dakota
Engagement and Persuasion

Mary Langley, M.D.

Assistant Professor of Clinical Psychiatry, University of Illinois College of
Medicine, Chicago, Illinois; Staff Physician (Inpatient Section), Veterans
Affairs West Side Medical Center, Chicago, Illinois
Posttramatic Stress Disorders and Addiction: What Are the Links?

Michael Levy, Ph.D.

Faculty Member, Zinberg Center for Addiction Studies, Harvard Medical
School, Boston, Massachusetts; Clinical Director, Center for Behavioral
Medicine, Southwood Community Hospital, Norfolk, Massachusetts
Group Therapy in Addictive and Psychiatric Disorders

Raye Z. Litten, Ph.D.

Treatment Research Branch, National Institute on Alcohol Abuse and
Alcoholism; Rockville, Maryland
*Experimental Pharmacological Agents to Reduce Alcohol, Cocaine, and Opiate
Use*

Craig McKenna, M.D.

Associate Professor of Clinical Psychiatry, Department of Psychiatry,
University of Illinois at Chicago, Chicago, Illinois; Chief, Consult-liaison
Psychiatry Section, Department of Psychiatry, Veterans Affairs West Side
Medical Center, Chicago, Illinois
*Neurocognitive Syndromes and Neuroimaging in Addictions; Substance-Induced
Psychiatric Disorders*

Laura J. Miller, M.D.

Assistant Professor, Department of Psychiatry, University of Illinois at
Chicago, Chicago, Illinois; Director, Women's Inpatient Treatment Service
and Director, Parenting Assessment Team, University of Illinois at
Chicago, Chicago, Illinois
Pharmacological Treatments for Addiction in Pregnant Populations

Norman S. Miller, M.D.

Associate Professor of Psychiatry and Neurology, Chief of Division of
Addiction Programs, Departments of Psychiatry and Neurology,
University of Illinois at Chicago, Chicago, Illinois
*Epidemiology of Comorbidity in Addiction Psychiatry; Generalized Vulnerability
to Drug and Alcohol Addiction; Intervention for Drug/Alcohol Addiction in
Acute Psychiatric Presentations; Anxiety Disorders and Addictions; Treatment of
Addictive and Depressive Disorders; Abstinence-Based Treatment and Depression*

Kenneth Minkoff, M.D.

Assistant Professor of Psychiatry, Cambridge Hospital Department of
Psychiatry, Harvard Medical School, Boston, Massachusetts; Medical
Director, Choate Integrated Behavioral Care, Woburn, Massachusetts
Integration of Addiction and Psychiatric Treatment

Robert E. Murray, M.D., Ph.D.
Assistant Professor, Department of Psychiatry, University of Tennessee,
School of Medicine, Memphis, Tennessee; Medical Director, Chemical
Dependency Center, Veterans Administration Medical Center, Memphis,
Tennessee
Treatment of Addiction and Psychotic Disorders

Catherine A. Nageotte, M.D., M.S.H.S.
Assistant Professor, Psychiatry, University of Illinois at Chicago, Chicago,
Illinois
*Treatment of Addiction in Adolescent Populations; Treatment of Adolescent
Addiction and Behavior Disorders*

Douglas L. Noordsy, M.D.
Assistant Professor of Psychiatry, Dartmouth Medical School, Lebanon,
New Hampshire; Psychiatrist, West Central Community Mental Health
Center, Lebanon, New Hampshire
Treatment of Comorbid Disorders with a Case Manager Approach

Ghanshyam N. Pandey, Ph.D.
Professor of Pharmacology in Psychiatry, The Psychiatric Institute, College
of Medicine, University of Illinois, Chicago, Illinois
*Neurochemical Findings in Alcoholism and Drug Addiction and Psychiatric
Comorbidity*

Subhash C. Pandey, Ph.D.
Assistant Professor of Biochemistry in Psychiatry, The Psychiatric Institute,
Department of Psychiatry, College of Medicine, University of Illinois at
Chicago, Chicago, Illinois
*Neurochemical Findings in Alcoholism and Drug Addiction and Psychiatric
Comorbidity*

Bradley M. Pechter, M.D.
Assistant Professor of Psychiatry, Department of Psychiatry, University of
Illinois at Chicago, College of Medicine, Chicago, Illinois
*Psychopharmacotherapy for the Addicted Borderline or Antisocial Patient;
Psychopharmacotherapy for the Dually Diagnosed: Novel Approaches*

Maureen Pennington, M.D., FRCP(C)
Lecturer, University of Western Ontario, London, Ontario, Canada;
Director, Addiction Rehabilitation Unit, St. Thomas Psychiatric Hospital,
St. Thomas, Ontario, Canada
Implementing a Dual-Diagnosis Program and Treatment Outcome

Kenzie Preston, Ph.D.
Treatment Branch, National Institute on Drug Abuse, Baltimore, Maryland
*Experimental Pharmacological Agents to Reduce Alcohol, Cocaine, and Opiate
Use*

Valerie D. Raskin, M.D.
Assistant Professor of Psychiatry, University of Illinois at Chicago,
Chicago, Illinois
Treatment of Addiction in Childbearing Populations

Richard K. Ries, M.D.

Associate Professor of Psychiatry, University of Washington, Seattle, Washington; Director of Outpatient Psychiatry, Harborview Medical Center, Seattle, Washington
Treatment of Addiction and Psychotic Disorders

Jennifer P. Schneider, M.D., Ph.D.

Medical Director, Kachina Center for Addiction Recovery, Tucson, Arizona
Addictive Sexual Disorders

Richard B. Seymour, M.A.

Instructor, Department of Psychology, John F. Kennedy University, Orinda, California; President and CEO, Westwind Associates, Sausalito, California; Consultant, Haight-Ashbury Free Clinics Inc, San Francisco, California
Treatment of Protracted Drug-Induced Syndromes

Andrew Edmund Slaby, M.D., Ph.D., M.P.H.

Clinical Professor of Psychiatry, New York University, New York, New York; Adjunct Clinical Professor of Psychiatry, New York Medical College, New York, New York; Board Member, American Suicide Foundation, New York, New York; President, Eastern Division of the American Suicide Foundation, New York, New York; Editorial Board Member, *Primary Psychiatry.*
Treatment of Addictive Disorders in Emergency Populations

Christopher Sinnappan, M.D.

Assistant Professor, Department of Psychiatry, University of Illinois at Chicago Medical Center, Chicago, Illinois
Treatment of Addictive and Depressive Disorders

David E. Smith, M.D.

Associate Clinical Professor of Occupational Health and Clinical Toxicology, University of California, San Francisco, California; Visiting Associate Clinical Professor of Behavioral Pharmacology, University of Nevada Medical School, Reno, Nevada; President and Founder, Haight-Ashbury Free Clinics Inc, San Francisco, California; President, American Society of Addiction Medicine, Chevy Chase, Maryland
Treatment of Protracted Drug-Induced Syndromes

Michael D. Stein, M.D.

Assistant Professor, Brown University School of Medicine, Providence, Rhode Island; Director of HIV Activities, Rhode Island Hospital, Providence, Rhode Island
Medical Disorders in Addicted Patients

Karen A. Stennie, M.D.

Resident, Department of Psychiatry, University of Florida, Gainesville, Florida
Eating Disorders and Addictions: Behavioral and Neurobiological Similarities

Robert M. Swift, M.D., Ph.D.

Associate Professor, Department of Psychiatry and Human Behavior, Brown University Medical School, Providence, Rhode Island; Psychiatrist-in-Chief, Roger Williams Medical Center, Providence, Rhode Island
Pharmacological Treatment of Alcoholism: Clinical Management

Mark C. Wallen, M.D.

Clinical Assistant Professor, Department of Mental Health Sciences, Hahnemann University, Philadelphia, Pennsylvania; Medical/Clinical Director, Livengrin Foundation, Bensalem, Pennsylvania
Addiction and Psychiatric Settings

William W. Weddington, M.D.

Associate Professor of Clinical Psychiatry, University of Illinois at Chicago, Chicago, Illinois; Chief, Addiction Psychiatry Service, Veterans Affairs West Side Medical Center, Chicago, Illinois
Pharmacological Interventions for Withdrawal Syndromes Other Than Alcohol and Nicotine

Joseph Westermeyer, M.D., Ph.D.

Professor of Psychiatry, University of Minnesota, Minneapolis, Minnesota; Chief of Psychiatry, Minneapolis Veterans Affairs Medical Center, Minneapolis, Minnesota
New and Experimental Psychosocial Therapies in Alcoholism and Addiction

William Yates, M.D.

Associate Professor of Psychiatry, University of Iowa College of Medicine, Iowa City, Iowa; Director, General Hospital Psychiatry, University of Iowa Hospitals and Clinics, Iowa City, Iowa
Genetic Factors in Human Drug Abuse and Addiction

PREFACE

The principles and practice of addictions have assumed central importance in the field of psychiatry. Addictive disorders affect a large patient population within psychiatry. Substantial interest has arisen and movement has occurred toward the diagnosis and treatment of comorbid addictive and psychiatric disorders. Many factors have contributed to the emergence of the principles and practices of addictions in psychiatry. First, the overall prevalence of addictive disorders has increased dramatically in recent decades, particularly in traditional psychiatric populations. More than 50% of psychiatric patients have substance-related disorders. Second, research in addictions has contributed to major shifts in diagnostic approaches that have been illustrated in the diagnostic and statistical manuals. Substance-related disorders have moved away from being subsumed under Personality Disorders in *DSM-I* and *DSM-II* to a relatively independent status in *DSM-III* and *DSM-IV*. Third, the growth of primary care medicine will probably secure addictions treatment as a standard of practice in managed care and capitation in patient populations. Fourth, advances in clinical skill and research knowledge have created a broad base for clinical principles and practices in addictions for the physician, particularly the psychiatrist and primary care physician. Fifth, the establishment of specialization in addiction psychiatry and addiction medicine has generated board certification standards and fellowships in addiction psychiatry and certification in addiction medicine.

Other factors beyond the objectives of the book have conspired to open new interest in developing strategies and practices for assessment and treatment of patients with addictive disorders, particularly in psychiatric and primary care settings. Sections and divisions of addiction psychiatry and addiction medicine are appearing in academic centers. Increased awareness and expansion of education and training in undergraduate medical education and residency programs are occurring throughout medical schools and departments.

A major focus of the book is addictive disorders in psychiatric patients. The organization is designed to highlight an integrative approach to the diagnosis and treatment of addictions in psychiatric populations. The theme of the book purposefully reflects the complex interactions between addictive and psychiatric disorders and attempts to show that a reductionist approach to either disorder is fraught with confusion. The adoption of sound principles and practices in management of addictions requires adequate clarity around essential points in diagnosis and treatment. Most of the acknowledged advances have been in diagnostic approaches. Effective treatment methods for addictive disorders have existed for decades, but only recently have they been employed by psychiatric staff. Further, modification of these treatment methods is indicated to provide integrated addictions treatment in psychiatric patients.

The scope and depth of *The Principles and Practice of Addictions in Psychiatry* are illustrated by the presentation of the book in sections: *I Etiology, II Neurobiology, III Diagnosis, IV Treatment Approach, V Treatment Process,* and *VI Pharmacological Treatments.* The authors represent the leadership in research principles and clinical practice in addictions. The approach of the book is eclectic and integrative in that it provides the biopsychosocial basis for addictive and psychiatric disorders for the psychiatrist, primary care physician, and other members of the multidisciplinary team who often participate in the care of patients with substance-related disorders.

The hope of the editor and one shared by the authors is that those who read this book will apply the knowledge and skills it presents to patient care and research studies for the ultimate benefit of patients. In no small measure will the common denominator of addictions across psychiatric populations provide coalescence around which professionals can rally to advance their missions and goals. Although the book thoughtfully depicts the history of where we have been in addictions, ultimately it is hoped that it will provide a vision of where we must go to continue our exciting adventure in this rapidly advancing field.

I am deeply grateful to my assistant, Jane Guttman, for her invaluable and exceptional work in the preparation of this book.

NORMAN S. MILLER, M.D.

CONTENTS

VI PHARMACOLOGICAL TREATMENTS

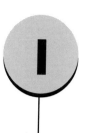

ETIOLOGY

The Integrated Psychology for Addiction Psychiatry

R. Jeffrey Goldsmith, MD

Alcoholism and drug addictions have occurred throughout the centuries, and observers have theorized about the etiology and dynamics for just as long. The disorders have intrigued and baffled the learned throughout the ages. More recently, the epidemic use and abuse of alcohol, tobacco, cocaine, marijuana, and other substances have challenged many physicians, psychologists, psychoanalysts, and psychotherapists to describe the motivation to use alcohol and drugs, as well as the dynamics that are acted out over and over again with family, friends, and therapists. These theories of behavior—these descriptions of the psyche—become important insofar as they shape the technology of treatment and the development of addiction psychiatry.

The last half of this century has seen a massive expansion of treatment and treatment paradigms, all of which are based on a description of alcoholic or addicted patients. Concurrently, research into the addictions has proceeded at an equally expansive rate, especially research into the biology of alcoholism and addictions. If these psychological descriptions are accurate, they contain important insights that must be retained and combined with the new biological understanding. Although medicine deals with the biopsychosocial model, operationalizing such a model is difficult and challenging. A new psychology—a psychology that integrates the old insights, the new biology, and family/group dynamics—would facilitate this challenge and forms the basis of addiction psychiatry.

Previous Psychologies

The twentieth century opened with the birth of psychoanalysis and a burgeoning of psychoanalytical theories, psychological systems based on the information gathered during sessions of free association and interpretations based on the theories of Freud, Jung, and others. Two of the early classics describing alcoholism and addiction were written by Glover[1] and Rado.[2] Glover emphasized the maladaptive aspect of an alcoholic patient's behavior and the flight from a real impasse into a world of fantasy. The regression into fantasy follows the layers of psychic development with alcoholism and the frequent intoxication "heading towards an infantile end, an oral regression." Projection is considered characteristic of all alcoholics. Ego development is described as the frustration of object relations with the subsequent investment of libido in the self, which produces a pathological narcissistic fixation. Once maladaptive heavy drinking begins, a vicious cycle of self-punishment, projected self-punishment, and punishment from the environment ensues, leading to escape drinking again.

Rado[2] had a different theory, focusing on the psychological motivation to use drugs. He interpreted drug cravings as a single disease, which he called *pharmacothymia*. He recognized a biological component, tolerance to euphoria, which he believed was crucial but unexplained, in the development of the pharmacothymic regimen, the state in which drugs are used to regulate a tense depression that worsens as guilt and environmental criticism are added as a consequence of each binge. Rado thought that the addictions were fundamentally a narcissistic disorder in which the self is invested with more than normal libido. He recognized the downward spiral of this situation, the desperate effort to escape the dysphoria through drugs, and the fear (based on tolerance) that the drugs, too, would fail. Additionally, Rado believed that the libidinal etiology of addictions was closely related to the oral level of development and homosexuality, the former resulting from a regressive or fixated level of development and the latter a developmental deviation.

During the 1940s and 1950s, Harry Tiebout was one of the prominent writers on the psychology of alcoholism. In his work,[3] he emphasized the role of psychological barriers, or unconscious defenses, in protecting the core self from a sense of nakedness or emptiness. The barriers are almost complete in alcoholics, shutting out stimuli from the environment and keeping in impulses from the core self. Normal people have barriers that screen out the hardest stimuli and keep in the impulses judged unacceptable, but these barriers are not as isolating as they are in alcoholics. For Tiebout, defiance was a critical trait among alcoholics not acknowledged by them until the barrier was understood. Defiance brings a sense of power, a "full" feeling that mobilizes energy, self-confidence, and empowerment, in contrast to an emptiness that is devoid of drive and of conviction. Defiance includes an outwardly directed aggression or hostility, whereas emptiness is characterized by a frozen, panic-stricken state. Tiebout recognized the self-deficits of self-care, self-protection, and self-esteem. The initial therapeutic task was to confront the defiance and the defensive nature of the barrier so the alcoholic would perceive reality and begin to suffer from the negative effects of alcoholism. Tiebout excelled in descriptions of the alcoholic's resistance to early and late treatment.[4] Although he used the language of the neo-Freudians, and later of ego psychology, he kept to the ideas of Alcoholics Anonymous (AA), which focused on the alcoholic's sense of self vis-à-vis alcohol.[5]

In the 1970s alcohol and drug use as well as alcoholism and drug dependence became epidemic and the demand for treatment of these disorders expanded. An understanding of the person who used the drugs became important because so many "experimenters" appeared, obscuring the line between healthiness and pathological dependence. Wurmser and Khantzian, more than any other theorists, provided the leading descriptions of drug addiction for the 1970s and 1980s.

Wurmser,[6] in his classic paper "Mr. Pecksniff's Horse?," laid down the principal elements of a drug addict's psychopathology. First and foremost, he thought that severe psychopathology was preexistent for those who develop a chronic dependence on drugs. He thought that it was crucial to understand these inner problems for effective treatment. Compulsiveness is the central concept for Wurmser, but he also recognized pathology in the formation of ideals. Another conceptual point is his emphasis on *complexity* of the problem list and, consequently, the treatment plan. He considered it naive to think that psychotherapy could be the only treatment, suggesting that "four to seven (or more) 'modalities' may have to be employed, concomitantly or sequentially." Wurmser[6] elegantly applies the psychoanalytical perspective to describe what he calls "the vicious circle in compulsive drug use." It begins with an acute narcissistic crisis, which leads to a regression resulting from an addict's inability to manage the intense affect. The defenses are mobilized, and much of the pain is externalized; however, the addict is left feeling defective and entitled as a compromise solution to the initial crisis. Drawing on Krystal[7] and Krystal and Raskin,[8] Wurmser further delves into the dynamics of affect regression and the breakdown of affect defense that are at the core of an addict's psychopathology. Drug use is an attempt to cope with a particular combination of painful feelings, a discovered solution to a difficult problem.

Khantzian[9] took a similar direction in his works, focusing on affect and drive defense, how a person handles intense affect and intense drives. He focused on Kohut's comment[10] that drugs act as a replacement for defects in the psychic structure, "helping" addicts cope with rage, shame, hurt, and loneliness. He designates these defects as ego impairments in self-care and self-regulation. Personal needs are repressed and disavowed in order to avoid the risk of narcissistic injury when wishes and wants are refused, disappointed, or ignored, leaving the addict feeling cut off, hollow, and empty. Treatment involved control over the addiction and the resultant destructive behavior through the use of institutions, prescribed drugs, and human relationships. Psychotherapy, for Khantzian, focused on the self-deficits because these left an addict vulnerable to the use of drugs, which in turn provided the motivation to use them for self-medication. "I believe a self-medication motive is one of the more compelling ones. There is both practical and heuristic value to consider that addicts are treating themselves for underlying psychiatric disorders and painful affect states." Elsewhere Khantzian elaborates, "It is too reductionist, however, to argue that physiologic or disease processes alone govern the complexities of a reliance on substances."[12]

Vaillant is one of the most influential psychodynamic theorists of the 1980s. His book *The Natural History of Alcoholism*[13] was the culmination of 30 years of prospective research into the etiology of alcoholism and recovery from it. As a psychoanalyst, he had every reason to favor a psychological explanation for alcoholism but argued eloquently in favor of the biological basis. His focus was less to describe the role of psychology than to warn the field that psychotherapy had an ancillary role in treatment. Affirming the disease concept as the organizing principle and renouncing the idea of the addictive personality were his most visible accomplishments. Through objective observation and a thorough review of the literature, he dispelled the old myths that impeded progress as long as experts gave them credibility.

The cognitive behaviorists, led by Beck,[14] were united with a different perspective. They explained maladaptive behaviors as products of aberrant beliefs about the self and the environment. Alcoholism and drug dependence are maladaptive coping mechanisms that can be minimized by strengthening problem-solving and coping skills. They focus more on relapse and the triggers that are associated with heavy drinking. Treatment is conceptualized as risk reduction through the anticipation of high-risk situations. By anticipating these risky moments, alternative strategies can be conceived, practiced, and implemented.

A few biopsychosocial models have been offered and do much to link different paradigms.[15, 16] They characterize the biology of addiction and the psychology of deficits as described by Wurmser and Khantzian. In addition, they point out family dynamics and group dynamic risks that increase the likelihood of alcohol or drug use. They describe the complexity of addictions and encourage multimodal treatments to respond to the diversity of problems.

Weaknesses and Strengths

For a better theory to be designed, the weaknesses must be understood and improved. Glover, Wurmser, and Khantzian leave biology out of their psychological systems. Glover omitted whatever biologies were known. Both Wurmser and Khantzian want their patients to be abstinent and to attend meetings of Alcoholics Anonymous if possible, but they both view compulsion (and addiction) as a function of psychopathology. Both describe pathological drug taking as an attempt to cope with overwhelming affect and drive states, focusing their psychotherapies on the recognition of these states and correction of the underlying deficits. By the mid-1980s, considerable knowledge had been gained about the genetics of alcoholism and the biology of tolerance, dependence, and drug reinforcement. Khantzian goes a step further to compare drug taking with a physician's prescribing medication for a painful psychiatric condition.[12]

The biological research and the psychosocial research just do not support this hypothesis. Animal studies have repeatedly demonstrated that certain drugs (such as cocaine or morphine), when injected into the nucleus accumbens and ventral tegmentum, respectively, lead to compulsive self-administration.[17] Furthermore, catecholamine depletion in these central nervous system areas is associated with reinforcement to use again, which can be attenuated by drugs such as bromocriptine.[18] Self-deficits and unhappy childhoods are irrelevant.

Research with human volunteers provides similar evidence for the biological motivation to use drugs. Self-administration studies by deWit and colleagues[19] revealed that (1) normal subjects do not like diazepam and do not want more, (2) anxious subjects do not want more diazepam despite feeling less anxious, (3) alcoholic subjects do want more diazepam, and (4) all subjects want more amphetamine. In more recent studies,[20] human subjects were given very small amounts of cocaine, which were identified the same as placebo (i.e., no euphoria). When offered microdoses (as low as 4 mg) of cocaine or placebo, the subjects thought they were selecting placebo; however, they consistently selected the microdoses of cocaine. This suggests that reinforcement may have nothing to do with getting high.

Other studies investigating the relationship between alcohol/drug use and mood observed that heavy drinking increased depression, even caused it, during acute intoxication.[21] Evidence showed that they drank a lot because they were depressed. Furthermore, when bipolar patients became depressed, many reduced their drinking and did not try to self-medicate.[22] Although almost all alcoholics report feeling depressed before detoxification—and about half tested in the moderate to severely depressed range—only about 10% met criteria for major depression according to the Diagnostic and Statistical Manual of Mental Disorders (DSM-III).[23] What seems more likely is that therapists become confused by the similarities and differences between mood, syndrome, and disorder when considering anxiety and depression.[24] Alcohol exaggerates both anxiety and depression, and alcoholics thus feel intense emotions, but the feelings often change quickly. In addition, alcohol and drugs *cause* organic mood and organic anxiety disorders. Although depression and anxiety are frequently associated with alcohol and drugs, they are most often a result of alcohol/drug use, not the motivation for it.

A second weakness of the studies is that they suggest the existence of an addictive personality, a prealcoholic personality. Vaillant's thorough review[13] of the leading prospective studies completely negates the previously held psychological myths. McCords' study,[25] a 15-year prospective study of teenagers, observed that men with oral tendencies and maternal encouragement of dependence were less likely to develop alcoholism. The men who developed alcoholism were outwardly more self-confident, less fearful, more aggressive, hyperactive, and more heterosexual. Robins[26] analyzed a 30-year study of disturbed juveniles. Those who developed alcoholism during the study period were *not more likely* to be impulsive, depressed, or unhappy premorbidly. In comparing the family life of future sociopaths and future alcoholics, they found no significant differences except that alcoholics received more consistent parental discipline.

A later study at the Institute of Human Development[27, 28] found that high-school boys who became alcoholic were characterized as "out of control, rebellious, pushing limits, self-indulgent and assertive"[27] but that the girls were "expressive, attractive, poised, and buoyant."[28] Loper and colleagues[29] reported that college students who later became alcoholic

were more compulsive, nonconforming, and gregarious than matched controls when assessed with a Minnesota Multiphasic Personality Inventory (MMPI). They also found that for a cohort of college students, the composite profile was within normal limits in college but pathologically elevated at the time when the men were hospitalized for alcoholism.

Vaillant's own 30-year study[13] found that bleak childhood environments, personality, instability in college, and evidence of premorbid personality disorder as adults all were correlated with oral-dependent behavior (pessimism, self-doubt, passivity, and dependence) but *not alcohol abuse*. In the college sample, an unhappy childhood led to adult mental illness, lack of friends, and low self-esteem but not alcoholism. Childhood environment seemed to predict use of tranquilizers and use of medicine for physical illness but not problem drinking in this nondelinquent sample. Parental alcoholism seemed to be relevant. Of 51 men with few childhood environmental weaknesses and parental alcoholism, 27% became alcoholic, but only 5% of 56 men with many environmental weaknesses but no parental alcoholism became alcohol dependent. In fact, alcoholism was most highly correlated with ethnicity and alcoholism in relatives.

High-Risk Youth

The work in prevention of teenage alcohol and drug use has added new data to the understanding of at-risk youth. Because the prevention research frequently investigates use rather than abuse/dependence, environmental factors are etiologically important. Most children are initiated to use of alcohol, tobacco, and drugs as adolescents, with the highest rates for initiation from 15 to 18 years of age for alcohol and marijuana.[30] Children who become involved with alcohol and drugs *before* adolescence may differ from those who begin later in adolescence, being more likely to engage in antisocial acts or severe aggression or to be shy or more likely to have a short attention span.[31] In addition, certain personality traits are associated with *preadolescent use*, including rebelliousness, sensation seeking, nonconformity with traditional values, high tolerance of deviance, resistance to traditional authority, strong need for independence, low self-esteem, and feeling a lack of control over one's life.

The first use of alcohol and drugs occurs in a social setting,[31] which makes peer pressure, positive group values toward using these substances, drug availability, pro-use norms in the community, parental lack of concern, and lax school policies risk factors for alcohol and drug use. Time in an unsupervised setting is also a risk factor. Children who are abused/neglected or handicapped, runaways, pregnant teens, dropouts, or the children of alcoholics/drug addicts are significantly at risk. Many of these factors cluster in alcoholic/addicted or abusive families. However, alcohol and drug use is not necessarily alcohol/drug dependence.

Longitudinal studies with adolescent and young adult subjects have reached conclusions that are consistent with the prospective studies reported by Vaillant. Newcomb and Bentler[32] reviewed several prospective studies in their book on adolescent drug use. They reported more life problems, especially deviant behavior, as a result of adolescent drug use (including marijuana use). Alcohol use seemed to produce deviant behavior among adolescents but not among young adults. Newcomb and Bentler's large prospective study of 1600 teenagers replicated this finding for alcohol and general drug use. Interestingly, alcohol use was associated with less social conformity in adulthood but not less deviant behavior. Newcomb and Bentler thought that evidence supported the concept of a teenage deviant behavior syndrome, of which drug use was part; however, they pointed out that the adult sequelae of this syndrome were varied and not uniform. In this study, the best predictors of alcohol and drug abuse problems as adults were teenage use and teenage deviant behavior.

When these studies are combined with the others, several important points emerge: (1) Familial alcoholism and drug addiction have a strong genetic influence in the development of alcoholism and addiction. (2) There is no prealcoholic or addictive personality type. (3) Teenage alcohol and drug use creates problems but does not predict addiction. More use causes more problems and heavy use as an adult. (4) Evidence suggests a teenage deviant behavior syndrome that includes drinking and drug use. Affected adolescents do grow up to have alcoholism and drug addiction along with their deviant behavior. This would be a subpopulation of the total alcohol and drug-dependent population.

Self-Psychology

Self-psychology relies on an experience near perspective, in which empathy is the definer of the field of relevant information and the empathic connection is the basis for its healing transformations.[33, 34] The self is considered the primary subjective experience, and the attainment and maintenance of a sense of cohesive wholeness (vital, dynamic, and capable) are a major psychological motivation.[35] Through the use of other people and things, the self borrows qualities, skills, and talents to experience wholeness. These relationships are called self–self-object (SSO) relationships, and as the name suggests, patients borrow from and incorporate the other into the self for the purpose of self-functioning and cohesion. These can be normal and healthy or pathological, depending on the person and the self-object. These significant others, the self-objects, provide critical self-regulatory functions, which individuals cannot yet achieve for themselves.[34] Repeated breaks with the self-object lead to frustration and an experience of disruption in the SSO relationship, which can lead to a sense of great need for a reliable and predictable self-object. Continued disruptions prevent a feeling of cohesion and often leave the person feeling shattered, fragmented, or unglued, producing suicidal, enraged/homicidal, or overwhelmed/panicky behaviors. Alcohol and drugs can be used as self-objects, as can many other things in our culture. They initially seem to be easy to control and predictable in their effects. They thus feel comfortable as self-objects, and development of a SSO relationship is facilitated.

Self-Psychology and Addiction Psychiatry

The challenge is to incorporate the biological, psychological, and sociocultural research findings with a psychology of the self. The biology happens to the self whether or not it was desired. This includes (1) the genetic predisposition to alcoholism and addiction, (2) tolerance, (3) the potential for withdrawal, (4) the reinforcing properties, which may be unrelated to euphoria, and (5) the various pharmacological effects of these drugs, especially with chronic use. An individual usually begins with tobacco, alcohol, and later marijuana.[30] Tolerance develops readily to the regular use of tobacco. For biologically predisposed individuals,[36] tolerance develops readily to alcohol, too, giving drinkers the illusion that they can control alcohol, even large amounts, better than can peers. With a social group that approves of drinking and encourages it, individuals feel good about themselves as drinkers. If they have the psychosocial desire to continue to drink heavily, the physical reinforcement for heavy drinking, and drug availability, then they will continue. They initially feel in control, but problems gradually arise from the repeated intoxicated behaviors[37] and the neurobiological changes.[38]

Families and friends now begin to give the drinker/drug user feedback. Some who prefer the drinking and drug-taking lifestyle reinforce these values as well as these behaviors. Some do not ascribe to the lifestyle and become alarmed by the behaviors, giving distressed or negative feedback. The self-objects who are opposed to excessive drinking and to drug taking disrupt the SSO relationship and stir frustration, resentment, guilt, shame, and so forth. The individual may seek new SSO relationships to maintain cohesiveness. Although the pro-alcohol/drug self-objects support the self's cohesiveness, the neurobiology of chronic use induces anxiety, depression, and loss of control. The self is confused and bewildered now, struggling to maintain control, terrified to see itself as out of control, addicted. Denial[39] is incited to preserve calm and self-esteem, but this is frequently assailed by the negative environmental feedback.

After many failed attempts to control the alcohol/drug use, the self may admit its failure and, in defeat, surrender to abstinence.[40] This releases the pent-up guilt, shame, self-reproach, and so forth that the denial has kept at bay. In addition, the self realizes that it can no longer trust itself because it was the self that approved the use in the first place. This is a traumatic experience to say the least. Where does the self turn for protection, guidance, self-soothing, a few good feelings? The hunger for self-objects is intense, and the history of frustration, distrust, and even traumatic relationships can be great. The road to recovery for many is stormy because of these contradictory impulses—the need for self-objects and the fear of trusting someone else.

Treatment must help alcoholic/addicted patients understand these experiences, how they came about, which were drug induced, and where to go for reliable and dependable help. Education about the biology is critical, as is the dialogue about guilt, shame, and self-reproach. Establishing SSO relationships that are growth promoting and healing is important. Patients need help in soothing themselves, learning new coping skills, and restoring self-esteem through positive feedback (mirroring). This can occur in group or individual therapy, Alcoholics Anonymous, a mentoring relationship, or

other setting. Khantzian and colleagues'[41] emphasis on self-soothing, self-esteem, and self-care is decidedly appropriate.

And what of the family? They also have their SSO relationships, which involve the alcoholic/addicted patient. Through repeated intoxications, an addict begins to frustrate the self-object needs and disrupt the SSO relationship. The family can try harder to maintain the SSO relationship by adapting (called *codependence* when this is extreme), can complain and manipulate the addict (also codependence in the extreme), withdraw and feel hurt/betrayed, or see the disease process as a function of the addiction and not the relationship. The latter is optimal but often only occurs after some combination of the first three. Recovery from codependence is frequently complicated by denial of the addiction among the family.

Denial of codependence is also common because an addiction, once recognized, is defined as the problem. When a family recognizes that they too suffer from the addictive process, then they can perceive codependence as a problem they have. The understanding of SSO relationships helps soothe the traumatic frustration, sense of betrayal, and hurt that many family members feel. They needed the addict for their own cohesiveness and were repeatedly disappointed by the unpredictable, intoxicated (or withdrawal) behaviors. They obviously need new and reliable SSO relationships. A person recovering from addiction will not be a reliable self-object for some time because of the many layers of healing that are necessary. Relapses may also occur. The first year or two of abstinence is not a stable period. Thus, a family's needs are similar to those of an alcoholic or addict. They need reliable and predictable self-objects so that they can establish self-esteem and a capacity to soothe themselves. They need to learn how to care for themselves and each other through discipline and the capacity to work, through enjoyment and the capacity to play and have fun, and through love and the capacity to trust and feel.

Conclusion

The concept of the integrated psychology is simple. The self experiences the disease process and reacts to it. The reaction may be adaptive or it may be maladaptive. The same is true for family members because they too experience the disease process and react to it. Recovery requires an understanding of the disease process—the neurobiology, the development of denial and intensification of guilt and shame, the traumatic awareness of being addicted, and the maladaptive family system dynamics that evolve as the illness progresses. For the many children of alcoholics who are now themselves addicted, an intergenerational element is worth mentioning, because recovery from addiction is different from codependence. With this understanding of the disease, an individual can effectively work on the problems. The neurobiology of addictions (which includes conditioned responses) becomes a biological given for a patient, the bottom line.

Working on the many problems that patients and their families bring into treatment requires stable SSO relationships. Appreciation of this and helping patients and their families establish such relationships through psychotherapy, improved interpersonal behavior, use of 12-step groups, and other means to establish the healing process. Understanding the dynamics of SSO relationships, their ups and downs, means to understand the vicissitudes of recovery. The difficulty of letting go of ineffective self-objects, the pain and turmoil when the SSO relationship is disrupted, and the healing that can occur within an adequate SSO relationship all are part of the recovery. Understanding these dynamics provides patients and therapists with a clearer idea of what to do next, where to put their energy and focus for effective treatment and long-term recovery.

REFERENCES

1. Glover EG: On the aetiology of alcoholism. J Subst Abuse Treat 1(1):120–123, 1984.
2. Rado S: The psychoanalysis of pharmacothymia (drug addiction). J Subst Abuse Treat 1:59–68, 1984.
3. Tiebout HM: Psychology and treatment of alcoholism. Q J Stud Alcohol 7:214–227, 1946–1947.
4. Tiebout HM: The problem of gaining cooperation from the alcoholic patient. Q J Stud Alcohol 8:47–54, 1947–1948.
5. Alcoholics Anonymous, 3rd ed. New York, Alcoholics Anonymous World Services, 1976.
6. Wurmser L: Mr. Pecksniff's Horse? In Blaine JD, Julius DA (eds): Psychodynamics of Drug Dependence. Rockville, MD, US Dept of Health, Education, and Welfare, 1977, pp 36–72.
7. Krystal H: The genetic development of affects and affect regression. Part I. Annu Psychoanal 2:93–126, 1974.
8. Krystal H, Raskin HA: Drug Dependence: Aspects of Ego Function. Detroit, Wayne State University Press, 1970.
9. Khantzian EJ: The ego, the self, and opiate addiction: Theoretical and treatment considerations. In Blaine JD, Julius DA (eds): Psychodynamics of Drug Dependence. Rockville, MD, US Dept of Health, Education, and Welfare, 1977, pp 101–117.
10. Kohut H: The Analysis of the Self. New York, International Universities Press, 1971.
11. Khantzian EJ: On the psychological predisposition for opiate and stimulant dependence. Psychiatry Letter 3(1):1–4, 1985.
12. Khantzian EJ: Self-regulation and self-medication factors in alcoholism and the addictions: Similarities and differences. In Galanter M (ed): Recent Developments in Alcoholism, vol VIII. New York, Plenum, 1990, pp 255–271.
13. Vaillant G: The Natural History of Alcoholism: Causes, Patterns, and Paths to Recovery. Cambridge, MA, Harvard University Press, 1983.
14. Beck AT, Wright FD, Newman CF, Liese BS: Cognitive Therapy of Substance Abuse. New York, Guilford Press, 1993.
15. Chiauzzi EJ: Preventing Relapse in the Addictions: A Biopsychosocial Approach. New York, Pergamon Press, 1991.
16. Donovan JM: An etiologic model of alcoholism. Am J Psychiatry 143(1):1–11, 1986.
17. Wise RA: The brain and reward. In Liebman JM, Cooper SJ (eds): The Neuropharmacology of Reward. Oxford, Oxford University Press, 1989.
18. Koob GF, Bloom FE: Cellular and molecular mechanisms of drug dependence. Science 242:715–723, 1980.
19. deWit J, Uhlenhuth EH, Hedeker D, et al: Lack of preference for diazepam in anxious volunteers. Arch Gen Psychiatry 43:533–541, 1986.
20. Fischman MW, Foltin RW: Self-administration of cocaine for humans: A laboratory perspective. In Fischman MW, Foltin RW (eds): Cocaine: Scientific and Social Dimensions. New York, John Wiley & Sons, 1992, pp 165–180.
21. Tamerin JS, Mendelson JH: The psychodynamics of chronic inebriation: Observations of alcoholics during the process of drinking in an experimental group setting. Am J Psychiatry 125:886–899, 1969.
22. Mayfield DG, Coleman LL: Alcohol use and affective disorder. Dis Nerv Sys 29:467–474, 1968.
23. Keeler MH, Taylor CI, Miller WC: Are all recently detoxified alcoholics depressed? Am J Psychiatry 136:586–588, 1979.
24. Schuckit MC, Monteiro MG: Alcoholism, anxiety and depression. Br J Addict 83:1373–1380, 1988.
25. McCord W, McCord J: Origins of Alcoholism. Stanford, Stanford University Press, 1960.
26. Robins LN: Deviant Children Grown Up: A Sociological and Psychiatric Study of Sociopathic Personality. Baltimore, Williams & Wilkins, 1966.
27. Jones MC: Personality correlates and antecedents of drinking patterns in adult males. J Consult Clin Psychol 36:61–69, 1971.
28. Jones MC: Personality antecedents and correlates of drinking patterns in women. J Consult Clin Psychol 36:61–69, 1971.
29. Loper RG, Kammeier ML, Hoffman H: M.M.P.I. characteristics of college freshman males who later became alcoholics. J Abnorm Psychol 82:159–162, 1973.
30. Yamaguchi K, Kandel DB: Patterns of drug use from adolescence to young adulthood: II. Sequences of progression. Am J Public Health 74(7):668–672, 1984.
31. Office of Substance Abuse Prevention: Prevention Plus 11. Rockville, MD, Office of Substance Abuse Prevention, 1989.
32. Newcomb MD, Bentler PM: Consequences of Adolescent Drug Use. Beverly Hills, Sage Publications, 1988.
33. Kohut H: How Does Analysis Cure? Chicago, University of Chicago Press, 1985.
34. Ornstein PH, Kay J: Development of psychoanalytic self psychology: A historical-conceptual overview. In Tasman A, Goldfinger SM, Kaufmann CA (eds): Re-

view of Psychiatry, vol IX. Washington, DC, American Psychiatric Press, 1990, pp 303–322.

35. Kohut H: Thoughts on narcissism and narcissistic rage. In Ornstein PH (ed): The Search for the Self-Selected Writings of Heinz Kohut: 1950–1978, vol 2. New York, International Universities Press, 1978, pp 615–658.

36. Anthenelli RM, Schuckit MA: Genetics. In Lowinson JH, Ruiz P, Millman RB, Langrod JG (eds): Substance Abuse: A Comprehensive Textbook, 2nd ed. Baltimore, Williams & Wilkins, 1992, pp 39–50.

37. Johnson VE: Intervention: How to Help Someone Who Doesn't Want Help. Minneapolis, Johnson Institute Books, 1986.

38. Tabakoff B, Hoffman PL: Alcohol: Neurobiology. In Lowinson JH, Ruiz P, Millman RB, Langrod JG (eds): Substance Abuse: A Comprehensive Textbook, 2nd ed. Baltimore, Williams & Wilkins, 1992, pp 152–185.

39. Goldsmith RJ, Green BL: A rating scale for alcoholic denial. J Nerv Ment Dis 176:614–620, 1988.

40. Tiebout HM: The act of surrender in the therapeutic process with special reference to alcoholism. Q J Stud Alcohol 10:48–58, 1949.

41. Khantzian EJ, Halliday KS, McAuliffe WE: Addiction and the Vulnerable Self: Modified Dynamic Group Therapy for Substance Abusers. New York, Guilford Press, 1990.

Epidemiology of Comorbidity in Addiction Psychiatry

Norman S. Miller, MD • James Fine, MD

The wide variability in prevalence rates reported for comorbidity of psychiatric and addictive disorders is attributable to differences in methods for investigating comorbidity of psychiatric and addictive disorders. The epidemiological data obtained for psychiatric conditions depend on the methods used in the study. The population sampled, the method, the perspective of the examiner, longitudinal perspectives, and treatment interventions are key parameters that determine the results at the outset.[1-6]

Methodology

In the Epidemiological Catchment Area Study, the rates for the combined psychiatric and alcohol and drug disorders in the general population were 8% male and 23.4% female for depressive disorders, 0.8% male and 3.1% female for bipolar disorders, 2.4% male and 7.2% female for schizophrenia, 14.6% male and 10.1% female for antisocial personality disorders, 2.1% male and 7.9% female for panic disorders, and 13.5% male and 33.1% female for phobic disorders. The prevalence rates for clinical psychiatric populations based on other studies are listed in Table 2–1.[2, 7, 8]

A ratio for the prevalence rates of the comorbidity for clinical psychiatric population versus the general population would yield the following perspective: 3.75 males, 1.28 females for depressive disorder; 62.5 males, 16.1 females for bipolar disorder; 20.8 males, 6.94 females for schizophrenic disorder; 5.5 males, 7.9 females for antisocial personality disorder; 14.3 males, 3.8 females for anxiety disorder; and 1.7 males, 0.69 females for phobic disorder. The corresponding ratios of the comorbidity for clinical addiction population to the general population are the following: 0.5 males, 0.17 females for depressive disorder; 1.0 males, 0.23 females for bipolar disorder; 0.45 males, 0.15 females for schizophrenic disorder, 0.28 males, 0.6 females for antisocial personality disorder; 1.0 males, 0.25 females for anxiety disorder; and 0.44 males, 0.18 females for phobic disorder. A comparison of the derived ratios for the psychiatric setting and addiction setting, respectively, with the general population clearly reveals the bias toward high rates of psychiatric diagnoses in addictive disorders in psychiatric clinical settings (Table 2–2).[2, 7, 8]

The principal methods pertain to clinical studies in treatment populations versus epidemiological studies in the general population and retrospective versus prospective acquisition of data. The rates vary markedly according to the particular method of study, with

Table 2–1. RATIOS OF COMORBIDITY PREVALENCE RATES COMPARED BY SETTING

Diagnosis: Comorbidity	Prevalence Rate: Psychiatric Setting	Prevalence Rate: Addiction Setting	Ratio of Psychiatric Setting to Addiction Setting
Depressive disorders	30	5.0	7.5
Bipolar disorders	50	0.8	62.5
Schizophrenia	50	1.1	27.3
Antisocial personality disorders	80	0.6	133.3
Anxiety disorders	30	3.0	15.0
Phobic disorders	23	6.0	38.3

higher rates of comorbidity for clinical populations and retrospective analysis. Studies have demonstrated that because of greater psychopathology in comorbid disorders, the likelihood is greater that these patients will reach the attention of a clinician and will use treatment facilities. This is readily apparent when comparing the rates for inpatients with the general population for the comorbidity of both categories of disorders.

The basic design of the data acquisition is important. The retrospective analysis typically yields higher, inflated rates for psychiatric symptoms and syndromes than does the prospective, longitudinal analysis to observe the stability of actual disorders over time. The principal reasons for this difference are that (1) alcohol and drugs produce psychiatric syndromes; (2) patients' self-reports tend to focus more on psychiatric symptoms than on alcohol and drug use, and patients deny alcohol and drug use as important in the genesis of psychiatric consequences; (3) patients and clinicians tend to view psychiatric symptoms as either independent of or a cause of alcoholism and drug use; and (4) longitudinal studies reveal that psychiatric syndromes in association with alcohol and drug disorders are more likely to be a result of alcohol and drug use and addiction.[9–11]

The cross-sectional analysis usually performed for addictive disorders in psychiatric populations typically does not allow a period for withdrawal, and abstinence is allowed before actual psychiatric diagnosis is attempted. The generally recommended period for observation before establishing independent psychiatric comorbidity independently from that arising from the pharmacological effects and acquired addiction is weeks to years. The time course is dependent on the diagnosis in question—that is, depressive and psychotic symptoms tend to resolve in days to weeks, whereas induced anxiety symptoms and personality changes resolve in months to years.[9–14]

It has been determined that depressive symptoms occur in 98% of alcoholic individuals at some point in their life histories and that one third meet criteria for persistent depression interfering with functioning for a period of 2 weeks or longer. The vast majority of these depressive syndromes resolve with abstinence and, especially, specific treatment of addictive disorders. Administration of low to moderate doses (three to five drinks) of alcohol can produce depressive symptoms in normal, healthy subjects under experimentally controlled conditions. Such alcohol administration in healthy women has been shown to produce mood disruptions that still can be measured days after the experiment. These and other studies show that continuous, heavy drinking produces a depressive syndrome of alcohol intoxication. This depressive syndrome is induced by other drugs such as stimulants, cannabis, sedative or hypnotic drugs, and opiates. In the case of depressive

Table 2–2. PREVALENCE RATES FOR COMORBIDITY IN THE PSYCHIATRIC SETTING COMPARED WITH THE GENERAL POPULATION (EPIDEMIOLOGICAL CATCHMENT AREA STUDY)

Diagnosis: Comorbidity	Prevalence Rate: Clinical Setting	Prevalence Rate: Nonclinical Male	Prevalence Rate: Nonclinical Female	Ratio: Clinical to Nonclinical
Depressive disorders	30	8	23.4	3.8/1.3
Bipolar disorders	50	0.8	3.1	62.5/16.1
Schizophrenia	50	2.4	7.2	20.8/6.9
Antisocial personality disorders	80	14.6	10.1	5.5/7.9
Anxiety disorders	30	2.1	7.9	14.3/3.8
Phobic disorders	23	13.5	33.1	1.7/0.7

disorders as well as anxiety disorders, studies show that only a small proportion of patients addicted to alcohol and drugs have enduring depressive and anxiety symptoms independent of the alcohol and drug disorders.[9, 11, 12]

An interesting phenomenon found in alcoholics and drug addicts is that abstinent alcoholics report drinking *because* of anxiety and depression when free of these symptoms on examination. When these same alcoholics are given alcohol under experimental conditions, anxiety and depression develop in proportion to the increases in the amount and duration of alcohol consumption to the point of suicidal thinking. On detoxification, the anxiety and depression as well as the suicidal thinking resolve, and the alcoholics do not relate the severe psychiatric symptoms to the alcohol, continuing to rationalize their drinking on the basis of anxiety and depression. This type of self-report of rationalization in alcoholics and drug addicts extends to other psychiatric symptoms such as hallucination and delusions in psychotic patients and in patients with personality difficulties.[11, 15, 16]

As demonstrated by these studies, if a retrospective observation occurs, particularly close to a recent episode of drinking or drug use, the self-reports often result in a high number of psychiatric symptoms. In the setting of alcohol and drug use, diagnoses lead to exaggerated rates of psychiatric disorders if not linked to the drinking and drug use. Moreover, self-reports by alcoholics and drug addicts minimize drinking and drug use, particularly the consequences associated with them. The minimization is greater the closer that these reports are to recent drinking or drug use. Although it may be accurate to assume that an alcoholic or drug addict interviewed in a treatment setting may yield fairly reliable data on frequency and duration of use of alcohol and drugs, the interpretation of why they use alcohol and drugs remains elusive to them until they have been abstinent for a prolonged period and have gained an understanding of their addictive use of these substances.[10, 17]

Prospective analyses reveal that emotional or psychological states and personality variables, in fact, do not predict the onset of drinking or alcoholism. These studies do not find that psychiatric diagnoses or symptoms precede or lead to higher rates of alcohol and drug addiction. When longitudinal follow-up occurs over time after the onset of addiction to alcohol and drugs in the abstinent, treated state, the psychiatric symptoms and personality abnormalities associated with addictive use and intoxication from alcohol and drugs resolve in many of those who are affected.[10, 17]

Populations Studied

Clinical populations generally yield rates that are higher for comorbidity than does the general population, based on the observation that individuals with multiple disorders tend to seek treatment. In clinical settings, the rates for a particular disorder also reflect the treatment provided, such that a general psychiatric setting contains higher rates of chronically mentally ill patients because of the orientation of the clinicians. Moreover, prevalence rates for co-occurrence are higher for inpatient than for outpatient treatment settings and are greater for public (community) than for private settings and for reimbursement-driven diagnoses in which a particular category of a disorder is reimbursed, such as psychiatric diagnoses, and not addictive disorders in psychiatric settings.[18-29]

Given these variables, the overall prevalence rates in clinical populations for addictive disorders in private and public psychiatric populations are approximately 50%; in other words, the likelihood of finding a substance use disorder diagnosis in a psychiatric patient is one in two. The actual prevalence rates for addictive disorders, according to psychiatric diagnostic categories, vary accordingly: 30% in depressive disorders, 50% in bipolar disorders, 50% in schizophrenic disorders, 80% in antisocial personality disorders, 30% in anxiety disorders, and 23% in phobic disorders[18, 21, 22, 27, 30] (see Table 2–1).

On the other hand, studies reveal that the prevalence rates for psychiatric disorders in addiction populations are considerably lower and are generally similar to those rates found in the general population for psychiatric disorders. These have been relatively well documented in addiction populations, accordingly: 4% for depressive disorders, 0.8% for bipolar disorder, 1.1% for schizophrenic disorders, 0.6% for antisocial personality disorder, 2% for anxiety disorders, and 6% for phobic disorders among those with a diagnosis of addictive disorders (see Table 2–1).[7, 8, 14]

Taking the ratio of these dramatically different rates yields the following perspective for psychiatric setting to addiction setting: 7.5 for depressive disorders, 62.5 for bipolar disorders, 27.3 for schizophrenic disorders, 133.3 for antisocial personality disorders, 15.0 for anxiety disorders, and 38.3 for phobic disorders.

Although these ratios are at first perplexing, they do provide an insight that psychiatric disorders are commonly diagnosed among those patients with addictive disorders (see Table 2–1).

Perspectives of the Examiner

What becomes apparent is that the perspective of the clinician or researcher is a key determinant in the assessment of prevalence rates for both categories of disorder. If the perspective is that addiction is an independent disorder and a genesis of psychiatric symptoms and syndromes, then exclusionary criteria are applied before making independent psychiatric diagnoses. As a result of excluding psychopathology that arises from the addictive disorders, the prevalence rates for psychiatric disorders in those patients with addictive disorders are generally in the range for those rates in the general population.

If the perspective is that psychiatric disorders or symptoms cause or lead to addictive use of alcohol and drugs, the prevalence rates for psychiatric disorders in addiction populations are high. The self-medication hypothesis remains a pervasive perspective that leads to a high rate of psychiatric diagnosis in addiction populations.[31] Although self-medication of an underlying or associated condition, often a psychiatric symptom of a disorder, is often cited in the literature as an explanation for alcohol and drug use, the hypothesis cannot be validated when tested. In fact, several studies show that addicts and alcoholics continue to use these substances despite worsening drug- and alcohol-induced psychiatric symptoms.[10–13, 17, 32]

The elevated rates for comorbid psychiatric and addictive disorders are obtained in the large epidemiological studies that begin the examination of comorbidity from the self-medication perspective. The prevalence rates are obtained by eliciting criteria through self-reports in alcoholics and drug addicts from 6 months before the interview in treatment settings, when the most severe use of alcohol and drugs typically occurs in the months leading to seeking treatment. Using such a retrospective analysis, the lifetime prevalence rates are 19.8% for any addictive disorder among persons with a mental disorder, 55% for any mental disorder among persons with alcohol disorders, and 64.4% for any mental disorder among persons with other drug disorders. The lifetime rates in epidemiological and clinical studies in psychiatric populations generally are obtained retrospectively and by interviewing a patient with bias when accepting the patient's report that psychiatric symptoms are the genesis of addictive alcohol and drug use.[16, 31]

A method used to allow for the comparison of base rates for psychiatric and addictive disorders is the odds ratio (OR), which is derived by taking the ratios for the combined comorbid disorders to the base rate of either the psychiatric or addictive disorder to derive the relative risk for their co-occurrence. Although the OR by itself does not assign causality, it does illustrate the degree of association of the disorders. ORs are influenced by either comorbid or independent prevalence rates, and association is reflected by the ultimate value of the OR; the higher the value of the ratio, the greater the association.[2, 7]

The following are published lifetime prevalence rates for combined community and institutional settings. The rate for any substance use or dependence with any unipolar major depression is 27% or OR 1.9, bipolar disorder is 60.7% or OR 7.9, schizophrenia is 47% or OR 4.6, antisocial personality is 83.6% or OR 29.6, anxiety disorder is 23.7% or OR 1.7, and phobic disorder is 22.9% or OR 1.6. The rate for any mental disorder with any alcohol disorder is 36.6% or OR 2.3 and with any other drug disorder is 53.1% or OR 4.5. The rate for any affective disorder among alcohol disorders is 13.4% or OR 1.9 and other drug disorder is 26.4% or OR 4.7; for schizophrenia among alcohol disorders is 3.8% or OR 3.3 and among drug disorders is 6.8% or OR 6.2; for antisocial personality is 14.3% or OR 21 and 17.8% or OR 13.4; and for anxiety disorder is 19.4% or OR 1.5 and 28.3% or OR 2.5, respectively.[2, 7]

The similar ratios for the two populations as denominators in either case (i.e., substance dependence or mental disorder) can be interpreted as a lack of differentiating those psychiatric symptoms and disorders induced by alcohol and drug disorders from those occurring independently. An example is the OR for antisocial personality, which is 29.6 for substance dependence among all patients with antisocial personality and 21.0 for antisocial personality disorders among all alcoholics. Certainly, the clinical data as well as longitudinal prospective data do not approximate these ratios for the number of antisocial personality disorders among all alcoholics, because most alcoholics do not have antisocial personality. Also, the comparison of ORs for substance dependence with any affective disorder is 2.6 versus 1.9

for affective disorder among alcoholics and 4.7 among drug addicts, thus leading to the erroneous conclusion that most alcoholics and drug addicts have independent affective disorders. The clinical data and longitudinal studies do not support these findings. Similar inflated ORs are found for the other disorders as well.[2, 7, 31]

Length of Follow-Up

The prevalence of psychiatric symptoms in the general population can be estimated to exceed that for psychiatric disorders by two- to threefold (see Table 2–1). The prevalence of psychiatric symptoms in addictive disorders can be estimated to exceed that for psychiatric disorders by seven- to eightfold (see Table 2–2). The pharmacological effects of alcohol and drugs in addition to the consequence of addictive disorders summate to induce the psychiatric symptoms in addictive disorders. It is important to note that the preponderance of psychopathology is not related to an independent psychiatric disorder.[17, 32]

Longitudinal follow-up is perhaps the only way ultimately to establish the stability of valid and reliable prevalence rates and ORs for the comorbidity of psychiatric and addictive disorders. Studies that examine the longitudinal changes in addictive disorders after detoxification find consistently that affective and anxiety symptoms diminish and resolve over time. A postintoxication period is not used in epidemiological studies and, therefore, in this way these studies are subject to artifactually elevated prevalence rates for psychiatric syndromes induced by drugs and alcohol. The lack of a careful longitudinal follow-up in clinical studies contributes to the false-positive rates of psychiatric comorbidity found among those with an alcohol or drug diagnosis.[9, 10, 17, 33]

Studies under laboratory conditions and in clinical populations de novo have demonstrated that subjects who are psychiatrically symptom free develop clearly definable psychiatric syndromes indistinguishable from those defined in DSM-III-R when exposed to alcohol and drugs. Cocaine infusions in human volunteers induce paranoid delusions as a pharmacological effect of cocaine; these delusions closely follow, in a dose-dependent manner, the blood levels of cocaine. Other studies with alcohol have demonstrated that severe depression develops with intoxication in otherwise symptom-free subjects and resolves with time. These affective changes have been correlated with blood alcohol levels and correspond to known pharmacokinetic characteristics of alcohol.[14]

Moreover, when clinical populations are examined over time, the psychiatric symptoms, such as anxiety and depression, and the severity and presence of these symptoms correspond to the periods of alcohol intoxication and diminish with periods of abstinence. Importantly, these ubiquitous psychiatric symptoms are correlated highly with the course and prognosis of the diagnosis of alcohol dependence and not with an independent psychiatric disorder, if observed over time. In general, similar results are found for the courses in other drug dependencies in which the psychiatric syndromes follow the course of drug use and are not reflective of independent psychiatric disorders.[9, 10, 12, 17]

The question of the length of follow-up has been examined for many drugs, including alcohol. For alcohol, 2 to 6 weeks is sometimes needed for the pharmacological effects to recede, although a normal but labile mood can appear within days in many alcoholics. A similar course for resolution of pharmacologically induced psychiatric symptoms due to cocaine has been documented by several investigators. For longer-acting drugs, such as benzodiazepines or methadone, the course may be protracted over weeks and months. A protracted withdrawal syndrome has been described and is related to the prolonged neurological effects of drugs in general. One remarkable characteristic is mood lability that may persist beyond resolution of major affective and anxiety symptoms.[17, 34]

Treatment Interventions

A differential response to treatment interventions can sometimes distinguish the comorbidity of psychiatric disorders from alcohol and drug disorders. Studies that use pharmacological treatments for alcoholics have not found a favorable response in either the psychiatric symptoms or addictive course. Antidepressants, neuroleptics, and antianxiety agents do not alleviate depression, psychosis, or anxiety in actively drinking alcoholics or alter the course of the alcoholism. Similarly, use of these medications does not result in alleviated depression, psychosis, and anxiety in actively using drug addicts or alter the course of the drug addiction. Preliminary studies of cocaine addicts suggest that certain therapeutic pharmacological agents (desipramine for cocaine and clonidine for heroin) have a beneficial effect in promoting abstinence in acute and subacute withdrawal in cocaine and heroin addicts in addition to psychosocial treatments. An analogous clinical practice is the use of benzodiazepines in the treatment of alcohol withdrawal in alcoholics. These therapeutic agents, however, do not have demonstrated efficacy in treating psychiatric comorbidity in addictive disorders as would be predicted if the genesis were psychiatric disorders.[17, 31]

In several treatment outcome studies, specific treatment of alcohol or drug addiction resulted in amelioration of the associated psychiatric syndromes and definitively altered the course of the addictive disorder. Abstinence from alcohol and drugs and specific treatment of the addictive disorder resulted in resolution or diminution of affective, anxiety, psychotic, and personality disturbance in the vast majority of the patients.[34, 35]

Summary

The conclusions from comprehensive analysis of studies of the comorbidity of psychiatric and addictive disorders during the past four decades indicate the following: (1) Prevalence rates for the psychiatric symptoms are somewhat greater than those for psychiatric disorders in the general population. (2) Prevalence rates for psychiatric symptoms generated by alcohol or drug use and addiction are much greater than those for concomitant independent psychiatric disorders in the addiction population. (3) Prevalence rates for addictive disorders are much greater than those for psychiatric disorders. When addictive disorders are considered as independent disorders (per DSM-III-R), the prevalence rates for comorbid psychiatric disorders are elevated modestly over those for the general population. (4) Prevalence rates for the comorbidity of addictive disorders in psychiatric populations are no greater than those for the general population, except for schizophrenia and antisocial personality disorder. When psychiatric disorders are considered as independent disorders (per DSM-III-R), the prevalence rates for addictive disorders are elevated for schizophrenia and antisocial personality disorder over those for the general population. (5) Prevalence rates for comorbid psychiatric disorders in addiction settings are influenced by patient selection but reflect actual prevalence rates for comorbidity of psychiatric and addictive disorders more closely than do those obtained in psychiatric settings. (6) Prevalence rates for comorbid addictive disorders in psychiatric settings are influenced by patient selection but reflect inflated rates for comorbidity of psychiatric disorders in addictive disorders.

REFERENCES

1. Mueser KM, Yarnold PR, Levinson DF, et al: Prevalence of substance abuse in schizophrenia: Demographic and clinical correlates. Schizophr Bull 16:31–56, 1990.
2. Regier DA, Farmer ME, Raw DS, et al: Comorbidity of mental disorders with alcohol and other drug abuse. JAMA 264:2511–2518, 1990.
3. Penick EC, Powell BJ, Nickel J, et al: Co-morbidity of extreme psychiatric disorder among male alcohol patients. Alcohol Clin Psychol Res 18(6):1289–1293, 1994.
4. Lehman AF, Myers CP, Corty E, Thompson JW: Prevaling and patterns of "dual diagnosis" among psychiatric inpatients. Compr Psychiatry 35(2):106–112, 1994.
5. Lehman AF, Herron JD, Schwartz RP, Myers CP: Rehabilitation for adults with severe mental illness and substance use disorders: A clinical trial. J Nerv Ment Dis 181(2):86–90, 1993.
6. Lehman AF, Myers CP, Corty E, Thompson J: Severity of substance use disorders among psychiatric inpatients. J Nerv Ment Dis 182:164–167, 1994.
7. Helzer JE, Pryzbeck TR: The co-occurrence of alcoholism with other psychiatric disorders in the general population and its impact on treatment. J Stud Alcohol 49:219–224, 1991.
8. Dixon LB, Dibietz E, Myers CP, et al: Comparison of DSM-III-R diagnosis and a brief interview for substance abuse among state hospital patients. Hosp Community Psychiatry 44:748–752, 1993.
9. Brown SA, Irwin M, Schuckit MA: Changes in anxiety among abstinent male alcoholics. J Stud Alcohol 52:55–61, 1991.
10. Schuckit MA, Montero MG: Alcoholism, anxiety, depression. Br J Addict 83:1373–1380, 1980.
11. Tamerin JS, Mendelson JH: The psychodynamics of chronic inebriation. Observations of alcoholics during the process of drinking in an experimental group setting. Am J Psychiatry 125:886, 1969.
12. Schuckit MA: Alcoholism and sociopathy—diagnostic confusion. Q J Stud Alcohol 34:157–164, 1973.
13. Schuckit MA, Irwin M, Brown SA: The history of anxiety symptoms among 171 primary alcoholics. J Stud Alcohol 31:34–41, 1990.
14. Weissman MM, Myers JK: Clinical depression in alcoholism. Am J Psychiatry 137:372–373, 1980.
15. Lehman AF, Myers P, Corty E: Assessment and classification of patients with psychiatric and substance abuse syndromes. Hosp Community Psychiatry 40:1019–1025, 1989.
16. Corty E, Lehman AF, Myers CP: Influence of psychoactive substance use on the reliability of psychiatric diagnosis. J Consult Clin Psychol 6:165–170, 1993.
17. Miller NS, Mahler JC, Belkin BM, et al: Psychiatric diagnosis in alcohol and drug dependence. Ann Clin Psychiatry 3:79–89, 1990.
18. Alterman AI, Erdlen FR, Murphy E: Alcohol abuse in the psychiatric hospital population. Addict Behav 6:69–73, 1981.
19. Brady K, Casto S, Lydrard RB, et al: Substance abuse in an inpatient psychiatric sample. Am J Drug Alcohol Abuse 17:389–398, 1991.

20. Caton CL, Gralnick A, Bender S, et al: Young chronic patients and substance abuse. Hosp Community Psychiatry 40:1037–1040, 1989.
21. Drake RE, Wallach MA: Substance abuse among the chronic mentally ill. Hosp Community Psychiatry 40:1041–1046, 1989.
22. Hekimian LJ, Gershon S: Characteristics of drug abusers admitted to a psychiatric hospital. JAMA 205:75–80, 1968.
23. Myers JK, Weissman MM, Tischler GL, et al: Six-month prevalence of psychiatric disorders in three communities. Arch Gen Psychiatry 41:959–967, 1984.
24. Craddock S, Hubbard R, Bray R, et al: Client Characteristics, Behaviors and In-Treatment Outcomes 1980 TOPS Admission Cohort. Rockville, MD, National Institute on Drug Abuse, 1982.
25. Pepper B, Kirshner MC, Ryglewicz H: The young adult chronic patient: Overview of a population. Hosp Community Psychiatry 32:463–474, 1981.
26. Rosenheck R, Massari L, Astrachan B, et al: Mentally ill chemical abusers discharged from VA inpatient treatment: 1976–88. Psychiatr Q 61:237–249, 1990.
27. Schwartz SR, Goldfinger SM: The new chronic patient: Clinical characteristics of an emergency subgroup. Hosp Community Psychiatry 32:470–474, 1981.
28. Sheets JL, Prevost JA, Reihman J: Young adult chronic patients: Three hypothesized subgroups. Hosp Community Psychiatry 33:197–203, 1982.
29. Woodward B, Fortgang J, Sullivan-Trainor M, et al: Underdiagnosis of alcohol dependence in psychiatric inpatients. Am J Drug Alcohol Abuse 17:373–388, 1991.
30. Drake RE, Osher EC, Wallach MA: Alcohol use and abuse in schizophrenia: A prospective community study. J Nerv Ment Dis 177:408–414, 1989.
31. Khantzian EJ: The self-medication hypothesis of addiction disorders: Focus on heroin and cocaine dependence. Am J Psychiatry 142:1259–1264, 1985.
32. Kosten TR, Kleber HD: Differential diagnosis of psychiatric comorbidity in substance abusers. J Subst Abuse Treat 5:201–206, 1988.
33. Vaillant GE, Milofsky E: The etiology of alcoholism: A prospective viewpoint. Am Psychol 37:494–503, 1982.
34. Miller NS, Ries RK: Drug and alcohol dependence and psychiatric populations: The need for diagnosis, intervention, and training. Compr Psychiatry 32:268–276, 1991.
35. Minkoff K: An integrated treatment model for dual diagnosis of psychosis and addiction. Hosp Community Psychiatry 40:1031–1036, 1989.

3

Generalized Vulnerability to Drug and Alcohol Addiction

Norman S. Miller, MD

The high prevalence of combined alcohol and drug use and addiction in alcoholics and drug addicts further supports mutual determinants of these disorders. Animal studies tend to support a genetic vulnerability to both drugs and alcohol. Environment continues to have a major role in determining exposure to alcohol and drugs, particularly as reflected by the widespread use of various drugs and alcohol in recent decades.

Neurochemical models are being developed to accommodate a common biological substrate for alcohol and drug addiction. Animal and human studies have identified interactive integrated brain mechanisms that are activated by various drugs and alcohol and have major roles in the onset and sustenance of drug/alcohol addictions.

The implications for treatment strategies are clear. Therapies directed at a single addiction will have limited efficacy because many alcoholics and drug addicts seeking treatment are multiply addicted. Moreover, the prognosis for the development of other drug and alcohol addictions in a particular individual addicted to a single drug is greatly influenced by the generalized vulnerability to drugs and alcohol.

Prevalence of Dependence in Treatment Populations

In treatment populations of adults and adolescents, between 70% and 90% of cocaine-addicts, 50% and 70% of opiate (heroin and methadone) addicts, 20% and 50% of benzodiazepine addicts, and 80% and 90% of cannabis addicts were alcoholics. Moreover, in other studies, 20% to 50% of opiate addicts were cocaine, benzodiazepine, and cannabis addicts.

Many studies of alcoholics and drug addicts in treatment populations have found that in both groups, alcohol is often the first drug used addictively. Moreover, more than two drug diagnoses were present in the majority of those addicted to alcohol, in addition to, in decreasing frequency, cannabis, cocaine, benzodiazepines, hallucinogens, and opiates. In adolescents and young adults, a triad of alcohol, marijuana, and cocaine addiction was a common occurrence.[2-4] The natural history of alcohol dependence is highly variable and age dependent as a young alcoholic begins using alcohol in early teenage years (ages 13 to 15) and progresses to addictive use of alcohol by the age of 15 or 16. A year or two after the onset of alcohol addiction, other drugs such as cannabis, cocaine, opiates, and hallucinogens are used addictively. The addictive use of sedative-hypnotic drugs does not appear to show an age effect, because they are used equally at all ages, but use is greater among women than among men by perhaps a ratio of 2:3.[5]

Prevalence of Use and Dependence in General Populations

The National Institute on Drug Abuse[6] conducted a national survey of high-school seniors for their drug and alcohol use. The survey consisted of interview responses of a nationally represented sample of students, usually interviewed over the telephone. Those students who had dropped out of school or who were chronically absent (approximately 20%) were not polled. As a result, sampling bias and underestimation may have occurred, because many of the dropout students may have had alcohol or drug problems that led to their poor academic outcome. In 1990, the lifetime use of alcohol by high-school seniors was 89.5%, marijuana 40.7%, cocaine 9.4%, heroin 1.3%, other opiates 8.3%, tranquilizers 7.2%, sedatives 5.3%, inhalants 18.5%, hallucinogens 9.4%, and cigarettes 64.4%. For these same drugs, reported use within the last year was 80.6%, 27.0%, 5.3%, 4.5%, 3.5%, 2.5%, 6.9%, and 5.9%, respectively (cigarettes not included). Use of these drugs within the year and the month prior to the survey was 57.1%, 15.0%, 1.9%, 0.2%, 1.5%, 1.2%, 1.0%, 2.7%, 2.2%, and 29.4%, respectively.

The Epidemiological Catchment Area (ECA) study, conducted in structured interviews using DSM-III criteria, found a lifetime prevalence of alcoholism to be almost 16% in the general population. The lifetime prevalence among men was 23.8% and among women was 4.6%. Approximately half the alcoholics met criteria for active alcoholism in the past year. Almost 40% of cases were diagnosable between the ages of 15 and 19 years, and 80% had begun by the age of 30 years. Men typically reported an earlier onset of alcoholism than did women. The average age of onset of alcoholism was 22 years in the men and 25 years in the women.[7, 8]

The prevalence of overall drug addiction among alcoholics in the ECA study of the general population was 30%. The prevalence of alcoholism among drug addicts was higher:

36% among cannabis addicts, 71% among sedative-hypnotic-tranquilizer addicts, 62% among amphetamine addicts, 64% among hallucinogen addicts, 67% among opiate addicts, and 84% among cocaine addicts.[7, 8]

The National Youth Polydrug study found that a sample of 2750 alcoholic youths regularly used a mean of 4.4 other drugs, most commonly marijuana and alcohol, 85% and 80%, respectively. Amphetamines were third in prevalence at 45%, followed by hashish 42%, barbiturates 40%, hallucinogens 40%, and phencyclidine 32%.[9]

A recent survey performed by the National Institute of Alcohol Abuse and Alcoholism (NIAAA) clinical research program in structured interviews showed results that corresponded to the ECA data. Regular drug use by alcoholics was reported by 48% of women and 51% of men. Of those alcoholics who used drugs, the alcoholic women used cannabis (80%), stimulants (67%), sedatives (47%), opiates (33%), and hallucinogens (27%), and the alcoholic men used cannabis (39%), stimulants (30%), sedatives (21%), opiates (19%), and hallucinogens (17%).[10]

Familial Studies

FAMILIAL ALCOHOLISM: ALCOHOLISM

The familial prevalence of alcoholism among male alcoholics has been well documented in large studies. The rate of familial alcoholism is 50% according to most studies, and if an alcoholic reported having one close relative who was alcoholic, he or she more often than a nonalcoholic reported having two or more relatives with alcoholism.[11–15]

Several studies have reported that younger alcoholics have alcoholic relatives more often than older alcoholics and that familial alcoholics show the first signs of dependence at a younger age than do nonfamilial alcoholics.[11, 14] Moreover, familial alcoholics tend to have an earlier age of onset and a more severe form of addiction with a more rapid fulminating course.[11, 14] Among 2215 male alcoholics treated for alcoholism, those with a family history of alcoholism responded less well to treatment than did those with no family history; furthermore, the greater the number of relatives with alcoholism, the worse the prognosis.[12]

FAMILIAL ALCOHOLISM: DRUG ADDICTION

Familial alcoholism among drug addicts is less studied, but some data are available. The rate of familial alcoholism was 50% among males and 80% for females in a retrospective study of 150 cocaine dependents. In a prospective study, the rate for familial alcoholism was 52% in male and 60% in female cocaine dependents.[4]

Opiate dependents with a parental history of alcoholism were more frequently diagnosed with concurrent alcoholism. In one study, 638 opiate dependents with a diagnosis of alcohol dependence had at least one parent with alcohol dependence in 21.3% of the families. Four hundred twenty-two opiate dependents without the diagnosis of alcohol dependence had a 12.5% rate of alcohol dependence in their families. Among the opiate dependents with alcohol dependence, those with parental alcoholism had more severe problems with alcohol.[16]

The results of this study are supportive of both familial and nonfamilial alcoholism in opiate addicts. Because alcoholism is high among opiate addicts, at rates of 50% to 75%, an increased rate of familial alcoholism among those opiate addicts with alcoholism may be significant.

FAMILIAL ALCOHOL AND DRUG USE/ADDICTION

Two hundred sixty-two adolescents, ages 13 through 17 years, and one of the parents of each adolescent were interviewed separately in a study on the impact of parental drug and alcohol use on adolescent behavior. The frequency of a parent's drinking directly correlated with greater drug and alcohol use in the offspring; 72% of the fathers and 77% of the mothers who took one or more drinks of beer or wine per day had offspring who used drugs and alcohol. Those parents who drank beer or wine less than once a month or not at all were much less likely to have adolescent children who used drugs and alcohol. A strong relationship was found between parental use of marijuana/hashish and adolescent drug and alcohol use. Eighty-one percent of the fathers and 78% of the mothers who used marijuana/hashish had children who used drugs and alcohol.[17]

In a longitudinal study, 82% of drinking families reared youths who also drank, whereas 72% of abstaining families produced abstainers. Not only did youths approximate parental behavior, but a generalization effect was noted, because youths used a greater variety of drugs than parents did.[18] Less consistent, however, is the evidence concerning which parent, father or mother, was more influential.

A high correlation between a father's alcohol use and the use of alcohol, marijuana, and other drugs by his offspring has been reported. Among African-Americans, a mother's alcohol use is correlated with juvenile drug and alcohol use.[19]

In a sample of 1380 youths who were examined between the ages of 12 and 18, data about the alcohol- and drug-using behaviors were obtained for a positive or negative history of alcoholism for offspring. The offspring with a family history of alcoholism were compared for early differences in patterns of alcohol and drug use with offspring without a family history of alcoholism (heavily drinking nonalcoholic families, high-stress families, and symptom-free families). No differences were found in several indicators of problem use (early onset of intoxication, frequent intoxication, and escape drinking). The analysis did, however, indicate that adolescent alcoholics with a history of familial alcoholism were more likely than family history–negative adolescents from symptom-free families to report experiencing problems/consequences relating to both drinking and drug use. Significantly, familial alcoholics had rates of self-reported alcohol or drug problems about twice that for nonfamilial alcoholics for both males and females.[20, 21]

Common Versus Specific Transmission of Drug and Alcohol Use and Dependence in Families

The questions of familial transmission of nonalcohol drug use/dependence in combination and for specific drug types, with and without alcohol use/dependence, have not been completely studied. Scherer and Mukherjee[22] (76 subjects) showed a high correlation between tranquilizer use in parents and both tranquilizer and cannabis use in offspring. Fawzy and colleagues[23] (262 subjects) found a 78% prevalence of drug use in adolescent children of parents who admitted to using marijuana and hashish. Annis[24] (539 subjects) found an association between alcohol use in parents and children as well as an association between the use of pain killers by parents and children. However, in this study, parental use of barbiturates was not associated with increased barbiturate use in children. In all of these studies, in children, predominant use of multiple types of drugs including alcohol was found to parallel that in their parents.

In a study of 6447 high-school students in Toronto in 1969, those students who used marijuana and LSD more than expected had parents who used both alcohol and tobacco. The study did not inquire about parental use of psychoactive drugs such as tranquilizers, barbiturates, and stimulants. In a follow-up study of these students, a positive association was noted between reported drug use by parents and their adolescents. This relationship held for parental use of psychoactive drugs, tranquilizers, barbiturates, stimulants, alcohol, and tobacco compared with adolescent use of psychoactive and illicit hallucinogens. Parents who were reported as frequent users of a psychoactive drug much more often had children who were using a hallucinogenic or psychoactive drug than parents who did not use these drugs. The relationship was very close when both parent and child were using the same drug (i.e., tranquilizers, barbiturates, or stimulants).[25]

In a study of 305 subjects with drug or alcohol abuse performed during a 1-year period, a positive family history of alcohol abuse in first-degree relatives was found in 60% and of drug abuse in 31% of the subjects. Significance was found for specificity; probands who were diagnosed as drug abusers were more likely to have a family history of drug abuse. Of the probands who had drug abuse, 18.5% had a positive first-degree family history of drug abuse only and 26% had a positive first-degree family history for both drug and alcohol abuse. Of the probands who had alcohol abuse only, 3% had a first-degree family history positive for drugs only and 14% had a positive family history for both drugs and alcohol. The relationship between drug abuse in parents and drug abuse in probands had the highest ratio and was more impressive than the relationship between alcohol abuse in parents and drug abuse in probands. In this study, 251 (82%) were male and 54 (18%) were female, and of importance is that in the majority of subjects, 177 (58%) were multiple drug addicts who met DSM-III criteria for both alcohol and drug abuse/dependence and were not pure drug abusers/dependents. Ninety-seven (35%) met criteria for alcohol abuse/dependence, and 27 (9%) met criteria for only nonalcoholic drug abuse/dependence.[26] Therefore, considerable overlap did exist between drug and alcohol abuse for probands and family members. Moreover, the rate of exposure to drugs in older family members such as parents was lower than that for the younger probands who were exposed to nonalcoholic drugs at a higher rate. In interviews of 32 alcoholics, 72 opiate addicts, and 42 alcoholic-opiate addicts, alcoholism to a significant extent tended to cluster in families, whereas alcoholism and opiate abuse did not occur in the same families significantly more or less often than expected by chance alone using the contingency chi-square analysis.[27] It is important to note that overlap of alcoholism and opiate addiction did exist between relatives and probands, however, and that the lower rate of opiate addiction among alcoholic parents may have been due to a low rate of exposure to opiates in this generation. Additionally, a more recent study examining this hypothesis failed to find specific intergenerational transmission of opiate use from parents to offspring independent of alcohol dependence.[28]

A study of younger drug addicts showed familial aggregation of drug abuse in 350 inpatients admitted for drug abuse in which 50% were opiate addicts, 33% were cocaine addicts, and the remainder (17%) were sedative-hypnotic addicts. The rate of familial drug abuse corresponded to the proband's drug of choice, from 16% of male relatives of cocaine addicts to 2% of male relatives of sedative-hypnotic addicts. In support of a common familial transmission of drug and alcohol abuse is that the rate of alcoholism was the same across all proband groups regardless of drug type, indicating a high association of familial alcoholism and drug abuse in the proband.[29] Further support for a common transmission is a study of 41 male veterans that found an association between family history status of alcohol and drug dependence. Family history status did not discriminate onset of type of drug or alcohol abuse (i.e., "pure" alcohol abuse versus mixed alcohol and drug abuse). Two thirds of the subjects had combined drug and alcohol abuse, and only one third met criteria for pure alcohol abuse or dependence. Thus, the distribution of alcohol or drug abuse in the proband was not related to the family history status.[30]

Genetic Studies

ADOPTION STUDIES: ALCOHOLISM

Several adoption studies showed that sons of alcoholics raised by adoptive parents became alcoholics significantly more often than sons of nonalcoholics raised by adoptive parents. Similar results of three separate adoption studies conducted in Denmark, Sweden, and Iowa (United States) and a half-sibling study revealed the following:

1. Sons of alcoholics were three to four times more likely to become alcoholics than were sons of nonalcoholics, whether the sons of alcoholics were raised by their alcoholic biological parent or by their nonalcoholic adoptive parents. The studies can be criticized on the basis of small numbers of subjects, criteria for diagnosis of alcoholism, and overlap between numbers of alcoholic parents of alcoholic and nonalcoholic adoptees. Nonetheless, the composite results and reliction in additional studies strongly support an inheritance factor in the development of alcoholism.[11, 31, 32]

2. Sons of alcoholics raised by nonalcoholic adoptive parents were no more susceptible to nonalcoholic adult psychiatric diagnoses than were sons of nonalcoholics raised by nonalcoholic adoptive parents. The Iowa study did find a higher rate of childhood conduct disorder in male offspring of alcoholics.[11, 31, 32]

3. No differences were found for female adoptees.[11, 31, 32]

4. Alcoholism and antisocial personality were genetically independent disorders for both males and females. The results of the Iowa study showed specificity of inheritance of antisocial and alcoholic condition, with two types of independent predispositions, one toward alcohol use and the other toward antisocial personality.[11, 31, 32]

ADOPTION: DRUG ADDICTION

An adoption study of genetic and environmental factors in drug abuse revealed that a biological background of alcohol problems predicted increased drug abuse in adoptees. Also, environmental factors, divorce, and psychiatric disturbance in the adoptive family were associated with increased drug abuse.[33]

TWIN STUDIES: ALCOHOLISM

A Finnish (11,500 twin pairs) and a Swedish (7500 male pairs) study showed drinking problems were greater in monozygotic twins than in dizygotic twins. Swedish (174 male pairs) and American (15,924 male twins) studies showed that a diagnosis of alcoholism was more concordant in monozygotic twins than in dizygotic twins. Only one study conducted in England, enrolling the smallest number of twin pairs (56 twin pairs) of all the studies, did not show a difference in alcohol behavior between monozygotic twins and dizygotic twins.[11]

A study of a U.S. treatment sample of 50 monozygotic and 64 dizygotic male twins and 31 monozygotic and 24 dizygotic female twins showed a significantly greater concordance rate for alcohol dependence in male and female twins and for alcohol abuse in males only.[34]

TWIN STUDIES: DRUG ADDICTION

In a U.S. study, only male monozygotic twins were significantly more concordant than dizygotic twins for other drug abuse/dependence and any substance abuse/dependence including alcohol dependence. However, the ratios of monozygotic to dizygotic concordance were comparable in the two sexes, suggesting that lack of significance in the female sample may be due to low statistical power.[35]

Common Biological Interactions in Addictive Drug/Alcohol Use

Several neurotransmitters may be involved in the various appetitive systems that underlie addictive behaviors. In studies, the major neurotransmitters identified in drug and alcohol addiction were the opioid peptides, dopamine, serotonin, and norepinephrine. These neurotransmitters had individual and interactive relationships in the reinforcement center and with the instinctual drive states. Together, this center and the drive states are thought to generate and underlie addictive use of drugs and alcohol.[36] Findings have suggested that the common denominator for a wide range of classes of addictive drugs is their ability to activate the dopaminergic fibers in the mesolimbic system.[36, 37]

The reinforcement center has been shown to contain dopamine neurons that project from their location in the ventral tegmentum to the mesolimbic system in the forebrain. Opiate receptors were found on these dopamine neurons, and stimulation with opiates activated this dopamine system. Self-administration studies have shown that stimulation of the mesolimbic area supports addictive use of heroin, cocaine, and ethanol. Blockade of dopamine receptors prevented self-administration of opiates and cocaine, and blockade of norepinephrine sites reduced alcohol intake. Also, antagonism with narcotic-blocking agents attenuated reinforcement behavior from cocaine, heroin, and ethanol administration.[38, 39]

Other neurotransmitters may be involved in drug and alcohol use and addiction by serving a modulatory function. In humans, administration of serotonin reuptake inhibitors (zimelidine, fluoxetine, citalopram) to nondepressed heavy alcohol consumers and alcoholics was associated with a reduction in the number of drinks consumed and an increase in abstinent days.[40] A possible rationale is the influence of serotonin on other neurotransmitter systems. Serotonin neurons in the hypothalamus project to the metencephalon neurons, which inhibit mesencephalic endogenous opiate peptides and projections of gamma-aminobutyric acid (GABA) neurons. GABA neurons interacted to inhibit dopamine neurons in the ventral tegmentum and other neurotransmitters and in doing so also performed widespread modulation functions.[41]

Theoretical Implications

The theoretical implications extend to concepts of generalized biological vulnerability for drug and alcohol addiction. The co-occurrence of multiple drug and alcohol addiction and their common transmission in the adoption, twin, and familial studies suggest a genetic predisposition inclusive of a wide range of drugs and alcohol.[42, 43] Although studies are inconclusive at this point, they do indicate that the genetic transmission for drugs may be similar to that for alcohol. Moreover, the genetic influence appears to be operative for both alcohol and drug addiction in the same individual and groups of ostensibly dissimilar individuals. These findings are consistent with the clinical observations that alcohol and drugs can be used interchangeably in the addictive mode and that distinct hierarchical combinations are apparent although alcohol is pervasive throughout subtypes.[44–48] It is important to examine current and future generations of alcoholics and drug addicts for transmission of specific or common drug types (alcohol) in adoption, twin, and family cases. It is important to continue to assess for combined alcohol and drug use/dependence in multiply addicted individuals for epidemiological, diagnosis, and treatment implications. It is also important to continue to elucidate common brain mechanisms that underlie generalized biological vulnerabilities and identify specific brain targets for subtypes of alcohol and drug addiction for future treatments.

More research studies distinguishing between genetic and environmental determinants are necessary. Investigations of genetic and familial patterns of generational transmission of drugs and alcohol in relation to environmental influences regarding exposure to alcohol and drugs are needed. In a simplified formula, the addiction rate can be equated to vulnerability plus exposure: Genetic factors pertain to vulnerability, whereas environmental factors relate to exposure. Prevention and treatment may be more easily accomplished by manipulation of the environment than genetic alteration for the immediate future, whereas knowledge of genetic factors will provide direction for therapeutic agents for addictive disorders and genetic counseling.[35]

Treatment Implications

The studies to date strongly suggest that treatment of alcohol and drug addiction must be aimed at both drugs and alcohol, in part, because of apparent genetically determined common biological mechanisms. The treatment of only a single drug addiction reduces the probability of achieving a successful outcome. Generally, it is advisable that alcoholics and drug addicts abstain from all drugs because of the potential for developing further addictions in addition to that of alcohol. Although not well documented, clinical experience confirms that cocaine addicts frequently return to cocaine use because of the use of alcohol or cannabis before using cocaine. Also, opiate addicts often return to use of alcohol or other drugs with or without returning to addictive use of opiates. Alcoholics may resort to using other drugs addictively, such as benzodiazepines, before eventually returning to alcohol use.

Both pharmacological and nonpharmacological treatments for drug and alcohol addiction benefit from a full appreciation and understanding of multiple drug and alcohol dependence and biological vulnerabilities.[49] Medications targeted for only drug or alcohol addiction have limited efficacy, as do the abstinence-based 12-step programs and behavioral, social, and cognitive therapies, if only alcohol or single drug types are the object of treatment.[1, 50]

REFERENCES

1. Miller NS: Special problems of the alcohol and multiple-drug dependent: Clinical interactions and detoxification. In Frances RJ, Miller SI (eds): Clinical Textbook of Addictive Disorders. New York, Guilford Press, 1991.
2. Schmitz J, DeJong J, Garnett D, et al: Substance abuse among subjects seeking treatment for alcoholism. Arch Gen Psychiatry 48:182–183, 1991.

3. Schnoll SH, Karrigan J, Kitchen SB, et al: Characteristics of cocaine abusers presenting for treatment. National Institutes of Health Drug Abuse Research Monograph Series 85:171–181, 1985.
4. Miller NS, Gold MS, Belkin BM: The diagnosis of alcohol and cannabis dependence in cocaine dependents and alcohol dependence in their families. Br J Addict 84:1491–1498, 1989.
5. Miller NS: The Pharmacology of Alcohol and Drugs of Abuse and Addiction. New York, Springer Verlag, 1991.
6. National Institute on Drug Abuse Capsules. US Dept of Health and Human Services. Press Office of the National Institute on Drug Abuse PHS, Washington DC, Alcohol and Drug Abuse and Mental Health Administration, 1990.
7. Helzer J, Burnam A: Epidemiology of alcohol addiction: United States. In Miller NS (ed): Comprehensive Handbook of Drug and Alcohol Addiction. New York, Marcel Dekker, 1991.
8. Robins LN, Helzer JE, Pryzbeck TR, et al: Alcohol disorders in the community: A report from the Epidemiologic Catchment Area. In Rose RM, Barrett J (eds): Alcoholism: Origins and Outcome. New York, Raven Press, 1988.
9. Watkins VM, McCoy CB: Drug use among urban Appalachian youths. In Watkins VM, McCoy CB (eds): Drug Abuse Patterns Among Polydrug Abusers and Urban Appalachian Youth (NIDA Services Research Report), DHHS Publication 80-1002. Washington, DC, US Government Printing Office, 1980.
10. Grant BF, Harford TC: Concurrent and simultaneous use of alcohol with cocaine: Results of a national survey. Drug Alcohol Depend 25:97–104, 1990.
11. Goodwin DW: Alcoholism and genetics: The sins of our fathers. Arch Gen Psychiatry 42:171–174, 1985.
12. Frances RJ, Timm S, Bucky S: Studies of familial and non-familial alcoholism. I. Demographic studies. Arch Gen Psychiatry 37:564–566, 1980.
13. Cotton NS: The familial incidence of alcoholism. J Stud Alcohol 40(1):89–116, 1979.
14. Miller NS, Gold MS: Research approaches to inheritance of alcoholism. J Subst Abuse Treat 9(3):157–163, 1988.
15. Jones RW: Alcoholism among relatives of alcoholic patients. Q J Stud Alcohol 33:810–813, 1972.
16. Kosten TR, Rounsaville BJ, Kleber HD: Parental alcoholism in opioid addicts. J Nerv Ment Dis 173(8):461–468, 1987.
17. Gfoerer J: Correlation between drug use by teenagers and drug use by older family members. Am J Drug Alcohol Abuse 13(1–2):95–108, 1987.
18. Kandel DB, Kessler RC, Marguiles RZ: Antecedents of adolescent initiation into stages of drug use: A development analysis. J Youth Adolesc 7:13–40, 1978.
19. Tec N: Parent-child drug abuse: Generational continuity or adolescent deviancy? Adolescence 9:351–354, 1974.
20. Pandina RJ, Johnson V: Serious alcohol and drug problems among adolescents with a family history of alcoholism. J Stud Alcohol 51(3):278–282, 1990.
21. Pandina RJ, Johnson V: Familial drinking history as a predictor of alcohol and drug consumption among adolescent children. J Stud Alcohol 50(3):245–253, 1989.
22. Scherer SE, Mukherjee BN: ''Moderate'' and hard drug users among college students: A study of their drug use patterns and characteristics. Br J Addict 66:315–328, 1971.
23. Fawzy FI, Coombs RH, Gerber B: Generational continuity in the use of substances: The impact of parental substance use on adolescent substance abuse. Addict Behav 8:109–114, 1983.
24. Annis HM: Patterns of intrafamilial drug use. Br J Addict 69:361–369, 1974.
25. Smart RG, Fejer D: 1972. Drug use among adolescents and their parents: Closing the generation gap in mood modification. J Abnorm Psychol 79(2):153–160, 1972.
26. Miller WH, Rinehart R, Cadoret RJ, et al: Specific familial transmission in substance abuse. Int J Addict 23(10):1029–1039, 1988.
27. Hill SY, Cloninger CR, Ayre FR: Independent familial transmission of alcoholism and opiate abuse. Alcohol Clin Exp Res 1:335–342, 1977.
28. Rounsaville BJ, Kosten TR, Weissman MM, et al: Psychiatric disorders in relatives of probands with opiate addiction. Arch Gen Psychiatry 48(1):33–42, 1991.
29. Mirin SM, Weiss RD, Griffin ML, et al: Psychopathology in drug abusers and their families. Compr Psychiatry 32(1):36–51, 1991.
30. Moss HB: Psychopathy, aggression, and family history in male veteran substance abuse patients: A factor analytic study. Addict Behav 14:565–570, 1989.
31. Svikis DS, Pickens RW: Methodological issues in family, adoption, and twin research. National Institutes of Health Drug Abuse Research Monograph Series 89:120–133, 1988.
32. Cloninger CR: Etiologic factors in substance abuse: An adoption study perspective. National Institutes of the Sciences Drug Abuse Research Monograph Series 89:52–72, 1988.
33. Cadoret RJ, Troughton E, O'Gorman TW, et al: An adoption study of genetic and environmental factors in drug abuse. Arch Gen Psychiatry 43:1131–1136, 1986.
34. Pickens RW, Svikis DS, McGue M: Heterogeneity in the inheritance of alcoholism: A study of male and female twins. Arch Gen Psychiatry 48:19–28, 1991.
35. Kendler KS, Neale MC, Heath AC, et al: A twin study of alcoholism in women. Am J Psychiatry 151(5):707–715, 1984.
36. Miller NS, Gold MS: Alcohol. New York, Plenum, 1991.
37. Wise RA: The brain and reward. In Liebman JM, Cooper SJ (eds): The Neuropharmacological Basis of Reward. Oxford, Oxford University Press, 1989.
38. Trachtenberg MC, Blum K: Alcohol and opioid peptides: Neuropharmacological rationale for physical cravings. Am J Drug Alcohol Abuse 13(3):365–372, 1987.
39. Blum K: A commentary on neurotransmitter restoration as a common mode of treatment for alcohol, cocaine and opiate abuse. Integrative Psychiatry 6:199–204, 1989.
40. Gorelick DA: Serotonin uptake blockers and the treatment of alcoholism. In Galanter MS (ed): Recent Developments in Alcoholism. New York, Plenum Press, 1988.
41. Kalivas PW, Widerlov E, Stanley D, et al: Enkephalin action on the mesolimbic system: A dopamine-dependent and dopamine-independent increase in locomotor activity. J Pharmacol Exp Ther 227:229–237, 1983.
42. Miller NS, Gold MS: Cocaine and alcoholism: Distinct or part of the spectrum. Psychiatry Ann 18(9):538–539, 1988.
43. Grant BF, Harford TC: Concurrent and simultaneous use of alcohol with sedatives and with tranquilizers: Results of a national survey. J Subst Abuse Treat 2:1–14, 1990.
44. Jekel JF, Allen DF: 1987. Trends in drug use in the mid-1980s. Yale J Biol Med 60:45–52, 1987.
45. Kaufman E: 1982. The relationship of alcoholism and alcohol abuse to the abuse of other drugs. Am J Drug Alcohol Abuse 9(1):1–17, 1982.

46. Needle R, Su S, Doherty W, et al: Familial, interpersonal, and intrapersonal correlates of drug use: A longitudinal comparison of adolescents in treatment, drug-using adolescents not in treatment, and non-drug-using adolescents. Int J Addict 23(12):1211–1240, 1988.

47. Kandel DB, Raveis VH: Cessation of illicit drug use in young adulthood. Arch Gen Psychiatry 46:409–416, 1989.

48. Freed EX: Drug abuse by alcoholics: A review. Int J Addict 8:451–473, 1973.

49. Kosten TR, Rounsaville BJ, Babor TF, et al: Substance abuse disorders in DSM-III-R. Br J Psychiatry 151:834–843, 1987.

50. Miller NS, Millman RB, Keskinen S: Outcome at six and twelve months post inpatient treatment for cocaine and alcohol dependence. Adv Alcohol Subst Abuse Treat 9(3–4):101–120, 1990.

BIBLIOGRAPHY

Cloninger RC, Bohman M, Sigvardson S: Inheritance of alcohol abuse: Cross-fostering analysis of adopted men. Arch Gen Psychiatry 38:861–868, 1981.

Devor EJ, Cloninger CR: Genetics of alcoholism. Annu Rev Genet 23:19–23, 1989.

George FR, Goldberg SR: Genetic approaches to the analysis of addiction processes. Trends Pharmacol Sci 10:78–83, 1989.

Kandel DB, Murphy D, Karus D: Cocaine use in young adulthood: Patterns of use and psychosocial correlates. National Institutes of Health Drug Abuse Research Monograph Series 85:76–111, 1985.

Kaufman E: The applications of biological vulnerability research to drug abuse prevention. National Institutes of Health Drug Abuse Research Monograph Series 89:174–180, 1988.

Meisch RA, George FR: Influence of genetic factors on drug-reinforced behavior in animals. National Institutes of Health Research Monograph Series 89:9–24, 1988.

Miller NS, Gold MS: A neuroanatomical and neurochemical approach to drug and alcohol addiction: Clinical and research considerations. In Miller NS (ed): Comprehensive Handbook of Drug and Alcohol Addiction. New York, Marcel Dekker, 1991.

Miller NS, Millman RB, Keskinen S: The diagnosis of alcohol, cocaine, and other drug dependence in an inpatient treatment population. J Subst Abuse Treat 6:37–40, 1989.

Pickens RW: Genetic vulnerability to drug abuse. National Institutes of Health Drug Abuse Research Monograph Series 89:41–51, 1988.

Schuckit MA: Biological vulnerability to alcoholism. In Miller NS (ed): Comprehensive Handbook of Drug and Alcohol Addiction. New York, Marcel Dekker, 1991.

Genetics of Alcoholism

Stephen H. Dinwiddie, MD

The observation that alcoholism clusters in families dates back to classical times and generally has been taken as sufficient demonstration of the hereditary nature of the illness. By comparison, the belief that social or environmental factors might be determinative is of much newer vintage.[1, 2] Advances in research techniques are now beginning to allow researchers to synthesize earlier findings and attempt to determine the ways in which constitutional and experiential factors interact to cause the disease. In this chapter, therefore, the evidence for the role of genetic influences in alcoholism is assessed and ways in which such factors might contribute to the disease reviewed.

Family Studies in Alcoholism

Despite use of different definitions of alcoholism, several ways of identifying proband cases, and different means of identifying the disorder among family members, it has been repeatedly demonstrated that alcoholism aggregates in families.[3] For example, Winokur and colleagues,[4] studying first-degree relatives of hospitalized alcoholics, found that 34% of male relatives and 9% of female relatives were themselves alcoholic. Ten years later, Reich and associates[5] found even higher rates: 54% of men and 17% of women, as compared with 20% and 4% of male and female relatives of nonalcoholics, respectively. A third study,[6] which like the study by Reich and coworkers made diagnoses based on explicit criteria and used structured interviews performed by raters blind to proband diagnosis, found 27% of male relatives and 6% of female relatives of alcoholics ascertained through an outpatient psychiatric clinic. These rates, again, were significantly higher than among relatives of nonalcoholic probands (17% and 2%, respectively, among men and women). Overall, reviewing studies such as these, it has been estimated that first-degree relatives of alcoholics may be as much as seven times more likely to develop alcoholism than those without such a family history.[7]

Men are more likely than women to develop alcoholism, whether one samples from the general population or from relatives of alcoholics. However, there appears to be no sex difference in its transmission. That is, male relatives of alcoholics are at higher risk than male relatives of nonalcoholics, and the same holds true for women, but the risk to the relative is about the same whether the alcoholic relative is male or female.

The fact that alcoholism clusters in families does not mean either that all cases of the disorder must be familial or that alcoholism must therefore be purely (or even partly) genetic in its etiology, nor does it mean that all cases of the illness must arise from the same factors. Nonetheless, risk for developing the illness among *biological* relatives of alcoholics is significantly higher than among relatives of nonalcoholics.[7] Moreover, familial cases of alcoholism, as opposed to sporadic ones, have been shown to be more severe, with earlier age of onset, more alcohol-related problems, and worse treatment outcome.[8-10] Such observations suggest (although they cannot establish) a biologically heritable component of the illness.

Although observed patterns of aggregation within families may suggest a genetic predisposition, they are at the same time inconsistent with a purely genetic illness at a single locus, either autosomal or sex linked, dominant or recessive. Nor, when one looks at studies including more distant relatives (e.g., half-siblings, grandparents, and so forth), are rates consistent with polygenic inheritance.[11-13]

Finally, evidence suggests that alcoholism has become more common over time, with younger cohorts demonstrating higher rates of alcoholism.[14] Although this finding is apparent in the general population, it is substantially amplified among those with an alcoholic family member. Analyzing data from a large family study, Cloninger[15] reported that consistent with earlier reported rates, men who were born between 1915 and 1924 and who were first-degree relatives of alcoholics themselves had a 26% risk of being diagnosed with alcoholism. That risk rose progressively in successive cohorts, up to 67% among those born after 1955—even though that group was still progressing through the age of risk.

Such a rapid change in prevalence is obviously inconsistent with fundamental genetic changes and underscores an important distinction: What is inherited is not the disease as such but rather the liability to develop it. Rather than being assigned a dichotomous affected/unaffected status, any individual can instead be conceptualized as being placed on a continuum of liability, with those above a given threshold exhibiting the disorder. Though such models typically assume multifactorial (genetic plus nongenetic liability factors) inheritance, one need not make any assumptions about the mechanism by which this liability is transmitted. In this way, findings such as the observed inconsistency in familial patterns of inheritance with known genetic patterns and change in risk over time can be reconciled. At any given degree of constitutional liability, the likelihood of expressing the disorder can be altered by experiential factors: Those with higher (inborn) liability may encounter protective factors and thus never manifest the illness. Conversely, those with lower loadings of liability factors, if exposed to an exacerbating environment, may nonetheless develop alcoholism.[16] (It should be kept in mind that any factor from

genomic imprinting to fetal alcohol exposure to social attitudes toward drinking may be "environmental" in this sense).

This finding also indicates that the distinction between familial and nonfamilial alcoholism, noted earlier, may be artifactual in nature. In the general population, there are regular relations between average alcohol consumption per capita and proportion of the population who are heavy drinkers (i.e., those most at risk for subsequently developing alcoholism).[17] If familial and nonfamilial alcoholism were etiologically distinct, an increase in per capita alcohol consumption (i.e., exposure) should be associated with an increase in sporadic (nonfamilial) alcoholism, whereas rates among relatives of alcoholics should stay relatively stable, except for the addition of a few cases accounted for by the increased exposure. By diluting the proportion of alcoholics with affected family members, an increase in average alcohol consumption should have the effect of making alcoholism appear less, rather than more, familial.

This does not appear to be the case. Instead, a substantial portion of the increase of alcoholism in younger cohorts appears to come from those with a positive family history. Thus, it is more consistent with the hypothesis that experiential factors (perhaps change in time over social attitudes toward drinking) have differentially increased the likelihood of developing alcoholism among those with transmissible liability factors.[18]

A second consideration that tends to undermine any genetic distinction between familial and nonfamilial alcoholism is the observation that reliability of diagnosis, as might be predicted, is higher among more severe cases (i.e., among those with higher numbers of alcohol-related problems). As noted by Cloninger,[15] more severe, more reliably diagnosed cases, which are likely to present as primary illness (rather than secondarily after other psychiatric disorders), can be shown to aggregate within families, whereas less-severe, probable, secondary cases do not. Because the definite, primary cases are likely to have earlier onset, as well, the distinction between familial and nonfamilial alcoholism may simply reduce to a difference in severity and aggregation of risk factors rather than be a reflection of predominantly different etiologic factors.

Adoption Studies of Alcoholism

Family studies show that alcoholism is transmissible or, more precisely, that the *liability* to the disorder aggregates in families, with exposure being one (presumably of many) necessary subsequent link in a causal chain leading to alcoholism. However, many things can be passed from one generation to the next without being genetic in nature, and studies of nuclear families cannot necessarily by themselves answer the question of what is inherited or how it is transmitted.

Although more elaborate family studies designed to contrast rates in more distant relatives (e.g., half-siblings, cousins, grandparents, and so forth) can be used to estimate the amount of genetic and shared environmental influences in risk for alcoholism, two techniques have traditionally been relied on to separate biologically heritable influences from postnatal factors. These are, of course, the twin study and the adoption study.

In theory, adoption, by severing connections between biological parent and child, should provide evidence about whether inheritance of a character is biological or cultural. Obviously, resemblance to the (absent) biological parent would suggest genetic inheritance, whereas resemblance to the adoptive parent would favor cultural inheritance. Unfortunately, adoption studies are made more difficult to interpret by factors such as nonrandom assignment of the adoptee (who may be "matched" to characteristics of the adoptive parents that resemble those of the biological parent as well), delayed separation from the birth mother, exposure to putatively nongenetic but congenital influences (e.g., maternal drinking during pregnancy), and the fact that birth parents are likely to be unrepresentative of subjects in general with a given disorder.

Despite these caveats, adoption studies generally support the role of biological factors in the transmission of alcoholism. One exception is the earliest such study,[19] which retrospectively compared 36 children of heavily drinking fathers with 25 offspring of normal parents, finding no difference in risk of alcohol-related difficulties in early adulthood.

Later, in a variant on the traditional adoption study, Schuckit and colleagues[20] studied half-siblings of alcoholics admitted to treatment, interviewing both the 69 subjects and 90 relatives. In that study, alcoholism in the biological parent was associated with alcoholism in the offspring, whereas exposure to alcohol abuse in the absence of genetic relationship was not.

Beginning in 1970, Goodwin and colleagues [2, 21–24] began a large-scale study of alcoholism among Danish adoptees, comparing them both with adoptees without a parental background of alcoholism and with subjects raised by alcoholic biological parents. In this study, alcoholism was rigorously defined, and probands were selected for early adoption without later contact with biological parents. Interview by a psychiatrist was performed blind to the subject's status. In this manner, 55 male adoptees were studied, and 20 of these were compared with 30 unadopted brothers, as were 49 female adoptees, who were compared with 81 nonadopted daughters of alcoholics. Further comparisons were made with matched control adoptees.

It was found that adopted-away sons of alcoholic parents were four times more likely than adopted-away sons of nonalcoholics to develop alcoholism, and the alcoholism tended to be more severe. Other psychiatric illness appeared not to be more prevalent. Finally, being raised by an alcoholic parent did not further increase the risk of alcoholism above that conveyed by biological factors: Rates of alcoholism did not differ between the adopted sons and their nonadopted brothers. By contrast, daughters of alcoholics appeared not to be at elevated risk: 2% of adopted-away daughters, compared with 4% among adoptive controls and 3% of nonadopted daughters, were diagnosed with alcoholism.

Similar results were reported in a study of adoptees in Iowa.[25] In that study, 45 adult adoptees and 84 of their adopted parents were interviewed; psychiatric problems in the biological parents were identified by record review. Six biological parents had alcohol-related problems. Two of the three adoptees with definite primary alcoholism (by Feighner's criteria) came from this group, versus only one child of the remaining 78 parents; by contrast, 7 adoptees (none from alcoholic biological backgrounds) had secondary alcoholism. Alcoholism in the child correlated with no other psychiatric illness in the biological parents.

A different approach was taken by Cloninger and colleagues,[26] who used a record-linkage approach to examine the heritability of alcohol abuse in a large sample. Looking at alcohol abuse (classified as none, mild, moderate, or severe, based on Temperance Board registration or treatment) among 862 Swedish men of known paternity adopted before the age of 3 years, the investigators demonstrated, first, that the biological backgrounds of the four groups was heterogeneous. They also found evidence for significant gene-environment interaction, with mild and severe abusers sharing similar biological backgrounds and differing primarily on exposure to exacerbating environmental factors. Adoptees with both prenatal and postnatal liability factors were about four times more likely to develop alcohol-related problems (27% vs. 6% of those from low-risk backgrounds). Interestingly, moderate abusers showed little evidence of postnatal influence; only 2% of those from low-risk biological backgrounds were classified as moderate abusers, versus 17% and 18%, respectively, of those from high-risk biological and low- or high-risk postnatal backgrounds.

A parallel analysis of 913 female adoptees[27] found similar results. Although rates of alcohol abuse were found to be much lower, women with congenital and postnatal risk factors were three times more likely to be classified as alcohol abusers than were those at low risk (7.7% vs. 2.3%). Based on these findings, Cloninger proposed two types of alcoholism: a rarer but highly heritable male-limited form and a more common form, milieu limited, which appeared to be more dependent on exacerbating environmental factors to be manifested.

Twin Studies in Alcoholism

Another way of separating and quantifying relative influences of constitutional and learned factors is to study twins. Excess concordance among monozygotic (MZ) twins, who share both genetic and many environmental influences, above that of same-sex dizygotic (DZ) twins (who presumably share many environmental factors plus on average half of their genes) argues for the presence of genetic influence on the trait in question.

As with adoption studies, twin studies cannot be accepted without certain caveats. Twins are a distinct population, with an elevated risk of birth complications and infant mortality; moreover, the assumption that MZ and DZ twins have equal common environmental influences has been questioned.[28] However, as in the case of adoption studies, results of twin studies of alcoholism generally support a role for heritable factors. With the exception of one small study,[29] studies to date have demonstrated an elevated proband-wise concordance (i.e., the likelihood of an alcoholic twin having an alcoholic co-twin) for MZ twins as compared with same-sex DZ twins. However, some intriguing differences between studies have arisen.

In an early study, Kaij,[30] examining concordance of male MZ and DZ twin pairs for Temperance Board registration, found significantly elevated proband-wise concordance among MZ twins (61% vs. 39% of DZ twin pairs for at least one registration). Interestingly, both rates were higher than in the general population.

Subsequent large record-linkage studies from Finland[31] and Sweden,[32, 33] comprising more than 16,000 twin pairs from Finland and nearly 13,000 from Sweden, used hospital records with discharge diagnoses of alcoholism, also finding elevated proband-wise concordance among MZ twins. In the Finnish study, concordances for MZ male twin pairs were 23.1% versus 10.8% for DZ males; in the Swedish study, rates were 13.2% and 7.9%, respectively. However, the low population prevalence as estimated by the criterion of treatment diminished the statistical power of these studies, such that although alcoholism was clearly highly familial, reanalysis could not confidently reject the hypothesis that concordance was entirely due to shared environmental influences.[34] Moreover, the decrement in statistical power is even more striking for women, because the population prevalence of alcoholism (however defined) is substantially lower than in men, thus leading to the need for astronomically large sample sizes in order to test adequately for (or confidently reject) the influence of genetic factors.[34]

A large record-linkage study in the United States, ascertaining 13,486 male twin pairs from Veterans Administration records, fared somewhat better and was more strongly consistent with the hypothesis of genetic effects.[35] In that study, proband-wise concordances of 26.3% for MZ and 11.9% for DZ twin pairs were found.

A more recent U.S. study[36, 37] used both direct interviews and mailed questionnaires. In that study, 404 twin pairs were ascertained through inpatient substance abuse treatment and assessed via questionnaire; a subsample of 169 pairs was directly interviewed by blind raters using a structured diagnostic assessment. Using DSM-III alcohol abuse or dependence criteria to assess alcoholism, the researchers found proband-wise concordances of 76% versus 53% for male MZ and DZ twin pairs and 39% and 42%, respectively, for female MZ and DZ twins. Although they found no evidence of genetic contribution to risk for alcoholism among women, evidence supported the role of genetic factors in the development of alcohol dependence in men. The researchers also found support for the existence of genetic heterogeneity, with more severe alcohol-related problems showing stronger evidence of genetic influence.

Sampling from hospitalized cases is likely to

identify severe cases of alcoholism differentially; in record-linkage studies in particular, rates of alcoholism identified tend to be far below estimates based on epidemiological samples. Thus, to an uncertain degree, such studies risk confounding influences of coexisting psychiatric or medical illness (e.g., end-organ disease) with genetic influences, specifically on the syndrome of alcoholism.[34]

An alternative, therefore, is to study cases derived from the general population, using either mailed questionnaires or interviews in person or via telephone. In general, mailed surveys have not supported the role of genetic factors. Prescott and colleagues,[38] surveying older volunteers and using Feighner's criteria for probable or definite alcoholism, found proband-wise concordances of 44.4% among male MZ twin pairs as compared with 15.4% among male DZ twins, but because of the small sample size, this was not a significant difference, and the magnitude was even smaller among women.

Similarly, Heath and coworkers[39] used self-report questionnaires in two cohorts of twins derived from a volunteer sample, the Australian National Health and Medical Research Council twin panel. Again using Feighner's criteria for alcoholism, among twins born in 1895 to 1964, no difference in concordance was found by zygosity in same-sex male or female twin pairs. In a younger cohort, born in 1964 to 1971, no differences emerged among male MZ versus DZ twin pairs, but among young women, proband-wise concordance was significantly higher, 52.9% among MZ and 34.2% among same-sex female DZ twin pairs.

At present, only one community-based study using interviews rather than mailed surveys, the Virginia Twin Register, has been reported, although results from two others (a sample of 3300 same-sex male twins, the Vietnam-era twin panel, and an expansion of the Australian Twin Survey drawing on 6000 twins) are pending.

In the Virginia sample,[40] 1030 like-sex twin pairs were ascertained from birth records and interviewed using standardized protocols and explicit diagnostic criteria. In that study, three different definitions of alcoholism were tested: a restrictive one, requiring DSM-III-R diagnosis of alcohol dependence plus manifestations of physiological dependence; intermediate (i.e., DSM-III-R alcohol dependence without requiring tolerance or withdrawal); or a broad definition that required only evidence of alcohol-related problems not limited to a single incident. Although prevalence differed based on each definition, proband-wise concordance was consistently higher for MZ than DZ twins: 26.2% versus 11.9% using the most restrictive definition, 31.6% versus 24.4% for the intermediate group, and 46.9% versus 31.5% using a broad definition. Although this pattern was consistent with the presence of genetic factors (indeed the investigators suggested that the heritability of liability to alcoholism was 50% to 60%), only for the broadest definition could the hypothesis of no genetic effects be very confidently rejected.

This study was subsequently extended by also interviewing 1468 parents of these twins.[41] Using the most restrictive definition of alcoholism, the researchers concluded that the data best fit a model in which the familial aggregation of alcoholism was due to genetic factors plus environmental influences unique to the individual, with no effect of shared environment due to parental alcoholism observed. The heritability of underlying alcoholism liability factors was estimated to be between 51% and 59%.

These findings are supported by preliminary results from the extension of the Australian Twin Survey. Administering a structured telephone interview to approximately 6000 Australian twins, Heath and associates[42] reported proband-wise concordance rates for DSM-III-R–defined alcohol dependence of 56.7% of MZ male twin pairs, versus 33.0% for DZ male twin pairs. For women, comparable rates were 28.9% for MZ and 15.8% among DZ twin pairs. This magnitude of difference is sufficient to reject the hypothesis of no genetic effects. Moreover, in examining unlike-sex pairs, it was found that the risk to male co-twins of affected female twins was substantial (60.0%, vs. 15.1% of women with affected male co-twins), suggesting that women require a more extreme genetic liability in order to manifest alcoholism. Using a multifactorial threshold model, the investigators estimated a heritability of alcoholism liability of 67%, with no significant gender difference.

Trait Markers

Taken as a whole, therefore, such studies strongly support the existence of biologically heritable factors that influence the risk of alcoholism. However, these factors are probably quite heterogeneous, and they potentially can affect the genesis and course of alcoholism at various levels. It is well to keep in mind that the clinical entity of alcoholism comprises a complex and changing mixture of behaviors (e.g., driving under the influence, fighting while intoxicated), subjective states (craving, guilt over consequences of drinking), social consequences (work impairment, divorce), physiological changes (tolerance, withdrawal states), and medical complications (cirrhosis, pancreatitis). Although specific manifestations of the illness differ widely between individuals, for the purposes of genetic analysis, this heterogeneous collection is typically lumped into the single phenotype of alcoholism, even though genetic factors may influence the ultimate phenotypical expression in various ways, ranging from influencing the probability of exposure to alcohol in the first place to determining specific forms of end-organ disease. Thus, more complete understanding of the genetics of alcoholism is predicated on better knowledge of characteristics ranging from the inheritance of personality to the genetic determination of specific metabolic pathways.

A corollary is therefore that for more complete understanding, components of the alcoholism phenotype should be separately investigated, at different points in the etiological pathway leading to alcoholism. Measurement at any given level may range from biochemical assay to psychological testing. For example, factors such as onset, quantity, and frequency of drinking may not be determinants of alcoholism per se but may influence risk of later developing alcohol-related problems and appear themselves to have genetic components.[31, 43] Similarly, personality characteristics are substantially influenced by genetic factors, and certain personality traits (such as unusually high or low levels of novelty seeking) may convey higher risk for developing alcoholism or specific kinds of alcohol-related difficulties.[44, 45] These characteristics, in turn, may be associated with differences in neurotransmitter and neurotransmitter metabolite differences in the cerebrospinal fluid of certain alcoholic subgroups, particularly those with early onset of problems and with violent behavior.[46, 47]

Such factors may be conceptualized as rather nonspecific risk or protective factors for alcoholism. At the other extreme, it is likely that certain kinds of end-organ diseases may be under relatively simple and specific genetic control. For example, Wernicke-Korsakoff syndrome may be associated with abnormal transketolase activity.[48] Conversely, a specific inherited deficiency in aldehyde dehydrogenase has been linked in some populations to the flushing response to alcohol and (presumably consequent) decreased alcohol intake; this unpleasant reaction may therefore act as a biological protective factor against development of alcoholism by limiting exposure.[49]

The genetics of other potential biological risk indicators can be studied without researchers' necessarily having specific knowledge of how those factors mediate (if they do) risk for alcoholism. In this manner, the power of other research techniques may be increased by allowing identification of at-risk individuals who have not developed the full phenotype of alcoholism, either because of protective factors or because they were ascertained early in the period of risk. Obviously, identification of such factors might also ultimately prove to be of clinical use by identifying at-risk individuals so that interventions aimed at primary prevention can be designed and evaluated.

One powerful method of identifying such risk indicators is to study high-risk populations (e.g., sons of alcoholics) before significant ethanol exposure has occurred. A number of studies have demonstrated population differences between young men with and without a family history of alcoholism on measures such as body sway and subjective intensity of intoxication. Endocrinological studies have also found population differences in response to thyrotropin-releasing hormone challenge as well as responses of adrenocorticotropic hormone, cortisol, and prolactin after administration of test doses of alcohol.[50, 51] Although the predictive value of some of these tests in identifying those who develop alcoholism remains to be determined, lessened subjective feelings of intoxication in response to a test dose of alcohol have been shown to be associated with a fourfold elevated risk of alcoholism later in life.[52]

Another technique that holds promise of identifying individuals at risk for alcoholism involves study of event-related potentials, characteristic electroencephalographic waveforms that occur in response to various stimuli. Because these may reflect heritable differences in attention and cognitive function, they may also prove to be a trait marker for heightened liability to alcoholism. Although a number of tasks and measures have been used to compare high- to low-risk subjects, the most reproducible finding appears to be reduction in voltage of one waveform (P3) after attentional tasks.[53]

GENETIC ASSOCIATION AND LINKAGE STUDIES

Studies of genetic markers for alcoholism have been limited until fairly recently by a lack of informative loci, but with the advent of more powerful methods for mapping the human genome has come the opportunity to test for association between many other markers and alcoholism. One technique by which this can be done is to study genetic linkage—that is, the degree to which the character of interest and a putative marker are cotransmitted within families. Although efforts are ongoing, to date no findings of genetic linkage have been replicated.

Another approach is to assess genetic association, which involves comparison of gene frequencies at a candidate locus between cases and matched controls. In 1990, Blum and colleagues[54] reported that 69% of a series of alcoholics, versus 20% of controls, carried the A1 allele at the dopamine D2 receptor (DRD2) locus. Unfortunately, although a number of replications have since been performed, definitive confirmation has remained elusive. Thus, clear evidence of genetic association with the alcoholism phenotype remains lacking.[34]

ANIMAL STUDIES

Although studies of aspects of the alcoholism phenotype in animals have progressed in parallel with clinical studies in humans, clinicians have as a rule taken surprisingly little notice of the results. The development of alcohol-preferring inbred strains of rodents[55] has led to the possibility of being able to separate out very specific components of alcohol and drug response, such as initial physiological and behavioral sensitivity to effects of ethanol and development of tolerance and withdrawal phenomena.[56] The ability to correlate such responses to studies of neurophysiology and receptor affinity has obvious importance in filling in the pathways from genes to behavior. More recent advances in the ability to perform reverse genetics (i.e., altering or eliminating specific genes so that resultant effects on phenotype can be studied) in rodents, combined with forward genetic techniques using high-efficiency mutagenesis to uncover previously unknown genes based on what alterations in phenotype are seen,[57] are likely to accelerate further the process of identification of specific genes involved in the multiple manifestations of alcoholism.

Conclusion

Although specific DNA sequences predisposing to alcoholism remain to be characterized, great progress has nonetheless been made from the initial observation that alcoholism clusters in families. It is now clear that genetic influences operate on many levels to influence liability to alcoholism and, if it develops, to help shape its ultimate expression. As a result, the specificity of such influences may differ greatly, ranging from genes coding for neurochemical susceptibility in brain, to individual enzymes important in an organ's metabolism of ethanol (and thus potentially implicated in end-organ disease), to general factors such as the heritable factors that help to determine personality, which might in turn influence factors such as exposure to alcohol or likelihood of changing behavior in response to adverse consequences. A complete understanding of the genetics of alcoholism must also account for how such factors interact with each other and influence their expression over time and how they reciprocally interact with environmental and experiential factors to produce the alcoholism phenotype.

Further advances in our understanding of the genetics of alcoholism are likely to come from integration of findings at a number of levels. Great progress has been made in development of animal models for numerous specific aspects of the alcoholism phenotype, such as alcohol preference, manifestation of tolerance and withdrawal phenomena, and control over rewarding aspects of alcohol intake. The availability of animal models allows researchers to use various extremely powerful techniques to relate such specific phenotypical features to genetic sequences and to characterize precisely the biological pathways by which they exercise their effects.

In humans, numerous methods of characterizing specific aspects of the alcoholism phenotype are now being used. Strategies involve, for example, ascertaining twins from general community samples and interviewing family members including spouses and offspring, or studying the extended pedigrees of identified alcoholic probands. Such studies, obviously, can be further extended into longitudinal projects that can both observe identified alcoholics and monitor individuals with high probability of alcoholism as they first enter the age of risk. By using a wide battery of assessments, including structured psychiatric interviews, personality assessments, neurophysiological studies, biochemical assays, and molecular genetic techniques such as linkage and association studies, the spectrum of factors influencing (positively or negatively) the risk for alcoholism can be separately evaluated and the manifold genetic influences on its inheritance characterized.

REFERENCES

1. Warner RH, Rossett HL: The effects of drinking on offspring: An historical survey of the American and British literature. J Stud Alcohol 36:1395–1420.
2. Goodwin DW: Alcoholism and heredity: A review and hypothesis. Arch Gen Psychiatry 36:57–61, 1979.
3. Cotton NS: The familial incidence of alcoholism. J Stud Alcohol 40:89–116, 1979.
4. Winokur G, Reich T, Rimmer J, Pitts FN: Alcoholism. III. Diagnosis and familial psychiatric illness in 259 alcoholic probands. Arch Gen Psychiatry 23:104–111, 1970.
5. Reich T, Rice J, Cloninger CR, Lewis C: The contribution of affected parents to the pool of affected individuals: Path analysis of the segregation distribution of alcoholism. In Robins L, Clayton P (eds): Social Consequences of Psychiatric Illness. New York, Brunner/Mazel, 1980, pp 91–113.
6. Guze SB, Cloninger CR, Martin R, Clayton PJ: Alcoholism as a medical disorder. Compr Psychiatry 27:501–510, 1986.
7. Merikangas K: The genetic epidemiology of alcoholism. Psychol Med 20:11–22, 1990.
8. Penick EC, Read MR, Crowley PA, Powell BJ: Differentiation of alcoholics by family history. J Stud Alcohol 39:1944–1948, 1978.
9. Frances RJ, Timm S, Bucky S: Studies of familial and nonfamilial alcoholism. I. Demographic studies. Arch Gen Psychiatry 37:564–566, 1980.
10. Frances RJ, Bucky S, Alexopoulos GS: Outcome study of familial and nonfamilial alcoholism. Am J Psychiatry 141:1469–1471, 1984.
11. Kaij L, Dock J: Grandsons of alcoholics: A test of sex-linked transmission of alcohol abuse. Arch Gen Psychiatry 32:1379–1381, 1975.
12. Saunders JB, Williams R: The genetics of alcoholism: Is there an inherited susceptibility to alcohol-related problems? Alcohol Alcohol 18:189–217, 1983.
13. Dawson DA, Harford TC, Grant BF: Family history as a predictor of alcohol dependence. Alcohol Clin Exp Res 16:572–575, 1992.
14. Helzer JE, Burnam A, McEvoy LT: Alcohol abuse and dependence. In Robins LN, Regier DA (eds): Psychiatric Disorders in America. New York, The Free Press, 1991, pp 81–115.
15. Cloninger CR: Recent advances in family studies of alcoholism. In Goedde HW, Agarwal DP (eds): Genetics and Alcoholism. New York, Alan R Liss, 1987, pp 47–60.
16. Reich T, Cloninger CR, Guze SB: The multifactorial model of disease transmission: I. Description of the model and its use in psychiatry. Br J Psychiatry 127:1–10, 1975.
17. Cloninger CR, Reich T, Sigvardsson S, et al: The effects of changes in alcohol use between generations on the inheritance of alcohol abuse. In Rose R (ed): Alcoholism: A Medical Disorder. New York, Raven Press, 1986, pp 49–74.
18. Reich T, Cloninger CR, van Eerdewegh P, et al: Secular trends in the familial transmission of alcoholism. Alcohol Clin Exp Res 12:458–464, 1988.
19. Roe A: The adult adjustment of children of alcoholic parents raised in foster-homes. Q J Stud Alcohol 5:378–393, 1944.
20. Schuckit MA, Goodwin DA, Winokur G: A study of alcoholism in half siblings. Am J Psychiatry 128:122–126, 1972.
21. Goodwin DW, Schulsinger F, Hermansen L, et al: Alcohol problems in adoptees raised apart from alcoholic biological relatives. Arch Gen Psychiatry 28:238–243 1972.
22. Goodwin DW, Schulsinger F, Moller N, et al: Drinking problems in adopted and nonadopted sons of alcoholics. Arch Gen Psychiatry 31:164–169, 1974.
23. Goodwin DW, Schulsinger F, Knob J, et al: Alcoholism and depression in adopted-out daughters of alcoholics. Arch Gen Psychiatry 34:751–755, 1977.
24. Goodwin DW, Schulsinger F, Knob J, et al: Psychopathology in adopted and nonadopted daughters of alcoholics. Arch Gen Psychiatry 34:1005–1009, 1977.
25. Cadoret RJ, Gath A: Inheritance of alcoholism in adoptees. Br J Psychiatry 132:252–258, 1978.
26. Cloninger CR, Bohman M, Sigvardsson S: Inheritance of alcohol abuse. Cross-fostering analysis of adopted men. Arch Gen Psychiatry 38:861–868, 1981.
27. Bohman M, Sigvardsson S, Cloninger CR: Maternal inheritance of alcohol abuse. Cross-fostering analysis of adopted women. Arch Gen Psychiatry 38:965–969, 1981.
28. Goodwin DW: Genetic factors in the development of alcoholism. Psychiatr Clin North Am 9:427–433, 1986.
29. Gurling HMD, Oppenheim BE, Murray RM: Depression, criminality and psychopathology associated with alcoholism: Evidence from a twin study. Acta Genet Med Gemellol 33:333–339, 1984.
30. Kaij L: Alcoholism in Twins: Studies on the Etiology and Sequels of Abuse of Alcohol. Stockholm, Almqvist and Wiksell, 1960.
31. Kaprio J, Koskenvuo M, Langinvainia H, et al: Genetic influences on use and abuse of alcohol: A study of 5638 adult Finnish twin brothers. Alcohol Clin Exp Res 11:349–356, 1987.
32. Allgulander C, Nowak J, Rice JP: Psychopathology and treatment of 30,344 twins in Sweden. I. The appropriateness of psychoactive drug treatment. Acta Psychiatr Scand 82:420–426, 1990.
33. Allgulander C, Nowak J, Rice JP: Psychopathology and treatment of 30,344 twins in Sweden. II. Heritability estimates of psychiatric diagnosis and treatment in 12,884 twin pairs. Acta Psychiatr Scand 83:12–15, 1991.
34. Heath AC, Slutske WS, Madden PAF: Gender differences in the genetic contribution to alcoholism risk and to alcohol consumption patterns. In Wilsnack RW, Wilsnack SC (eds): Gender and Alcohol. Rutgers, NJ, Rutgers University Press (in press).
35. Hrubeck Z, Omenn GS: Evidence for genetic predisposition to alcoholic cirrhosis and psychosis: Twin concordances for alcoholism and its biological end points by zygosity among male veterans. Alcohol Clin Exp Res 5:207–215, 1981.
36. Pickens RW, Svikis DS, McGue M, et al: Heterogeneity in the inheritance of alcoholism: A study of male and female twins. Arch Gen Psychiatry 48:19–28, 1991.
37. McGue M, Pickens RW, Svikis DS: Sex and age effects on the inheritance of alcohol problems: A twin study. J Abnorm Psychol 101:3–17, 1992.
38. Prescott CA, Hewitt JK, Truett KR, et al: Genetic and environmental contributions on alcohol abuse in a community sample of older twins. J Stud Alcohol 55:184–202, 1994.
39. Heath AC, Bucholz KK, Dinwiddie SH, et al: The contribution of genetic factors to risk of alcohol problems in women. Presented at Behavior Genetics Association Annual Meeting, Sydney, Australia, July 13–16, 1993.
40. Kendler KS, Heath AC, Neale MC, et al: A population-

based twin study of alcoholism in women. JAMA 268:1877–1882, 1992.

41. Kendler KS, Neale MC, Heath AC, et al: A twin-family study of alcoholism in women. Am J Psychiatry 151:707–715, 1994.

42. Heath AC, Madden PAF, Bucholz KK, et al: Genetic contribution to alcoholism risk in women. Presented at Research Society on Alcoholism Annual Meeting, Maui, Hawaii, June 18–23, 1994.

43. Heath AC, Martin NG: Teenage alcohol use in the Australian Twin Register: Genetic and social determinants of starting to drink. Alcohol Clin Exp Res 12:735–741, 1988.

44. Plomin R, Owen MJ, McGuffin P: The genetic basis of complex human behaviors. Science 264:1733–1739, 1994.

45. Cloninger CR: Neurogenetic adaptive mechanisms in alcoholism. Science 236:410–416, 1987.

46. Limson R, Goldman D, Roy A, et al: Personality and cerebrospinal fluid monoamine metabolites in alcoholics and controls. Arch Gen Psychiatry 48:437–441, 1991.

47. Linnoila M, DeJong J, Virkkunen M: Family history of alcoholism in violent offenders and impulsive firesetters. Arch Gen Psychiatry 46:613–616, 1989.

48. Blass JD, Gibson GE: Abnormality of a thiamine-requiring enzyme in patients with Wernicke-Korsakoff syndrome. N Engl J Med 297:1367–1370, 1977.

49. Agarwal DP, Goedde HW: Human aldehyde dehydrogenases: Genetic implications in alcohol sensitivity, alcohol-drinking habits and alcoholism. In Cloninger CR, Begleiter H (eds): Genetics and Biology of Alcoholism, Banbury Report 32. Plainview, NY, Cold Spring Harbor Laboratory Press, 1991, pp 105–129.

50. Schuckit MA: Biological markers in alcoholism. Prog Neuropsychopharmacol Biol Psychiatry 10:191–199, 1986.

51. Loosen PT, Prange AJ: TRH in alcoholic men: Endocrine responses. Psychosom Med 41:584–585, 1979.

52. Schuckit MA: Low level of response to alcohol as a predictor of future alcoholism. Am J Psychiatry 151:184–189, 1994.

53. Begleiter H, Porjesz B: Potential biological markers in individuals at high risk for developing alcoholism. Alcohol Clin Exp Res 12:488–493, 1988.

54. Blum K, Noble EP, Sheridan PJ, et al: Allelic association of human dopamine D2 receptor gene in alcoholism. JAMA 263:2055–2060, 1990.

55. McClearn GE, Rodgers DA: Differences in alcohol preference among inbred strains of mice. Q J Stud Alcohol 20:691–695, 1959.

56. Crabbe JC, Belknap JK, Buck KJ: Genetic animal models of alcohol and drug abuse. Science 264:1715–1723, 1994.

57. Takahashi JS, Pinto LH, Vitaterna MH: Forward and reverse genetic approaches to behavior in the mouse. Science 264:1724–1733, 1994.

Genetic Factors in Human Drug Abuse and Addiction

Remi J. Cadoret, MD • William Yates, MD •
Eric Devor, PhD

Drug abuse and addiction are a complex of behaviors caused by diverse potential etiological factors ranging from variability in an individual's metabolic response to a substance to the psychosocial variables that led the individual to take the drug in the first place. In this vast array of causes leading from use to abuse and drug addiction, there is ample opportunity for expression of genetic factors. This chapter presents evidence implicating genetic influences in drug abuse in humans. Current psychiatric nomenclature defines drug abuse as a less severe syndrome than drug dependence (addiction). In this chapter we will use drug abuse to designate the full syndrome of problems (including drug dependence) that occur with the use of illicit drugs. Although the study of genetic factors in drug abuse is relatively recent, older studies of genetic factors in alcoholism have suggested the involvement of similar factors in drug abuse. Research into alcoholism has shown that genetic factors interact in a number of different ways with alcohol, ranging from control of alcohol metabolism to control of quantity and frequency of drinking and to a role in alcohol-related behavior such as tolerance and intoxication.

These studies of genetic factors in alcoholic behavior have used several methodological approaches that have been applied to behavior related to drugs. The two main approaches in humans have been the twin study and the adoption study. The twin study contrasts monozygotic with dizygotic twins to examine the role of genes in determining the resemblance of one twin to the other. The adoption study examines adoptees separated at birth from biological parents and determines their resemblance to biological parents. In both the twin and adoption methods, environmental effects responsible for causing twin adoptee behaviors can be estimated. In the twin paradigm, environmental effects are usually estimated from mathematical models, whereas in the adoption paradigm, environmental effects are usually estimated from correlations of adoptee outcome with specific features of the environment. In the sections that follow, results of applying the twin and adoptee methods to drug behavior are presented separately, as well as more details about the methodology and limitations of each approach.

Advances in molecular biology have also been applied to the question of genetic influence on substance abuse. It is now possible to chemically define genes that might be involved in substance-related behavior leading to addiction. These studies range from determination of genes that code for enzymes metabolizing alcohol or drugs to genes that code for neurotransmitters and attempt to relate these specifically defined genes to addictive behavior. These studies are presented in a separate section.

Family and Twin Studies of Drug Abuse

The first step in examining possible genetic effects of a particular illness is determining whether the illness aggregates in families. Although family studies cannot confirm a genetic effect, failure to find familial association is inconsistent with a genetic effect. Clinical experience supports a strong multigenerational component of drug abuse. Family studies of drug abuse have been conducted during at least the past 30 years, and these studies support the clinical experience of familial aggregation for drug abuse as well as alcoholism.

Early family studies of drug abuse were summarized by Croughan.[1] These early studies demonstrated high rates of alcoholism and drug abuse in the relatives of probands with opioid addiction. Early studies are limited by

a lack of attention to structured family history methods, by the application of variable criteria for the diagnosis of drug abuse and dependence, and by failure to use control samples from other psychiatric populations and the general population.

RECENT FAMILY STUDIES OF DRUG ABUSE

Family studies since 1988 have used increased proband sample sizes with more focus on specific proband drug classes. Structured diagnostic interviews and direct structured interviews of family members have been increasingly used. Additionally, comparisons with controls including general population samples have been made. Table 5–1 summarizes some of the more recent family studies of probands with a drug abuse or drug dependence diagnosis.

Meller and colleagues[2] conducted a family study of 305 probands admitted for treatment of alcohol and drug abuse.[2] Thirty-five percent of the subjects had an alcohol problem only, 58% had both an alcohol and drug problem,

Table 5–1. RECENT FAMILY AND TWIN STUDIES OF THE GENETICS OF DRUG ABUSE

Family Studies Author	Proband N	Drug Class	Findings
Meller et al[2]	305	Multiple drugs	• Drug abuse probands have a higher family rate of drug abuse than do probands with alcoholism alone
Mirin et al[3]	350	Multiple drugs Drug of choice	• Opioid and cocaine choice probands more likely to have positive FH of drug abuse in male relatives than probands with a sedative-hypnotic drug of choice
Rounsaville et al[4]	201	Opiates	• Opioid addicts had increased rates of antisocial personality, alcoholism, depression, and drug abuse
Chaudhry et al[5]	129	Opiates	• FH of drug abuse predicted early onset of proband abuse
Stabenau[6]	219	Multiple drugs	• FH drug abuse predicted drug abuse • FH drug abuse plus antisocial personality predicted combined alcohol and drug abuse
Luthar et al[7]	201	Opiates	• 64% of opioid abusers' siblings had drug abuse diagnosis
Luthar and Rounsaville[8]	298	Cocaine	• Sibling drug abuse rates four to six times higher than rates in the general population
Luthar et al[9]	499	Opiates/cocaine	• Limited evidence for specificity of drug abuse/alcoholism aggregation in families
Kosten et al[10]	201	Opiates	• Drug use and increased sensation seeking noted in siblings of opiate abusers

Twin Studies Author	Twin Pairs	Drug Class	Findings
Grove et al[11]	32	Multiple drugs	• Significant heritability of drug-related problems in monozygotic twins
Pickens et al[12]	169	Multiple drugs	• Significant genetic contribution to drug abuse in male but not in female twins

FH, family history.

and 9% had a drug abuse problem only. Probands with a drug problem only reported a 45% rate of drug abuse in their families, compared with a rate of only 17% for family drug abuse in probands only abusing alcohol. Log-linear analysis demonstrated that the strongest association with proband drug abuse was a parent with a drug abuse diagnosis.

Mirin and coworkers conducted a large psychiatric study of the families of drug-dependent patients.[3] Comparisons between drug abusers were made based on the patient's drug of choice. Of 350 probands in the study, 186 endorsed opioids as their drug of choice, 120 endorsed cocaine, and 44 endorsed sedative-hypnotics. Male relatives of the opioid- and cocaine-choosing probands had higher rates of drug abuse than male relatives of the probands choosing sedative-hypnotics. This study suggests that family risk factors may be specific to the drug class preferred by an index proband.

Rounsaville and associates conducted a large study of family members linked to a proband with opiate addiction.[4] Compared with controls, family members of the opiate proband group had high rates of alcoholism, drug abuse, depression, and antisocial personality. Interestingly, rates of depression in family members were increased if the probands themselves had a depressive disorder. Concurrent antisocial personality (ASP) in the opiate-abusing proband did not seem to increase the risk of familial psychopathology.

Chaudhry and colleagues studied the effect of family history of opium use on the phenomenology of proband opiate use in a series of opiate addicts in Pakistan.[5] He demonstrated a link between a positive family history (FH) and a younger age of onset of opiate use in the probands. This link confirmed similar results from studies in the United States. In Pakistan, opiate use is not associated with pervasive personal or family problems, apparently because of the cultural attitude differences concerning the use of opium in Pakistan compared with the United States. Despite these cultural differences, evidence for a genetic effect in opiate use appears to be present across nations and continents.

Stabenau used an FH study to examine whether the risk for alcohol and drug abuse is a unitary phenomenon or a more complex one.[6] Using a sample of untreated alcohol and drug abuse and control probands, subjects were categorized into those with alcoholism alone, those with alcoholism plus a drug abuse or dependence diagnosis, those with drug abuse alone, and those without a drug abuse or alcohol abuse diagnosis (controls). Using a logistic regression, the proband group was compared with a set of predictor variables including gender, age, years of education, FH of alcoholism, FH of drug abuse, FH of ASP, and ASP in the proband. A family history of drug abuse was the best predictor of proband drug abuse. ASP diagnosis in the proband predicted alcohol abuse/dependence. ASP and FH of drug abuse additively predicted combined alcohol abuse/dependence and drug abuse/dependence in the proband. This study supports some independent risk factors for drug abuse/dependence from the risk factors for alcohol abuse/dependence.

Luthar and colleagues interviewed 132 siblings of probands with opiate addiction.[7] Eighty-five (64%) of the siblings were found to have abused opiates. Siblings were more likely to abuse opiates if they were younger than their probands, had high scores on sensation seeking, had tried drugs as a teenager, and associated with peers using drugs.

Luthar and Rounsaville performed a similar sibling analysis starting with probands with cocaine abuse.[8] Drug problems were identified in 40% of male siblings and 22% of female siblings. These rates were five to six times higher than expected from those estimated from the Epidemiological Catchment Area study. Siblings with drug misuse had high rates of other psychiatric disorders including alcoholism, major depression, and ASP. High rates of sibling drug misuse and ASP were found for both opiate- and cocaine-abusing probands. Major depression and alcoholism often occurred after the development of drug misuse. This study suggests that interventions that prevent drug abuse in high-risk populations may serve to reduce other secondary psychiatric disorders.

Luthar and associates, in a separate manuscript, reported several factors that appeared to modify family risk for drug abuse.[9] Paternal alcoholism predicted drug abuse in blacks but not in whites. Additionally, drug abuse risk in children increased sequentially when neither, one, or both parents were affected with alcoholism. There appeared to be little evidence for specificity for aggregation of alcoholism or drug abuse in the families in this study.

Kosten and coworkers examined the role of sensation seeking in the siblings of opiate addicts.[10] One hundred thirty-three siblings of opiate addicts participated in a cross-sectional family study. Siblings with drug problems demonstrated high scores on sensation seeking—these high scores correlated with the high scores of the opiate-abusing probands. Siblings without drug problems had lower sensation-seeking scores. This study suggests a mechanism of genetic risk for opiate abuse. Additionally, sensation-seeking scores correlated highly with early age of onset of drug use.

Limitations of the family study method need consideration. This is particularly true for drug abuse. Major cross-generational differences in popularity and availability of drugs such as cocaine and opioids significantly affect individual risk. Thus, a genetic risk for cocaine abuse will not be manifested in an environment where cocaine is not available. This period effect on disease rates is particularly important for family studies of drug abuse compared with major depression, schizophrenia, or even alcoholism. Additionally, family studies are unable to separate family environmental effects from genetic effects. Specific genetic and environmental effects can be examined using the more complex twin and adoption study paradigms.

Despite these methodological problems, the family studies reviewed here continue to demonstrate high familial rates for drug abuse problems for both opiates and cocaine. This is especially true for siblings of probands with drug abuse. Although family studies do not confirm a genetic basis for risk in families, they do provide support for continuing research using adoption and twin models. Two twin studies have examined genetic factors in the risk for drug abuse.

TWIN STUDIES

Twin studies use a comparison of monozygotic and dizygotic concordance rates to estimate the genetic effect (or heritability) for medical and psychiatric disorders. The twin study paradigm has been powerful in determining the genetic effects of medical conditions such as hypertension and obesity. Twin studies have also been used for investigating various psychiatric disorders. Although twin studies have been used more frequently in alcoholism, two twin studies of drug abuse provide insight into possible genetic mechanisms in drug abuse.

Recent Twin Studies of Drug Abuse

Grove and colleagues examined a series of 32 monozygotic twins for concordance in a series of DSM-III axis I disorders and ASP.[11] This twin sample was confined to twins reared apart to limit the effect of environmental factors on outcome. Twins were recruited from a

nonclinical sample and as expected demonstrated low rates for DSM-III disorders that were comparable to general population rates. Item counts were obtained for alcohol-related problems, drug-related problems, childhood antisocial behavior, and adult antisocial behavior. Both the drug scale scores and the antisocial scale scores demonstrated significant heritability. This twin sample was interviewed at a fairly young age and is being observed for later interview to pick up emergent alcohol and drug abuse problems.

Pickens and coworkers examined the genetic influence on alcoholism and other drug abuse in a sample of 81 monozygotic and 88 dizygotic same-sex twin pairs.[12] Heritability was demonstrated for alcohol abuse and alcohol dependence (DSM-III) diagnoses for males, but it was only demonstrated for the diagnosis of alcohol dependence in females. Similarly, other drug dependence demonstrated a genetic effect with higher rates in monozygotic twins than in dizygotic twins. Heritability estimates were 0.31 for drug abuse in males and 0.22 for females. Interestingly, shared environmental factors were found to account for high level of risk variance in drug abuse for male twins, whereas nonshared environmental factors accounted for the most variance in the female twin population.

These two twin studies also suggest that genetic factors have a role in the risk of drug abuse. Further twin studies using a specific drug of abuse (such as cocaine) are needed to better understand the complex role of genetics in drug abuse vulnerability.

Evidence for Genetic Factors in Drug Abuse/ Dependence from Adoption Studies

This section describes two adoption studies conducted at the University of Iowa to determine genetic and environmental factors in drug abuse/dependence. In the two studies described here, adoptees separated from biological parents at birth and placed with nonrelatives were interviewed as adults to determine their psychiatric and substance use/abuse history. In the first study, genetic factors were assessed from information in adoption agency records about biological parents' substance use or other relevant psychiatric conditions such as antisocial behavior; in the second study, substance abuse/dependence and ASP in biological parents were diagnosed from hospital or prison records of biological parents. Environmental influences to which the adoptee was exposed were assessed from several sources: (1) the adoptee, (2) both adoptive parents, and (3) the adoption agency record of the preplacement life of the adoptee. In both studies reported here, the adoptive parents were given an extensive structured interview that asked about environmental factors such as marital problems, psychiatric substance use/abuse, or behavioral problems in family members and socioeconomic level of the adoptive family, discipline used, rural or urban home, or home broken by death or divorce of adoptive parents. In the second study, further information about adoptive parents' behavior or psychiatric problems was obtained by administration of a structured psychiatric interview (Diagnostic Interview Schedule). In both studies, a case-control approach was used. For each adoptee from a biological background with psychopathology, a control adoptee was selected whose biological background was free of psychopathology (as determined from available records) and matched by age, sex, adoption agency, and age of biological mother. Genetic effects were defined by comparisons between the outcome of the control adoptees compared with the adoptees from biological parents with documented psychopathology.

In order to detect and measure the genetic effect on substance abuse/dependence and to distinguish it from any environmental effect, a multivariate analysis was used (log-linear modeling) to allow for simultaneous consideration of a number of relevant genetic and environmental factors and determination of the relative importance of each in the causation of substance abuse/dependence. This multivariate procedure also allowed for control of a condition that is unique to adoption studies and that could alter adoptee outcome in a way that makes an environmental effect resemble a genetic effect. This unique condition is selective placement, and it occurs when information about an adoptive environment is used to place an adoptee in a situation that would be correlated with the biological parents' environment—for example, placing a child of an alcoholic parent into a home with an alcoholic adoptive parent. In this extreme example, genetic and environmental factors are confounded by the selective placement. In the log-linear analysis, selective placement based on information about biological parents' substance abuse/dependence is controlled by forcing into the model a correlation between the

biological parent's condition and an environmental factor found to affect adoptee outcome. This relationship then acts like a covariate to adjust the outcome-environment correlation.

RESULTS OF THE FIRST STUDY

Adoptees from two private adoption agencies were used. Enrolled in the study were 242 male adoptees, of whom 28 (11.6%) had drug abuse/dependence; of the 201 females, 12 (6.0%) were drug abusers or addicts. The number of individuals abusing marijuana was 38/40, followed by amphetamines (15/30) and hallucinogens (21/40). The median number of drug types abused was three per individual. In order to have enough observations to fit log-linear models, the sexes were combined, and the resulting best-fit model developed from the data is shown in Figure 5–1, which is adapted from the original publication.[13]

A combination of genetic and environmental factors was found to predict drug abuse/dependence in the sample: (1) An alcohol problem (ranging from heavy drinking to treated alcoholism) in biological parents predicted not only adoptee alcohol abuse but drug abuse in adoptees who were *not* antisocial (odds ratio = 6.7 for this group). (2) Antisocial biological relatives (mostly convicted felons) predicted adoptee ASP, which in turn was highly correlated (odds ratio = 18.8) with drug abuse. (3) An environmental effect, such as a disturbed adoptive parent (parent with alcohol or antisocial problem, divorce or separation), predicted increased drug abuse in adoptees (odds ratio = 2.8). This environmental effect was independent of the genetic factors noted earlier even when controlling for selective placement based on those genetic factors. These results suggested *two* genetic factors in drug abuse: (1) a direct effect from alcoholic biological parents to offspring; (2) an indirect effect from antisocial biological parents to offspring who are antisocial and who, as a part of their antisocial behavior, become involved in substance use and abuse. A third independent factor in drug abuse is the environmental factor of a disturbed adoptive family. Similar environmental factors have been reported from family studies,[14–18] but the direction of the effect is unclear: whether a disturbed parent is a result of having a child with drug abuse/dependence or whether an already disturbed parent or marital situation leads to drug abuse/dependence. Some idea of direction of effect can be obtained from the temporal ordering of events. Examining the 14 drug abusers in this study with a

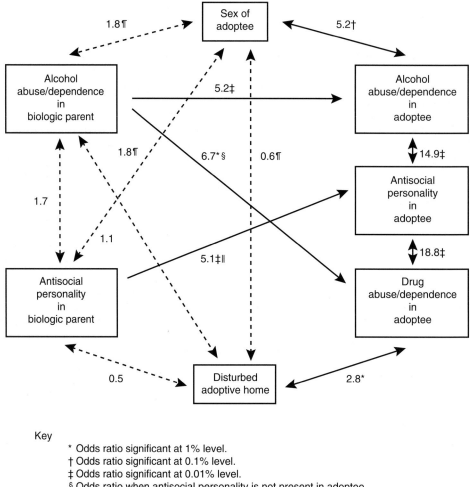

Key

      * Odds ratio significant at 1% level.
      † Odds ratio significant at 0.1% level.
      ‡ Odds ratio significant at 0.01% level.
      § Odds ratio when antisocial personality is not present in adoptee.
      ‖ Odds ratio when alcohol abuse/dependence is not present in biological parents.
      ¶ Odds ratio when sex is male.
    ⎯⎯▶ Relationship found in data.
   - - -▶ Relationship forced into model to control for selective placement.

Figure 5–1. Log-linear interaction diagram of genetic and environmental factors with adoptee outcome (n = 443).

parental psychiatric problem, parental divorce, or separation, in nine cases the parent or marital problem preceded the abuse, in three the abuse followed the marital problem, in one case the events occurred simultaneously, and in the remaining case there was insufficient information to make a determination of temporal order. Thus, the temporal order suggests that marital and parental problems manifested earlier than the drug abuse, but causality is still not clear because of the possibility that conduct disorder problems manifested earlier by a large proportion of the drug abusers could have adversely influenced parental health and marital adjustment.

That significant socially deviant behavior occurred in drug-abusing individuals is attested by a further study of the male sample in which

the 28 drug abusers/dependents were investigated for factors that determined transitions from no drug use to drug use and from use without abuse to abuse/dependence.[19] In this study, social factors such as having an antisocial sibling and consorting with friends that the adoptive parents disapproved of led to drug use. Genetic factors (alcohol problem in a biological parent) facilitated the transition from drug use to abuse/dependence. Two individual factors predicted both transition from no use to use and from use to abuse/dependence. One factor was adoptee aggressiveness; the second was conduct disorder symptoms. Although conduct disorder symptoms in the adoptee could have resulted from drug-seeking and drug-taking behavior, aggressiveness was often noted earlier in the adoptee life cycle. No genetic correlations were found in this first study between aggressiveness and any psychiatric condition in a biological parent.

The second adoption study was designed to confirm the three factors (two genetic and one environmental) noted earlier and to determine the roles of aggressiveness and conduct disorder and their correlations with genetic and environmental factors. The methodology of the second study was improved as mentioned in the introduction to this section, and a more elaborate measure of aggressiveness was added.[20] The environmental effect of family disturbance was better specified from the Diagnostic Interview Schedule interviews given to the adoptive parents (to detect alcoholism, depression, and anxiety states) and from structured interviews of adoptee and adoptive parents inquiring about marital problems, separation, and divorce. A count of the number of the foregoing conditions per family was made to construct a variable for the log-linear analyses.

RESULTS OF THE SECOND STUDY

This study obtained subjects from four different adoption agencies. A total of 95 male and 102 female adoptees was studied. Data

were analyzed separately for males and females, and results for males are presented first.

Forty-one of the 95 males (43%) were drug abusers or addicts as defined by DSM-III-R criteria. The best-fitting log-linear model is shown in Figure 5–2. The model shows the two hypothesized genetic pathways to drug abuse: the direct one from biological parent alcohol abuse/dependence to adoptee drug abuse/dependency (odds ratio = 2.8) and the second from antisocial biological parent via aggressiveness and ASP in the adoptee to drug abuse/dependence. The factor of a disturbed adoptive home enters the model by predicting an increase in ASP in the adoptee and acts to increase the probability of drug abuse by its effect on the ASP factor. In general, the model for males confirms the hypotheses predicted from the first study.

In the female sample, 17 of 102 (16.7%) were drug abusers or addicts. However, because only five female adoptees met criteria for ASP, conduct disorder (23 individuals of 102) was substituted in the model. The best-fitting model is shown in Figure 5–3. The model shows the hypothesized relationship between antisocial biological background and drug abuse through intervening variables of aggression and conduct disorder. A disturbed adop-

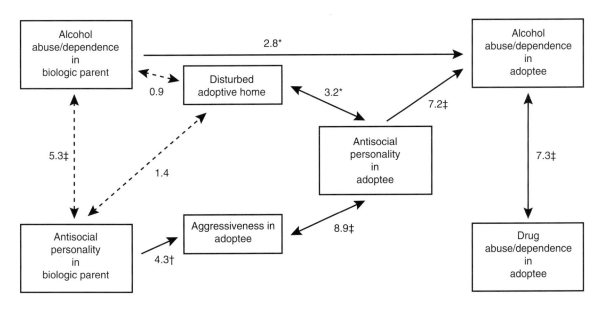

Key

* Odds ratio significant at 5% level.
† Odds ratio significant at 1% level.
‡ Odds ratio significant at 0.1% level.
——→ Relationship found in data.
- - -→ Relationship forced into model to control for selective placement.

Figure 5–2. Log-linear interaction diagram of male sample (n = 95).

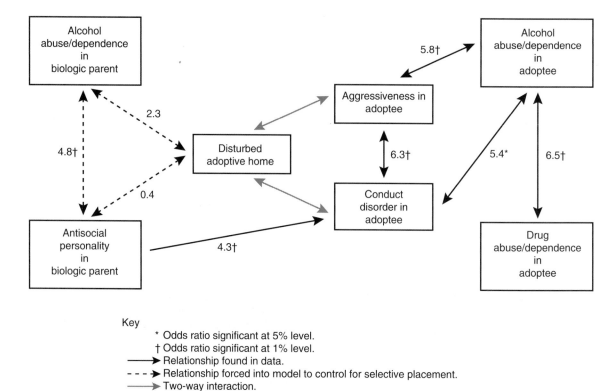

Key

  * Odds ratio significant at 5% level.
  † Odds ratio significant at 1% level.
 ——▶ Relationship found in data.
 - - -▶ Relationship forced into model to control for selective placement.
 ——▶ Two-way interaction.

Figure 5–3. Log-linear interaction diagram of female sample (n = 102).

tive home interacts with both adoptee aggression and conduct disorder in the following fashion: In the presence of a disturbed adoptive home, both aggression and conduct disorder are more likely to occur in the same individual, with a result of increased chance of drug abuse/dependence for that individual. In this model, the direct effect between alcoholic biological parent and adoptee drug abuse/dependence was not found. However, in a previous study of alcoholism in women adoptees, Cutrona and colleagues found that family conflict in early life and psychopathology in adoptive parents increased the chance of alcohol abuse/dependence among women who had at least one alcoholic biological parent.[21] The researchers also found that women who reported low social support and who had an alcoholic biological parent were more likely to become alcoholic.[22] This finding in female alcoholics suggested that gene-environment interaction might have a role in female drug abuse. In the present study of females, disturbed adoptive home *did not* interact with alcoholic biological background to increase the chance of drug abuse in the female adoptee; however, social support reported by the adoptee *did* show significant interaction with a biological parent's alcoholism. In the presence of alcoholism in a

biological parent, reported low social support was associated with a significantly increased chance of drug abuse.

SUMMARY OF ADOPTION STUDIES

The Iowa adoption studies confirm the importance of a genetic factor in drug abuse whose origin is a biological parent with ASP. This biological background leads to intervening variables of conduct disorder and aggressiveness, which in turn lead to drug abuse. A second genetic influence is a direct effect of an alcoholic biological parent on adoptee drug abuse/dependence. The latter effect has been found in two independent studies and appears to be more of a factor in male substance abuse. Environmental factors broadly characterized as disturbed parenting also have a role in drug abuse, although the direction of effect is undetermined. In the second study, their effect appears to be mainly on behavior associated with the antisocial biological factor. There is some suggestion that gene-environment interaction may have a role, especially in women, in that certain environmental factors increase substance abuse in the presence of a genetic background of alcoholism.

Molecular Genetics of Substance Abuse

The so-called molecular revolution of the past two decades has profoundly affected every aspect of biomedical research. The development and availability of techniques through which individual genes can be examined directly at the DNA sequence level has led to a large number of major advances in the understanding of the processes involved in disease development. Included among these is identification of the genes involved in disorders such as cystic fibrosis,[23] muscular dystrophy,[24] and Huntington's disease.[25] Also included, however, is the realization of a profound distinction between what may be termed *unitary disease*, in which a genetic basis can be ascribed to mutations occurring in a single major gene, and what must be termed *complex diseases*, in which a genetic basis involves the presence of multiple gene loci as well as interactions both among these loci themselves and between specific genes and their biological and nonbiological milieu. It is in this second group of disorders that substance abuse must be classified.

Devor described a heuristic developmental genetic model of complex, multifactorial diseases.[26] This model is composed of five distinct levels through which genetic risk is translated into an observed disease state. If, as seems likely, substance abuse can be thought of as a complex multifactorial disorder, then this model provides a reasonable heuristic framework for a discussion of its molecular genetics. Briefly, the evidence suggesting a genetic basis for substance abuse implies the existence of genes that confer *primary risk* for developing the disorder. That is to say that there are primary substance abuse genes that contribute to risk either individually or in concert and that any individual risk genotype is derived from a finite pool of specific gene loci that segregate independently in the human genome. Thus, the presence of any combination of these primary risk genes is essentially random. However, whenever two or more of these primary risk genes are present in any one individual, the possibility of *primary gene-gene interactions* exists.

Primary gene-gene interactions depend on which specific risk genes are present, and these interactions could range from simple additive effects in which each gene adds to overall risk without regard to which other genes are present, to true nonlinear epistatic effects in which the increase in risks is either greater than or less than a simple sum, and it does depend on

which specific genes are present. Beyond this is a second level of gene-gene interactions that recognize the fact that a primary risk genotype exists in a developmental milieu composed of the rest of the genome. This *secondary gene-gene interaction* level involves genes that are *not* directly involved in disease risk but rather serve to modify the baseline risk. This may occur as unique effects in which these secondary genes may exert a unique effect, affecting one or a few primary risk genotypes, or they may exert a common effect, affecting most or all primary risk genotypes. It must be pointed out here that such secondary interactions may serve to further *increase* risk conferred by the primary genotype or they may be protective and *decrease* risk.

The potential role of nongenetic and even nonbiological factors in modifying the entire relevant risk genotype is explicitly recognized in the form of *genotype-environmental interactions*. As with the secondary gene-gene interactions, these effects may be unique or specific to a small number of genotypes by acting through, for example, one particular secondary interaction pathway, or they may be ubiquitous in affecting most or all possible genic combinations. The overall consequence of this interactive developmental model is to produce precisely the types of epidemiological and clinical variations observed in substance abuse—for example, age-of-onset and gender differences, differences in response to treatment, ranges of severity, and ultimately the spectrum of degree of familiality.

At this point, it may be tempting to adopt the view that the problem of identifying specific molecular effects in substance abuse is simply too complex. However, the practical experiences from the study of the genetics of alcoholism, a disorder to which the foregoing developmental model also applies, suggest that there are relatively few distinct phenotypes and that the levels of interactions or the actual numbers of primary risk genes and secondary modifying loci are relatively small and therefore manageable.[27–28] If the same can be said of substance abuse in general, then the systematic molecular study of potential primary and secondary risk genes will, in fact, lead to an understanding of the processes involved. Although no specific primary substance abuse risk genes have to date been identified, encouraging progress has been made on a number of different fronts. Some of these are discussed next.

Tabakoff and colleagues reported that the activity of the membrane-bound enzyme adenylate cyclase (AC) was significantly lower in the platelets of alcoholics than in controls when assayed in the presence of cesium fluoride (CsF).[29] This finding was verified by Devor and associates in an independently ascertained sample of alcoholic families.[30] It was also noted in that replication study that many of the first-degree relatives of alcoholics also showed deficits in CsF-stimulated platelet AC activities. This finding suggested the possibility of significant genetic control of AC activity and, consequently, a primary genetic defect at the root of the alcoholism finding. Subsequent analysis by Devor and coworkers determined that stimulated AC activity was indeed regulated by a single major gene locus, and the candidate locus identified was the alpha subunit of the stimulatory G-protein, GNAS.[31] This suggestion was supported by a study of alcoholics by Ozawa and colleagues in which the levels of G_s in the platelet membranes of affectees were significantly decreased compared with controls, and these decreases were correlated with decreased CsF-stimulated AC activity.[32] Further, a site-directed mutagenesis study of GNAS by Itoh and Gilman demonstrated that specific mutations introduced in the gene would decrease and even extinguish AC activity *in vitro*.[33]

The potential role of AC activity in other substance abuse has been eloquently demonstrated in an animal model by Nestler and colleagues.[34, 35] They have shown the presence of a genetic difference in AC regulation in response to cocaine administration in two lines of rats. In the drug-preferring Lewis strain, AC activity in the nucleus accumbens (NAc) is increased compared with the nonpreferring Fisher 344 strain. In addition, dopamine synthesis in the ventral tegmental area (VTA) and levels of the *inhibitory* G-protein (GNAI) in the NAc are decreased in the Lewis strain compared with the Fisher 344 line. As depicted in Figure 5–4, all these phenomena are causally linked through the D1 and D2 dopamine receptors. As seen, the activity of AC can be up-regulated through the D1 dopamine receptor via GNAS and down-regulated through the D2 dopamine receptor via GNAI. In addition, decreased levels of both tyrosine and dopamine can lead to D1 dopamine receptor hypersensitivity and a resultant increase in AC activity.[36, 37] Thus, the list of potential candidate genes suggested by the phenomena of increased and decreased AC activity in alcoholism and cocaine abuse includes the tyrosine-to-dopamine pathway enzymes such as tyrosine hydroxylase and dopamine beta-hydroxylase, the D1 and D2 dopamine receptors, and the

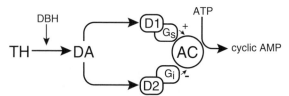

Figure 5–4. A graphic representation of dopamine receptor–mediated regulation of adenylate cyclase (AC). The upper pathway represents AC stimulation through the dopamine D1 receptor via the stimulatory G-protein, and the lower pathway represents AC inhibition through the dopamine D2 receptor via the inhibitory G-protein. AC function is measured by the rate at which ATP is converted to cyclic AMP in vitro. The level of dopamine (DA) at the synapse is largely determined by the activity of tyrosine hydroxylase (TH) and to a lesser extent by dopamine-β-hydroxylase (DBH).

two G-protein subunits GNAS and GNAI. Of these, of course, the one that has received the most attention and controversy is the D2 dopamine receptor gene, DRD2.

The dopaminergic neurotransmitter system has been implicated in reward and reinforcement phenomena in a number of studies.[38, 39] The current interest in the DRD2 gene itself was stimulated by the finding by Blum and colleagues of an association of a DNA sequence variant near the DRD2 gene with severe alcoholism.[40] This finding led to a spate of DRD2 association studies in both alcoholism and other substance abuse. The results of these studies are mixed, and the controversy about the role of DRD2 continues unabated.[41–43] As regards substance abuse apart from alcoholism, it must be noted that DRD2 is only one of a family of related genes that includes DRD3 and DRD4, and the latter gene has also been implicated in alcoholism by George and associates.[44] However, it is the DRD3 gene that appears to show a relationship to cocaine abuse.[45–47] Thus, the dopamine receptor candidate gene story continues to play out, and it remains to be seen what, if any, part these specific genes play in substance abuse. Moreover, it remains to be seen whether these and other genes will fit the characteristics of primary risk genes or secondary modifier genes as defined in the developmental genetic model of Devor.[26] Clearly, the impact of molecular genetics on the study of substance abuse is only just being felt, and the early results are already leading to many interesting and potentially important lines of investigation.

Summary

Evidence from family, twin, and adoption studies is compatible with both genetic and environmental etiologies of drug abuse. The adoption studies suggest the possibility of more than one genetic factor: one that originates in antisocial parents and leads to drug abuse through aggressiveness and conduct disorder and a second that comes from alcoholic parents and correlates directly with drug abuse. There is some suggestion that the latter factor might interact in females with the environmental factor of low social support. That other environmental factors are relevant to drug abuse and act independent of the genetic factor is evident from both the twin and adoption studies. The adoption studies have shown that a disturbed adoptive home is associated with an increased chance of drug abuse and with increased aggressiveness and conduct disorders.

At present, not enough detail is known about the physiology of addiction to suggest a specific genetic hypothesis that would lead to candidate genes that could be studied. The same statement applies to the complex psychosocial behavior that leads to substance use/abuse/dependence.

REFERENCES

1. Croughan JL: The contributions of family studies to understanding drug abuse. In Robins LN (ed): Studying Drug Abuse. New Brunswick, NJ, Rutgers University Press, 1985, pp 240–264.
2. Meller WH, Rinehart R, Cadoret RJ, Troughton E: Specific familial transmission in substance abuse. Int J Addict 23:1029–1039, 1988.
3. Mirin SM, Weiss RD, Griffin ML, Michael JL: Psychopathology in drug abusers and their families. Compr Psychiatry 32:36–51, 1991.
4. Rounsaville BJ, Kosten TR, Weissman MM, et al: Psychiatric disorders in relatives of probands with opiate addiciton. Arch Gen Psychiatry 48:33–42, 1991.
5. Chaudhry HR, Arria A, Tarter R, et al: Familial history of opium use and reported problems among opium addicts in Pakistan. Br J Addict 86:785–788, 1991.
6. Stabenau JR: Is risk for substance abuse unitary? J Nerv Ment Dis 180:583–588, 1992.
7. Luthar SS, Anton SF, Merikangas KR, Rounsaville BJ: Vulnerability to drug abuse among opioid addicts' siblings: Individual, familial, and peer influences. Compr Psychiatry 33:190–196, 1992.
8. Luthar SS, Rounsaville B: Substance misuse and comorbid psychopathology in a high-risk group: A study of siblings of cocaine misusers. Int J Addict 28:415–434, 1993.
9. Luthar SS, Merikangas KR, Rounsaville BJ: Parental psychopathology and disorders in offspring. A study of relatives of drug abusers. J Nerv Ment Dis 181:351–357, 1993.
10. Kosten TA, Ball SA, Rounsaville BJ: A sibling study of sensation seeking and opiate addiction. J Nerv Ment Dis 182:284–289, 1991.
11. Grove WM, Eckert ED, Heston L, et al: Heritability of substance abuse and antisocial behavior: A study of monozygotic twins reared apart. Biol Psychiatry 27:1293–1304.
12. Pickens RW, Svikis DS, McGue M, et al: Heterogeneity in the inheritance of alcoholism. Arch Gen Psychiatry 48:19–28, 1991.
13. Cadoret RJ, Troughton E, O'Gorman T, Heywood E: An adoption study of genetic and environmental factors in drug abuse. Arch Gen Psychiatry 43:1131–1136, 1986.
14. Egger GJ, Webb RAJ, Reynolds I: I: Early adolescent antecedents of narcotic abuse. Int J Addict 13:773–781, 1978.
15. Haastrup S, Thomsen K: The social backgrounds of young addicts as elicited in interviews with their parents. Acta Psychiatr Scand 48:146–173, 1972.
16. Rosenberg CM: Young drug addicts: Background and personality. J Nerv Ment Dis 148:65–73, 1969.
17. Rosenberg CM: Young drug addicts: Addiction and its consequences. Med J Aust 1:1031–1033, 1968.
18. Ball DS, Trethowan WH: Amphetamine addiction. J Nerv Ment Dis 133:489–496, 1961.
19. Cadoret RJ: Genetic and environmental factors in initiation of drug use and the transition to abuse. In Glantz M, Pickens R (eds): Vulnerability to Drug Abuse. Washington, DC, American Psychological Association, 1992.
20. Loney J, Langhorne JE, Paternite C: An empirical basis for subgrouping the hyperkinetic/minimal brain dysfunction syndrome. J Abnorm Psychol 87:431–441, 1978.
21. Cutrona CE, Cadoret RJ, Suhr JA, et al: Interpersonal variables in the prediction of alcoholism among adoptees: Evidence for gene-environment interactions. Compr Psychiatry 35:171–179, 1994.
22. Cutrona CE: Unpublished communication.
23. Riordan JR, Rommens JM, Kerem B, et al: Identification of the cystic fibrosis gene: Cloning and characterization of complementary DNA. Science 245:1066–1073, 1989.
24. Monaco A, Neve R, Colletti-Feener C, et al: Isolation of the candidate cDNAs for portions of the Duchenne muscular dystrophy gene. Nature 323:646–650, 1986.
25. The Huntington's Disease Collaborative Group: A novel gene containing a trinucleotide repeat that is expanded and unstable on Huntington's disease chromosome. Cell 72:1–20, 1993.
26. Devor EJ: Why there is no gene for alcoholism. Behav Genet 23:145–151, 1993.
27. Babor TF, Hoffman M, Del Boca FK, et al: Types of alcoholics. I. Evidence for an empirically derived typology based on indicators of vulnerability and severity. Arch Gen Psychiatry 49:599–608, 1992.
28. Cloninger CR: Neurogenic adaptive mechanisms in alcoholism. Science 236:410–416, 1987.
29. Tabakoff B, Hoffman PL, Lee JM, et al: Differences in platelet enzyme activity between alcoholics and nonalcoholics. N Engl J Med 318:134–139, 1988.
30. Devor EJ, Cloninger CR, Hoffman PL, Tabakoff B: Adenylate cylase activity in the families of alcoholics is controlled by a single major gene. In Kalant H, Khanna JM, Israel (eds): Advances in Biomedical Alcohol Research. Oxford, Pergamon Press, 1991, pp 157–160.
31. Devor EJ, Cloninger CR, Hoffman PL, Tabakoff B: A genetic study of platelet adenylate cyclase activity: Evidence for a single major locus effect in fluoride-stimulated activity. Am J Hum Genet 49:372–377, 1991.
32. Ozawa H, Katamura Y, Ashizawa T, et al: Platelet adenylate cyclase activity in long-term abstinent alcoholics. Alcohol Alcohol 27:69, 1992.
33. Itoh H, Gilman AG: Expression and analysis of $G\alpha s$ mutants with decreased ability to activate adenylylcyclase. J Biol Chem 266:16226–16231, 1991.
34. Nestler EG: Molecular mechanisms of drug addiction. J Neurosci 12:2439–2450, 1992.
35. Beitner-Johnson D, Guitart X, Nestler EJ: Common in-

tra-cellular actions of chronic morphine and cocaine in dopamine brain reward regions. Ann N Y Acad Sci 654:70–87, 1992.

36. Henry DJ, White FJ: Repeated cocaine administration causes persistent enhancement of D1 dopamine receptor sensitivity within the rat nucleus accumbens. J Pharmacol Exp Ther 258:882–890, 1991.

37. Peris J, Boysen SJ, Cass WA, et al: Persistence of neurochemical changes in dopamine systems after repeated cocaine administration. J Pharmacol Exp Ther 253:38–44, 1990.

38. Kobb GF, Bloom FE: Cellular and molecular mechanisms of drug dependence. Science 242:715–723, 1988.

39. Wise RA, Rompre PP: Brain dopamine and reward. Annu Rev Psychol 40:191–225, 1989.

40. Blum K, Noble EP, Sheridan PG, et al: Allelic association of human D2-dopamine receptor gene alcoholism. JAMA 263:2055–2060, 1990.

41. Uhl GR, Persico AM, Smith SS: Current excitement with D2-dopamine receptor gene alleles in substance abuse. Arch Gen Psychiatry 49:157–160, 1992.

42. Kidd KK: Associations of disease with genetic markers: Deja vu all over again. Am J Med Genet (Neuropsych Genet) 48:71–73, 1993.

43. Gelernter J, Goldman D, Risch N: The A1 allele at the D2 dopamine receptor gene and alcoholism: A reappraisal. JAMA 269:1673–1677, 1993.

44. George SR, Cheng R, Nguyen T, et al: Polymorphism of the D4 dopamine receptor alleles in chronic alcoholism. Biochem Biophys Res Commun 196:107–114, 1993.

45. Caine SB, Koob GF: Modulation of cocaine self-administration in the rat through D-3 dopamine receptors. Science 260:1814–1816, 1993.

46. Levesque D, Diaz J, Pilon C, et al: Identification, characterization, and localization of the dopamine D3 receptor in rat brain using 7-[3H]hydroxy-N,N-di-n-propyl-2-aminotetralin. Proc Natl Acad Sci U S A 89:8155–8159, 1992.

47. Schwartz JC, Giros B, Martres M-P, Sokoloff P: The dopamine receptor family: Molecular biology and pharmacology. Semin Neurosci 4:99–108, 1992.

Familial and Genetic Studies of Comorbidity of Addictive and Psychiatric Disorders

Laura J. Bierut, MD •
Stephen H. Dinwiddie, MD

Illnesses are often studied in "pure" forms without comorbid diseases; patients, however, rarely present with pure illnesses. Instead, clinicians are faced with patients who have multiple illnesses. This comorbidity complicates diagnostic evaluations, prognostication, and treatment results.

Comorbidity is the occurrence of two or more illnesses in the same person. A narrow definition of comorbidity is the simultaneous coexistence of two or more active diseases. More broadly, comorbidity is the co-occurrence of any illnesses during a person's lifetime, and diseases need not be simultaneously active. The broad definition of comorbidity is used in this chapter.

One strategy to understand the relationship between multiple diseases in an individual is to study the occurrence of these illnesses in families. Different patterns of familial occurrence imply different relationships between the illnesses. Clarifying the interactions between multiple diseases aids in the diagnosis, prognosis, and treatment of individual patients.

Comorbid Mental Disorders and Addiction

Addiction and mental illnesses are often comorbid. In clinical populations, addiction and mental illnesses occur more frequently than expected by chance whether subjects are selected from substance abuse centers[1] or inpatient psychiatric units.[2] This increased comorbidity in clinical settings is partially explained by Berkson's bias: Individuals who are afflicted with multiple disorders are more likely to receive treatment.[3] A spurious association between diseases may thus be observed in clinical samples because either disease may cause a patient to seek treatment.

Bias due to treatment seeking, however, cannot fully explain the increased association between addiction and other mental illnesses. General population surveys consistently show increased comorbidity. In the Epidemiological Catchment Area (ECA) study, individuals with alcoholism were found to have a 36.6% lifetime prevalence of another nonaddictive mental dis-

Table 6–1. COMORBID PSYCHIATRIC DISORDERS WITH ADDICTION: LIFETIME PREVALENCE AND (ODDS RATIO)

	Lifetime Prevalence	Affective Disorder	Anxiety Disorder	Schizophrenia	Antisocial Personality Disorder	Any Nonaddictive Mental Disorder
Alcohol addiction	13.5%	13.4% (1.9)	19.4% (1.5)	3.8% (3.3)	14.3% (21.0)	36.6% (2.3)
Drug addiction	6.1%	26.4% (4.7)	28.3% (2.5)	6.8% (6.2)	17.8% (13.4)	53.1% (4.5)

Some statistics adapted from Regier DA, Farmer ME, Rae DS, et al: Comorbidity of mental disorders with alcohol and other drug abuse. JAMA 264(19):2511–2518, 1990.

order, twice the rate observed in those without alcoholism (Tables 6–1 and 6–2).[4] The risk of comorbid mental illness is even greater in persons with drug addiction, which is associated with a 53.1% lifetime rate of nonaddictive mental disorder, more than four times the expected rate. Similarly, the National Comorbidity Survey (NCS), which was designed to evaluate the comorbidity of substance use disorders and other psychiatric disorders, demonstrates concentrated comorbidity, with one sixth of the population having a history of three or more disorders.[5]

The percentage of individuals with a comorbid illness is not the best measure of the increased risk. Instead, the magnitude of this risk can be better computed by an odds ratio. An odds ratio is an estimate of the risk ratio or relative risk of a disorder given the presence or absence of another illness. For instance, in the ECA study,[4] the odds ratio of having an anxiety disorder given the presence or absence of alcoholism is 1.5, meaning that alcoholics are 1.5 times more likely to be diagnosed with an anxiety disorder than are nonalcoholics. Other illnesses with lower population prevalences and thus fewer individuals with comorbid illnesses nonetheless might be associated with higher odds ratios. For instance, the presence of alcoholism increases the likelihood of a lifetime history of an affective disorder and schizophrenia (odds ratios = 1.9 and 3.3, re-

spectively), and antisocial personality disorder is associated with the highest odds ratio (21.0). An odds ratio takes into account the population prevalence of both illnesses and allows for meaningful comparisons of increased risk across disorders with different baseline rates. It also gives a crude estimate of the magnitude of interaction between diseases. Such findings clearly show that addictive and psychiatric disorders do not simply co-occur randomly. Instead, one illness must cause the other or both processes must share at least some etiological factors.

Family and Genetic Studies

The facts that addiction and mental illness co-occur more commonly than expected by chance and that these illnesses are familial allow researchers to evaluate their interrelationships by using the family rather than the individual as the unit of analysis. By using family, adoption, and twin studies, researchers can evaluate three possible relationships between disorders: Diseases co-occur by chance, one illness causes another, or common factors contribute to both disorders. A common factor may be either genetic or environmental.

By using the family study technique, it can be shown that if two disorders co-occur in an individual by chance, as when illnesses have a

Table 6–2. COMORBID ADDICTION WITH PSYCHIATRIC DISORDERS: LIFETIME PREVALENCE AND (ODDS RATIO)

	Lifetime Prevalence	Alcohol	Drug	Any Substance
Affective disorder	8.3%	21.8% (1.9)	19.4% (4.7)	32.0% (2.6)
Anxiety disorder	14.6%	17.9% (1.5)	11.9% (2.5)	23.7% (1.7)
Schizophrenia	1.5%	33.7% (3.3)	27.5% (6.2)	47.0% (4.6)
Antisocial personality disorder	2.6%	73.6% (21.0)	42.0% (13.4)	83.6% (29.6)
Any nonaddictive mental disorder	22.5%	22.3% (2.3)	14.7% (4.5)	28.9% (2.7)

Some statistics adapted from Regier DA, Farmer ME, Rae DS, et al: Comorbidity of mental disorders with alcohol and other drug abuse. JAMA 264(19):2511–2518, 1990.

hereditary link with different sides of the family, the familial pattern of inheritance shows independence of these disorders. The rate of illness for each disease in family members of a patient with comorbid illnesses is equal to the rate of disease in families of individuals affected with just one illness.

A different familial pattern occurs when one illness causes another. In such cases, one illness is dependent on the other for its expression and so occurs only in the presence of the first illness. Relatives should have an increased rate of the first illness or both illnesses in combination compared with nonaffected families, but the rate of the pure second disease in the relatives should not be elevated.

Finally, if two disorders have a common etiological factor, either illness may be expressed in family members of a comorbid proband, and rates of both diseases in family members should be elevated. In addition, families of probands with one illness should also have elevated rates of both disorders because the specificity of transmitting each illness is lost.

These family patterns can demonstrate the relationship of illnesses but this familial clustering may be due to either environmental factors or genetic factors or both. Adoption and twin studies of comorbidity are then needed to separate environmental and genetic factors. Keeping these considerations in mind, we review the more common comorbid combinations of addictive and psychiatric illnesses.

Alcoholism and Depression

FAMILY STUDIES

Both alcoholism and depression are familial; when studied in pure forms, without comorbid disorders, each illness is transmitted independently. Depression but not alcoholism is more common in families of pure depressed probands;[6, 7] alcoholism but not depression is more common in families of pure alcoholic probands.[8] Family studies thus support the independent transmission of these illnesses.

However, as clinicians well know, patients frequently present with both alcoholism and depression. Therefore, family studies have been extended to study probands afflicted with both disorders. Illnesses are typically classified as primary or secondary, a purely temporal distinction[9] that orders the time of onset between two diseases and implies no etiological link.

Many studies have examined rates of alco-holism and affective disorders in families of alcoholics. Comparisons between families of probands with primary alcoholism and secondary depression and families of probands with primary alcoholism and no secondary depression have shown that rates of alcoholism in relatives of both proband groups are similar.[10–14] A study by Guze and colleagues,[10] which included a nonalcoholic control group, also confirms that alcoholism is more common in relatives of alcoholics than in relatives of controls (15.3% vs. 8.7%, $P = 0.001$). Thus, the rate of alcoholism in families of alcoholics is elevated, and the additional diagnosis of depression in probands does not further increase or decrease this rate.

These families of probands with primary alcoholism have been studied for affective disorders. Only one study has shown an increased rate of affective disorders in siblings of probands with primary alcoholism and secondary depression compared with siblings of nondepressed alcoholics (28% vs. 14%, $P < 0.05$),[11] and in that study no other class of family members had an elevated rate of affective disturbance. In all other studies, rates of depression in relatives of probands with alcoholism and secondary depression have not been found to be significantly greater than rates in relatives of probands with alcoholism and no secondary depression.[10, 12–14]

Thus, the combination of primary alcoholism and secondary depression shows distinct patterns of inheritance for each disease: Alcoholism is strongly familial with and without secondary depression, but depression as a secondary illness does not show significant familial clustering. This pattern is most consistent with alcoholism leading to the development of depression.

The converse relationship, that of primary depression and secondary alcoholism, has also been evaluated. In a study by Merikangas and colleagues,[7] families were divided into three groups: relatives of unaffected community controls, relatives of primary depressed probands, and relatives of primary depressed probands with comorbid alcoholism, and a total of 1331 relatives were evaluated. Rates of depression in these three groups increased in a statistically significant stepwise manner (5.6%, 13.4%, and 23.7%, respectively). Thus, primary depression had strongly familial transmission, and the presence of alcoholism in probands with primary depression further increased the risk of depression in relatives.

Next, the rate of alcoholism was examined in these same families. A significantly increased rate of alcoholism was found in relatives of alcoholic probands with primary depression (19.5%) compared with relatives of depressed-only probands or relatives of community controls (11.9% and 9.0%, respectively). The rate of alcoholism in families with depression only was not significantly different from the baseline community rate. Thus, alcoholism diagnosed as a secondary illness showed familial clustering.

Studies of alcoholism and depression using a primary-secondary dichotomy have yielded evidence of two different interactions between the diseases. Primary alcoholism with secondary depression has a significant familial clustering of alcoholism but not depression, a pattern of inheritance most consistent with alcoholism's causing the depression. On the other hand, primary depression with secondary alcoholism had a familial aggregation of both diseases consistent with independent transmission of these disorders or common etiological factors.

Another method to study comorbidity of alcoholism and depression has been proposed by Winokur.[15] In this scheme, depression may be subdivided into two forms, pure depression and depressive spectrum disorder. Depressive spectrum disorder is identified by major depression in a proband along with a family history of alcoholism or antisocial personality disorder. Individuals categorized in this way differ in that those with depressive spectrum disorder have a younger age of onset of depressive symptoms, a remitting course, and more interpersonal difficulties. The family pattern of inheritance also differs: pure depression is transmitted to both men and women in families, but the rate of alcoholism is not elevated. On the other hand, in families with depressive spectrum disorder, female relatives have high rates of depression and male relatives have high rates of alcoholism.[15]

To test the utility of depressive spectrum disorder, a family study of primary depression and secondary alcoholism examined gender differences in the expression of both diseases in 619 relatives.[16] Consistent with the study by Merikangas and colleagues,[7] relatives of probands with primary depression and secondary alcoholism had a higher rate of alcoholism than did relatives of probands with only primary depression (28.7% vs. 10.3%), and the rate of depression in relatives of the comorbid group was greater than in relatives of the pure depressed group (44.8% vs. 32.0%).

Rates of illness were further analyzed for each sex. Female relatives of probands with both illnesses showed no significant increased rates of alcoholism than did female relatives of probands with depression only (8.0% vs. 5.4%). The rate of depression was higher in female relatives of depressed and alcoholic probands than in females of depressed probands (58.0% vs. 40.3%), although because of small sample size this did not reach statistical significance.

Male relatives showed a different pattern of inheritance of these diseases. Male relatives of probands with primary depression and secondary alcoholism had a significantly greater rate of alcoholism than did male relatives of depressed-only probands (56.0% vs. 16.7%), and rates of depression were not markedly different (27.0% vs. 21.4%).

Thus, the greater rate of depression in families of probands with primary depression and secondary alcoholism was mostly due to the elevated rate of depression in female relatives, and the increased rate of alcoholism was expressed in the male relatives. If confirmed, this familial pattern would support the mechanism of a shared etiological factor causing alcoholism in men and depression in women in families of probands with both disorders.

Family studies therefore support familial forms of pure alcoholism, pure depression, and a mixture of alcoholism and depression but cannot differentiate between cultural and genetic inheritance in families. Adoption studies and twin studies can help sort out the genetic and environmental contributions.

ADOPTION STUDIES

Adoption studies are a natural experiment separating genetic inheritance and environmental exposure. Resemblance of an adoptee to biological parents supports the role of biological factors, whereas resemblance to adoptive parents argues for cultural inheritance. Adoption studies to date support a genetic component in the development of pure alcoholism and pure depression, with adopted-away children having elevated rates of the same illness that affected their biological but not their adoptive parents.

Adoption studies have also examined the co-occurrence of alcoholism and depression. In one study, biological relatives of 71 adoptees with a history of an affective disorder had significantly greater rates of both depression (2.1% vs. 0.3%, $P < 0.05$) and alcoholism (5.4% vs. 2.0%, $P < 0.05$)[17] than did biological relatives of control adoptees.

A similar study compared biological relatives of 56 adoptees with affective disorder with relatives of 59 adoptees with substance abuse and relatives of adoptees with no psychiatric illness.[18] In contrast to the previous study, a greater rate of substance abuse was found in biological mothers of adoptees with affective disorder than in biological relatives of control adoptees (7.1% vs. 0.9%, $P < 0.025$), but otherwise, no correlation between biological parents and adoptee was found.

An adoption study by Goodwin and colleagues[19] took a different approach. In this study, psychiatric illness in 55 adopted-away children with a biological parent diagnosed with alcoholism was compared with that in control adoptees, and no differences emerged. Thus, results of adoption studies are mixed, possibly partly because of the limited power to study comorbid diseases in these small samples.

TWIN STUDIES

Like adoption studies, twin studies generally support a genetic component in the development of pure alcoholism and depression. By examining the occurrence of a second illness in a co-twin, this approach can be extended to evaluate comorbidity.

In a small study by Gurling and associates,[20] twin pairs derived from a treatment registry were evaluated for depression and alcoholism. This study was somewhat anomalous in that it did not show an elevated concordance of alcoholism in monozygotic twins compared with dizygotic twins. A high rate of depression was noted in both alcoholic and nonalcoholic twins, but the sample was not analyzed further in terms of the relationship of this comorbidity.

A much larger study by Kendler and co-workers,[21] derived from a general population sample of more than 2000 female twins, found rates of depression and alcoholism of 31% and 8.8%, respectively. As shown in other epidemiological studies, comorbidity for alcoholism and depression was increased (odds ratio = 3.62). In addition, the liability to develop alcoholism in one twin was significantly correlated with the liability to develop depression in the other twin. Using twin analysis, this study demonstrated shared genetic factors that influenced the joint predisposition to alcoholism and depression.

In summary, the studies of alcoholism and depression in families support at least three types of interactions between the two diseases: Alcoholism and depression can be independently transmitted, alcoholism can cause depression, and alcoholism and depression can

share some common etiological factors. In an individual case, any one of these mechanisms may hold true. Examining the pattern of addiction and psychiatric illness in relatives can aid in distinguishing between these mechanisms.

Alcoholism and Anxiety

Cross-sectional studies of patients with alcoholism and anxiety show variable patterns of onset for these disorders. Although agoraphobia and social phobia most commonly precede the onset of alcoholism by several years, panic disorder and generalized anxiety disorder often follow its development.[22] Thus, it has been proposed that phobias predispose one to alcoholism whereas alcoholism predisposes an individual to panic disorder and generalized anxiety disorder.

Although family studies are potentially a powerful method of testing these hypotheses, few studies have directly examined the comorbidity of alcoholism and anxiety states. Noyes and colleagues[23] examined 919 family members of probands with anxiety neurosis (similar to panic disorder) and no secondary mental illness, finding significantly higher rates of both anxiety neurosis (18% vs. 3%, $P < 0.001$) and alcoholism (6% vs. 4%, $P < 0.05$) than in relatives of controls.

A similar family study of 41 probands with panic disorder and no secondary illness was performed,[24] confirming the familial aggregation of panic disorder: a 17.3% rate of panic disorder in 278 first-degree relatives of probands with panic disorder versus a 1.8% rate in 262 first-degree relatives of surgical controls. These relatives also had a higher rate of alcoholism than did controls (6.1% vs. 3.8%), but this did not reach statistical significance.

A family history study by Munjack and Moss[25] compared 68 agoraphobic subjects, 35 miscellaneous phobic subjects, and 10 social phobic subjects. Various rates of family history of alcoholism were found (26.5%, 8.6%, and 20.0%, respectively), with a trend toward statistical significance ($P < 0.1$) for the agoraphobic group compared with the other phobias combined. Thus, different subtypes of phobia may have different relationships with alcoholism.

The family study of 1331 relatives by Merikangas and colleagues[7] of depression and alcoholism was extended to anxiety. Relatives of probands with primary depression and secondary alcoholism had a significantly higher rate of anxiety disorders than did relatives of depressed probands without secondary alcoholism (19.5% vs. 11.7%, $P < 0.001$).[7] This sample was further analyzed to estimate the combined genetic and environmental transmissibility of alcoholism and anxiety in these depressed probands. Confirming previous findings, alcoholism had significant independent (of anxiety disorder) transmission factors, but it also shared some transmission factors with anxiety.[26]

Overall, as with the interactions between alcoholism and depression, the relationship between alcoholism and anxiety is highly complex and heterogeneous.

Alcoholism and Drug Dependence

A natural question when studying alcoholism and drug dependence is whether this overlap represents one disease or several separate diseases. Given the close relationship between alcoholism and other drug dependence, it might appear that all these entities are manifestations of one disorder. In fact, family studies can show differences between these illnesses.

A study by Luthar and colleagues[27] interviewed 133 siblings of opiate-addicted probands. Studying siblings minimized secular trends of increasing drug and alcohol use that have occurred in younger generations. A nonsignificant increase was noted in alcoholism among siblings of probands with opiate dependence and alcoholism compared with siblings of probands with just opiate dependence (46.9% vs. 42.3%).

A similar study by Kosten and associates[28] examined 877 first-degree relatives of opiate-dependent probands. This study, however, demonstrated a significant increase of alcoholism in relatives of probands with both diseases compared with relatives of nonalcoholic opioid addicts (30% vs. 19%, $P < 0.01$).

These findings were extended to other drug use by Mirin and associates,[29] who examined 1478 first-degree relatives of probands dependent on opiates, cocaine, and sedative-hypnotics. Relatives of individuals with drug addiction and alcoholism again had a higher rate of alcoholism than did relatives of nonalcoholic individuals with drug addiction (24.3% vs. 14.0%). These data were not further analyzed by specific drug addiction.

Although there is significant overlap in the transmission of alcoholism and drug addiction, these studies argue for at least some independent features of alcoholism and drug dependence transmitted in families.

Addiction and Other Psychiatric Disorders

Other psychiatric disorders accompany addiction more frequently than expected by chance. Alcoholism and schizophrenia, alcoholism and bipolar affective disorder, and alcoholism and antisocial personality disorder significantly co-occur.[4] Other studies also suggest a connection between alcoholism and eating disorders and between alcoholism and tobacco dependence. However, family transmission of these comorbid conditions awaits further study.

Complicating Factors in Genetic Studies of Comorbidity

A number of factors complicate the interpretation and comparison of family, adoption, and twin studies of comorbidity. Some of these factors are unique to comorbidity, others are unique to family studies, and others may bias any type of study.

Diagnostic reliability is a particular concern when studying co-occurrence of addiction and psychiatric illness. The presence of one illness can confuse diagnosis of another. In individuals with current substance dependence, mood and psychotic disorders are less reliably diagnosed.[30] Thus, a diagnostic evaluation of an individual with two or more disorders may be less accurate than an evaluation of a subject with a single disease. Diagnostic reliability is also dependent on severity of illness; more severe illnesses are diagnosed more reliably.[10] Reliability has a significant impact on studies of primary and secondary disorders because these categorizations may change during different assessment periods.[10]

Another complication is variability between studies in ascertaining cases. Use of hospital discharge diagnoses or registry listings may be biased, because only those who received treatment are identified and untreated but ill individuals are counted as unaffected. Use of an informant to describe illness among relatives (the family history method) avoids reliance on registries and has been shown to have high specificity, but sensitivity remains low.[31] This means that if an individual is identified as ill, it is likely true, but many family members with a disease are missed. A more accurate approach, although time consuming and expensive, is direct interview of family members. However, even using the family interview technique, potentially informative subjects are unavailable for interview owing to refusal, incapacitation, inaccessibility, or death. In such cases, researchers again must rely on less accurate assessments.

Addiction and psychiatric illness have been changing over time. These temporal trends include differences in rates of illnesses, ages of onset, and exposure to alcohol and drugs. Rates of mental illnesses such as addiction, affective disorders, and anxiety disorders appear to be increasing in younger generations;[32] therefore, comparisons between generations in a family are difficult to interpret. Moreover, age of onset for addiction is decreasing,[33] further complicating comorbidity studies using a primary-secondary classification. Age of onset for one illness may decrease faster than age of onset for another disorder, and a previously secondary illness may become primary. Finally, availability and accessibility of drugs such as alcohol and cocaine have changed over time. Transmission of illnesses or lack of transmission and apparent genetic relationships can appear to change drastically merely as a result of exposure or nonexposure to these drugs.

Etiological heterogeneity may also obscure significant relationships between illnesses. Many diagnostic categories, such as major depression, anxiety syndromes, and alcoholism, probably represent an end stage of several different disease processes. This potential difficulty is made worse by grouping several illnesses into a single category. For instance, anxiety disorder often represents phobias, panic disorder, and obsessive-compulsive disorder, whereas researchers may lump under the rubric of affective disorder bipolar I, bipolar II, unipolar major depression, and dysthymia. Similarly, drug abuse is often a combination category of any illicit drug disorder and may range from any use with or without associated problems to severe addiction. This combining of illnesses may blur significant relationships between disorders.

Neither addictive nor psychiatric disorders are equally represented among men and women. For instance, men are more commonly affected with addiction and women more often have anxiety and affective disorders. However, in many analyses, because men and women are analyzed together, potential differences in comorbidity between the sexes are not observed.

All of these factors complicate the study of comorbidity, hamper comparisons across different studies over time, and may distort potentially significant findings.

Conclusions

Comorbidity of addiction and psychiatric disorders is a common problem, and given increasing rates of addiction and psychiatric illnesses in younger generations, an increase in comorbidity is to be expected. Family studies can help us better understand the relationships between these comorbid diseases.

Family studies of comorbid addiction and psychiatric illnesses have shown that several interactions are occurring between these illnesses. At times, disorders randomly occur; at other times, one illness causes another or a common etiological factor has a role. In an individual patient, any one of these interactions may explain the presence of comorbidity.

Future studies of these illnesses are attempting to unravel genetic and environmental factors involved in their development. These studies involve further clarification of the clinical presentation of the disorders singly or in combination, identification of biological markers to recognize a disorder, and possibly the development of animal models of these diseases. Genetic linkage studies that search for DNA sequences that are transmitted in tandem with the predisposition to these disorders are under way.

These studies and future studies will help us trace the underlying aspects of addiction and psychiatric disorders and will assist us in identifying genetic and environmental factors. As our knowledge of these diseases improves, we will have the opportunity to improve treatment and possibly to prevent the occurrence of these illnesses.

REFERENCES

1. Hesselbrock MN, Meyer RE, and Keener JJ: Psychopathology in hospitalized alcoholics. Arch Gen Psychiatry 42:1050–1055, 1985.
2. Crowley TJ, Chesluk D, Dilts S, Hart R: Drug and alcohol abuse among psychiatric admissions. A multidrug clinical-toxicologic study. Arch Gen Psychiatry 30(1):13–20, 1974.
3. Berkson J: Limitations of the application of four-fold table analysis to hospital data. Biometrics 2:47–53, 1946.
4. Regier DA, Farmer ME, Rae DS, et al: Comorbidity of mental disorders with alcohol and other drug abuse. JAMA 264(19):2511–2518, 1990.
5. Kessler RC, McGonagle KA, Zhao S, et al: Lifetime and 12-month prevalence of DSM-III-R psychiatric disorders in the United States. Arch Gen Psychiatry 51:8–19, 1994.

6. Gershon ES, Liebowitz JH: Social, cultural and demographic correlates of affective disorders in Jerusalem. J Psychiatr Res 12(1):37–50, 1975.
7. Merikangas KR, Leckman JF, Prusoff BA, et al: Familial transmission of depression and alcoholism. Arch Gen Psychiatry 42:367–372, 1985.
8. Cloninger CR, Reich T, Wetzel R: Alcoholism and affective disorders: Familial associations and genetic models. In Goodwin DW, Erickson CK (eds): Alcoholism and Affective Disorders: Clinical, Genetic and Biochemical Studies. New York, SP Medical & Scientific Books, 1979, pp 57–86.
9. Robins E, Guze SB. Classification of affective disorders: The primary-secondary, the endogenous-reactive, and the neurotic-psychotic concepts. In Williams TA, Katz MM, Shield JA Jr (eds): Recent Advances in the Psychobiology of the Depressive Illnesses. Proceedings of a Workshop Sponsored by the NIMH. US Government Printing Office, 1972.
10. Guze SB, Cloninger CR, Martin R, Clayton PJ: Alcoholism as a medical disorder. Compr Psychiatry 27(6):501–510, 1986.
11. O'Sullivan K, Whillans P, Daly M, et al: A comparison of alcoholics with and without coexisting affective disorder. Br J Psychiatry 143:133–138, 1983.
12. Schuckit M: Alcoholic patients with secondary depression. Am J Psychiatry 140(6):711–714, 1983.
13. Cadoret R, Winokur G: Depression in alcoholism. Ann N Y Acad Sci 233:34–39, 1974.
14. Yates WR, Petty F, Brown K: Factors associated with depression among primary alcoholics. Compr Psychiatry 29(1):28–33, 1988.
15. Winokur G: Unipolar depression: Is it divisible into autonomous subtypes? Arch Gen Psychiatry 36:47–52, 1979.
16. Coryell W, Winokur G, Keller M, et al: Alcoholism and primary major depression: A family study approach to coexisting disorders. J Affect Disord 24:93–99, 1992.
17. Wender PH, Kety SS, Rosenthal D, et al: Psychiatric disorders in the biological and adoptive families of adopted individuals with affective disorders. Arch Gen Psychiatry 43:923–929, 1986.
18. von Knorring A-L, Cloninger CR, Bohman M, Sigvardsson S: An adoption study of depressive disorders and substance abuse. Arch Gen Psychiatry 40:943–950, 1983.
19. Goodwin DW, Schulsinger F, Hermansen L, et al: Alcohol problems in adoptees raised apart from alcoholic biological parents. Arch Gen Psychiatry 28:238–243, 1973.
20. Gurling HMD, Oppenheim BE, Murray RM: Depression, criminality and psychopathology associated with alcoholism: Evidence from a twin study. Acta Genet Med Gemellol 33:333–339, 1984.
21. Kendler KS, Heath AC, Neale MC, et al: Alcoholism and major depression in women: A twin study of the causes of comorbidity. Arch Gen Psychiatry 50:690–698, 1993.
22. Kushner MG, Sher KJ, Beitman BD: The relation between alcohol problems and the anxiety disorders. Am J Psychiatry 147(6):685–695, 1990.
23. Noyes R Jr, Clancy J, Crowe RE, et al: The familial prevalence of anxiety neurosis. Arch Gen Psychiatry 35(9):1057–1059, 1978.
24. Crowe RR, Noyes R, Pauls DL, Slyman D: A family study of panic disorder. Arch Gen Psychiatry 40(10):1065–1069, 1983.
25. Munjack DJ, Moss HB: Affective disorder and alcoholism in families of agoraphobics. Arch Gen Psychiatry 38:859–872, 1981.
26. Merikangas KR, Risch NJ, Weissman MM. Comorbidity and cotransmission of alcoholism, anxiety and depression. Psychol Med 24:69–80, 1994.
27. Luthar SS, Anton SF, Merikangas KR, Rounsaville BJ. Vulnerability to substance abuse and psychopathology among siblings of opioid abusers. J Nerv Ment Dis 180:153–161, 1992.
28. Kosten TR, Koston TA, Rounsaville BJ: Alcoholism and depressive disorders in opioid addicts and their family members. Compr Psychiatry 32:521–527, 1991.
29. Mirin SM, Weiss RD, Griffin ML, Michael JL: Psychopathology in drug abusers and their families. Compr Psychiatry 32:36–51, 1991.
30. Bryant KJ, Rounsaville B, Spitzer RL, Williams JB: Reliability of dual diagnosis. Substance dependence and psychiatric disorders. J Nerv Ment Dis 180(4):251–257, 1992.
31. Lavori PW, Keller MB, Endicott J: Improving the validity of FH-RDC diagnosis of major affective disorder in uninterviewed relatives in family studies: A model base approach. J Psychiatr Res 22(4):249–259, 1988.
32. Robins LN, Helzer JE, Weissman MM, et al: Lifetime prevalence of specific psychiatric disorders in three sites. Arch Gen Psychiatry 41:949–958, 1984.
33. Reich TR, Cloninger CR, Van Eerdewegh P, et al: Secular trends in the familial transmission of alcoholism. Alcohol Clin Exp Res 12(4):458–464, 1988.

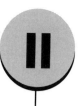

NEUROBIOLOGY

7

The Neurobiology of Addictive Disorders: The Role of Dopamine, Endorphin, and Serotonin

Mark S. Gold, MD

According to a recent Robert Wood Johnson healthcare report (Substance Abuse: The Nation's Number One Health Problem. Prepared by Institute for Health Policy, Brandeis University, for the Robert Wood Johnson Foundation, Princeton, NJ, October 1993), substance abuse is the nation's leading health problem (Fig. 7–1). According to this report, more deaths and disabilities result from substance abuse each year than from any other preventable cause. Of the two million U.S. deaths each year, one in four is attributable to use of alcohol, illicit drugs, or tobacco. This report also notes a direct link to crime and arrests, with one half to two thirds of homicides and serious crimes involving alcohol and nearly one half of men arrested for homicide and assault testing positive for an illegal drug. Substance abuse contributes to family problems: One in four Americans reports that alcohol has been a cause of family trouble, and alcohol abuse plays a part in one of three failed marriages. Education and prevention activities have been successful in reducing occasional drug use, reducing cigarette smoking, and decreasing alcohol-related traffic fatalities, but the plateau of benefits from these approaches is near. Treatment services are the missing link in a society in which increasing social stigma, prohibition, and drug education/prevention have had marked effects on most groups of users with the exception of addicts or regular and heavy users. Experts estimate that for every 1000 employees, 60 are chemically dependent, 3 are receiving treatment, and 57 are not being treated.

Treatment

Psychopharmacological approaches that have been developed during the past decade are designed to treat addictive disorders and are targeted at reversal of the signs and symptoms of withdrawal, such as methadone or clonidine for opiate withdrawal or the nicotine patch for cigarette smokers.[1, 2] Many of these treatments were developed after basic and clinical investigations led to new theories of neurobiological mechanisms for a particular drug or drug-specific abstinence state.[3, 4] This has been particularly true of theories of opiate reward and withdrawal and the opioid–locus coeruleus connection,[4] the dopamine (DA) hypothesis of reward,[5] and chronic cocaine self-administration and DA deficiency theory.[2] New treatments directed at reversal of postabstinence

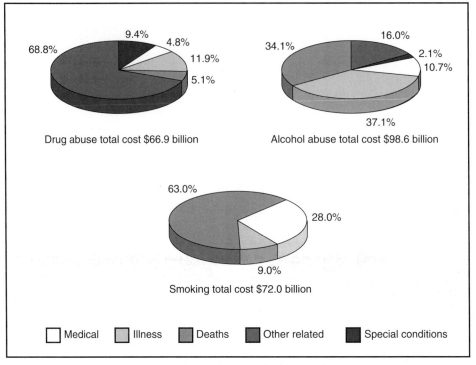

Figure 7–1. Economic costs of substance abuse.

craving, such as desipramine for cocaine abstinence, are based on the assumption that successful craving reduction in some way reduces drug use or relapse.[3] Antiopioid treatment with naltrexone has been rediscovered long after the early success in the treatment of addicted physicians and other addicts.[6] Clinical observations of reduced alcohol relapse in naltrexone-treated alcoholics have been replicated in experimental studies,[7, 8] causing renewed interest in treatments that directly reduce drug taking and endorphin theories of reward.[9] With naloxone and naltrexone studies of animals and humans, neurobiological mechanisms of drug reward must be expanded beyond DA to include endorphins. Independently, basic studies have linked specific serotonin reuptake inhibitors (SSRIs) with drinking behavior in animals and psychiatrists' observations that these SSRIs that are used to successfully treat obsessive-compulsive illness might be useful in alcoholism or cocaine dependence. Serotonergic treatments are being tried in various laboratory and human addiction paradigms. Thus, both serotonin (5-HT) and endorphin influences on addiction must be included in any common theory of neuroanatomical or unified DA neurobiology of addiction.[3, 10]

What Is Necessary for a Drug to Be a Drug of Abuse?

Neurobiological theories should stem from important and clinically relevant questions. What do drugs of abuse have in common? This question seems to be an important place to start. The numerous and often obvious differences between the various drugs of abuse have been the focus of attention in the past. Whether phencyclidine piperdine or amphetamine or cocaine produces a paranoid psychosis but not a classical abstinence syndrome whereas opiates do not produce psychosis but rather a classical abstinence syndrome appears less relevant to their propensity for abuse. Among other attributes, all drugs of abuse appear to have important similarities in various experimental paradigms (Table 7–1).

Previously suggested[1, 3, 10] was the need to reevaluate target signs and symptoms in developing pharmacological treatment and to reconsider the relative importance and significance of withdrawal intensity, treatment of withdrawal and craving, and other subjective measures in relapse and focus instead on modifying drug reward. Drug reward appears primary and

Table 7-1. SIMILARITIES OF ALL DRUGS OF ABUSE

All drugs of abuse
- Are voluntarily self-administered by animals
- Acutely enhance brain reward mechanisms
- Produce a "rush" or "high"
- Affect brain reinforcement circuits either through basal neuronal firing and/or basal neurotransmitter discharge
- Have their reinforcement properties significantly attenuated by blockade of the brain reinforcement system (either through lesions or pharmacological methods)
- Appear capable of increasing (directly or indirectly) dopamine release in the nucleus accumbens *and* producing sizable increases as the animal *waits* for or anticipates the opportunity to self-administer the drug

necessary in supporting the chronic relapsing course of nicotine, alcohol, and other drug dependencies—the nation's most preventable cause of death (Fig. 7–2). A clearer understanding of the basic mechanisms that support drug taking—which change with drug use and which may be modified by genetic and environmental factors—should produce far more effective treatments than currently available.

Cocaine: The Importance and Anatomy of Drug Reward

Experience with cocaine use, dependence, binges, and recidivism has provided insights that have helped to define more clearly the relative importance of withdrawal versus drug reward in supporting drug taking.[1, 3, 10] Cocaine's unique effects, its propensity for stimulating its own taking and undermining survival drives, have for the past decade been the subject of intense study by neurobiologists. Although cocaine has numerous effects influencing multiple neurotransmitter systems, its effects on dopaminergic neurons and neurotransmission appear to be the critical component in cocaine's reinforcing properties.[2, 5, 11–19] Thus, the cocaine epidemic has focused research attention on the putative neuroanatomy of cocaine reward and on drug reward in general. Cocaine self-administration appears to be dependent on the brain's dopaminergic system, which projects from the ventral tegmental area to the nucleus accumbens, which is now viewed as the central feature of the cocaine and DA hypothesis and by implication the core of the endogenous drug reward system. Data supporting such a hypothesis are extensive[2, 3, 5, 10, 11–19] and are summarized in Tables 7–2 and 7–3.

Starting with the hypothesis that activation of DA systems in the mesocorticolimbic areas of the brain is responsible for the motor and reinforcing effects of cocaine, DA activation has been described as essential in most if not all drug reinforcement. A wealth of evidence implicates the nucleus accumbens and DA in incentive motivational effects of drugs as well as of food, sex, and other natural incentives.[20, 21] On the basis of this evidence that mesotelencephalic DA systems mediate the subjective pleasure produced by food, electrical brain stimulation, and sex, drug taking could be

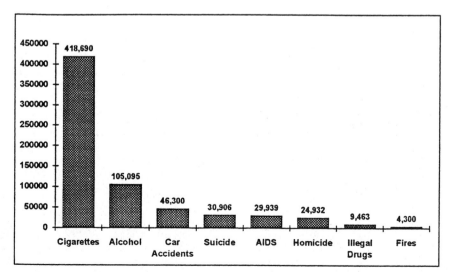

Figure 7-2. Causes of death. (From Centers for Disease Control. US Dept of Health and Human Services.)

Table 7-2. COCAINE AND THE
DOPAMINERGIC SYSTEM—1

- Cocaine produces large increases in extracellular dopamine in the nucleus accumbens
- Increased extracellular dopamine is greater in the nucleus accumbens than other forebrain dopamine loci
- Increased extracellular dopamine is dose dependent
- Cocaine levels in extracellular loci are closely related to extracellular dopamine levels
- Dopamine increases are identical if self-administered or administered by the investigator
- Lower extracellular dopmaine is necessary for reward with chronic cocaine exposure

thought of as taking on the attributes of a drive state such as sex—a drive that is activated by the rewarding activity. Pleasure is normally activated by an encounter with a natural incentive, such as when a hungry person eats food. Therefore, cocaine and other drugs of abuse, which have effects on DA, reward, and the nucleus accumbens that resemble those associated with naturally occurring reward for survival behavior, might persist in confounding the natural behavior-brain reward programs. This may explain the perception and attributes of cocaine or tobacco, depending whether the clinician asks the addict or the loved one or employer. Drug reward or a particular drug experience is commonly explained by addicts in terms such as "hunger," "taste," and "sex." This may not be coincidence at all and may reflect the similarities between sites of natural and drug reward. The nucleus accumbens and DA may be critically important in food, drinking, and sex reward as well.[20, 21]

The bingelike pattern of cocaine taking and the predominance of drug taking for brain reward rather than to reverse withdrawal have led to large numbers of studies attempting to link all illicit drug taking with DA and new

Table 7-3. COCAINE AND THE
DOPAMINERGIC SYSTEM—2

- Dopamine synthesis rate decreases with chronic cocaine use
- Cocaine self-administration produces an initial burst of dopamine in the nucleus accumbens
- Nicotine, opiates, ecstasy, and other drugs increase extracellular dopamine levels in the terminal loci of the mesotelencephalic dopamine system
- Drugs that are self-abused by humans are self-administered by animals and produce extracellular dopamine levels in the terminal projection loci of the mesotelencephalic dopamine system
- Naloxone blocks the increased extracellular dopamine levels produced by opiates and tetrahydrocannabinol

attempts to consider drug seeking and taking as acquired primary drives. Such efforts explain the persistence of addictive drug use and the difficulties in psychopharmacological and psychological treatment on the basis of the neurobiology of cocaine's effects and phenomenology of binge use and relapse. It thus appears likely that drugs stimulate their own taking by interacting with brain systems normally reserved for rewarding survival behaviors. If giving up cocaine becomes analogous to giving up food, water, or sex, then treatment certainly takes on a tremendous challenge.[1]

Cocaine Abstinence

Withdrawal need not be filled with counselors, nausea, or vomiting, although until the mid-1980s, organized psychiatry discounted the possibility that cocaine use was associated with an abstinence syndrome of any consequence on discontinuation of chronic administration.[10] Observations of humans[2, 11] and more recently animal studies[22] support the concept of a cocaine abstinence state. Although severe cocaine abuse is characterized by binges alternating with abstinence, the occurrence of a withdrawal dysphoria with neurovegetative symptoms that occurs within hours after a binge is accepted by cocaine users and psychiatrists as "the crash."[11, 13] In humans, the acute abstinence state is of variable intensity and symptoms but generally includes irritability, anxiety, and depression, which can be and often are self-medicated with cocaine. The concept previously presented postulates[3] a commonalty of all drugs of abuse taken for euphoria production, generating during abstinence an affective or dysphoric withdrawal state related to DA/the nucleus accumbens and an autonomic withdrawal state related to the locus coeruleus. Other brain systems may be found to have an important role but are mediated primarily through these systems.[23] This model led to a proposal that cocaine, rather than simply producing increases in DA availability, with chronic use causes DA to become unavailable. Support for this hypothesis in humans is outlined in Table 7-4.

Although a DA theory may explain symptoms or complaints common to cocaine abstinence and many other drug abstinence states that naturally share anhedonia, boredom, depression, and other common features, DA depletion cannot explain the hypertension, tachycardia, nausea, diarrhea, sweating, sense of impending doom, or panic commonly asso-

Table 7–4. CLINICAL SUPPORT FOR THE DOPAMINE DEPLETION THEORY

- Several studies of chronic cocaine abusers have demonstrated substantially elevated prolactin levels
- Elevated prolactin levels persist for at least 1 month after stopping cocaine
- Positron emission tomography (PET) studies found marked decrease D_2 receptor density persisting for at least 2 weeks after stopping cocaine
- Athletes and others complain of parkinsonian symptoms
- Clinical efficacy of bromocriptine and other dopamine agonists in reversing acute abstinence complaints
- Withdrawal anhedonia is reversed by intracranial electrical stimulation

ciated with opiate withdrawal and locus coeruleus hyperactivity. On the basis of a DA depletion hypothesis, research was conducted using bromocriptine, a DA agonist widely used without abuse in the treatment of infertility, amenorrhea-galactorrhea, and Parkinson's disease. Bromocriptine reversed many of the physiological and affective features of cocaine abstinence and has also shown promise in reducing cocaine craving and withdrawal dysphoria. The original report has been supported by studies of humans[24, 25] and cocaine withdrawal in rats, and bromocriptine reduces cocaine self-administration in rats[26] and monkeys. Bromocriptine or bromocriptine-like medications (pharmacological treatments that enhance DA neurotransmission) may be useful in alleviating the affective and motivational aspects of cocaine and other drug withdrawal states, and clonidine might be useful in reversing the autonomic features common to many other withdrawal syndromes.[2, 3]

New behavioral models in animals[11, 23, 26, 27] and characterization of the cocaine receptor appear to offer promise for identifying new treatments that might prevent relapse or cocaine euphoria. The fact that not all DA uptake inhibitors exert reinforcing properties similar to cocaine suggests that once the neuronal DA transporter is purified and cloned, new nonaddicting treatments for human cocaine addicts might be developed.

Other Potential Treatments for Dependence on Cocaine and Other Drugs

Although initial study focused on DA depletion and its reversal, other potential treatments came from the bench to the bedside or vice versa. Serotonergic agents[23] such as fluoxetine, ritanserin, and sertraline have effects on human drinking and in animal models, but studies of these SSRIs in cocaine craving and cocaine responding in animals generally show effects only at doses that suppress behaviors maintained by food and other reinforcers. SSRIs may still prove to be important new treatments for cocaine addicts. One lesson from the literature on eating suggests that SSRIs such as fluoxetine suppress carbohydrate with no change in fat or protein intake, but 5HT manipulations work only at special times in circadian and developmental stages, not at all times. Opiate antagonists work in a different system and more generally to stop fat intake regardless of circadian or developmental issues. SSRIs may require administration at a particular point in time, whereas whole opioid antagonists may have efficacy at any time.

Alcohol-preferring animals find low doses of alcohol extremely reinforcing and have greater increases in nucleus accumbens DA release after drinking or in anticipation of being allowed to self-administer alcohol. In these animals, ethanol drives the system toward normal. Interesting data reported by T. K. Lee at meetings of the American Society of Addiction Medicines in 1994 suggest that these animals have neurobiological deficits in DA and serotonin systems and a significantly decreased number of D2 receptors and decreased 5-HT projections from the raphe. Serotonergic function appears to be critical in alcohol use, depression, and aggression and is a prime candidate for mediating the overlap between these behaviors. Linnoila and coworkers (ASAM 1994) found a number of interesting interactions between levels of the serotonin metabolite cerebrospinal fluid 5-hydroxyindoleacetic acid (5-HIAA) and various behaviors and traits. 5-HIAA production appears to be a meaningful and highly heritable biological trait related to ongoing function within the environment. For example, low-5-HIAA monkeys raised with parental neglect when given ethanol in adolescence "drink like fish ... the monkeys have to be protected from their drinking." In all rearing conditions, low-5-HIAA monkeys drink excessively. Linnoila has found that low 5-HIAA levels correlate with a number of personality indices observed in human studies, with the most striking associations with chronic irritability, low-grade chronic somatic anxiety, dysphoria, violence (acting or lashing out), alcohol-related problems, and suicide attempts. However promising these and other data are for 5-HT and alcohol dependence, hydroxytryptamine agents have not been well studied in human alcohol dependence to date.

Desipramine has been reported to reduce cocaine craving and promote abstinence, but it has little or no effect on cocaine self-administration in animals or humans.[12] Reports on anticraving and compounds from carbamazepine to methylphenidate to mazindol[12, 13] suggest that cocaine abuse can be modified by a wide range of compounds without therapeutic efficacy. A specific compound that alters cocaine reward/taking is needed to improve clinical treatment outcomes.

Addiction Psychiatry: Negative Versus Positive Reward

Neurobiological theories form an important but often competing foundation for the field of addiction psychiatry. Although each theory has something for everyone, a theory should be able to explain the essential features of addictive illness. Competing theories should explain the five hallmarks of addictive behavior and the target to be "treated" by any biological approach to drug addiction: (1) drug craving, (2) drug relapse, (3) increased desire for the drug and concurrent decreased pleasure from drugs, (4) spontaneous remission, and (5) compulsive addictive drug use regardless of withdrawal or the consequences of use.

When treating addictions ranging from nicotine dependence with the nicotine patch to opiate dependence with methadone or clonidine, clinicians have observed a dissociation between abstinence complaints and return to drug taking. Why do people still smoke today in spite of all of the information about dangers? Why have most smokers not only tried to quit but tried to quit within the past year? They are addicted to nicotine. Some 45 million Americans have successfully stopped smoking, but nearly 70% of America's remaining smokers say that they are definitely addicted. A cigarette is a successful and efficient delivery system, and a bolus of nicotine reaches the brain in 7 seconds or less. With 20 to 30 uses a day, a powerful physiological dependence with complex conditioning occurs, making discontinuation difficult. Smoking is a habitual behavior that is physically addicting. Nicotine has a direct effect on the brain and reward pathways; it stimulates the desire to repeat the behavior. Smokers link the activities of daily life to smoking. Many cannot imagine talking on the phone or drinking a cup of coffee without a cigarette. They have difficulty conducting the activities of daily living without a cigarette. Of people who attempt to stop smoking every year in the United States, only 2% to 3% succeed at 1 year. Therefore, from a public health perspective, if 5% succeed and we identify every patient who smokes and start each on an attempt to quit, our success rate will be improved by starting so many patients in a cessation program. Seventy percent of smokers visit a clinician every year, offering opportune moments for diagnosis, motivational interviewing, and initiation of smoking cessation—all of which need to be maximized by physicians. In most studies, 50% of relapses to smoking occur in the first 2 weeks. Physicians should plan to see and talk to their patients more during these critical times. Cigarette smoking while visiting with friends, while drinking a beer, or after sex, according to smokers, increases the pleasure of these activities. Smoking also reduces the negative affect and physiological symptoms from withdrawal, including hunger and irritability. Treatment of withdrawal using gum, clonidine, or the patch is associated with the low response rate common to other drug addictions. Cigarette smoking during patch administration again calls into question the value of the negative reinforcement theory—that drugs are taken to relieve or avoid withdrawal.[3] Historically, this theory, with its emphasis on the aversive consequences of drug discontinuation or the drug withdrawal syndrome, has been the central focus of neurobiological research. Many of the new treatments developed during the past decade have successfully reversed the autonomic or affective components of a particular drug abstinence state but have had less dramatic effects on recidivism.

Negative Reinforcement Theories: Drugs Are Taken to Reverse Withdrawal Pain and Discomfort

Negative reinforcers could sustain behavior such as drug seeking and taking not because of the state that they produce but because of the state that they reverse. Drug use according to this model is thus maintained by the aversive symptoms associated with withdrawal and reversed by the drug. Although the focus of considerable investigation, the neurobiology of abstinence and withdrawal behavior is a new subject for comprehensive study. Much has been learned about drug withdrawal syndromes, but much remains unknown (Table 7–5).

The abstinence syndrome associated with use of alcohol, heroin, cocaine, benzodiazepines, and other drugs of abuse include physical signs and symptoms peculiar to each drug of abuse but with many common features including anxiety, anhedonia, dysphoria, depression, craving, and reversal of this syndrome by the drug of abuse. Antiwithdrawal treatment appears to be steadily improving but is independent of successful abstinence and recovery. Successful detoxification with the patch or methadone does not suggest success during the early or later stages of abstinence. This is important evidence for the relative importance of abstinence or pain/discomfort versus positive reward in supporting addictive drug use. Cocaine may produce a negative affective state and a variable physical abstinence syndrome, but the rewarding aspects of cocaine use are clearly more important and impressive[2, 3, 10] and related to the attachment of the person to the drug. One result of the negative reinforcement theory is that by focusing on withdrawal or craving, pharmacological treatments may be found to be successful and to be abysmal failures at the same time. Clinicians recognize that maximal periods of drug self-administration or binges in humans do not coincide with periods of maximal withdrawal distress.[3] Jaffe[14] has even said that "there is little corre-

lation between the visibility or physiological seriousness of withdrawal signs and their motivational force" in maintaining addictive behavior. Experimental work demonstrated the persistence of drug taking when former heroin addicts who showed no withdrawal symptoms on naloxone challenge worked at high rates of lever pressing to receive a low-dose injection of morphine.[15] The theory of negative reinforcement also is inadequate for explaining why many drugs that produce withdrawal syndromes are not typically self-administered for nonmedical purposes (e.g., clonidine, opioid agonists, imipramine). Finally, treatment professionals recognize the ever-present possibility of relapse even after an extended period of abstinence from drugs, long after acute or protracted withdrawal.

One major addition to the negative reinforcement theories is conditioned abstinence. Conditioned stimuli themselves after paired association with drug administration may produce symptoms of withdrawal with accompanying increases in dopaminergic transmission as if the drug were actually taken. The nucleus accumbens has an important role in the conditioned locomotor responses to cocaine and logically should be expected to play such a part in opiate and other addictions. DA neurons do not discharge when an animal actually eats the food or when an animal would experience sensory pleasure but change firing as the stimulus becomes more salient or attention grabbing. The ability of drugs to elevate DA neuro-

Table 7–5. FEATURES OF VARIOUS DRUG WITHDRAWAL SYNDROMES IN HUMANS

Features	Withdrawal Syndrome				
	Nicotine	Alcohol/Sedative	Opioids	Amphetamine/Cocaine	Caffeine
Pharmacological specificity	Yes	Yes	Yes	Yes	Yes
Animal models	Yes	Yes	Yes	Yes	Yes
Associated with tolerance	?	Yes	Yes	Yes	Yes
Precipitated withdrawal	No	Not tested	Yes	Not tested	Yes
Acute physical dependence	?	Yes	Yes	?	Not tested
Related to dose and duration	?	Yes	Yes	Not tested	Yes
Cross-dependence	Not tested	Yes	Yes	Not tested	Not tested
Symptom stages	Not tested	Yes	Yes	?	No
Gradual reduction decreases	Yes	Yes	Yes	Not tested	Not tested
Protracted withdrawal	No	Yes	Yes	?	Not tested
Conditioned withdrawal	?	Yes	Yes	?	Not tested
Influenced by instructions	Yes	Yes	Yes	Not tested	Not tested
Nonpharmacological treatment effective	Not tested	Yes	Not tested	Not tested	Not tested
Genetic effects	?	Yes	Not tested	Not tested	Not tested
Neonatal withdrawal	No	?	Yes	?	No

From Hughes JR, Higgins ST, Bickel WK: Nicotine withdrawal vs. other drug withdrawal syndromes: Similarities and dissimilarities. Addiction (in press).

transmission beyond that which normally occurs may be the feature of drugs that makes them such potent incentives, causing stimuli to be perceived as brighter and more attractive.

Cocaine and Conditioning

Cocaine users describe intense craving for cocaine when cocaine is made available to them or merely when the word *cocaine* is uttered in conversation. Seeing places where they used cocaine, smelling cocaine, seeing a cocaine pipe, seeing a friend with whom they used cocaine, hearing a song that they heard while using cocaine, and numerous other casual smells, sights, and sounds can trigger an intense reaction in individuals who used cocaine in the past but are now abstinent. In such circumstances, previous users report tasting cocaine, craving cocaine, sweating, feeling short of breath and faint, smelling cocaine, and feeling a little of the cocaine euphoria, among other self-reports. Even the presentation of cocaine paraphernalia after weeks or months of abstinence can produce intense cravings and withdrawal-like symptoms. In experimental studies of humans, individuals with a history of cocaine use show greater physiological reactivity in response to cocaine cues than do cocaine-naive individuals. The greater responses were also demonstrated to cocaine stimuli rather than powerful opiate cues. Cocaine-related stimuli elicit conditioned physiological and subjective states in cocaine users.[28] These clinical situations and problems remind us of classical conditioning and the clear importance of linking cocaine to all sorts of cues. The neural system that normally says to an organism, "pay attention, and pay attention to this now," or attributes salience to incentive stimuli and becomes sensitized to drugs of abuse is the mesotelencephalic DA system. Sensitization results in an increase in the responsiveness of the DA system to activating stimuli such that activating stimuli produce a greater increase in DA neurotransmission in sensitized than nonsensitized individuals.

Positive Reinforcement

An alternative neurobiological theory in addiction psychiatry explains drug seeking, drug taking, and the resistance of addiction to rational thinking or treatment by invoking positive reinforcement. Simplistically, drugs are taken because they stimulate their own taking. Positive reinforcement could be expanded to include host preference or other factors that cause drug reward to be greatest in certain individuals—for example, in those who have used the drug before, those raised in a certain environment, or those with a genetic predisposition for drug self-administration. Self-administration data support the theory that drugs are taken because of the state they induce and not because they alleviate any unpleasant state.[2, 3]

With repeated drug use, the act of drug taking and drug-associated stimuli gradually become more and more attractive and able to control behavior. Wanting the drugs becomes sensitized, and drug use takes on the characteristics of an acquired drive to the extreme of an obsessive-compulsive illness with prominent obsessive craving and compulsive drug seeking and drug taking. The positive reinforcement theory is little more than drugs that stimulate their own taking. In explaining drug use, *positive* can also imply that drug taking equals euphoria or pleasure. This is problematic because nicotine is highly addictive but does not produce marked euphoria. Similarly, opiates may induce vomiting or cigarettes nausea, but both are taken again anyway. Many addictive drugs produce strong aversive or even profoundly dysphoric effects. Addicts report that they are miserable, that their life is in ruins, and that the drug is not even that good anymore, but they still somehow are motivated to look for it and use it.

Cocaine, Dopamine, and Acquired Dopamine-Endorphin-Serotonin Neuroanatomy and Neuropharmacology of Drug Reward and Treatment

Cocaine has been a particularly useful model because of the intensity of the euphoria, persistence of the attachment to the drug, rapidity of addiction, and compulsive and bingelike features associated with its use. Although cocaine reward has been linked to the DA system and the DA transporter, other brain systems also contribute to its rewarding effects.[2, 3, 10] The serotonergic system, a recent focus for obsessive-compulsive disorder research and therapy, appears to have an important role in cocaine reward.[22] Opioid systems have been the focus of much investigation since their discovery, and early hypotheses of an important role in endogenous reward have been buoyed by evidence of an important role in cocaine reward. These data and studies suggesting that opioid systems are essential in the reinforcing properties of opiates, alcohol, and other drugs suggest a critical role for endorphins in positive reinforcement per se and that opiate antagonists such as naltrexone may have considerable clinical promise in humans.

Host Factors

Alcohol and other drugs may be more rewarding for those who are born with or who acquire greater DA release in anticipation of drug availability. Alcohol-preferring rats are clearly different from non–alcohol-preferring rats in behavior and neurochemistry (Table 7–6).

In humans, genetic or host factors appear equally important. Kendler asks why drunkards beget drunkards,[37] to paraphrase Hippocrates. Twin studies in the literature and Kendler's work suggest that genetic influences are the single most important answer to this question for both men and women. Heritability of 50% to 60% for alcoholism means that for all the risks that influence the probability of alcoholism, at least half are directly attributed to genetics. The genetic predisposition and contribution to the development of alcoholism are similar to the contributions reported for

Table 7–6. ANIMAL MODEL FOR HUMAN ALCOHOLISM

Alcohol-Preferring Rats (P) vs. Nonpreferring Rats (NP)	
P Animals	NP Animals
Low doses produce positive reinforcing effects	Do not sense the positive reinforcing effects
Low aversive effects to alcohol	High aversive effects to low doses of alcohol
Tolerance to high doses of alcohol	Hangover effects
Less sensitive to impairing effects	Motor performance impaired
Excessive ethanol self-administration	
Born with: 1. Decreased number of D2 receptors 2. Decreased serotonin projections from the raphe 3. Increased anticipatory ventral tegmental area and nucleus accumbens dopamine	

other factors—height is 95%, serum cholesterol 40%, blood pressure 40% to 50%, and adult-onset diabetes 50%. In addition to genetic data gathered for more than a decade, Schuckit has studied the effects of alcohol in sons of alcoholic men compared with subjects without a family history of alcoholism using 454 male staff at the University of California, San Diego. Individuals who were relatively insensitive to a moderate alcohol dose in subjective response and body sway were significantly more likely to be abusing alcohol or to be dependent at long-term follow-up by their own history and that reported by significant others. A low level of response to alcohol at age 20 years was associated with a fourfold greater likelihood of future alcoholism in both the sons of alcoholics and the comparison subjects. Fifty-six percent of the sons of alcoholics with the lesser alcohol response developed alcoholism during the subsequent decade. Schuckit clearly separated the risk for development of alcoholism from the risk of development of other psychiatric disorders with this paradigm of sensitivity to the intoxicating effects of alcohol.[38] Insensitivity was highly significant for young men with a positive family history for alcoholism.

The basic science literature is quite supportive of these data. For example, rats bred for alcohol preference appear less sensitive to the effects of alcohol than other rats. A number of family, adoption, and twin studies have identified important genetic influences on the risk for the development of alcoholism.[29] Morphine and cocaine exert common chronic actions on tyrosine hydroxylase in dopaminergic brain reward regions. Both morphine and cocaine have other common actions in the nucleus accumbens, increasing levels of adenylate cyclase and cyclic adenosine monophosphate (cyclic AMP)–dependent protein kinase and decreasing levels of inhibitory G-protein. One particularly interesting finding in these strains is that chronic morphine up-regulates the cyclic AMP pathway in the locus coeruleus in both rat strains, thereby explaining the similar acquisition and demonstration of physical or autonomic opiate withdrawal signs. Although the overall severity of withdrawal was similar between the two strains, different types of behaviors predominated. Lewis rats show greater withdrawal than Fischer rats with respect to those behaviors mediated by the locus coeruleus, yet chronic morphine up-regulation occurs in the nucleus accumbens in only the Fischer rats, suggesting an explanation for the lower self-administration by Fischer rats. Similarly, chronic morphine increases levels of tyrosine hydroxylase in the locus coeruleus in both rat strains but, again, in the ventral tegmental area in Fischer rats only.[30]

Endogenous Opioids, Drug and Alcohol Reward

Endogenous opioids have been suggested as primary mediators of opioid reward and most recently alcohol reward. Early data from laboratory studies linking alcohol to endorphins were inconsistent. The endogenous opioid system does appear to alter ethanol-induced behavior. Naloxone potentiates the progressive increase in the latency of visual evoked potentials during acute alcoholic intoxication in cats, perhaps by increasing opiate receptor sites. Blockade of opiate receptors by nalorphine eliminated the effects of acute alcohol intoxication on the activity of neurons in the ventromedial hypothalamus. Animals show a differential ethanol-induced release of beta-endorphin concentration and a greater release of the peptide under basal conditions, suggesting a genetic basis for the differential ethanol consumption.[31] Ethanol increases beta-endorphins in the hypothalamus and in the plasma of monkeys after 2 to 4 weeks of chronic ingestion.[32] In humans, plasma beta-endorphin levels were found to be below normal in alcoholics entering treatment, returning to normal during 5 weeks of treatment.[33] Antiopiates have been used in the treatment of alcohol dependence in humans, with the principal finding of two groups suggesting that when naltrexone was taken and the alcoholic drank[7] or when naltrexone was coupled with adjunctive therapy, the likelihood that a lapse in abstinence would become a full-blown relapse was reduced.[8]

Evidence suggests that opioid and serotonergic influences, rather than occurring independently, exert their effects through the mesolimbic DA system. In addition, serotonin may have its major role in the mediation of reward directly through the modulation of the mesolimbic DA system. Similarly, the endogenous opioid system appears to have specific modulatory effects on DA release in the nucleus accumbens. Naloxone or naltrexone attenuation of many drugs of abuse in self-administration and human paradigms is consistent with the modulatory role of opioids. Naltrexone has been directly demonstrated to reverse ethanol-induced increases in extracellular DA but not 5-HT.[34] DA neurons appear to discharge under conditions consistent with an attribution of incentive salience, suggesting that DA functions

to give survival meaning to a particular occurrence.[35] Opiate antagonists or SSRIs could attenuate perceived reward by modifying the extent or timing of DA increase produced in the nucleus accumbens by the drug or drug availability. Mu and kappa opioid receptor antagonists have been shown to modify basal DA release within the nucleus accumbens,[36] suggesting that tonically active endogenous opioid systems may actually regulate mesolimbic DA neurons. Naltrexone could reduce relapses in abstinence from alcohol and other drugs by altering the organismic significance attributed to the drug event and ultimately the endogenous reward produced by ethanol and other drugs. If endogenous opioid systems have such an important role in ongoing survival behavior reward and attribution of salience, then chronic treatment with naltrexone may have antidrug reward but subjectively unpleasant or other unrewarding effects that may limit medication compliance or the duration of antagonist treatment.

Prevention

What is prevention, and is it relevant to a practicing clinician or neurobiologist? It is generally believed by clinicians that education is prevention. For example, when asked about their prevention activities, many physicians and health providers describe lectures and patient education sessions. During the past decade, a science of prevention has emerged because of objective measures and scientific methods applied to prevention and control interventions. Studying a group of fifth- or sixth-grade students for the next decade, scientists will gain a much better idea of the natural history of nicotine dependence or smoking initiation and what can be done to prevent it. Primary prevention is not a waste of time. It is worthwhile not just to teach the facts about drugs but to teach social skills for resisting drugs and ways to reduce the effects of social influence. Physicians have an important role as well. They are well-respected authorities on disease and treatment. Their efficacy as primary prevention providers is limited by the fact that the length of the interaction with patients is too short, the typical format too didactic/authoritarian, and the frequency between interactions too infrequent for maximizing effect. Although a police officer may have considerable credibility in describing what is happening on the streets and the association between drugs and crime, physicians in many communities are the experts in prevention, disease, addiction, and public health. As experts, physicians may need to become familiar with certain facts in the science of prevention. First, knowledge and imparting of information are not prevention. It is now clear that a child or an adult can be taught about the effects of cigarette smoke on health or any bodily function and learning can be proved by a posttest, yet smoking rates remain unchanged. Second, changing attitudes about cigarettes or drugs may have slightly better effects on smoking behavior—especially in those who have not started—yet attitude change appears to be independent of behavior change. Third, among nonfamily/nongenetic or host factors, a child's group of friends and their cigarette or drug use rates appear to be quite important determinants. Students generally overestimate the number of the people their age who smoke, drink, or use drugs. This overestimation creates the widespread belief that such behavior is normative and acceptable. If a child's best friend smokes cigarettes or uses drugs, peer influence factors will continuously pressure the child to try them, to use them, and to fit in. Peer environments are diverse within the same school and even within the same family in the same school. Prevention, organized and delivered in the context of a multiweek course at school with periodic "boosters," appears to work by reducing the impact of social influ-

ence, teaching positive resistance skills, and supporting the use of these skills. Physicians need to understand the power of prevention activities in reducing cigarette smoking, to recognize the differences between fact training and attitude training and prevention, and to provide expert advice to the school, police, Drug Abuse Resistance Education, or other providers on the value of prevention efforts and methods. Trained as scientists, physicians are also experts on the need for baseline use and longitudinal follow-up data to evaluate a program that a school has implemented. This role for physicians is different from the traditional role of assessing cigarette or drug use, detailing the history, evaluating for consequences, and starting a discontinuation program.

Conclusion

The various drugs of abuse—opiates, stimulants, alcohol, nicotine, cannabinoids, and cocaine—have distinct and apparently different primary sites of neurotransmitter action. They directly interact with different receptors or other cell surface proteins. With continued understanding of the cellular basis and postreceptor intracellular targets for drug reward and the possibility that drug rewards and other rewards are separable, new pharmacological treatments that focus on the positive aspects of

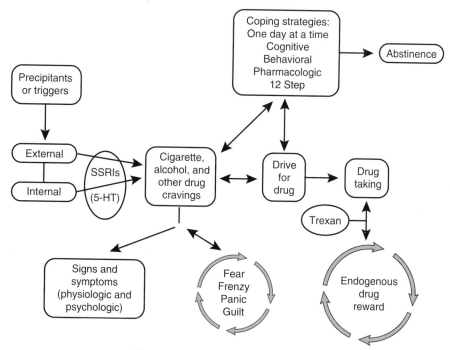

Figure 7–3. Reward versus abstinence.

the drug-taking experience and that reduce drug reward and drug taking may be possible. While we search for an elusive magic bullet or vaccine, we are left to develop new treatments or to improve the efficacy of existing methods to reduce drug reward and encourage abstinence (Fig. 7–3).

Pharmacological treatments that reduce the attachment between a person and his or her drugs could easily be understood as augmenting psychosocial treatments, which have their own positive and rewarding qualities. Antiopioids and SSRIs might be understood to work primarily in preventing drug reward and interfering with cue-provoked events. Other explanations are possible and await research in this area. Pharmacological treatments might work in the same brain area as Alcoholics Anonymous, through a different mechanism, and have additive or even potentiating effects. It was previously stated that prevention is the single most effective treatment for addiction. From Figure 7–3, it is clear that in terms of drug use, triggers, physiological and psychological consequences, and so on do not occur in nonusers. The natural history of addiction is as a chronic, relapsing disorder. Prevention is the ideal treatment, inoculating our population against the effects of drug self-administration and offering unlimited access to endogenous reward. Treatments that focus on reducing the likelihood of relapse after detoxification may redefine the neurobiology of addiction and lead to a new understanding of the persistence of drug taking and new treatments. Use of drugs and alcohol and addictive disorders remain an enormous public health problem in 1995. Understanding the neurobiology of drug use and addiction and development of new treatments for these diseases are, appropriately, a national priority.

REFERENCES

1. Gold MS: Is there a treatment or treatments for drug abuse or addiction? Contemp Psychol 38:1119–1120, 1993.
2. Dackis CA, Gold MS: New concepts in cocaine addiction: The dopamine depletion hypothesis. Neurosci Biobehav Rev 9:469–477, 1985.
3. Gold MS, Miller NS: Seeking drugs/alcohol and avoiding withdrawal: The neuroanatomy of drive states and withdrawal. Psychiatr Ann 22:430–435, 1992.
4. Gold MS: Opiate addiction and the locus coeruleus. Psychiatr Clin North Am 16:61–73, 1993.
5. Wise RA, Rompre PP: Brain dopamine and reward. Annu Rev Psychol 40:191–225, 1989
6. Washton AM, Gold MS: Successful use of naltrexone in addicted physicians and business executives. Adv Alcohol Subst Abuse 4(2):89–96, 1984.
7. Volpicelli JR, Alterman AI, Hayashida M, O'Brien CP: Naltrexone in the treatment of alcohol dependence. Arch Gen Psychiatry 49:876–880, 1992.
8. O'Malley SS, Jaffe AJ, Chang G, et al: Naltrexone and coping skills therapy for alcohol dependence. Arch Gen Psychiatry 49:881–887, 1992.
9. Gold MS, Byck R: Endorphins, lithium and naloxone: Their relationship to pathological and drug induced manic euphoric states. National Institute of Drug Abuse Research Monograph Series 19:192–209, 1978.
10. Gold MS: Drugs of Abuse: A Comprehensive Series for Clinicians, vol III. Cocaine. New York, Plenum, 1993.
11. Gold MS: Cocaine (and crack). In Lowinson JH, Ruiz P, Millman RB (eds): Clinical Aspects in Substance Abuse: A Comprehensive Textbook, 2nd ed. Baltimore, Williams & Wilkins, 1992, pp 205–221.
11a. Linnoila M: Facts About Tobacco, Alcohol and Other Drugs. 4:3, 1995.
12. Meyer RE: New pharmacotherapies for cocaine dependence . . . revisited. Arch Gen Psychiatry 49:900–904, 1992.
13. Gawin FH. Cocaine addiction: Psychology and neurophysiology. Science 251:1580–1586, 1991.
14. Jaffe JH: Current concepts of addiction. In O'Brien CP, Jaffe JH (eds): Addictive States. New York, Raven Press, 1992, pp 1–21.
15. Lamb RJ, Preston KL, Schindler C, et al: The reinforcing and subjective effects of morphine in post-addicts: A dose-response study. J Pharmacol Exp Ther 259:1165–1173, 1991.
16. Fischman MW, Foltin RW: Self-administration of cocaine by humans: A laboratory perspective. In Bock GR, Whelan J (eds): Cocaine: Scientific and Social Dimensions. CIBA Foundation Symposium 166. Chichester, UK, Ciba Foundation, 1992, pp 165–180.
17. Kuhar M, Ritz M, Boja J: The dopamine hypothesis of the reinforcing properties of cocaine. Trends Neurosci 14:299–302, 1991.
18. Johanson C-E, Fischman MW: The pharmacology of cocaine related to its abuse. Pharmacol Rev 41:3052, 1989.
19. Wise RA, Bozarth MA: A psychomotor stimulant theory of addiction. Psychol Rev 94(4):469–492, 1987.
20. Yoshida M, Yokoo H, Mizoguchi Y, et al: Eating and drinking cause increased dopamine release in the nucleus accumbens and ventral tegmental area in the rat: Measurement by in vivo microdialysis. Neurosci Let 139:73–76, 1992.
21. White NM, Milner PM: The psychobiology of reinforcers. Annu Rev Psychol 43:443–471, 1992.
22. Markou A, Koob GF: Post cocaine anhedonia: An animal model of cocaine withdrawal. Neuropsychopharmacology 4:17–26, 1991.
23. Sellers EM, Higgins GA, Sobell MB: 5-HT and alcohol abuse. Trends Pharmacol Sci 13:69–75, 1992.
24. Nunes EV, McGrath PJ, Stewart JW, Quitkin FM: Bromocriptine treatment for cocaine addiction. Am J Addict 2:169–172, 1992.
25. Moskovitz H, Brookoff D, Nelson L: A randomized trial of bromocriptine for cocaine users presenting to the emergency department. J Gen Intern Med 8:1–4, 1993.
26. Izenwasser S, Rosenberger JG, Cox BM: Inhibition of 3H-dopamine and 3H-serotonin uptake by cocaine: Comparison between chopped tissue slices and synaptosomes. Life Sci 50:541–547, 1992.
27. Markou A, Weiss F, Gold LH, et al: Animal models of drug craving. Psychopharmacology 112:163–182, 1992.
28. Ehrman RN, Robbins SJ, Childress AR, O'Brien CP: Conditioned responses to cocaine-related stimuli in cocaine abuse patients. Psychopharmacology 107:523–529, 1992.

29. Schuckit MA: Low level of response to alcohol as a predictor of future alcoholism. Am J Psychiatry 151:184–189, 1994.

30. Guitart X, Kogan JH, Berhow M, et al: Lewis and Fischer rat strains display differences in biochemical, electrophysiological and behavioral parameters: Studies in the nucleus accumbens and locus coeruleus of drug naive and morphine-treated animals. Brain Res 611:7–17, 1993.

31. De Waele JP, Papachristou DN, Gianoulakis C: The alcohol-preferring C57BL/6 mice present an enhanced sensitivity of hypothalamic B-endorphin system to ethanol than the alcohol-avoiding DBA/2 mice. J Pharmacol Exp Ther 261:788–797, 1992.

32. Kornet M, Goosen C, Thyssen JHH, Van Ree JM: Endocrine profile during acquisition of free-choice alcohol drinking in rhesus monkeys. Alcohol 27:403–410, 1992.

33. Vescovi PP, Coiro V, Volpi R, et al: Plasma β-endorphin but not met-enkephalin levels are abnormal in chronic alcoholics. Alcohol 27:471–475, 1992.

34. Benjamin D, Grant ER, Poherecky LA: Naltrexone reverses ethanol-induced dopamine release in the nucleus accumbens in awake, freely moving rats. Brain Res 621:137–140, 1993.

35. Robinson TE, Berridge KC: The neural basis of drug craving: An incentive-sensitization theory of addiction. Brain Res Rev 18:247–291, 1993.

36. Spanagel R, Herz A, Shippenberg TS: Opposing tonically active endogenous opioid systems modulate the mesolimbic dopaminergic pathway. Proc Natl Acad Sci U S A 89:2046–2050, 1992.

37. Kendler KS: Facts About Tobacco, Alcohol, and Other Drugs. 3:3, 1994.

38. Schuckit MA: Low level of response to alcohol as a predictor of future alcoholism. Am J Psychiatry 151:184–189, 1994.

8

Neurochemical Findings in Alcoholism and Drug Addiction and Psychiatric Comorbidity

Subhash C. Pandey, PhD • John M. Davis, MD • Ghanshyam N. Pandey, PhD

Alcoholism represents a major public health concern. Alcohol abuse and dependence are serious problems that affect both adult and teenage populations.[1] Alcohol-dependent persons represent a heterogeneous population in terms of psychiatric comorbidity and differences in genetics, personality, family characteristics, and social status.[1] Alcoholism is a biologically based disease in which biology and behavior interact in complex ways. Evidence suggests that alcohol-drinking behavior may be caused by abnormalities in several central neurotransmitters, including serotonin (5HT) and dopamine (DA).[2] Serotonergic abnormalities have been hypothesized for most of the major psychiatric disorders (e.g., depression, anxiety, and obsessive-compulsive disorder).[3, 4] Serotonergic abnormalities have been also reported in alcoholism.[3, 4] It has been shown that augmentation of 5HT neurotransmission attenuates alcohol consumption whereas depletion enhances it.[4] Thus, 5HT may represent a common denominator for various behavioral disorders such as depression, aggression, anxiety, and alcoholism.

Changes in the serotonergic and the dopaminergic systems are associated with states of alcohol intoxication and withdrawal. These changes may be related to alterations in neurotransmitter turnover or receptor sensitivity or in second-messenger systems (e.g., phosphoinositide-signaling system and cyclic adenosine monophosphate [cyclic AMP] second-messenger system). A number of neuroendocrine studies have suggested an abnormal serotonergic system in aggression, depression, and alcoholism.[5, 6] It has also been suggested that drug addiction (cocaine) exerts its mood effects by modulating the dopaminergic and serotonergic systems in the brain.[7] This chapter discusses serotonergic and dopaminergic abnormalities along with the second-messenger system in alcoholism and drug addiction, as well as ways in which the observed neurochemical findings of psychiatric disorders and drug/alcohol abuse might interact and relate to each other.

Prevalence of Comorbidity

Prevalence studies indicate that the majority of alcoholics display anxious or mixed anxious and depressive symptoms. Weissman and colleagues[8] reported that 70% of alcoholics meet criteria for another psychiatric disorder at some point in their lifetime and that 50% of those with a history of alcohol abuse or dependence also meet criteria for major depression or bipolar affective disorder. Depression is a common psychiatric symptom among alcoholics. Because transient depression often is secondary to alcohol withdrawal, it is not appropriate to attribute such symptoms to major depression without ruling out alcohol abuse. Like depression, anxiety is common in alcoholics. Several studies have shown high comorbidity rates between alcoholism and anxiety disorders. Alcohol-related phenomena such as withdrawal symptoms overlap with anxiety symptoms. It has been shown that patients often report drinking alcohol to lower anxiety; however, little evidence supports self-medication as a primary comorbidity mechanism. Several investigators have presented data showing that comorbidity rates vary for specific anxiety disorders. For example, panic disorder complicated by agoraphobia, social phobia, and obsessive-compulsive disorder is more often comorbid with an alcohol disorder than are simple phobias, panic disorder uncomplicated by agoraphobia, and agoraphobia without panic attacks.[9, 10]

The Epidemiological Catchment Area study has estimated that the measured prevalence of alcohol abuse is increased in patients with mental illness in general but is particularly increased in patients with schizophrenia or mania. This study found that the lifetime prevalence of alcohol dependence is 24% in schizophrenia, 27.6% in "any" bipolar disorder, and almost 15% in any affective disorder. Thus, the likelihood of alcohol dependence is increased 3.8 times in schizophrenic patients. In other words, the chance of alcohol dependence in schizophrenic individuals is 3.8 times greater than in the rest of the population, and the chance of alcohol dependence in any bipolar disorder is 4.6 times greater than in the rest of the population.[11]

A close relationship exists between antisocial personality disorders and alcoholism. It has been shown that antisocial personality disorder may promote antisocial alcohol consumption patterns, and alcoholism may promote behavioral disinhibition during alcohol drinking that results in antisocial behavior. According to several studies, it is hypothesized that alcoholics are a high-risk group for suicide, and the lifetime risk for suicide has been estimated to be 15-fold that for the general population.[12]

Several causal models have been proposed for the association between psychiatric disorders and alcohol use disorders. Depression, anxiety, and antisocial personality disorders all may be associated with alcohol use disorder through different mechanisms. It is possible that alcoholism may lead to depression in some patients and may follow from depression in others. The family/genetic study as a method for evaluating comorbidity mechanisms suggests the common factor model, which indicates that alcohol and psychiatric disorders share a common etiology. The self-medication hypothesis for comorbidity mechanisms suggests that individuals with psychiatric symptoms are motivated to drink alcohol to relieve these symptoms.[1] Despite these causal models, efforts to understand neurochemical mechanisms may have implications for the etiology, treatment, and prevention of alcohol and psychiatric disorders in comorbid individuals.

Serotonergic Abnormalities in Alcoholism and Other Psychiatric Disorders

A large body of literature that has emerged suggests an important role for 5HT in the regulation of alcohol intake and the development of alcoholism.[4, 13] One hypothesis that has been put forward is that genetically determined low brain levels of 5HT may be related to a predisposition to alcoholism. 5HT has also been implicated in depression, obsessions, compulsions, and anxiety.[3, 14] It has been shown that these behaviors co-occur with alcoholism with a high frequency. Furthermore, 5HT has also been implicated in the control of impulsive, aggressive, and suicidal behavior. In clinical studies of aggression, suicide, and impulsivity, lower levels of cerebrospinal fluid (CSF) 5-hydroxyindoleacetic acid (5HIAA) have been reported by several investigators. Aggressive, impulsive, and suicidal behavior also tends to co-occur with alcohol use and dependence.[14] An interesting aspect concerning the neurochemical effects of alcohol and the development of tolerance is that depletion of brain 5HT impairs the acquisition of tolerance to ethanol, whereas activation of 5HT brain neurotransmission facilitates development of tolerance and increases consumption of ethanol.[15] The role of 5HT in the modulation of alcohol intake and the development of alcoholism has been derived from both clinical and preclinical studies.

Clinical Studies in Alcohol/Drug Abuse and Other Psychiatric Disorders

Abnormalities in 5HT neurotransmission in alcoholism can be demonstrated by studying the levels of 5HT or 5HIAA, the uptake of 5HT, 5HT receptor subtypes, and the 5HT receptor-linked phosphoinositide-signaling system (Fig. 8–1). A common method of assessing the central 5HT function in alcoholics is measurement of CSF 5HIAA levels. CSF 5HIAA has been proposed as a valid marker for general changes in 5HT metabolism in the central nervous system (CNS). It has been shown that CSF 5HIAA levels positively correlate with 5HIAA levels in the cortex of postmortem human brain.[16] Several studies have found lower levels of CSF 5HIAA in abstinent alcoholics than in controls.[4] Low levels of CSF 5HIAA could be interpreted as lower rates of degradation and thus increased 5HT synaptic availability. Other explanations may be low CSF 5HIAA, which could indicate low 5HT synthesis and thus low brain 5HT content. The tryptophan hydroxylase enzyme is primarily responsible for the synthesis of 5HT. An abnormality in the gene coding for this enzyme has been reported in alcoholic

impulsive offenders, and this has been associated with low CSF levels of 5HIAA and suicide attempts in these individuals.[17] Researchers found that 5HIAA levels in the CSF varied depending on whether subjects were drinking alcohol or undergoing withdrawal. It has been shown that intoxicated alcoholics have normal CSF 5HIAA levels, but during withdrawal, the levels become abnormally low. These studies suggest the possibility that low CSF levels of 5HIAA may indicate inherently low 5HT activity in alcoholics.[18] Evidence shows that depressed and suicidal depressed subjects suffer from impaired 5HT function, as demonstrated by low CSF 5HIAA levels.[19] Both of these problems are more common in alcoholics than in nonalcoholics.

Several investigators measured urinary 5HIAA levels in alcoholics and observed that urinary 5HIAA levels are lower in alcoholics than in normal controls. Because urinary 5HT level likely reflects 5HT metabolism in the periphery rather than the CNS, the decreased urinary 5HIAA levels in alcoholics may be suggestive of decreased tryptophan in the periphery and thus reduced tryptophan availability in the brain.[4] These studies also suggest decreased serotonergic function in alcoholics.

The blood platelet has been suggested as a

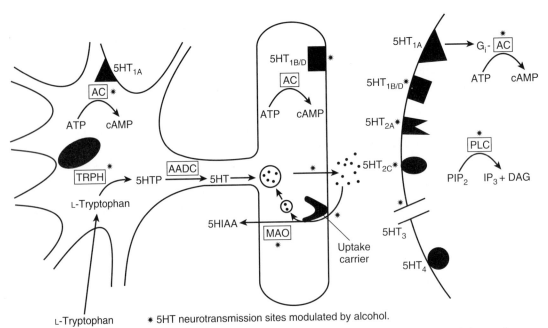

L-Tryptophan   * 5HT neurotransmission sites modulated by alcohol.

Figure 8–1. Various steps involved in presynaptic and postsynaptic 5HT neurotransmission and possible sites affected by alcohol exposure. AC, adenylate cyclase; cAMP, cyclic adenosine monophosphate; 5HT, serotonin; MAO, monoamine oxidase; G_i, inhibitory G-protein; PIP_2, phosphatidylinositol 4,5-biphosphate; IP_3, inositol triphosphate; DAG, diacylglycerol; PLC, phospholipase C; 5HIAA, 5-hydroxyindoleacetic acid; 5HTP, 5-hydroxytryptophan; AADC, aromatic L-amino acid decarboxylase; TRPH, tryptophan hydroxylase.

model for the CNS neuron because of similarities in uptake, storage, and release of 5HT in the tissues of both.[20] Also, in both tissues, $5HT_{2A}$ receptors are linked to the phosphoinositide system.[21] Several investigators have shown reduced concentration and uptake of 5HT in platelets of alcoholics as compared with normal controls.[4] Friedman and colleagues[22] studied 5HT metabolism in 35 inpatient alcoholics and reported that this group converted significantly more tryptophan than 5HT to kynurenine. These studies further suggest a deficiency in the 5HT system in alcoholics. In three separate postmortem studies, the presence of alcohol in the blood at autopsy was related to decreased $5HT_{1A}$ receptors in the cortex and increased 5HT uptake sites in the hippocampus.[4] Thus, acute ethanol exposure may facilitate 5HT reuptake in the hippocampus and decrease $5HT_{1A}$ receptor function in the cortex. It has been shown that $5HT_{2A}$ receptors are not changed in the brain of alcoholics post mortem.[4] Decreased function of the $5HT_{2A}$ receptors has also been shown in platelets of recently detoxified alcoholics, as assessed by a decrease in $5HT_{2A}$ receptor-mediated phosphoinositide turnover.[23]

Serotonergic mechanisms have been studied by neuroendocrine strategies. Using this strategy, 5HT function in psychiatric patients and alcoholic subjects has been studied by the administration of various 5HT agents. It has been shown that fenfluramine-induced prolactin response is decreased in patients with depression. Coccaro and associates have studied fenfluramine-induced prolactin release in patients with affective and personality disorders. They observed that a decrease in fenfluramine-induced prolactin release in these patients may be related to a history of suicide attempts as well as impulsive aggression in patients with personality disorders.[6] It has been shown that 5-hydroxytryptophan and L-hydroxytryptophan–induced prolactin release is blunted in patients with depression. It has also been shown that the direct-acting $5HT_{2A/2C}$ receptor agonist (MK-212)–induced plasma prolactin response and L-5-hydroxytryptophan–induced cortisol are significantly decreased in male alcoholic subjects.[5] These neuroendocrine studies thus provide evidence that 5HT function is altered in the brain of patients with depression, suicidal behavior, impulsive aggression, and alcohol abuse. It appears from the previously described clinical studies that abnormal function of the 5HT system may be responsible for the comorbidity of these psychiatric disorders with alcohol use.

When oral doses of L-tryptophan (1 to 4 g) are administered, there is evidence of increased 5HT synthesis. Three of four double-blind studies of tryptophan in mania suggest that tryptophan has antimanic properties. Tryptophan shows promise of being an effective treatment.[24, 25] Because serotonin may be involved in both mania and alcoholism, serotonin may be the link that explains this comorbidity.

The evidence suggests that whatever the commonality that causes the comorbidity of alcoholism and mania, it is not linked through the antimanic mechanism of action of the properties of lithium. Fawcett and his coworkers,[26] in a placebo-controlled lithium efficacy study of alcoholism, found the number who remained abstinent in the two groups (lithium vs. placebo) to be virtually equal (i.e., the number who remained completely abstinent at 12 months was 18 of 51 on lithium and 17 of 53 on placebo). Dorus and colleagues studied lithium versus placebo in a large number of alcoholic patients.[27] No significant differences were found between the lithium group and the placebo group in either depressed or nondepressed alcoholics, whether investigating the number completely abstinent, the number of alcohol-related hospitalizations, the number of drinks taken, or the addiction severity index.

Preclinical Studies in Alcohol Dependence

Despite a relatively large body of evidence on the role of 5HT in the regulation of alcohol intake, the functional significance of 5HT neurotransmission and its relationship to alcohol intake and dependence needs to be fully elucidated. Animal models provide insight into the mechanism by which alcohol acts on the brain to cause dependence. Researchers used various methods to induce animals to consume alcohol and then examined changes in 5HT neurotransmission in the brain of the alcohol-treated animals.[13] Because alcohol dependence may represent a distinct pathological state, it is important to use animal models that approximate human alcohol dependence. The majority of evidence that 5HT neurotransmission may be involved in alcohol preference is derived from studies of strains of alcohol-preferring and nonpreferring rats.[28] It is clear that 5HT neurotransmission is a complex process and that alcohol can affect this at any number of points (see Fig. 8–1). At this time, it is difficult to draw any firm conclusions about the effect of alcohol on 5HT neurotransmission; however, overall evidence suggests that acute ethanol facilitates whereas chronic ethanol administration inhibits 5HT functioning in the rat brain.[13] It has been shown that 5HT release is decreased by chronic ethanol treatment in the rat brain. A number of studies found increased 5HT uptake after chronic ethanol administration, suggesting decreased availability of 5HT in the synapse.[13]

The existence of several 5HT receptor subtypes has been proposed, and various laboratories have examined the possible role of specific 5HT receptor subtypes in alcohol tolerance and dependence. The $5HT_2$ receptor family currently consists of the $5HT_{2A}$, $5HT_{2B}$, and $5HT_{2C}$ receptors.[29] Activation of these receptors leads to generation of intracellular second messengers such as inositol triphosphate, diacylglycerol (see Fig. 8–1), and calcium.[29] These are molecules that regulate membrane and intracellular processes at a distance from the reception of extracellular signals. Second-messenger formation involves a family of membrane protein known as *G-protein*, which couple different neurotransmitter receptors to effectors (e.g., phospholipase C [PLC] enzyme).[21] Acute or chronic ethanol ingestion can modify second-messenger formation by alteration in either neurotransmitter receptors or postreceptor sites (e.g., G_q-protein or PLC). Several investigators have shown that $5HT_{2A}$ receptors are not changed in the brain of mice or rats exposed to alcohol.[21] The function of $5HT_{2A}$ receptors is decreased however, as demonstrated by measuring the 5HT-stimulated inositol phosphate (second messenger) formation in rat brain chronically treated with ethanol.[21] These studies suggest that changes in postreceptor events such as in Gq-protein or PLC may be responsible for the decreased function of $5HT_{2A}$ receptors in rat brain after chronic ethanol administration.[21] Pharmacological blockade of the $5HT_{2A}$ receptor with $5HT_{2A}$ receptor antagonists (ritanserin, amperozide) has been shown to decrease alcohol consumption in both animals and alcoholic subjects.[13]

The role of $5HT_{2A}$ receptors in alcohol withdrawal has also been studied by several investigators. It was observed that ethanol withdrawal after chronic ethanol consumption, unlike ethanol consumption itself, results in down-regulation of $5HT_{2A}$ receptors in the rat brain.[30] The decrease in $5HT_{2A}$ receptors is also associated with a decrease in the 5HT-stimulated phosphoinositide hydrolysis system in the rat brain after ethanol withdrawal. It is not clear how the changes in $5HT_{2A}$ receptors are related to ethanol withdrawal symptoms, but they may be important in producing some of the manifestations of anxiogenic behavior during ethanol withdrawal.[31] Anxiety is a symptom of ethanol withdrawal that occurs early and persists for an extended period in the rat model.[31] Behavioral studies in rats suggest that reduced function of $5HT_{2A}$ receptors is involved in producing anxiety related to ethanol withdrawal.[31] Thus, both behavioral and neurochemical studies suggest that decreased function of $5HT_{2A}$ receptors may be involved in the development of ethanol withdrawal symptoms after chronic ethanol administration.

It was also observed that chronic ethanol administration causes up-regulation of $5HT_{2C}$ receptors in the choroid plexus but no change in the cortex and the hippocampus brain regions of rats. It was also observed that up-regulation of $5HT_{2C}$ receptors is associated with an increase in 5HT-stimulated phosphoinositide hydrolysis in the rat choroid plexus.[32] Some evidence suggests that the choroid plexus receives serotonergic innervation that originates in the raphe nuclei and is distributed supraependymally throughout the ventricles.[33] It is possible that 5HT released from these fibers has a hormonal or neuromodulatory effect on the choroid plexus by interacting with the $5HT_{2C}$ receptors. It has been shown that alcoholic patients have lower levels of 5HIAA in the CSF, which may be due to lower levels of 5HT in the CSF.[18] It is quite likely that supersensitive $5HT_{2C}$ receptors and this receptor-mediated phosphoinositide hydrolysis in the choroid plexus may reflect postsynaptic adaptation caused by the loss of 5HT input during chronic ethanol consumption. This result also suggests that 5HT activity in the brain may be decreased during ethanol consumption and may be involved in alcohol dependence.

Behavior studies of both animals and alcoholic subjects suggest the possible involvement of $5HT_{2C}$ receptors in the etiology of alcoholism. Animal studies showed that m-chlorophenyl piperazine (mCPP) has a higher affinity for $5HT_{2C}$ and $5HT_{2A}$ than for $5HT_{1A}$ and $5HT_{1B/D}$ receptors.[34] It has been shown that type II alcoholics who received mCPP have expressed the urge to drink alcohol whereas type I alcoholics have not.[35] The differential "urge to drink alcohol" response to mCPP observed in type I and type II alcoholics supports the notion that $5HT_{2A/2C}$ receptors may be involved in the etiology of only type II alcoholism. It has been shown that during ethanol withdrawal, rats are more sensitive to the anxiogenic properties of mCPP, leading to the suggestion that chronic ethanol administration may result in up-regulation of $5HT_{2C}$ receptors.[31] It has been shown that a $5HT_{2A/2C}$ receptor antagonist (mianserin) caused the blockade of anxiogenic properties occurring during ethanol withdrawal.[31] Sanna and colleagues[36] have shown that the concentration of ethanol that can be reached in the brain during alcohol intoxication inhibits the function of $5HT_{2C}$ receptors expressed in *Xenopus* oocytes. Thus, it appears from all these results that the function of $5HT_{2C}$ receptors is altered by alcohol and that the phosphoinositide system linked to $5HT_{2A/2C}$ second messenger receptors may represent targets for the action of this drug.

One way to better understand the biological basis of genetic vulnerability to alcohol would be to study animal lines that have been selectively bred for alcohol-drinking and alcohol-seeking behavior. Animal lines such as alcohol-preferring (P) and alcohol-nonpreferring (NP) rats have been established by Lumeng and colleagues.[37] The P line of rats has been well characterized[28] and has satisfied the criteria for a suitable animal model of alcoholism. It appears that P rats consume ethanol for its CNS positive-reinforcement properties, which leads to the development of tolerance and dependence. It has been shown that levels of 5HT and 5HIAA are decreased along with decreased $5HT_{1B}$ and $5HT_{2A}$ receptors and increased $5HT_{1A}$ receptors in several brain regions of P rats as compared with NP rats.[28] It has also been shown that $5HT_{2C}$ and $5HT_3$ receptor subtypes are not changed in the brain of P rats as compared with NP rats. If the lower levels of 5HT/5HIAA in the brain of P rats are involved in promoting alcohol-drinking behavior, then increasing the extracellular (synaptic) concentration of 5HT and treatment with 5HT agonists should decrease alcohol intake. It has been shown that systematic administration of fluoxetine, $5HT_{1A}$ agonists, $5HT_{2A}/5HT_{2C}$ agonists, and $5HT_{2A}$ antagonists results in an attenuation of alcohol consumption in the P rats.[28]

All these results suggest that a deficient 5HT system is involved in promoting alcohol intake. If 5HT is involved in regulating alcohol drinking, then alcohol itself might be expected to alter the activity of the 5HT system in P rats. Neurochemical evidence suggests that systemic ethanol can increase the activity of the 5HT system in some brain regions of P rats.[28] These results of studies of specific types of rats and data of CSF 5HIAA in alcoholics suggest the possibility that alcohol intoxication may be an attempt to self-medicate by persons who either have inherently low 5HT levels or who have developed low 5HT levels as an adaptation to chronic heavy alcohol use.

Dopaminergic Abnormalities in Alcohol and Drug Abuse: Clinical and Preclinical Evidence

Many of the behavioral effects produced by ethanol also appear to be due to its action on the dopaminergic system.[2] Several studies have shown that ethanol modulates the release, metabolism, and synthesis of DA. It has been shown that ethanol also modulates DA receptor sensitivity[38] (D_1, D_2 receptor subtypes) as well as DA-stimulated adenylate cyclase (AC) activity.[39, 40] In the striatum, a brain region that has been implicated in motor and cognitive brain circuitry, DA was reported to stimulate AC activity through DA receptors and their interaction with G_s-protein (a stimulatory G-protein). It has been shown by several investigators that ethanol potentiates the effects of DA-stimulated AC activity in the rat striatum.[39, 40] Several investigators have also shown alteration in D_1 and D_2 receptors after chronic ethanol treatment in the rat brain.[38] It has been shown that DA may mediate the reinforcing properties of alcohol. Fadda and colleagues[41] observed that voluntary ingestion of ethanol in Sardinian alcohol-preferring rats can increase levels of the DA metabolite 3,4-dihydroxyphenylacetic acid in the caudate nucleus, medial prefrontal cortex, and olfactory tubercle. It has been shown that DA concentration as well as D_2 receptors in some brain regions of P rats are lower than in NP rats.[42] The suggestion that D_2 receptors in the nucleus accumbens are an important factor in controlling the high alcohol intake in P rats is also supported by the results of pharmacological manipulation. Levy and coworkers[43] observed that microinjection of the D_2 antagonist sulpiride directly into the nucleus accumbens of P rats significantly increases alcohol intake. Imperato and Dichiara[44] reported that low doses of alcohol increased DA release in the nucleus accumbens of freely moving rats. Overall, data from animal studies suggest an involvement of the mesolimbic DA system in mediating the action of alcohol.

An interesting new finding suggests that the effects of alcohol on the DA system in the accumbens and the olfactory tubercle may possibly involve the 5HT system. It has been shown that alcohol enhances $5HT_3$ receptor activity in these brain regions.[45] Furthermore, $5HT_3$ receptors have been found in DA-rich areas (nucleus accumbens and olfactory tubercle) to stimulate the release of DA. These data suggest an interaction between the DA system and $5HT_3$ receptors in mediating the action of alcohol.

In clinical studies, an allelic association of the human D_2 receptor gene in alcoholism has been reported.[46, 47] This finding has been replicated by many laboratories but with some exceptions. Another study reported reduced D_2 receptor number in the caudate nuclei of subjects with A_2/A_2, A_2/A_1, and A_1/A_1 combinations.[48] These results suggest a role of D_2 receptor gene variants in the predisposition to alcoholism. Furthermore, evidence shows that DA activity is decreased in alcoholics experiencing withdrawal symptoms, compared with persons not undergoing withdrawal. It is possible that decreased DA activity may be responsible for the development of alcohol withdrawal symptoms and that alcohol use may increase DA production and block the withdrawal symptoms.[49] Pharmacological agents that mimic DA, such as bromocriptine, can relieve withdrawal symptoms.[50] These results thus suggest that similarly to the 5HT system, the DA system also has an important role in mediating the action of alcohol in the brain.

Serotonergic and Dopaminergic Abnormalities in Drug Abuse

Cocaine is a potent euphoriant that has become a growing medical and social problem. It has been suggested that depressive symptoms occurring after the abrupt discontinuation of cocaine are common and may lead to self-medication with cocaine and the perpetuation of cocaine addiction. Cocaine has been shown to alter the metabolism of 5HT and other neurotransmitters in a number of ways. A link between the involvement of the serotonergic system and the CNS effects of cocaine is derived from the observation that both the inhibition of 5HT synthesis and receptor blockade potentiate the motor activity induced by cocaine in rats. It has been shown that enhanced 5HT synthesis antagonizes the motor activity induced by cocaine in rats.[51] Javaid and associates[52] reported that chronic treatment with cocaine does not alter the $5HT_{1A}$ or the $5HT_{2A}$

receptors in different parts of the rat brain. Cunningham and colleagues[53] reported a significant decrease in $5HT_{1A}$ receptors in the central medial amygdala. These groups also reported increased 5HT uptake binding sites as measured by [^{3}H]-imipramine binding in several regions of the rat brain after chronic administration of cocaine. It was suggested that modifications of autoregulatory 5HT mechanisms secondary to alterations in the 5HT uptake system may contribute to the development of sensitization to cocaine abuse.

The psychotropic effects of cocaine are usually attributed to its ability to block the reuptake of DA into mesocortical or mesolimbic neurons rather than its ability to block the reuptake of 5HT.[7] The euphoric effect of cocaine may be caused by blocking the synaptic reuptake of DA and increasing the availability of DA at dopaminergic synapses in the brain. It has been shown that chronic use of cocaine leads to DA depletion, and cocaine is thought to precipitate psychosis by stimulating DA neurotransmission.[7] The neurochemical findings support the DA depletion hypothesis. It has been shown that brain DA levels are decreased and DA receptors are supersensitive in cocaine-dependent rats.[7] In a clinical situation, the levels of the DA metabolite homovanillic acid are decreased in cocaine-dependent patients.[54] The dopamine deficiency state may become manifested with chronic use or withdrawal, and this is clinically associated with depression and intense cocaine craving. Studies showed that about one third of cocaine-dependent patients meet criteria for major depression after cocaine detoxification.[55] The DA depletion hypothesis is also supported by the efficacy of pharmacological agents that have DA agonist properties, including bromocriptine and amantadine, in relieving depression and craving associated with cocaine withdrawal.[56] It is tempting to suggest that although cocaine euphoria may result from the acute stimulation of DA neurotransmission, cocaine craving states result from the depletion of synaptic DA.

Summary

Advances in neuroscience research have been crucial to our understanding of the neurobiology of alcohol tolerance and dependence as well as drug addiction. Neuroscience research has also provided insight into the molecular mechanisms by which alcohol and cocaine interact with various neurotransmitter systems, including 5HT and DA neurotransmission. Both clinical and preclinical research suggest that deficient 5HT and DA systems are involved in alcohol abuse. It has been concluded from various studies that cocaine euphoria may result from the acute stimulation of DA neurotransmission, whereas cocaine craving states result from the depletion of synaptic DA. In searching for molecular mechanisms that might explain alcohol's effects on the brain, investigators have shown great interest in understanding processes that might be common to several neurotransmitter systems. In this regard, the AC and the phosphoinositide second-messenger system have been receiving much attention. In this context, it is interesting to mention that not only neurotransmitter receptors but steps beyond the receptors, such as G-protein (proteins G_s, G_i, and G_q) and effector enzymes (AC and PLC), are modulated by alcohol exposure and involved in alcohol tolerance and dependence. The research on postreceptor sites is provocative because it indicates that alcohol exposure can affect gene expression and basic cellular signaling processes that may have a role in maintaining tolerance and dependence. Together, basic animal studies and clinical research have pointed the way for exciting breakthroughs in our understanding of the neurobiology of alcoholism and drug addiction.

REFERENCES

1. Epidemiology of alcohol use and alcohol related consequences. In Eighth Special Report to the U.S. Congress on Alcohol and Health. PHS National Institute of Alcohol Abuse and Alcoholism, 1993, pp 1–35.
2. Hoffman PL, Tabakoff B: Ethanol's action on brain biochemistry. In Tarter RE, VanThiel DH (eds): Alcohol and the Brain: Chronic Effects. New York, Plenum, 1985, pp 19–68.
3. Tollefson GD: Anxiety and alcoholism: A serotonin link. Br J Psychiatry 159:34–39, 1991.
4. LeMarquand D, Pihl RO, Benkelfat C: Serotonin and alcohol intake, abuse and dependence: Clinical evidence. Biol Psychiatry 36:326–337, 1994.
5. Lee MA, Meltzer HY: Neuroendocrine responses to serotonergic agents in alcoholics. Biol Psychiatry 30:1017–1030, 1991.
6. Coccaro EF, Siever LJ, Klar HM, et al: Serotonergic studies in patients with affective and personality disorders: Correlates with suicidal and impulsive aggressive behavior. Arch Gen Psychiatry 46:587–599, 1989.
7. Galloway MP: Neurochemical interactions of cocaine with dopaminergic systems. Trends Pharmacol Sci 9:451–455, 1988.
8. Weissman MM, Meyers JK, Harding PS: Prevalence and psychiatric heterogeneity of alcoholism in a United States urban community. J Stud Alcohol 41:672–681, 1980.
9. Brown SA, Inaba RK, Gillin C, et al: Alcoholism and

10. Himle JA, Hill EM: Alcohol abuse and the anxiety disorders: Evidence from the epidemiologic catchment area survey. Journal of Anxiety Disorders 5(3):237–245, 1991.
11. Regier DA, Farmer ME, Rae DS, et al: Comorbidity of mental disorders with alcohol and other drug abuse: Results from the Epidemiological Catchment Area (ECA) study. JAMA 264:2511–2518, 1990.
12. Virkkunen M, DeJong J, Bartko J, et al: Psychobiological concomitants of history of suicide among violent offenders and impulsive fire setters. Arch Gen Psychiatry 46:604–606, 1989.
13. LeMarquand D, Pihl RO, Benkelfat C: Serotonin and alcohol intake, abuse and dependence; Findings of animal studies. Biol Psychiatry 36:395–421, 1994.
14. Benkert O, Wetzel H, Szegedi A: Serotonin dysfunction syndromes: A functional common denominator for classification of depression, anxiety, and obsessive-compulsive disorder. Int Clin Psychopharmacol 8(Suppl 1):3–14, 1993.
15. Ferriera L, Soares Da Silva P: 5-Hydroxytryptamine and alcoholism. Hum Psychopharmacol 6:521–524, 1991.
16. Stanley M, Traskman-Bendz L, Dorovini-Zis K: Correlations between aminergic metabolites simultaneously obtained from human CSF and brain. Life Sci 37:1279–1286, 1985.
17. Nielsen DA, Goldman D, Virkkunen M, et al: Suicidality and 5-hydroxyindoleacetic acid concentration associated with a tryptophan hydroxylase polymorphism. Arch Gen Psychiatry 51:34–38, 1994.
18. Ballenger J, Goodwin FK, Major LF, et al: Alcohol and central serotonin metabolism in man. Arch Gen Psychiatry 36:224–227, 1979.
19. Asberg M, Traskman L, Thoren P: 5-HIAA in the cerebrospinal fluid: A biochemical suicide predictor? Arch Gen Psychiatry 33:1193–1197, 1976.
20. Rotman A: Blood platelets in psychopharmacological research. Prog Neuropsychopharmacol Biol Psychiatry 7:135–151, 1983.
21. Pandey SC, Davis JM, Pandey GN: Phosphoinositide system-linked serotonin receptor subtypes and their pharmacological properties and clinical correlates. J Psychiatry Neurosci 20:215–225, 1995.
22. Friedman MJ, Krstulovic AM, Severinghaus JM, et al: Altered conversion of tryptophan to kynurenine in newly abstinent alcoholics. Biol Psychiatry 23:89–93, 1988.
23. Simonsson P, Alling C: The 5-hydroxytryptamine stimulated formation of inositol phosphate is inhibited in platelets from alcoholics. Life Sci 42:385–391, 1988.
24. Chouinard G, Young SN, Annable L: A controlled clinical trial of L-tryptophan in acute mania. Biol Psychiatry 20:546–557, 1985.
25. Prange AJ, Wilson IC, Lynn CW: L-Tryptophan in mania: Contribution to a permissive hypothesis of affective disorder. Arch Gen Psychiatry 30:56–62, 1974.
26. Fawcett J, Clark DC, Aagesen CA, et al: A double-blind, placebo-controlled trial of lithium carbonate therapy of alcoholism. Arch Gen Psychiatry 44:248–256, 1987.
27. Dorus W, Ostrow DG, Anton R, et al: Lithium treatment of depressed and nondepressed alcoholics. JAMA 262:1646–1652, 1989.
28. McBride WJ, Murphy JM, Yoshimoto K, et al: Serotonin mechanisms in alcohol drinking behavior. Drug Dev Res 30:170–177, 1993.
29. Hoyer D, Clarke DE, Fozard JR, et al: International union of pharmacology classification of receptors for

5-hydroxytryptamine (serotonin). Pharmacol Rev 46:157–203, 1994.

30. Pandey SC, Piano MR, Schwertz DW, et al: Effect of ethanol administration and withdrawal on serotonin receptor subtypes and receptor-mediated phosphoinositide hydrolysis in rat brain. Alcohol Clin Exp Res 16:1110–1116, 1992.

31. Wallis CJ, Rezazadeh SM, Lal H: Role of serotonin in ethanol abuse. Drug Dev Res 30:178–188, 1993.

32. Pandey SC, Dubey MP, Piano MR, et al: Modulation of $5HT_{1C}$ receptor and phosphoinositide system by ethanol consumption in rat brain and choroid plexus. Eur J Pharmacol (Mol Pharmacol Sect) 247:81–88, 1993.

33. Richards JG, Guggenheim R: Serotonergic axons in the brain: A bird's eye view. Trends Neurosci 5:4, 1982.

34. Hoyer D: Functional correlates of serotonin $5HT_1$ recognition sites. J Recept Res 8:59–89, 1988.

35. George DT, Wozniak K, Linnoila M: Basic and clinical studies on serotonin, alcohol and alcoholism. In Naranjo CA, Sellers EM (eds): Novel Pharmacological Intervention for Alcoholism. New York, Springer-Verlag, 1990, pp 92–104.

36. Sanna E, Dildy-Mayfield JE, Harris RA: Ethanol inhibits the function of 5-hydroxytryptamine type 1C and muscarinic M_1G protein-linked receptors in *Xenopus* oocytes expressing brain mRNA: Role of protein kinase C. Mol Pharmacol 45:1004–1012, 1994.

37. Lumeng L, Hawkins TD, Li TK: New strains of rats with alcohol preference and nonpreference. In Thurman RG, Williamson JR, Drott H, Chance B (eds): Alcohol and Aldehyde Metabolizing Systems, vol. 3. New York, Academic Press, 1977, pp 537–544.

38. Hamdi A, Prasad C: Bidirectional changes in striatal D_1-dopamine receptor density during chronic ethanol intake. Life Sci 52:251–257, 1992.

39. Rabin RA, Molinoff PB: Activation of adenylate cyclase by ethanol in mouse striatal tissue. J Pharmacol Exp Ther 216:129–134, 1981.

40. Luthin GR, Tabakoff B: Activation of adenylate cyclase by alcohol requires the nucleotide-binding protein. J Pharmacol Exp Ther 228:579–587, 1984.

41. Fadda F, Mosca E, Colombo G, et al: Effect of spontaneous ingestion of ethanol on brain dopamine metabolism. Life Sci 44:281–287, 1989.

42. McBride WJ, Chernet E, Dyr W, et al: Densities of dopamine D_2 receptors are reduced in CNS regions of alcohol preferring P rats. Alcohol 10:387–390, 1993.

43. Levy AD, Murphy JM, McBride WJ, et al: Microinjection of sulpiride in to the nucleus accumbens increases ethanol drinking in alcohol-preferring (P) rats. Alcohol Alcohol Suppl 1:417–420, 1991.

44. Imperato A, Dichiara G: Preferential stimulation of dopamine release in the nucleus accumbens of freely moving rats by ethanol. J Pharmacol Exp Ther 239:219–228, 1986.

45. Carboni E, Acouas E, Frau R, et al: Differential inhibitory effects of a $5HT_3$ antagonist on drug-induced stimulation of dopamine release. Eur J Pharmacol 164:515–519, 1989.

46. Blum K, Noble EP, Sheridan PJ, et al: Allelic association of human dopamine D_2 receptor gene in alcoholism. JAMA 263:2055–2060, 1990.

47. Blum K, Noble EP, Sheridan PJ, et al: Association of the A_1 allele of the D_2 dopamine receptor gene with severe alcoholism. Alcohol 8:409–416, 1991.

48. Noble EP, Blum K, Ritchie T, et al: Allelic association of the D_2 dopamine receptor gene with receptor binding characteristics in alcoholism. Arch Gen Psychiatry 48:648–654, 1991.

49. Tabakoff B, Hoffman PL, Petersen R: Advances in neurochemistry. A leading edge of alcohol research. Alcohol Health & Research World 14:138–143, 1990.

50. Borg S, Weinholdt T: Bromocriptine in the treatment of the alcohol-withdrawal syndrome. Acta Psychiatr Scand 65:101–111, 1982.

51. Pradhan SN, Bhattacharya AK, Pradhan S: Serotonergic manipulation of the behavioral effects of cocaine in rats. Commun Psychopharmacol 2:481–485, 1978.

52. Javaid JI, Sahni SK, Pandey SC, et al: Repeated cocaine administration does not affect 5HT receptor subtypes (5-HT_{1A}, $5HT_2$) in several brain regions. Eur J Pharmacol 238:425–429, 1993.

53. Cunningham KA, Paris JM, Goeders NF: Chronic cocaine enhances serotonin autoregulation and serotonin uptake binding. Synapse 11:112–116, 1992.

54. Extein I, Dackis CA: Brain mechanisms in cocaine dependency. In Washton AM, Gold MS (eds): New York, Guilford Press, 1987, pp 73–84.

55. Mirin SM, Weiss RD, Sollogub A, et al: Affective illness in substance abusers. In Mirin SM (ed): Substance Abuse and Psychopathology. Washington, DC, American Psychiatric Press, 1984, pp 57–77.

56. Dackis CA, Gold MS. Bromocriptine as treatment of cocaine abuse. Lancet 1:1151–1152, 1985.

9

Neurocognitive Syndromes and Neuroimaging in Addictions

Craig McKenna, MD

Psychoactive substance addiction is the most prevalent psychiatric disorder, according to the Epidemiological Catchment Area Study,[1] and cognitive impairment is a common complication in addictions. The most common substances associated with consistently documented neurocognitive sequelae, in order of frequency, include alcohol, marijuana, cocaine and other stimulants, hallucinogens, benzodiazepines, and opiates.[2] Depending on the specific substance(s), the dose, the route of administration, and other idiopathic subject factors (e.g., preexistent brain, liver, or renal disease), these agents cross the blood-brain barrier and may exert toxic effects on brain chemistry and metabolism. These syndromes most frequently are metabolic as a result of acute intoxication or withdrawal states and, as such, are reversible. In some instances of chronic use, however, especially with ethanol, structural alterations may occur and may become persistent and permanent. These effects and complications of addiction may be manifested in what is best characterized as neurocognitive syndromes in that substance-induced brain disease causes cognitive impairment. Individuals with neurocognitive impairment may present with various degrees of severity, ranging from full-fledged clinical disorders such as dementia or the amnestic syndrome to more subtle, subsyndromal impairment.

In addition to the immediate diagnostic and morbidity issues involved in addicted patients with neurocognitive impairment are long-term treatment implications. A number of studies have found that cognitive impairment in alcohol-addicted patients may have treatment implications.[3-9] Most addiction programs are cognitively based and require intact cognitive abilities including attention and concentration, memory and learning, abstraction, generalization, and anticipation. These are fundamental to the learning-in-treatment of sobriety maintenance and to relapse prevention in alcohol rehabilitation. This is becoming more fully appreciated in the literature, and various researchers are offering their approaches to cognitive impairment in alcoholics.[10-12] Thus, careful attention to cognitive assessment is imperative in the assessment of addicted patients, from both a diagnostic and treatment perspective.

A current trend found in addicted patients is dual addiction and polyaddiction.[2, 13] This may result in clinical presentations with various permutations of substance intoxication and withdrawal interactions with cognitive sequelae, further complicating assessment. This trend challenges the diagnostic acumen of clinicians evaluating patients with such complicated neurocognitive syndromes.

Neuroimaging in Addiction

Neuroimaging techniques such as positron emission tomography (PET) and single-photon emission computerized tomography (SPECT) as probes of brain metabolism and blood flow are being applied in the study of addictions and associated neurocognitive complications.

PET and SPECT are used to examine the regional distribution of radiotracers. These radiotracers are incorporated into compounds of biological interest in order to describe the chemistry of the biological process being studied. In all cases, an attempt is made to label a chemical compound with a radioisotope such that the tracer principle is maintained (i.e., that the basic pharmacology of the compound is not changed and has not altered the biological process being studied). These attempts often require low-atomic-weight isotopes, such as ^{11}C, ^{18}F, and ^{13}N, because the smaller masses of these positron emitters are less likely to perturb their pharmacological properties. In contrast, larger isotopes, such as ^{99m}Tc and ^{123}I, which are typically available for SPECT, must be placed in a special chemical environment that makes the radiolabeled complex relatively lipophilic and neutral while retaining the biological properties of the unlabeled ligand. The corresponding stable atoms are prevalent in biological tissues and can often be substituted in ligands to allow imaging of the radioactive form of the compound.

A reliable correlation exists between PET and SPECT, in that when alterations are reported in glucose metabolism or regional cerebral blood flow (CBF) with PET scanning, similar findings are anticipated with SPECT CBF imaging. Strategies using functional tracers such as fluorine-18 or carbon-11 deoxyglucose to measure regional brain metabolism or oxygen-15 or butanol to measure CBF have been used to investigate patterns of regional brain functional abnormalities. Radioligands to label receptors, enzymes, or neurotransmitter metabolism have also been applied to the investigation of neurochemical changes in addictions.

The rationales for using neuroimaging methods as functional indices are based on the following assumptions:[14, 15] (1) Adenosine triphosphate, an energy-supplying substrate needed for many processes in the brain, is supplied by glucose metabolism; (2) glucose normally is the sole substrate for oxidative metabolism in the adult brain; and (3) blood flow is coupled to oxidative metabolism. Thus, there is a mutual reciprocity between CBF and cerebral metabolic rate (CMR). In normal nonpathological states, CMR dictates CBF, by which blood flow adjusts to metabolic demand. During increased brain activity, regionally increased CMR gives rise to increased blood carbon dioxide levels, which in turn induce relative vasodilation, resulting in increased CBF. In periods of relative inactivity, decreased regional CMR effectively lowers the level of blood carbon dioxide, which allows for relative vasoconstriction and subsequently lowering of CBF. Two major processes modulate this reciprocity: abiotrophy (aging processes) in the brain and cerebrovascular disease. For this reason, interpretation of neuroimaging findings in addicted patients with these concomitant processes is more complicated and requires sophisticated analysis.

In a normal brain, CBF and CMR serve as indices of brain function reflected in behavioral effects. Psychoactive substances can influence CBF through several mechanisms. Metabolic effects, blood gases such as carbon dioxide, and direct cerebrovascular effects are the three predominant mechanisms responsible for the acute effects of drugs on CBF.[16]

Neuroimaging in the addictions is still in its infancy, and few conclusions are justified given limitations of the technology such as problems of spatial and temporal resolution. In addition, although information about the important effects of age and cerebrovascular disease on hemodynamic function has been well developed, these factors have yet to be successfully incorporated into the study of the effects of psychoactive substances on CBF. Experimental methods for teasing apart the intricacies of cause and effect have improved, as has the ability to select an appropriate control group to avoid subclinical effects associated with social or recreational substance use.

Despite such limitations, neuroimaging studies in the addictions and associated neurocognitive complications are important for a number of reasons. Such studies may be helpful in elucidating pathophysiological neurobiological mechanisms in the neuropsychiatric syndromes to be described in this chapter. In the area of dual diagnosis, research may also help explain how idiopathic psychiatric disorders such as schizophrenia and depression may be related to addictive disorders and identify the neurobiological correlates of subjects who are at increased risk for addiction. Psychoactive drugs that support compulsive self-administration behavior also share the property of producing a positive mood state. The relationship between euphoria and reward mechanisms in addiction and regional CBF is an area of fruitful research. Although PET studies to date have not identified a particular brain region or system that is critical to the production of drug-induced euphoria, it is notable that most drugs of addiction reduce cerebral glucose metabolism in doses that produce euphoria. Therefore, the effects of these agents on glucose metabolism may be fundamentally related to drug-induced reward, and these effects may be a useful marker of addiction liability.

Ethanol

Ethanol is the most commonly used legal substance, and alcohol-induced neurocognitive syndromes are the most prevalent. Pharmacologically, ethanol is an aliphatic alcohol and as an organic solvent is readily distributed in total body water. It readily crosses the blood-brain barrier, dissolving in the cell membrane, and exerts a recognized part of its effects through the gamma-aminobutyric acid (GABA) complex. As a central nervous system (CNS) depressant, it has physiological dependent and tolerance properties.

Ethanol may induce acute and chronic neurocognitive syndromes. Acutely, ethanol may directly and indirectly induce delirium by several mechanisms. Chronic alcohol abuse, combined with other associated morbidity factors, may cause persistent and chronic cognitive impairment.

COGNITIVE IMPAIRMENT SYNDROMES

Subsyndromal Cognitive Impairment

The most common cognitive impairments induced by alcohol are subsyndromal rather than full-fledged syndromes such as dementia or the amnestic disorder known as the Wernicke-Korsakoff syndrome. Grant and colleagues[17] proposed the term *intermediate-duration organic mental disorder associated with alcoholism* to be used to describe such subclinical neurocognitive states in recently sober alcoholics. Such deficits may be noted on bedside cognitive testing and are readily apparent on neuropsychological testing, a very sensitive and specific indicator of cerebral integrity.[18] Neuropsychological testing surpasses the clinical neurological examination, electroencephalogram, and neuroradiological procedures[19] in detecting

cognitive impairment. Further, neuropsychological testing is reflective and predictive of adaptive functioning in various patient groups.[20] Therefore, identifying cognitive impairment may have implications for how alcohol-dependent patients adapt to life, including addiction treatment, which becomes an integral part of their lives.

Approximately 45% to 70% of alcohol-dependent patients have specific deficits in the following cognitive domains: attention, memory acquisition and new learning of associations between stimuli, calculation, abstraction, visuospatial skills including perceptual-motor speed and accuracy, concept formation, cognitive flexibility, set maintenance and set shifting, the ability to follow complex commands, and problem solving.[21-24] These findings have transcultural stability and are therefore very generalizable. Further, such neuropsychological deficits are specifically related to direct and indirect effects of alcohol on the brain and are not an artifact of depressive or anxiety symptoms commonly affecting alcoholics.

Age-related effects of cognitive impairment exist in alcoholics older than 45 years. These patients consistently have more frequent and severe cognitive impairment.[25, 26]

Neuropsychological data also demonstrate other specific deficiencies. Alcoholics consistently perform more poorly than normal controls on the categories, trails B, and tactual performance tests of the Halstead-Reitan neuropsychological test battery. When these deficits are examined more closely to determine the reasons for the poor performance, it appears that alcoholics use inefficient problem-solving strategies, may shift problem-solving sets too soon, or persist in using the same problem-solving set long after it is clearly ineffective. They also may use weak or inappropriate encoding strategies to learn new information, which makes later recall of the information extremely difficult. Other researchers have pointed to problems in visuospatial orientation, as well as attention and concentration difficulties.[27]

Regional Brain Vulnerabilities

The brain has selective neurocognitive vulnerabilities to the effects of alcohol.[28] General intelligence, as conventionally assessed by the Wechsler Adult Intelligence Scale, is most often spared and reported to be average or even slightly above. Verbal IQs among alcoholics are comparable to age- and education-matched controls. In contrast, performance IQ is significantly impaired, as are specific subtests of the Wechsler Adult Intelligence Scale, including block design, picture arrangement, object assembly, and digit symbol. Visuospatial functions involving abstracting and problem solving, as well as information handling requiring complex sensorimotor coordination, are vulnerable to the effects of alcohol. In addition, learning and memory in the visuospatial domain seems to be more vulnerable than in the verbal domain. Less complex sensory or motor functions and functions that are mainly dependent on long-term memory (vocabulary) are generally less sensitive.

There is evidence of a graded vulnerability from anterior to posterior.[29] In two studies, regional vulnerability has been ranked, from most to least: frontal-temporal-parietal-occipital. These results are consistent with the nature of neuropsychological impairments in alcoholics.

Severity

Various degrees of cognitive impairment are noted in alcohol-dependent patients. In a Veterans Administration population, Shelly and Goldstein[30] found the following breakdown in terms of degrees of severity of cognitive impairment in 150 alcoholics referred for treatment: severe 6.7%, moderate 52%, mild 30.7%, and minimal or none 15.3%.

Cognitive Recovery

Studies examining the reversibility and recovery of cognitive impairment in alcoholics have had mixed results. In general, with sobriety, improvement occurs within 3 weeks as an individual progresses from inebriation through withdrawal and into a state of sobriety.[31] During abstinence, improvement appears to continue, but the extent and course of recovery are not well understood. Some researchers have not observed dramatic recovery[32] and find that alcoholics do not improve to normal levels on all tasks. Some neuropsychological tasks do not reveal improvement to normal levels during test periods of 1 month, 2 months, or even 1 year.[33] In addition, some evidence suggests continuing short-term memory impairments in younger alcoholics.[25] Older alcoholics demonstrate the worst course of recovery.[25, 26, 34, 35] These findings are consistent with the view that after a critical age (approximately 40 years), synergism between alcohol abuse and aging produces apparent behavioral deficits. Further, these findings are convergent with the neurobiological concepts of reduced brain plasticity and the existence of critical periods of brain vulnerability in older patients, thus implying a worse prognosis for aging alcoholics.

Selectivity is observed in the recovery of specific cognitive domains.[31] Existing verbal abilities (vocabulary) are not found to be impaired during immediate sobriety. Most other abilities, especially when any new learning is involved, remain impaired during the first week or two of abstinence. Visuospatial abstraction and problem solving, short-term memory, and simple sensory perception show persistent impairment, particularly in older alcoholics. It is possible that with prolonged abstinence, some of these abilities may be recovered. In general, the more novel, complex, and rapid information processing that a task requires, the longer it takes to recover.

Two types of recovery processes have been hypothesized and described by Goldman and colleagues.[25] One is a neurobiologically based, time-dependent recovery process that may be related to the decreased edema, collateral neural sprouting, and so forth. Another is an activation-related recovery process dependent on experience (learning), which may have implications for specialized cognitive interventions. In accordance with the activation-related recovery process, some evidence suggests that cognitive training and practice experience (remedial mental exercises) can facilitate recovery from impairment.[36–38] This may have important clinical implications for improving cognitively impaired alcoholics' performance in addiction treatment.

Morphological Reversibility

At least eight independent studies have confirmed the finding that computed tomography (CT) abnormalities in some alcoholics normalize after periods of abstinence or greatly reduced drinking.[29] The occurrence of ventricular and sulcal enlargement in alcoholics and the potential reversibility of these abnormalities are difficult to reconcile with the concept of cerebral atrophy. The term *atrophy*, as conventionally used by neuropathologists, designates disturbances of neurons that lead to their gradual degeneration and death. To speak of CT abnormalities of the brain and their reversibility as reversible atrophy takes unwarranted license with the term and does nothing to enhance our understanding of the process. With our current knowledge, it is preferable to refer to ventricular enlargement and sulcal widening as such, rather than as cerebral atrophy.

The finding of reversible cortical abnormalities is paralleled by increased tissue density in the caudate and thalamus. This is consistent with previous reports of increases in tissue density in abstinent alcoholics and suggests that the observed changes are not simply a result of a reabsorption of displaced water and electrolytes from extracellular space. Reports of elevated tissue density in frontal white matter suggest that the hypothesis of fluid reabsorption may need to be revived as part of the explanation of morphological plasticity in the brains of recently abstinent alcoholics. Such changes may involve structural alterations such as axonal sprouting, dendritic arborization, and revascularization of tissue. The overall increase in tissue density that seems to occur in abstinent alcoholics makes reabsorption of displaced fluid improbable.

Etiology

The causes of subsyndromal cognitive impairment in alcoholic patients are varied, multiple, and complex, involving[39] developmental (native and congenital) deficits, such as minimal brain dysfunction and mental retardation, and acquired deficits such as from alcohol and other drug toxicity, head trauma, medical complications, and nutritional deficiencies. Although the causal role of duration of alcohol abuse and current drinking practices in these deficits has not been clearly established, recent evidence suggests that maximal quantity drunk per occasion and the frequency of those occasions are predictive of neuropsychological deficits.

Pathophysiology

Two complementary models can be used to view the developmental pathophysiology in the chronic alcohol-related cognitive impairment syndromes, the generalized/diffuse model, and the genetically based threshold vulnerability model.[40, 41]

The generalized/diffuse model posits that alcohol addiction results in both cortical and subcortical changes that lead to different impairments that may have different rates and courses of recovery. Within this model, two different morphological syndromes exist. An early, more acute and less permanent cortical process (cortical atrophy—visible widening of cortical sulci) is related to visuospatial and abstracting deficits and may be antecedent to al-

coholism. A later, more insidious, and longer-lasting central (dilated lateral ventricular system) process is associated with neuropsychological deficits of memory, particularly in middle-aged or older alcoholics.

The genetically based vulnerability threshold model of the etiology of brain damage is a more valid alternative to a dose-dependent model. In this model, for example, ventricular dilation is related to alcohol consumption exceeding some genetically determined threshold and is expressed as deficits in memory and general intellectual abilities. There might be no relationship up to a threshold level to exposure, but above that level the expected relationship between drinking habits and signs of brain damage might occur. This hypothetical threshold level probably varies between individuals, owing to constitutional characteristics.

Thus, findings suggest that the more common deficits of abstracting and visuospatial abilities can be dissociated from the problems of memory that tend to be identified in older alcoholics. Thus, in alcoholism, two neuropsychological syndromes of different etiology may tend to develop in parallel.

Table 9–1 provides a basic simplification and summary of the neuropsychological findings in alcoholics.

Implications for Addiction Treatment

Particularly in the first weeks of abstinence during treatment, cognitive impairment may make it difficult for some alcoholics to benefit from the educational and skill development sessions that are important components of many treatment programs. Reduced abstraction abilities may contribute to a patient's inability to generalize and to abstract principles of treatment and to apply them in terms of maintaining sobriety and coping with problems of everyday living, necessitating a more

Table 9–1. SUMMARY OF NEUROPSYCHOLOGICAL FINDINGS IN ALCOHOLICS

- Prolonged, excess ingestion of alcohol is associated with brain damage.
- Atrophy (cortical and subcortical) is the major brain change found in alcoholics.
- The brain changes in alcoholics are associated with neuropsychological deficits.
- Neuropsychological deficits in alcoholics are varied with respect to extent and recoverability.
- Neuropsychological deficits associated with alcoholism may be factors in the adaptive functioning of alcoholics.

concrete, tangible approach. Cognitive functions are important to group psychotherapy in terms of patients' ability to generalize, ability to reason by analogy, approach toward change in psychotherapy, and attitude toward planning change in their future lives.

Becker and Jaffe[42] reported that alcoholics who were tested soon after beginning abstinence were unable to recall treatment-related information presented in a film that was part of the regular treatment program. An implication of such findings is that information presented to alcoholics during the period of impairment in the early weeks of abstinence may need to be repeated at later stages in the treatment program.

It may be necessary to modify and adapt the cognitive component of treatment, including the exposure to treatment materials. Material may need to be presented repeatedly and in modified form to compensate for poor attention, concentration, and retention in memory. Educational materials may need to be simplified, and programmed learning texts could be developed to ensure learning of one concept before proceeding to the next. Spaced rather than massed practice may enhance learning, and providing the same information through multiple sensory modalities might also help. Alternatively, presentation of treatment-related information may be delayed until tests indicate some improvement in cognitive function.

Thus, programs should include some degree of flexibility to accommodate the varied cognitive capacities between patients. This may represent an indicated need for special treatment matching in cognitively impaired persons.

As an essential component to addiction treatment, staff attitudes and expectations may need to be modified in the presence of cognitive impairment. Patients whose behaviors may be interpreted psychodynamically as denial or resistance may, instead, have comprehension or memory problems interfering with their cooperation. Learning difficulties may be interpreted as motivational problems instead of cognitive deficits. Staff may assume insensitive or punitive postures with regard to such patients. Likewise, when demands are put on such patients beyond their cognitive limitations, they may feel frustrated and helpless. Such emotional reactions may interfere with treatment compliance and may contribute to relapse.

Neuroimaging

Neuroimaging is usually performed on addicted patients with an identified brain disease.

However, Volkow and colleagues[43] examined relatively purely alcoholic patients with no neurological symptoms and with minimal or no brain morphological changes and found decreased brain glucose metabolism. This sample, in all likelihood, closely approximates a sample of patients with subsyndromal cognitive impairment. Although preliminary and needing replication, this study demonstrates brain metabolic correlates in a group of healthy alcoholics.

The neuropsychological findings in older alcoholics are supported by neuroimaging techniques. Berglund and associates[44] examined alcoholics older than 45 years and found significantly decreased CBF values. This is also in agreement with CT scan studies reporting a strong relationship between atrophy and age in alcoholic patients older than 50 years. This study also found that in many alcoholics older than 45 years, at least 7 weeks is required to partially normalize their brain dysfunction, whereas in younger alcoholics a shorter period is needed. Reversibility of the change in CBF (as well as in cognitive dysfunction) with abstinence and appropriate treatment suggests that part of the decrease in CBF may be due to primary metabolic dysfunction instead of secondary metabolic impairment from permanent structural brain damage.

ACUTE SYNDROMES

Delirium

Alcohol Intoxication Delirium. Alcohol intoxication delirium is one of the most frequent alcohol-induced cognitive impairment states. The DSM-IV[45] criteria for alcohol intoxication delirium are given in Table 9–2.

The development of alcohol intoxication delirium is most dependent on the rate of increase of blood alcohol concentration, although other important factors include the absolute alcohol level and the time during which it is maintained. Consequently, the induction of alcohol intoxication delirium is affected by a number of basic factors: the total dose of alcohol consumed, the speed and pattern of drinking, the presence or absence of food in the stomach and the effects of physiological or pharmacological alteration of gastric motility, the presence of other drugs, and coexisting disease. Wide variations in initial and acquired tolerance of the nervous system modify the degree of effect on the brain produced at any given ethanol concentration. In addition, the effects of intoxication are greater with a rising than a falling blood alcohol level.

Table 9–2. DSM-IV CRITERIA FOR SUBSTANCE INTOXICATION AND WITHDRAWAL DELIRIUM

A. Disturbance of consciousness (i.e., reduced clarity of awareness of the environment) with reduced ability to focus, sustain, or shift attention.
B. A change in cognition (such as memory deficit, disorientation, language disturbance) or the development of a perceptual disturbance that is not better accounted for by a preexisting, establishing, or evolving dementia.
C. The disturbance develops during a short period of time (usually hours to days) and tends to fluctuate during the course of the day.

For intoxication delirium:
D. There is evidence from the history, physical examination, or laboratory findings of either (1) or (2):
  (1) The symptoms in criteria A and B developed during substance intoxication.
  (2) Medication use is etiologically related to the disturbance.

For withdrawal delirium:
E. There is evidence from the history, physical examination, or laboratory findings that the symptoms in criteria A and B developed during or shortly after a withdrawal syndrome.

Note: This diagnosis should be made instead of a diagnosis of substance withdrawal only when the cognitive symptoms are in excess of those usually associated with the withdrawal syndrome and when the symptoms are sufficiently severe to warrant independent clinical attention.

From the American Psychiatric Association: Diagnostic and Statistical Manual of Mental Disorders, 4th ed. Washington, DC, American Psychiatric Association, 1994.

In general, a close correlation is noted between blood levels of ethanol and brain levels, and thus blood alcohol concentrations correlate with the degree of intoxication.[46] Thus, the signs and symptoms of alcohol intoxication delirium are directly proportional to the blood alcohol concentration, and this correlation is shown in Table 9–3. Behaviorally, individuals with alcohol-induced delirium are usually hyperactive and disinhibited with initial and low doses of alcohol and become hypoactive and drowsy or lethargic with high doses, especially when rapidly acquired.

Alcohol concentration varies between different types of alcoholic beverages, with the equivalence being 1 drink = 1.5 oz 90 proof (45% alcohol) = 4 oz wine = 12 oz beer = 10 g alcohol. One drink raises the blood concentration approximately 15 mg/dl; therefore, five beers or shots within 1 hour raise the blood alcohol to the legal limit of 100 mg/dl. The metabolic rate of alcohol is about one drink per hour,[47] and therefore it takes approximately 3 hours for the blood level to increase from 100 mg/dl to 50 mg/dl.

Pathophysiology. Polysynaptic integrating neuronal pathways in the reticular activating system and heteromodal associational areas of the frontal and parietal cortices and cerebellum are preferentially sensitive to the effects of alcohol.[48–50] In general, alcohol acts as a CNS depressant. However, at lower concentrations, inhibitory polysynaptic influences are inhibited, resulting in cortical disinhibition with the associated changes in mood and cognitive function.[46] At increasingly greater levels of intoxication, depression of excitatory presynaptic influences, potentiation of presynaptic inhibition, or direct depression of impulse propagation results in delirium leading to coma or death due to respiratory depression.

The precise molecular mechanisms responsible for ethanol intoxication are unknown. Be-

Table 9–3. SIGNS AND SYMPTOMS OF ALCOHOL INTOXICATION CORRELATED WITH BLOOD ALCOHOL LEVELS

Blood Alcohol Level (mg/dl)	Behavioral Signs and Symptoms
25–100	• Incoordination • Increased reaction time • Alteration in mood, personality, judgment
100–200	• Ataxia, nystagmus • Dysarthria • Impaired reflexes and motor coordination • Confusion
200–300	• Nausea, vomiting • Diplopia, sluggish pupils • Marked ataxia • Severely disturbed sensory perception
300–400	• Severe dysarthria and ataxia • Stupor (arousable unresponsiveness) • Amnesia (blackouts)
400–500	• Perception obliterated • Coma (unarousable unresponsiveness) • Stage I anesthesia
>500	• Respiratory center paralysis • Acidosis • Death

cause ethanol is a very weak drug, which acts at concentrations thousands of times higher than other misused drugs such as cocaine, opiates, or phencyclidine, it is unlikely to interact with specific high-affinity receptors in the brain. Rather, ethanol is thought to dissolve into the plasma membrane, resulting in a more general perturbation of the hydrophobic regions of membrane lipids and proteins. One of the most likely sites of ethanol's intoxicating effect is a complex of membrane proteins containing a receptor for the inhibitory neurotransmitter GABA and associated chloride ion channel. Barbiturates and benzopiazepines, which interact with receptor sites linked to this complex, produce clinical syndromes of intoxication resembling that produced by ethanol. Ethanol modifies GABA-activated neurotransmission by stimulating ion flux through chloride channels activated by GABA,[51] resulting in hyperpolarization.

Studies have suggested that ethanol may alter the fluidity of neural membranes in a manner similar to general anesthetics.[52] Effects of alcohol on key neurotransmitters have also been proposed to explain intoxication.

Alcohol Withdrawal Delirium. Alcohol withdrawal delirium is a cognitive complication of withdrawal that occurs in fewer than 5% of alcohol-dependent patients.[47] The DSM-IV criteria for this syndrome are listed in Table 9–2.

Alcohol withdrawal delirium usually occurs within 48 hours after an individual abruptly stops or cuts back on his or her drinking and may occur as the blood alcohol level is falling. Consumption of large amounts of ethanol over a few days or of smaller amounts of ethanol at frequent intervals and for prolonged periods induces a state of physical dependence. When the concentration of ethanol in the brain declines, the emergence of clinical features of withdrawal, including delirium, may result. Most individuals who undergo withdrawal have a 5 to 15-year history of heavy drinking and have been drinking 10 to 15 drinks (100 to 150 g/day) for 1 to 4 weeks before onset of withdrawal.

There are actually two specific phases of alcohol withdrawal, minor and major.[47] Early, minor withdrawal occurs within 6 to 8 hours of the last drink and may actually develop at a time when the blood ethanol concentration has not reached zero. Signs and symptoms are typically most pronounced at 24 to 36 hours and include hyperactive autonomic signs such as tachycardia, hypertension, and temperature (mild), as well as diaphoresis, tremor, facial flushing, anorexia, nausea, and insomnia. Minor withdrawal usually resolves within 48 to 72 hours, and the majority of patients have only autonomic hyperactivity. In some patients, cognitive and mental status examination may reveal hyperalertness, impairment in attention and concentration, psychomotor agitation, and hallucinatory phenomena consistent with delirium.

The early withdrawal phase is the most likely time for seizures to occur (usually 7 to 30 hours after cessation of drinking in approximately three fourths of patients who have seizures). In addition, as many as one third of patients with alcohol withdrawal seizures progress into major alcohol withdrawal delirium. The importance of pharmacological prophylaxis with benzodiazepines when signs or a history of withdrawal exists is thus emphasized.

Major withdrawal is technically what is referred to as *delirium tremens*. One to 10% of patients with minor withdrawal progress into major withdrawal, which may be viewed as a continuation and amplification of minor withdrawal. Major withdrawal generally occurs within 4 days after reduction or cessation of ethanol intake, and it typically persists for 1 to 6 days, averaging 3 days. Patients in major withdrawal tend to be more floridly delirious, with impaired consciousness, attention, and concentration, as well as autonomic hyperactivity, psychomotor agitation, and visual illusions and hallucinations.

Patients in major withdrawal may complain of insomnia, nightmares, and restlessness, which may be related to disturbances in rapid-eye-motion sleep. Patients may also complain of confusion, and 25% of patients experience illusions and hallucinations.[52] The frequency of hallucination type in terms of sensory modality is, in decreasing order, visual, auditory, tactile, gustatory, and olfactory.[53] Patients may also have delusions referenced to the hallucinations.

Twenty years ago, the mortality rate due to major withdrawal was 10% to 20%. This has been reduced to 1% with the prompt administration of sedative drugs cross-tolerant to alcohol, such as benzodiazepines, to prevent progression from minor into major withdrawal. In addition, the treatment of associated medical disorders such as seizures, arrhythmias, and dehydration has contributed to reduced mortality.

Pathophysiology. Brain metabolic changes during withdrawal could represent fluid and electrolyte changes, neuronal and neurotransmitter adaptation, or remyelination and neuronal plasticity. However, the model of neuronal and neurotransmitter adaptation is consistent with many of the acute clinical features of alcohol withdrawal and is discussed here.

Alcohol is a CNS depressant, and when its intake is stopped or decreased, the CNS rebounds into a hyperadrenergic state. Alcohol withdrawal can be suppressed by resumption of drinking or by administration of benzodiazepines, beta-adrenergic receptor antagonists, or alpha-2-adrenergic receptor agonists. The ability of sympatholytic drugs to attenuate symptoms suggests a role for the hyperactivity of adrenergic neurons in the genesis of the withdrawal syndrome.

More specifically, the locus caeruleus (LC) is a group of brainstem nuclei that are the main source of adrenergic neurotransmitters for the brain. A wide variety of dependence-producing drugs, with apparently little in common pharmacologically, share common withdrawal effects associated with the LC.[54] Support for a shared withdrawal pathway also stems from similarities in withdrawal treatment in that opiates, benzodiazepines, nicotine, and alcohol all have had their withdrawal treated effectively by clonidine, a medication that suppresses LC hyperactivity.

The LC normally is activated by pain, blood loss, and cardiovascular collapse but not by nonthreatening stimuli. Numerous studies have chronicled ethanol's ability to suppress LC activity,[55] with significant evidence supporting the role of alpha-2 adenoreceptors in the pathogenesis of alcohol addiction. An alpha-2 agonist, clonidine, has been shown to be effective in treating alcohol withdrawal.[56] Administration of the alpha-2 antagonist yohimbine has been found to reverse the LC inhibition of ethanol.[57] This finding suggests that the alpha-2 receptors are involved in LC inhibition and in the development of ethanol tolerance and even withdrawal.

Wernicke's Thiamine Deficiency Delirium. It is estimated that the Wernicke-Korsakoff syndrome constitutes 3% of all alcohol-related disorders. This syndrome may be regarded as two facets of the same disease process.[58, 59] The term *Wernicke's disease* has traditionally been applied to the symptom complex triad that consists of ophthalmoparesis or nystagmus, ataxia, and an acute apathetic-confusional state. These symptoms may also occur singly, but more often they occur in various combinations. Korsakoff's syndrome specifically refers to a deficit of memory and learning in an other-

wise nonintoxicated, alert, and responsive patient.

The Wernicke phase of the Wernicke-Korsakoff syndrome is manifested primarily by delirium (acute confusional state), ataxia, lateral gaze palsy, nystagmus, and a number of other less frequent signs. In clinically based studies, only one third of the patients with acute Wernicke's syndrome present with the classical clinical triad. The remainder may have partial or subclinical versions of the syndrome. Cognitive impairment highlights the presentation of this syndrome, and the majority of patients are profoundly disoriented, indifferent, and inattentive.

With treatment, the mode of recovery of the classic Wernicke's features are palsies first, ocular ataxia later, and finally delirium and cognitive impairment. Without treatment, progression with further morbidity and mortality may occur.

Approximately 80% of alcoholic patients recovering from Wernicke's delirium initially manifest the disturbance of Korsakoff's syndrome, which is characterized by apathy and marked deficits in anterograde and retrograde memory with other intellectual abilities preserved. In terms of cognitive morbidity and recovery, of the survivors in one study,[58] 80% to 90% developed Korsakoff's syndrome. In this group, complete or practically complete clinical recovery occurred in 21% of patients, significant recovery in 25%, slight improvement in 28%, and no improvement in 26% (required chronic institutionalization).

In the foregoing study,[58] consisting of 216 patients, 37 deaths occurred during the early stages of the illness (1 to 21 days after the onset, average 8 days), generating a mortality rate of 17%. It seems logical to assume that in the patients who died in the early phase of the disease, the classical brain lesions and the general nutritional depletion contributed to the patients' deaths. Thus, if left untreated, patients may progress through stupor and coma to death.

The clue to Wernicke's delirium is the presence of confusion and delirium accompanied by neurological features such as ataxia and ophthalmological features (lateral gaze palsy, nystagmus). Although atypical presentations can occur, delirium and confusion are the initial presenting features in 66% of cases.[59] Therefore, cognitive impairment is the most consistent and reliable finding.

Additionally, it is important to emphasize that once treatment is provided, delirium or cognitive impairment is usually the last sign to resolve and may take weeks. It is imperative that all alcoholics with delirium receive thiamine and other B vitamins for metabolic support of the brain, and follow-up cognitive assessment is advised.

Wernicke's syndrome is distinguished from alcohol withdrawal delirium by the latter, exhibiting psychomotor agitation, sleeplessness, vivid hallucinations, and signs of autonomic nervous system overactivity (profuse sweating, dilated pupils, tachycardia, and fever in the absence of infection). Besides the cognitive and neurological features in Wernicke's delirium, patients behaviorally are usually hypoactive and apathetic[58, 59] and have few hallucinations.

Pathophysiology. Wernicke's delirium is caused by a mix of etiological factors, including the toxic effects of alcohol, nutritional deficiencies, and a possible genetic transketolase enzyme deficiency in some patients. Wernicke's delirium and its response to thiamine represent the recovery of primarily a biochemical process, although patients may be left with a residual structural lesion.

At the molecular biochemical level, thiamine, as thiamine pyrophosphate, is a cofactor for three critical enzymes of cerebral carbohydrate catabolism: pyruvate decarboxylase, alpha-ketoglutarate dehydrogenase, and transketolase.[60] Thiamine deficiency can, therefore, impair cerebral glucose utilization by inhibiting the tricarboxylic acid cycle and the hexose monophosphate shunt. Because the CNS depends almost entirely on the metabolism of carbohydrate for its energy, this results in decreased production of adenosine triphosphate, acetyl coenzyme A, and the reduced form of nicotinamide-adenine dinucleotide phosphate. As a consequence, lipid incorporation into myelin is reduced and marked alterations occur in the biosynthesis and turnover of several putative neurotransmitters, including serotonin, acetylcholine, and amino acids. Thus, a deficiency of thiamine produces a diffuse decrease in the use of glucose by the cerebrum. Thiamine may also function in axonal conduction and synaptic transmission.

Repeated subclinical episodes of thiamine deficiency and accumulation of lesions over time, rapid development of irreversible lesions during a single acute Wernicke's episode, or inadequate treatment of patients with low-affinity transketolase variants may lead to Korsakoff's syndrome.

It is apparent that Wernicke's delirium and Korsakoff's amnesia are not separate diseases. Rather, the changing cognitive, ocular, and ataxic signs and the transformation from a global confusional state to an amnestic syndrome represent successive stages in the process of recovery from a single disease. The pathological brain changes in patients who die in the acute stages of Wernicke's disease are essentially the same as the changes in patients who die in the chronic stages with a Korsakoff's amnestic state.

Neuroimaging

Acute Effects of Alcohol Administration. The effects of acute ethanol administration on cerebral glucose utilization and blood flow have been studied in human volunteers with PET.[14] In one study,[61] glucose metabolism generally declined in response to ethanol, with variable effects at the lower dose and particularly marked decrements in the frontal cortex.

In another study,[62] the researchers reported an overall reduction of glucose metabolism of approximately 15%, with relative sparing of the basal ganglia and corpus callosum. The effect was more pronounced in alcoholics than in normal controls, and the pattern of metabolic inhibition in both groups paralleled the distribution of benzodiazepine receptors in the human brain. In comparison with studies showing reduced glucose metabolism, other studies have found increased cortical blood flow.[16] The dissociation between the effects of ethanol on glucose metabolism and CBF may reflect direct vascular effects of ethanol.

Most human studies suggest that cerebral vasodilation occurs with small doses of alcohol and that higher doses produce cerebral vasoconstriction.[14] Confusion exists in the literature because of differences in the types of subjects studied and the doses of alcohol used. Ethanol can produce CBF changes in opposite directions through different mechanisms. As a well-known cerebral depressant, alcohol, like other sedatives, should reduce CBF as a result of its effect on brain function. PET scan studies showing reduced glucose metabolism after ethanol support this possibility. However, in small doses, ethanol has a disinhibiting effect that may produce an increase in CBF, at least in certain brain regions (subcortical). Alcohol is vasoactive and induces vasodilation in the periphery, and such a mechanism may also be operant in the cerebral vascular bed. Acetaldehyde, a byproduct of alcohol metabolism, is a vasodilator, and individuals differ in the amount of acetaldehyde produced after a standard dose of ethanol.

In another method of study,[62] pharmacological challenge can be used to accentuate and demonstrate particular defects associated with addiction. In this method, six alcoholics were compared with six controls before and after 1 g of acute ethanol administration. This study revealed a greater response to alcohol in alcoholic than in normal individuals. The alcoholics showed a greater decrease in brain metabolism than did the normal subjects on acute alcohol administration. Because the pattern of regional decrease in brain glucose metabolism paralleled the known regional concentration of benzodiazepine receptors in the human brain, it was hypothesized that the accentuated response to the actions of alcohol in the alcoholics was due to hypersensitization of the benzodiazepine GABA receptor complex. Whether accentuated response to alcohol represents a basic difference between normals and alcoholics or whether it represents a state of alcohol withdrawal is an issue that needs to be clarified.

Interpretation of neuroimaging data on the acute effects of alcohol has certain limitations. Because of the possibility of intravascular effects associated with alcohol intoxication and known uncoupling, the CBF data on acute intoxication are rather moot. In addition, the many various studies are confounded by dissimilar patient populations. Furthermore, in interpreting results, it must be kept in mind that the data are usually presented as group average metabolic values. Despite average values in metabolism similar to those in normal subjects, individual assessment reveals some patients with markedly decreased glucose metabolism throughout the brain.[14]

Withdrawal: Neuroimaging Findings. Eisenberg[63] found a reduction in CBF and cerebral oxygen and glucose metabolism in six patients with delirium tremens. Another study[64] examined patients with mild alcoholic delirium, patients with acute delirium tremens, and nondelirious patients and found statistically significant differences in CBF and cerebral metabolism among the three groups. Berglund and Risberg and colleagues[65, 66] examined 13 withdrawal periods in 12 alcoholic patients and found a significant reduction in global CBF, which was most marked in patients with clouded sensoria after an extended binge, during the first 2 days of withdrawal. Auditory and visual hallucinations were associated with elevated CBF in temporal, parietal, and occipital regions. They found an inverse correlation between degrees of confusion and CBF.

Hemmingsen and coworkers[67] measured regional CBF in 12 patients with alcohol withdrawal during the acute state and after recovery. The overall finding was that CBF in patients with hallucinations and psychomotor agitation was significantly greater during withdrawal than recovery. The findings suggest a type of acute brain syndrome characterized by CNS hyperexcitability. Figure 9–1 demonstrates the CBF tomograms and CT findings in two study patients during and after alcohol withdrawal. In summary, in most cases of alcohol withdrawal, CBF seems to decrease. However, an increase is noted in hallucinating and agitated patients. Much variability in CBF occurs during withdrawal. This is not surprising in view of the multiplicity of withdrawal symptoms and variations in severity from patient to patient, as well as complicating issues such as concomitant Wernicke's syndrome and polysubstance abuse. These methodological issues present some limitations in the interpretations of the neuroimaging data.

TRANSIENT ALCOHOL-INDUCED AMNESTIC STATES (BLACKOUTS)

Blackouts represent a transient, time-limited anterograde memory deficit acquired during intoxication. During a blackout, a patient is ostensibly alert and consciously behaving but later, with sobriety, is unable to remember his or her behavior during the episode.[51] Blackouts have been experimentally related to a rapid rise in the blood alcohol level but not to memory functioning in the sober state.[68]

During a blackout, encoding of episodic memory (memory related to real-time sensory-perceptual processing of experiential episodes) is impaired. When sober, these individuals have intact memory, distinguishing the blackout as a transient rather than persistent amnestic state. Unlike patients with Korsakoff's syndrome, their capacity for future learning is maintained.

Neuroimaging

Berglund and colleagues[68] measured regional CBF during an alcoholic blackout in a 61-year-old man with a blood alcohol of 380 mg/dl and found the mean flow level to be elevated by about 30% to 60% compared with repeated studies during long-term abstinence. A trend for CBF in temporal areas to be more elevated during the blackout is of interest in light of the well-known coupling between this area and memory functions. The blackout state might thus be linked to temporal lobe hyperfunction causing transient dysfunction in memory encoding.

PATIENT 3   PATIENT 7

CEREBRAL BLOOD FLOW TOMOGRAMS

During acute alcohol withdrawal reaction   During acute alcohol withdrawal reaction

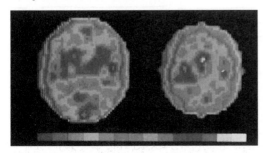   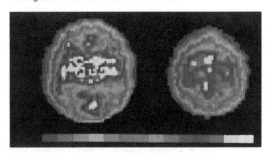

After recovery (8 days later)   After recovery (5 days later)

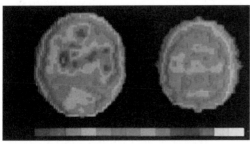   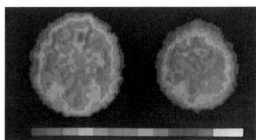

Slice 2   Slice 3   Slice 2   Slice 3

CT SCANS

7 days after admission   5 days after admission

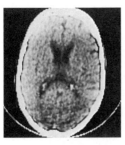 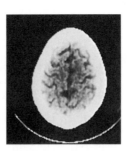   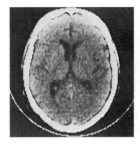 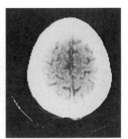

Figure 9–1. Cerebral blood flow tomograms and computed tomography scans for two patients with acute alcohol withdrawal reactions. The mean hemispheric cerebral blood flow for patient 3 was 69.0 ml/100 g/min during withdrawal and 62.0 ml/100 g/min after recovery. The cerebral blood flow for patient 7 was 78.5 ml/100 g/min during withdrawal and 50.5 ml/100 g/min after recovery. (From Hemmingsen R, Vorstrup S, Clemmesen L: Cerebral blood flow during delirium tremens and related clinical states studied with xenon-133 inhalation tomography. Am J Psychiatry 145:1384–1390, 1988.)

CHRONIC SYNDROMES

Ten percent of alcoholics exhibit a severe and chronic full-fledged cognitive impairment syndrome.[24, 28] These syndromes have been historically conceptualized in the literature as the alcohol amnestic disorder (Korsakoff's syndrome) and alcoholic dementia. The DSM-IV criteria for these syndromes are listed in Tables 9–4 and 9–5, respectively.

Alcohol-Induced Persisting Amnestic Disorder

Korsakoff's syndrome is the most distinctive and specific alcohol-induced chronic cognitive impairment syndrome. Unlike delirium and dementia, in which global and diffuse impairment occur, Korsakoff's syndrome exhibits discrete cognitive impairment as an amnestic disorder. Cognitive impairment is primarily in short-term memory and new learning, with various degrees of long-term memory deficits. Most individuals who have Korsakoff's findings have had previous episodes of Wernicke's syndrome. They may have a rather sharp temporal gradient or cutoff in their long-term memory demonstrative of the point at which the critical mass of neurons was lost and beyond which new memories are able to be formed.

In addition to memory deficits, these patients may exhibit both confabulation and apathy. Confabulation is the unwitting production

Table 9–4. DSM-IV CRITERIA FOR SUBSTANCE-INDUCED PERSISTING AMNESTIC DISORDER

A. The development of memory impairment as manifested by impairment in the ability to learn new information or the inability to recall previously learned information.

B. The memory disturbance causes significant impairment in social or occupational functioning and represents a significant decline from a previous level of functioning.

C. The memory disturbance does not occur exclusively during the course of delirium or a dementia and persists beyond the usual duration of substance intoxication or withdrawal.

D. There is evidence from the history, physical examination, or laboratory findings that the memory disturbance is etiologically related to the persisting effects of substance use (e.g., a drug of abuse, a medication).

Code (specific substance)-induced persisting amnestic disorder: (229.1 alcohol; 292.83 sedative, hypnotic, or anxiolytic; 292.83 other [or unknown] substance)

From the American Psychiatric Association: Diagnostic and Statistical Manual of Mental Disorders, 4th ed. Washington, DC, American Psychiatric Association, 1994.

Table 9–5. DSM-IV CRITERIA FOR SUBSTANCE-INDUCED PERSISTING DEMENTIA

A. The development of multiple cognitive deficits manifested by both:
  (1) memory impairment (impaired ability to learn new information or to recall previously learned information)
  (2) One (or more) of the following cognitive disturbances:
    (a) Aphasia (language disturbance)
    (b) Apraxia (impaired ability to carry out motor activities despite intact motor function)
    (c) Agnosia (failure to recognize or identify objects despite intact sensory function)
    (d) Disturbance in executive functioning (i.e., planning, organizing, sequencing, abstracting)

B. The cognitive deficits in criteria A1 and A2 all cause significant impairment in social or occupational functioning and represent a significant decline from a previous level of functioning.

C. The deficits do not occur exclusively during the course of a delirium and persist beyond the usual duration of substance intoxication or withdrawal.

D. There is evidence from the history, physical examination, or laboratory findings that the deficits are etiologically related to the persisting effects of substance use (e.g., a drug of abuse, a medication).

Code (specific substance)-induced persisting dementia: (291.2 alcohol; 292.82 inhalant; 292.82 sedative, hypnotic, or anxiolytic; 292.82 other [or unknown] substance)

From the American Psychiatric Association: Diagnostic and Statistical Manual of Mental Disorders, 4th ed. Washington, DC, American Psychiatric Association, 1994.

of fictitious responses or narrative to compensate for memory deficits. Confabulation is due to impairments in memory and self-reflection and criticism due to subcortical and frontal lobe brain disease, respectively.[69] Apathy is a lack of motivation, emotion, and drive, primarily related to disease in frontolimbic circuits.

In terms of anatomical location, the pathology of Korsakoff's syndrome is primarily in the midline structures, including the diencephalon, the mamillary bodies, and the dorsomedial nucleus of the thalamus. Lesions are also found with regularity throughout the brainstem and cerebellum, as well as in the cerebral cortex. New evidence suggests that the orbitobasal frontal lobe is also involved.[28]

Alcohol-Induced Persisting Dementia

Alcoholic Dementia in Controversy. Some alcoholics with profound amnesia do not fit the clinical or psychometric definitions of Korsakoff's amnesia, because they do not have preserved intelligence. In fact, they have a global loss of cognitive ability generally referred to as *dementia*.

Some investigators[70] believe, however, that

the concept of a nonkorsakovian alcoholic dementia lacks a distinctive, defined pathology. They further emphasize that a direct toxic effect of alcohol on cerebral cortical neurons in humans has been postulated but remains to be proved. Alcohol can cause neuronal death in experimental animals, however, and it seems likely that similar mechanisms may operate in humans.

Courville[71] described in a monograph the neuropathological changes in chronic alcoholics who did not exhibit the clinical picture of the Wernicke-Korsakoff syndrome. The primary lesions were widespread cortical atrophy preferentially affecting the frontal lobes, together with ventricular enlargement and meningeal thickening. Microscopically, neuronal loss, disruption of cortical laminae, pigmentary degeneration, and glial proliferation were the main findings.

There is little doubt that the neuropathological changes described by Courville coexist in some cases with the lesions found in the Wernicke-Korsakoff syndrome. The large majority of patients who have come to autopsy with the clinical diagnosis of primary alcoholic dementia have shown the lesions of the Wernicke-Korsakoff syndrome, the clinical features of which had not been recognized during life. However, traumatic lesions of various types and degrees of severity were sometimes added. In addition, isolated cases have shown the lesions of anoxic encephalopathy, acute and chronic hepatic encephalopathy, communicating hydrocephalus, Alzheimer's disease, Marchiafava-Bignami disease, ischemic infarction, or some other disease unrelated to alcoholism. The clinical material can almost always be accounted for by one or a combination of these disease processes, and there may be no need to invoke a separate entity such as alcoholic dementia due to the toxic effect of alcohol on the brain.

Further, the nature of the cerebral changes responsible for the radiographic findings of sulcal widening and ventricular enlargement in young alcoholics has never been delineated. It may be that light-microscopic methods are inadequate to disclose the lesions.

In view of this information, many researchers believe that the concept of a primary alcoholic dementia must remain ambiguous until such time as its morphological basis is established.

In Support of Alcoholic Dementia. Other researchers[34, 59] believe that the term *alcoholic dementia* does not denote any specific etiological determinant other than a history of excessive alcoholic beverage consumption. They view the term *dementia* as a descriptive label designating a decline in intellectual ability from a previous level and referring to a specific pattern of cognitive impairment without reference to prognosis. The course may be progressive, static, or remitting.

The heterogeneity of the cognitive deficits among alcoholics can be interpreted to indicate that the category of dementia may be overly inclusive or encompassing. Thus, these researchers would endorse that when a clear and general loss of cognitive capacity is observed, the use of the descriptive term *alcoholic dementia* is quite justified. However, it must be emphasized that it is not justified to view such persons as representing the end stage of the subsyndromal deficiencies in abstraction and problem-solving ability often noted in alcoholics, because these deficiencies clearly do not involve a global loss of cognitive ability. Hence, to refer to persons with such circumscribed functional deficits as having a dementia is to make unjustified etiological assumptions and involves somewhat unorthodox and permissive use of the term *dementia*.

A Clinical Resolution. As discussed, the existence of a specific alcohol-induced dementia is controversial owing to semantic and definitional issues, overlap of clinical findings with Korsakoff's syndrome, multiple causes of cognitive impairment, and methodological problems including diagnostic criteria and population samples.

The most accurate resolution of this dilemma is to state that definite and discrete, irreversible subcortical brain changes due to thiamine deficiency are consistent with Korsakoff's syndrome. In addition, some alcoholics show evidence of diffuse cortical changes described by some as dementia due to multiple causes, and some of the changes may be reversible. It has now been recognized, however, that these two disorders are not mutually exclusive and that some features of each often coexist in the same patient.[22–24, 27] In the midst of such academic controversy, maintaining a clinical perspective is important. The significant clinical issue is the existence of global and diffuse cognitive impairment in dementia versus more focal and discrete impairment in Korsakoff's syndrome. This further translates into the preservation of intelligence in Korsakoff's syndrome and its decline in alcoholic dementia. In addition, alcoholic dementia tends to be characterized by selective right-sided cerebral findings and executive cognitive impairment.

A number of other clinical and epidemiological features are associated with Korsakoff's syndrome as compared with alcoholic dementia.[59] Korsakoff's syndrome appears a decade earlier, is relatively more common in men, has an acute onset and a shorter drinking history, and ophthalmoplegia can usually be detected at its outset. In addition, it has a poor outcome once established.

There seems to be enough evidence to argue for the distinctiveness of both syndromes in terms of clinical features, notwithstanding putative etiological and pathophysiological overlap with Korsakoff's syndrome. From a pragmatic standpoint, the salient issue in both syndromes is that the cognitive impairment is clinically significant and severe enough to interfere with an individual's ability to function. Figure 9–2 demonstrates the distinguishing features of alcoholic dementia and Korsakoff's syndrome.

Perhaps subsequent research, aimed at delineating the role and impact of the various etiological determinants (craniocerebral trauma, psychopathology, nutrition, hepatic disease, hypertension), will lend further validation to the concept of alcoholic dementia and perhaps reveal subtypes of dementia according to neuropsychological presentation.

NEUROIMAGING FINDINGS IN CHRONIC ALCOHOLICS

Chronic alcoholism is associated with reduced CBF and CMR.[14, 16] This decrease in CBF in chronic alcoholism is not likely due to asso-

ciated loss of brain tissue. Reversibility of the change in CBF, as well as in cognitive dysfunction, with abstinence and appropriate treatment, suggests that part of the decrease in CBF may be due to brain dysfunction.

Shimojyo and colleagues[72] found a 38% reduction in CBF and cerebral metabolism during the acute stages of Wernicke-Korsakoff encephalopathy, which persisted for 5 to 28 days after abstinence. Several other studies have yielded similar findings, and one demonstrated an increase in CBF after abstinence and treatment with thiamine.

There is some uncertainty about whether all alcoholics with various degrees of dementia show reduced CBF. In a review, Berglund[73] concluded that the average 30- to 40-year-old alcoholic is likely to have normal CBF values, whereas alcoholics with delirium tremens and hepatic cirrhosis are more likely to have reduced CBF.

Cocaine

Cocaine is a psychostimulant whose use has increased dramatically during the past 10 years, especially with the introduction of the freebase smoking technique of administration. Cocaine is well known for its capacity to induce psychiatric syndrome in both the intoxication and withdrawal states. Findings of cognitive impairment have been described in cocaine users.

There currently is no evidence of a unique,

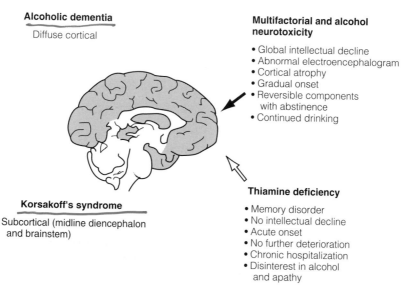

Alcoholic dementia
Diffuse cortical

Korsakoff's syndrome
Subcortical (midline diencephalon and brainstem)

Multifactorial and alcohol neurotoxicity

- Global intellectual decline
- Abnormal electroencephalogram
- Cortical atrophy
- Gradual onset
- Reversible components with abstinence
- Continued drinking

Thiamine deficiency

- Memory disorder
- No intellectual decline
- Acute onset
- No further deterioration
- Chronic hospitalization
- Disinterest in alcohol and apathy

Figure 9–2. Comparison profile of alcohol-induced persistent dementia and amnestic syndrome. (Adapted from Martin PR, Adinoff B, Weingartner H, et al: Alcoholic organic brain disease: Nosology and pathophysiologic mechanisms. Prog Neuropsychopharmacol Biol Psychiatry 10:147–164, 1986.)

full-fledged cognitive impairment syndrome associated with cocaine use. However, a number of studies suggest that memory, psychomotor speed, problem solving, and abstraction abilities are often affected by chronic cocaine addiction, at least during the acute phase of withdrawal.[74–76] This does not appear to be attributable to withdrawal-related depression; however, many of these studies are complicated by addiction to multiple substances, including alcohol.

Three sound studies[77] indicate a strong association between the chronic use of cocaine and deficiencies in short-term auditory recall, memory and concentration, nonverbal abstracting and problem solving, and reaction time. All researchers state that the results of these findings are at best preliminary and that future studies with larger populations and prospective designs are required.

The results of a study[78] of exclusively and specifically cocaine-dependent patients indicate that memory, visuospatial abilities, and concentration were most affected by cocaine use within 72 hours of testing. Although the course trajectory was one of improvement, after 2 weeks of abstinence, the cocaine-dependent group failed to demonstrate the expected degree of neuropsychological recovery in comparison with the control group on measures of psychomotor speed, memory, and concentration. As in cognitively impaired alcoholics, important treatment implications may arise from these findings.

COCAINE-INDUCED DELIRIUM

Cocaine intoxication in high doses, especially with the peak plasma levels associated with smoking and intravenous administration, may cause a delirium syndrome.[79] This delirium typically is of the hyperkinetic type, with agitation, restlessness, and emotional lability. It may have other features indicative of cocaine intoxication such as dyskinesias including tics, dystonic reactions, and chorea, as well as compulsively repeated nonpurposeful behavior (stereotypical behavior). Patients may also experience hallucinations and delusions in association with the delirium.

NEUROIMAGING

Acute Effects

London[14] used PET to examine the effects of 40 mg of cocaine hydrochloride given intravenously to eight polydrug addicts in a double-blind, placebo-controlled crossover study. Most brain regions showed decrements in glucose metabolism after the drug was given. Figure 9–3 illustrates the effects of cocaine on cerebral glucose metabolism.

Chronic Effects

Human studies show reduced cerebral glucose metabolism after cocaine use. Volkow[80] studied regional CBF with PET and showed marked disruption of CBF in chronic cocaine abusers. These defects were more frequently localized in the frontal cortex and left hemisphere. The decreases in CBF were interpreted as representing vascular pathology secondary to the chronic use of cocaine. These findings are in accordance with the well-known vasoactive properties of cocaine.

Investigation of CBF in cocaine addicts with SPECT has shown similar findings to those reported using PET. Cocaine addicts tested with SPECT show widespread defects in accumulation of the tracers in the brain, suggestive of vascular pathology.[14] In addition, it should be noted that a high incidence of cerebrovascular accidents following cocaine abuse has been reported.[16] The reasons for the deranged blood flow to the brain in cocaine addicts and its relation to the cerebrovascular disorders are unclear. The various explanations include activation of vasoconstrictive cerebral sympathetic fibers, vasoconstriction mediated through other neurotransmitters, cerebral vasculitis, and sudden increase in perfusion pressure.

Limitations in many of these studies include the small number of studies, the limited number of participants, and the difficulty in satisfactorily imaging most subcortical structures of interest with PET.

Marijuana

ACUTE EFFECTS

Marijuana has clear-cut acute effects on cognition, affecting perceptual-motor coordination, reaction time, eye tracking, and sensory and perceptual functions. In addition, impairments in more complicated and integrated behavior such as oral communication and automobile driving skills have been demonstrated.[74] In high doses, marijuana may induce delirium.

CHRONIC EFFECTS

After numerous studies spanning many years, it is still unclear whether marijuana pro-

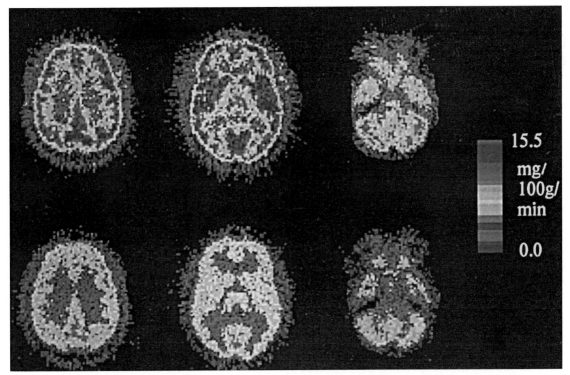

Figure 9–3. Effect of cocaine on cerebral glucose utilization. All images shown are of the same research volunteer. Rates of cerebral glucose utilization, color coded as indicated on the bar, are shown at three levels of brain from superior (left) to inferior (right). The images above were obtained in the placebo condition; those below were obtained after the intravenous injection of 40 mg of cocaine hydrochloride. (From London ED: Imaging Drug Action in the Brain. Boca Raton, FL, CRC Press, 1993.)

duces cognitive deficits that persist beyond the period of acute drug effects.[77] Clinical evidence suggests that there are persistent effects but that they are reversible after several months of abstinence.

NEUROIMAGING

Acute Effects

In one study,[14] after marijuana use, CBF decreased in inexperienced smokers but increased in experienced smokers, in comparison with the two measurements in the control subjects. The influence of the vasodilative effect of marijuana on CBF is unclear at the moment.

Chronic Effects

Mild to moderate users of cannabis with no significant physical or psychiatric complications show normal CBF. However, heavy users of marijuana show a decrease in CBF, which tends to return to normal with abstinence. Only two studies on the subject are available, and no firm conclusions can be drawn.

Opiates

Cognitive impairment is a common, acute effect of opioid use and may be manifested as mental clouding, confusion, delirium, visual hallucinations, and in rare instances psychosis with acute agitation. The mechanism of action of this effect is thought to be the effect of these drugs on opiate receptors in cortical neurons as well as in hypothalamic and temporal regions.

The information available about the long-term cognitive effects of opiate use remains unclear.

NEUROIMAGING

Neuroimaging is limited to reports. London[14] evaluated the effects on cerebral glucose metabolism of 30 mg of morphine sulfate given intramuscularly to 12 polydrug users. Morphine reduced glucose use by 10% in the whole brain and by about 5% to 15% in the telencephalic areas of the cerebellar cortex.

Sedative-Hypnotics, Phencyclidine, Hallucinogens

Sedative-hypnotics may induce delirium in both the intoxication and withdrawal states. Phencyclidine and hallucinogens may also induce delirium in the intoxication state.

The benzodiazepines are a special group of sedative-hypnotic-anxiolytic medications, all of which cause memory deficits; the pattern of deficits is that of an anterograde amnesia. The distinction between episodic and semantic memory is important when discussing this deficit. Episodic memory represents the memory of specific events. It includes information about when the events occurred, preceding and subsequent events, and the context of the events. Semantic memory includes stored knowledge of facts, language, procedures, and rules. These are organized and schematized in a way that allows for interpretation and encoding of ongoing events.

The most consistently demonstrated effect of the benzodiazepines across multiple studies is a dose-dependent anterograde impairment in the acquisition of newly learned information into episodic memory.[81, 82] This can be demonstrated on both visual and verbal tasks. These deficits are apparent within minutes after the presentation of test material. Benzodiazepines do not alter retrieval function from episodic memory for information learned before or during drug exposure. Similarly, benzodiazepines do not impair recall from semantic memory.

The amnestic effects of the benzodizepines may be localized neuroanatomically to the amygdala, a structure densely populated with GABA receptors and believed to be involved in the mediation of anxiety as well.

At the neurophysiological level, the amnestic findings are linked to the benzodiazepines, through GABA. GABA is the major inhibitory neurotransmitter in the brain; the GABA receptor complex spans the neuronal membrane and includes the GABA recognition site, the chloride ion channel, and a specific benzodiazepine receptor-binding site. In the presence of GABA, the benzodiazepines increase chloride conductance through the membrane by increasing the ability of GABA to open the chloride channel, thereby hyperpolarizing the neuronal membrane and rendering it less excitable.

Significantly, reports have shown that GABA antagonists facilitate long-term potentiation in low doses, and this may explain the effects of GABA (and the benzodiazepines) on memory.

In addition, benzodiazepine receptor antagonists, such as flumazenil, block the amnestic effects of the benzodiazepines.

The benzodiazepines also produce impairments in other aspects of cognition, particularly attention, concentration, and psychomotor speed and performance.

Summary

The overall summary of the cognitive and neuroimaging findings in the drug-induced cognitive impairment syndromes yields vague and tentative information owing to research problems including methodological and analytical flaws, insufficient sample size, lack of appropriate controls, separation of acute from chronic effects, polysubstance addiction, and antisocial personality and other psychopathology in the samples.

A number of methodological issues must be addressed for an improved quality of research to generate accurate, valid, and reliable findings:

1. Baseline evaluation. One important factor in providing an accurate assessment of the possible effects of long-term drug use is to have knowledge of the user's premorbid cognitive capacity before exposure to drugs.
2. Controls and reliability. It is essential to have control groups and conditions in which the groups receive nearly identical testing on repeated occasions.
3. Observed subjects and length of abstinence. Polysubstance users are probably the most convenient group of individuals to study because of ease of availability, but without knowledge of the drug(s) used and sobriety status, very little information about the effects of one specific drug class compared with another can be learned. Researchers ideally should observe a user for a period with repeated urine testing to confirm abstinence, to determine the drug of use and the pattern of use, and to obtain as much information as possible about the pattern of use and dose. The best studies have the longest periods of abstinence in a protected environment where drugs are not available. Recovery of function may occur weeks or months after last exposure to drugs.
4. Age range. One must control for the effects of aging. If all of the subjects are very young, subtle cognitive deficits may be missed. If subjects are too old, however, acute or chronic physical conditions that

cause cognitive deficits may be impossible to differentiate from long-term drug effects.

5. Choice of test. It is essential to match the appropriate test to the dependent cognitive variables being assessed.

These standards are difficult to achieve, but many studies that have failed to attend to these issues have involved large expenditures of effort with little or no new knowledge as the outcome.

At the clinical level, it is important to have an appreciation of substance-induced cognitive impairment syndromes for the differential diagnostic assessment as well as the implications for addiction treatment.

The reversible cognitive impairment syndromes are treatable only if recognized during clinical assessment. Especially with alcohol, without recognition and treatment, the disease may continue to progress, with increased cognitive morbidity beyond the point of reversibility and accompanying psychosocial complications. Once Korsakoff's syndrome or dementia has been established, cognitively based 12-step programs may have little to offer these patients because of their inability to learn, retain, and apply treatment principles.

Patients with reversible substance-induced cognitive impairment syndromes may need treatment modifications to maximize and optimize the cognitive assimilation of treatment. This may include delaying the cognitively based aspect of treatment, grading the cognitive demands of treatment exposure in accordance with a patient's limitations, significantly modifying educational materials and exposure, or a combination of these.

ACKNOWLEDGMENT

The author would like to thank Gwendolyn Armster for assistance in manuscript preparation.

REFERENCES

1. Regier DA, Farmer ME, Rae DS, et al: Comorbidity of mental disorders with alcohol and other drug abuse: Results from the Epidemiologic Catchment Area (ECA) study. JAMA 264(19):2511–2518, 1990.
2. Miller NS, Ries RK: Drug and alcohol dependence and psychiatric populations: The need for diagnosis, interventions, and training. Compr Psychiatry 32(3):268–276, 1991.
3. Gregson RAM, Taylor GM: Prediction of relapse in men alcoholics. J Stud Alcohol 38(9):1749–1761, 1977.
4. Abott MW, Greson RAM: Cognitive dysfunction in the prediction of relapse in alcoholics. J Stud Alcohol 42(3):230–243, 1981.
5. Berglund M, Leijonquist H, Horlen M: Prognostic sig-nificance and reversibility of cerebral dysfunction in alcoholics. J Stud Alcohol 38(9):1761–1769, 1977.
6. Goldman MS: Cognitive impairment in chronic alcoholics. Am Psychol 38:1045–1054, 1983.
7. O'Leary MR, Donovan DM, Chaney EF, et al: Cognitive impairment and treatment outcome with alcoholics: Preliminary findings. J Clin Psychiatry 40:397–398, 1979.
8. Erwin JE, Hunter JJ: Prediction of attrition in alcoholic aftercare by scores on the embedded figures test and two piagetian tasks. J Consult Clin Psychol 52(3):354–358, 1984.
9. Chaney EF, O'Leary MR: Skill training with alcoholic. J Consult Clin Psychol 46(5):1092–1104, 1978.
10. Meek PS, Clark HW, Solana VL: Neurocognitive impairment: The unrecognized component of dual diagnosis in substance abuse treatment. J Psychoactive Drugs 21(2):153–160, 1989.
11. Miller L: Neuropsychological assessment of substance abusers: Review and recommendations. J Subst Abuse Treat 2:5–17, 1985.
12. Gillen RW, Kranzler HR, Kadden RM, et al: Utility of a brief cognitive screening instrument in substance abuse patients: Initial investigation. J Subst Abuse Treat 8:247–251, 1991.
13. Miller NS, Mirin SM: Multiple drug use in alcoholics: Practical and theoretical implications. Psychiatr Ann 19(5):248–255, 1989.
14. London ED: Imaging Drug Action in the Brain. Boca Raton, FL, CRC Press, 1993.
15. Shaw TG: Discussion: Alcohol and brain function: An appraisal of cerebral blood flow data. Changes in brain structure and function. In Parsons OA, Butters N, Nathan PE (eds): Neuropsychology of Alcoholism, Implications for Diagnosis and Treatment. New York, Guilford Press, 1987, pp 129–149.
16. Mathew RJ, Wilson WH: Substance abuse and cerebral blood flow. Am J Psychiatry 148(3):292–305, 1991.
17. Grant I, Reed R, Adams KM: Diagnosis of intermediate-duration and subacute organic mental disorder in abstinent alcoholics. J Clin Psychiatry 48(8):319–323, 1987.
18. Lezak MD: Neuropsychological Assessment, 2nd ed. New York, Oxford University Press, 1983.
19. Goldstein S, Deysach R, Kleindkecht R: Effect of experience and amount of information on identification of cerebral impairment. J Consult Clin Psychol 41:30–34, 1973.
20. Heaton RK, Pendleton MG: Use of neuropsychological tests to predict adult patient's everyday functioning. J Consult Clin Psychol 49(6):807–821, 1981.
21. Parsons OA, Leber WR: The relationship between cognitive dysfunction and brain damage in alcoholics: Causal, interactive or epiphenomena? Alcohol Clin Exp Res 5:326–343, 1981.
22. Eckardt MJ, Martin PR: Clinical assessment of cognition in alcoholism. Alcohol Clin Exp Res 10(2):123–127, 1986.
23. Tabakoff B, Petersen RV: Brain damage and alcoholism. The Counselor 6(5):13–16, 1988.
24. Alcohol Alert, Alcohol and Cognition. National Institute on Alcohol Abuse and Alcoholism, PH 258, 4:1–3, 1989.
25. Goldman MS, Williams DL, Kliz DK: Recoverability of psychological functioning following alcohol abuse: Prolonged visual-spatial dysfunction in older alcoholics. J Consult Clin Psychol 51(3):370–378, 1983.
26. Forsbers LK, Goldman MS: Experience-dependent recovery of visuospatial functioning in older alcoholic persons. J Abnorm Psychol 94(4):519–529, 1985.
27. McCrady BS, Smith DE: Implications of cognitive im-

pairment for the treatment of alcoholism. Alcohol Clin Exp Res 10(2):145–149, 1986.

28. Parsons OA, Nixon SJ: Neurobehavioral sequelae of alcoholism. Neurol Clin 11(1):205–217, 1993.

29. Wilkinson DA: Discussion: CT Scan and Neuropsychological Assessment of Alcoholism. Changes in Brain Structure and Function: 76–102.

30. Shelly CH, Goldstein G: An Empirically Derived Typology of Hospitalized Alcoholics. Empirical Studies of Alcoholism. Cambridge, MA, Ballinger, 1976, pp 195–229.

31. Goldman MS: The role of time and practice in recovery of function in alcoholics. In Parsons OA, Butters N, Nathan PE (eds): Neuropsychology of Alcoholism: Implications for Diagnosis and Treatment. New York, Guilford Press, 1987, pp 191–321.

32. Carlsson C, Claeson L, Petterson L: Psychometric signs of cerebral dysfunction in alcoholics. Br J Addict 68:83–86, 1973.

33. Ellenberg L, Rosenbaum G, Goldman M, et al: Recoverability of psychological functioning following alcohol abuse: Lateralization effects. J Consult Clin Psychol 48(4):503–510, 1980.

34. Harper CG, Kril JJ: Neuropathology of alcoholism. Alcohol Alcohol 25(23):207–216, 1990.

35. Schuckit MA: A clinical review of alcohol, alcoholism, and the elderly patient. J Clin Psychiatry 43(10):396–399, 1982.

36. Godfrey HPD, Spittle BJ, Knight RG: Cognitive rehabilitation of amnesic alcoholics: A twelve month follow-up study. N Z Med J 98(784):650–661, 1985.

37. Goldman MS: Neuropsychological recovery in alcoholics: Endogenous and exogenous processes. Alcohol Clin Exp Res 10(2):136–144, 1986.

38. Goldman MS: The role of time and practice in recovery of function of alcoholics. In Parson OA, Butters N, Nathan PE (eds): Neuropsychology of Alcoholism: Implications for Diagnosis and Treatment. New York, Guilford Press, 1987, pp 191–321.

39. Tarter RE, Edwards KL: Multifactorial etiology of neuropsychological impairment in alcoholics. Alcohol Clin Exp Res 10(2):128–135, 1986.

40. Parson OA: Neuropsychological consequences of alcohol abuse: Many questions. In Parsons OA, Butters N, Nathan PE (eds): Neuropsychology of Alcoholism: Implications for Diagnosis and Treatment. New York, Guilford Press. 1987.

41. Bergman H: Brain dysfunction related to alcoholism: Some results from the KARTAD project. In Parsons OA, Butters N, Nathan PE (eds): Neuropsychology of Alcoholism: Implications for Diagnosis and Treatment. New York, Guilford Press. 1987.

42. Becker JT, Jaffe JH: Impaired memory for treatment-relevant information in inpatient men alcoholics. J Stud Alcohol 45(4):339–343, 1984.

43. Volkow ND, Hitzemann R, Wang GJ, et al: Decreased brain metabolism in neurologically intact healthy alcoholics. Am J Psychiatry 149(8):1016–1022, 1992.

44. Berglund M, Hagstadius S, Risberg J, et al: Normalization of regional cerebral blood flow in alcoholics during the first 7 weeks of abstinence. Acta Psychiatr Scand 75:202–208, 1987.

45. American Psychiatric Association: Diagnostic and Statistical Manual of Mental Disorders, 3rd ed (Revised). Washington, DC, American Psychiatric Association, 1987.

46. Arieff AI, Griggs RC: Metabolic Brain Dysfunction in Systemic Disorders. Boston, Little, Brown & Co, 1992.

47. Sellers EM, Kalant H: Alcohol intoxication and withdrawal, medical intelligence, drug therapy. N Engl J Med 294(14):757–762, 1976.

48. Mesulam MM: Principles of Behavioral Neurology. Philadelphia, FA Davis, 1986.

49. Perrin RG, Hockman CH, Kalant H, Livingston KE: Acute effects of ethanol on spontaneous and auditory evoked electrical activity in cat brain. Electroencephalogr Clin Neurophysiol 36:19–31, 1974.

50. Hyvarinen J, Laakson M, Roine R, et al: Effect of ethanol on neuronal activity in the parietal association cortex of alert monkeys. Brain 101:701–715, 1978.

51. Charness ME, Simon RP, Greenberg DA: Medical progress: Ethanol and the nervous system. N Engl J Med 321(7):442–454, 1989.

52. Mitchell MC: Alcoholism and associated medical problems. In The Principles and Practice of Medicine. Norwalk, CT, Appleton Lange, 1984, pp 1483–1490.

53. Lipowski ZJ: Delirium: Acute Brain Failure in Man. Springfield, IL, Charles C Thomas, 1980.

54. Gold MS, Miller NS: Seeking drugs/alcohol and avoiding withdrawals: The neuroanatomy of drive state and withdrawal. Psychiatr Ann 22(8):430–435, 1992.

55. Strahlendorf JC, Strahlendorf HK: Response of locus coeruleus neurons to direct application of ethanol. Neurosci Abstr 7:312, 1984.

56. Baumgartner GR, Rowen RC: Clonidine vs chlordiazepoxide in the management of acute alcohol withdrawal syndrome. Arch Intern Med 147:1223–1226, 1987.

57. Verbanck P, Seutin V, Massotte L, Dresse A: Yohimbine can induce ethanol tolerance in an in vitro preparation on rat locus coeruleus. Alcohol Clin Exp Res 15:1036–1039, 1991.

58. Victor M, Adams RD, Collins GH: The Wernicke-Korsakoff Syndrome and Related Neurologic Disorders Due to Alcoholism and Malnutrition. Philadelphia, FA Davis, 1989.

59. Strub RL, Black FW: Organic Brain Syndromes: An Introduction to Neurobehavioral Disorders. Philadelphia, FA Davis, 1981.

60. Martin PR, Adinoff B, Weingartner H, et al: Alcoholic organic brain disease: Nosology and pathophysiologic mechanisms. Prog Neuropsychopharmacol Biol Psychiatry 10(2):147–164, 1986.

61. de Wit H, Metz J, Wagner N, Cooper M: Behavioral and subjective effects of ethanol: Relationship to cerebral metabolism using PET. Alcohol Clin Exp Res 14:482–489, 1990.

62. Volkow ND, Hitzemann R, Wolf AP, et al: Acute effects of ethanol on regional brain glucose metabolism and transport. Psychiatry Res 35:39–48, 1991.

63. Eisenberg S: Cerebral blood flow and metabolism in patients with delirium tremens (abstract). Clin Res 16:71A, 1968.

64. Marx P, Neundorfer B, Potz G, et al: Cerebral blood flow and amino acid metabolism in chronic alcoholism. In Harper M, Jennett B, Miller D, et al (eds): Blood Flow and Metabolism in the Brain. Edinburgh, Churchill Livingstone, 1975.

65. Berglund M, Hagstadius S, Risberg J, et al: Normalization of regional cerebral blood flow in alcoholics during the first seven weeks of abstinence. Acta Psychiatr Scand 75:202–208, 1987.

66. Berglund M, Risberg J: Regional cerebral blood flow during alcohol withdrawal. Arch Gen Psychiatry 38:351–355, 1981.

67. Hemmingsen R, Vorstrup S, Clemesen L, et al: Cerebral blood flow during delirium tremens and related clinical states studied with xenon-133 inhalation tomography. Am J Psychiatry 145:1384–1390, 1988.

68. Berglund M, Prohovnik I, Risberg J: Regional cerebral blood flow during alcoholic blackout. Psychiatry Res 27:49–54, 1989.

69. Cummings JL: Clinical Neuropsychiatry. Orlando, FL, Grune & Stratton, 1985.
70. Victor M: Persistent altered mentation due to ethanol. Neurol Clin 11(3):639–661, 1993.
71. Courville CB: Effects of Alcohol on the Nervous System of Man. Los Angeles, San Lucas Press, 1955.
72. Shimojyo S, Scheinbert P, Reinmut O: Cerebral flow and metabolism in the Wernicke-Korsakoff syndrome. J Clin Invest 46(5):849–854, 1967.
73. Berglund M: Cerebral blood flow in chronic alcoholics. Alcoholism 5:295–303, 1981.
74. Manschreck TC, Schneyer ML, Weisstein CC, et al: Freebase cocaine and memory. Compr Psychiatry 4:369–375, 1990.
75. Herning RI, Glover BJ, Koppel B, et al: Cognitive deficits in sustaining cocaine users. NIDA Res Monogr 101:167–178, 1990.
76. O'Malley SS, Gawin FH: Abstinence symptomatology and neuropsychological impairment in chronic cocaine abusers. NIDA Res Monogr 101:179–190, 1990.
77. Weinrieb RM, O'Brien CP: Persistent cognitive deficits attributed to substance abuse. Neurol Clin 11(3):663–691, 1993.
78. Berry J, VanGorp WG, Herzberg DS, et al: Neuropsychological deficits in abstinent cocaine abusers: Preliminary findings after two weeks of abstinence. Drug Alcohol Depend 32:231–237, 1993.
79. Miller NS, Gold MS, Millman RB: Cocaine: General characteristics, abuse and addiction. NY State J Med 89:290–295, 1989.
80. Volkow ND, Fowler JS: Neuropsychiatric disorders: Investigation of schizophrenia and substance abuse. Semin Nucl Med 22(4):254–267, 1992.
81. Barbee JG: Memory, benzodiazepines, and anxiety: Integration of theoretical and clinical perspectives. J Clin Psychiatry 54(Suppl):10, 1993.
82. Wolkowitz OM, Weingartner H, Thompson BS, et al: Diazepam-induced amnesia: A neuropharmacological model of an "organic amnestic syndrome." Am J Psychiatry 144:1, 1987.

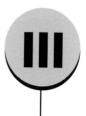

DIAGNOSIS

Substance-Induced Psychiatric Disorders

Craig McKenna, MD

Psychiatric symptoms in patients with addiction are most commonly associated with acute intoxication and withdrawal syndromes, either with or without delirium, and commonly include psychotic, mood, or anxiety symptoms. These symptoms most often are subclinical and do not qualify as a full-fledged symptom-based psychiatric disorder. However, psychoactive substances can induce specific psychiatric symptom-based clinical disorders. These include psychotic, mood, anxiety, personality, and sensory-perceptual disorders. Tables 10–1 to 10–5 provide the DSM-IV[1] diagnostic criteria for substance-induced psychiatric disorders, respectively, in the order of their discussion.

Most of these disorders have subtypes that denote the predominant symptom. Also, in most cases, onset specifiers of either intoxication or withdrawal are required to identify which of these substance-induced states exists in association with the psychiatric symptom. These clinical syndromes generally are time limited and remit with addiction treatment and sobriety. However, without treatment and with continued substance use, these syndromes may progress and substantially contribute to the psychosocial complications and morbidity associated with addiction.

The diagnosis of substance-induced psychiatric disorders should be made only instead of a diagnosis of substance intoxication or withdrawal when the psychiatric symptoms are in excess and when the symptoms are sufficiently severe to warrant independent clinical attention. The history, physical examination, or laboratory findings must provide evidence of intoxication or withdrawal. In addition, the diagnosis of a substance-induced psychiatric disorder is not justified if the psychiatric symptoms occur only during the course of a delirium. Cognition, in general, should be minimally impaired in patients with substance-induced psychiatric disorders. If a primary cognitive impairment syndrome exists, this may relegate the psychiatric symptom to a secondary status as a complication of the primary syndrome.

The onset and course of substance-induced psychiatric disorders are variable. After cessation of substance use, the washout/withdrawal period and central nervous system (CNS) normalization can be protracted. As a result, the onset of psychiatric symptoms can occur as late as 4 to 6 weeks after the last episode of substance use.[2] In most patients, psychiatric syndromes resolve within 4 to 6 weeks of sobriety, but in a smaller group, symptoms may persist after this acute stage. In a minority of patients, symptoms may persist beyond 3 to 6 months and become chronic. In consideration of these temporal factors and clinical probability, it is prudent to wait a minimum of 4 to 6 weeks before diagnosing an addiction-independent psychiatric disorder.

Table 10–1. DSM-IV CRITERIA FOR SUBSTANCE-INDUCED PSYCHOTIC DISORDER

A. Prominent hallucinations or delusions. *Note*: Do not include hallucinations if the person has insight that they are substance induced.
B. There is evidence from the history, physical examination, or laboratory findings of either (1) or (2):
  (1) The symptoms in criterion A developed during or within a month of substance intoxication or withdrawal.
  (2) Medication use is etiologically related to the disturbance.
C. The disturbance is not better accounted for by a psychotic disorder that is not substance induced. Evidence that the symptoms are better accounted for by a psychotic disorder that is not substance induced might include the following: The symptoms precede the onset of substance use (or medication use); the symptoms persist for a substantial period of time (e.g., about a month) after cessation of acute withdrawal or severe intoxication or are substantially in excess of what would be expected given the type or amount of the substance used or the duration of use; or there is other evidence that suggests the existence of an independent non–substance-induced psychotic disorder (e.g., a history of recurrent non–substance-related episodes).
D. The disturbance does not occur exclusively during the course of a delirium.
Note: This diagnosis should be made instead of a diagnosis of substance intoxication or substance withdrawal only when the symptoms are in excess of those usually associated with the intoxication or withdrawal syndrome and when the symptoms are sufficiently severe to warrant independent clinical attention.
Specify type:
With delusion: This subtype is used if delusions are the predominant symptom
With hallucinations: This subtype is used if hallucinations are the predominant symptom
Specify (see table on p. 177 in DSM-IV for applicability to substance):
With onset during intoxication: If criteria are met for intoxication with the substance and the symptoms develop during the intoxication syndrome
With onset during withdrawal: If criteria are met for withdrawal from the substance and the symptoms develop during or shortly after a withdrawal syndrome

From the American Psychiatric Association: Diagnostic and Statistical Manual of Mental Disorders, 4th ed. Washington, DC, American Psychiatric Association, 1994, pp 314–315.

Table 10–2. DSM-IV CRITERIA FOR SUBSTANCE-INDUCED MOOD DISORDER

A. Prominent and persistent disturbance in mood predominates in the clinical picture and is characterized by either (or both) of the following:
  (1) Depressed mood or markedly diminished interest or pleasure in all, or almost all, activities
  (2) Elevated, expansive, or irritable mood
B. There is evidence from the history, physical examination, or laboratory findings of either (1) or (2).
C. The disturbance is not better accounted for by a mood disorder that is not substance induced. Evidence that the symptoms are better accounted for by a mood disorder that is not substance induced might include the following: The symptoms precede the onset of the substance use (or medication use); the symptoms persist for a substantial period (e.g., about a month) after the cessation of acute withdrawal or the duration of use; or there is other evidence that suggests the existence of an independent non–substance-induced mood disorder (e.g., a history of recurrent major depressive episodes).
D. The disturbance does not occur exclusively during the course of a delirium.
E. The symptoms cause clinically significant distress or impairment in social, occupational, or other important areas of functioning.
Note: This diagnosis should be made instead of a diagnosis of substance intoxication or substance withdrawal only when the mood symptoms are in excess of those usually associated with the intoxication or withdrawal syndrome and when the symptoms are sufficiently severe to warrant independent clinical attention.
Specify type:
With depressive features: If the predominant mood is depressed
With manic features: If the predominant mood is elevated, euphoric, or irritable
With mixed features: If symptoms of both mania and depression are present and neither predominates
Specify (see table on p. 177 in DSM-IV for applicability by substance):
With onset during intoxication: If the criteria are met for intoxication with the substance and the symptoms develop during the intoxication syndrome
With onset during withdrawal: If criteria are met for withdrawal from the substance and the symptoms develop during or shortly after a withdrawal syndrome

From the American Psychiatric Association: Diagnostic and Statistical Manual of Mental Disorders, 4th ed. Washington, DC, American Psychiatric Association, 1994, pp 374–375.

Table 10–3. DSM-IV CRITERIA FOR SUBSTANCE-INDUCED ANXIETY DISORDER

A. Prominent anxiety, panic attacks, or obsessions or compulsions predominate in the clinical picture.
B. There is evidence from the history, physical examination, or laboratory findings of either (1) or (2):
    (1) The symptoms in criterion A developed during or within 1 month of substance intoxication or withdrawal medication
    (2) Metication use is etiologically related to the disturbance.
C. The disturbance is not better accounted for by an anxiety disorder that is not substance induced. Evidence that the symptoms are better accounted for by an anxiety disorder that is not substance induced might include the following: The symptoms precede the onset of the substance use (or medication use); the symptoms persist for a substantial period (e.g., about a month) after cessation of acute withdrawal or severe intoxication or are substantially in excess of what would be expected given the type or amount of the substance used or the duration of use; or there is other evidence suggesting the existence of an independent non–substance-induced anxiety disorder (e.g., a history of recurrent non–substance-related episodes).
D. The disturbance does not occur exclusively during the course of delirium.
E. The disturbance causes clinically significant distress or impairment in social, occupational, or other important areas of functioning.
Note: This diagnosis should be made instead of a diagnosis of substance intoxication or substance withdrawal only when the anxiety symptoms are in excess of those usually associated with the intoxication or withdrawal syndrome and when the anxiety symptoms are sufficiently severe to warrant independent clinical attention.
Specify:
With generalized anxiety: If excessive anxiety or worry about a number of events or activities predominates in the clinical presentation
With panic attacks: If panic attacks predominate in the clinical presentation
With obsessive-compulsive symptoms: If obsessions or compulsions predominate in the clinical presentation
With phobic symptoms: If phobic symptoms predominate in the clinical presentation
Specify (see table on p. 177 in DSM-IV for applicability by substance):
With onset during intoxication: If the criteria are met for intoxication with the substance and the symptoms develop during the intoxication syndrome
With onset during withdrawal: If criteria are met for withdrawal from the substance and the symptoms develop during or shortly after a withdrawal syndrome

From the American Psychiatric Association: Diagnostic and Statistical Manual of Mental Disorders, 4th ed. Washington, DC, American Psychiatric Association, 1994, pp 443–444.

Table 10–4. DSM-IV CRITERIA FOR SUBSTANCE-INDUCED PERSONALITY CHANGE

A. A persistent personality disturbance that represents a change from the individual's previous characteristic personality pattern. (In children, the disturbance involves a marked deviation from normal development or a significant change in the child's usual behavior patterns lasting at least 1 year.)
B. There is evidence from the history, physical examination, or laboratory findings that the disturbance is the direct physiological consequence of a general medical condition.
C. The disturbance is not better accounted for by another mental disorder (including other mental disorder due to a general medical condition).
D. The disturbance does not occur exclusively during the course of a delirium and does not meet criteria for a dementia.
E. The disturbance causes clinically significant distress or impairment in social, occupational, or other important areas of functioning.
Specify type:
Labile type: If the predominant feature is affective lability
Disinhibited type: If the predominant feature is poor impulse control as evidenced by sexual indiscretions, etc.
Aggressive type: If the predominant feature is aggressive behavior
Apathetic type: If the predominant feature is apathy and indifference
Paranoid type: If the predominant feature is suspiciousness or paranoid ideation
Other type: If the predominant feature is not one of the above, e.g., personality change associated with a seizure disorder
Combined type: If more than one feature predominates in the clinical picture
Unspecified type

From the American Psychiatric Association: Diagnostic and Statistical Manual of Mental Disorders, 4th ed. Washington, DC, American Psychiatric Association, 1994, pp 173–174.

Table 10–5. DIAGNOSTIC CRITERIA FOR HALLUCINOGEN PERSISTING PERCEPTION DISORDERS (FLASHBACKS)

A. The reexperiencing, after cessation of use of a hallucinogen, of one or more of the perceptual symptoms that were experienced while intoxicated with the hallucinogen (e.g., geometrical hallucinations, false perceptions of movement in the peripheral visual fields, flashes of color, intensified colors, trails of images of moving objects, positive afterimages, halos around objects, macropsia, and micropsia).

B. The symptoms in criterion A cause clinically significant distress or impairment in social, occupational, or other important areas of functioning.

C. The symptoms are not due to a general medical condition (e.g., anatomical lesions and infections of the brain, visual epilepsies) and are not better accounted for by another mental disorder (e.g., delirium, dementia, schizophrenia) or hypnopompic hallucinations.

From the American Psychiatric Association: Diagnostic and Statistical Manual of Mental Disorders, 4th ed. Washington, DC, American Psychiatric Association, 1994, p 234.

Etiology

All individuals are vulnerable to the development of psychiatric symptoms from various drugs at different doses and frequency intervals. For clinical purposes, however, a biopsychosocial interactional model is appropriate and useful in understanding specific etiology when evaluating substance-induced psychiatric disorders.[3]

Biological factors include preexistent organicity, especially in organs (liver, kidney) responsible for the metabolism of drugs as well as in the brain itself, the target organ of psychoactive substances. These factors allow for longer half-lives and increased sensitivity of the brain. Other biological variables include pharmacological characteristics of the particular substance; the dose, frequency, and pattern of use; polysubstance interactions; and kindling,[4] a form of neurobiological sensitization that may occur with intoxication[5] and withdrawal states.[6] Kindling renders the CNS more susceptible to abnormal activation, which may be manifested at a biochemical level as neurotransmitter system alterations and at the clinical level as a particular symptom complex.

Psychological factors include premorbid personality vulnerabilities and deficits, preexistent psychiatric disorders, emotional state, expectations, and novice versus experienced user status. Social factors include social stress and peer pressure. These and other various biopsychosocial factors interact to produce a substance-induced psychiatric disorder in any particular individual, in a particular setting, at a specific time. An important clinical caveat is that once an individual has experienced a substance-induced psychiatric disorder, that individual is more susceptible to subsequent episodes.

Dual Diagnosis

In contradistinction to substance-induced psychiatric disorders as a complication of addiction is the problem of dual diagnosis,[7] noted in addicted patients who have an additional, independent psychiatric disorder such as schizophrenia, major depression, and so forth. The National Institute of Mental Health's Epidemiologic Catchment Area Study[8] uncovered unexpectedly high comorbidity rates in reference to anxiety, mood, and psychotic disorders. For those with alcohol addiction, 37% also have diagnosable psychiatric disorders including anxiety disorder (19%), mood disorder (13%), and schizophrenia (4%). More than half the people addicted to drugs other than alcohol have at least one comorbid mental disorder as indicated by the following percentages: anxiety disorder 28%, mood disorder 26%, and schizophrenia 7%.

One of the singular most important diagnostic problems in the course of assessment for addictions is screening to identify patients with a dual diagnosis. These patients are well known to have a poorer prognosis[9] than patients with exclusive substance addiction, with a higher incidence of hospitalization, medication noncompliance, criminality, homelessness, and suicide. Because of such complicated diagnostic and morbidity issues, patients identified as having a dual diagnosis require specialized treatment for a successful outcome.[10]

Addicted patients who present with psychiatric symptoms require careful and meticulous diagnostic assessment. Distinguishing between a substance-induced psychiatric disorder and a primary idiopathic psychiatric disorder may be a daunting and challenging task. Some practical clinical guidelines in evaluating such complicated cases include consideration of the following factors: temporal onset and sequence of development of psychiatric symptoms versus addiction, past psychiatric history, course during sobriety, atypical features, type of substance and dose, and associated clinical features. More specifically, the probability of a primary idiopathic psychiatric disorder (independent non–substance induced) is increased if a patient has a history of prior psychiatric symptoms that are not substance related or psychiatric symptoms preceding the onset of substance use; if the symptoms persist beyond the acute withdrawal period (4 to 6 weeks); if the symptoms are unusual or in excess, as would be expected given the substance type, use frequency, and dose amount; if the substance-specific physiological and behavioral features of intoxication or withdrawal are absent; and if the onset of symptoms is before age 45 years.

In one study that examined the dual-diagnosis identification problem, McKenna[11] found the following variables predictive of dual diagnosis in a sample of addicted patients: history of sexual abuse, psychiatric symptoms during subacute sobriety, emotionally motivated substance use rationale, anxiety-panic with subacute sobriety, sober periods less than 1 year, onset of addiction after 20 years of age, and use of four different substances. Further studies, using different samples and a more longitudinal design, would be helpful in replicating and further validating these findings. The aim of such research is to provide earlier identification and treatment of patients with a dual diagnosis without having to wait the requisite 4 to 6 weeks before a definitive, addictions-independent psychiatric diagnosis can be made.

Substance-Induced Psychotic Disorder

ALCOHOL

Alcohol may cause hallucinations or delusional symptoms in either the intoxication or withdrawal state. Psychotic symptoms are most frequently related to withdrawal and may, in fact, be a variant of withdrawal.

A large number of alcoholic patients report psychotic symptoms. In a study by Schuckit,[12] 43% of a sample of alcoholics reported psychotic symptoms including both delusions and hallucinations. This included 22% who had hallucinations only, 9% who reported only mind control, 3% who related only feelings of being influenced, and 9% whose complaints consisted of combinations of symptoms.

Acute hallucinosis is usually auditory with unpleasant voices but may also be visual or tactile. The hallucinations may initially have a formless organic quality, such as cackling, knocking, whispering, or roaring sounds. Once a patient hears voices, such formed hallucinations are usually unpleasant and derogatory, dealing with threats against the patient or family. Individuals may also experience delusions of a persecutory nature that are often thematically consistent and referenced to the auditory hallucinations.

Alcohol-induced psychotic symptoms often have a compelling quality and affect patients profoundly. Patients generally take their hallucinations and delusions very seriously and respond with fear, anxiety, depression, or a feeling of despair.

Alcohol hallucinosis may be confused with the hallucinations in idiopathic psychotic disorders such as schizophrenia. However, there are a number of differentiating features.[13] Classically, alcohol hallucinosis occurs after several years of drinking, and the majority of patients are in their 40s and 50s. Alcohol hallucinosis starts acutely and may begin while a patient is drinking or after a period of abstinence lasting from a few hours to a week or longer. The majority of cases start within 2 days after the last drink and may be the only evidence of a withdrawal reaction. The hallucinosis may subside spontaneously or eventually progress to a full-fledged withdrawal. Most patients recover spontaneously within 1 to 6 days, although some cases may persist for a few weeks, and a minority may last for years.[14] No family history of schizophrenia or premorbid schizoid-schizotypal personality traits is usually elicited in patients with alcohol hallucinosis. Table 10–6 lists a number of these and other representative factors distinguishing between alcohol and schizophrenic hallucinosis.

Several researchers have further attempted to characterize the hallucinosis in alcoholism compared with that in schizophrenia. Cutting[15] characterizes the hallucinations in alcohol hallucinosis as well localized and usually only one voice. The speaker of the voice is often identified, and meaningful noise and drowsiness cause the voices to increase. In general, sensory qualities of the hallucinations are prominent, suggesting that unlike the voices heard by schizophrenic patients, these voices are false perceptions of environmental sounds.

Albert and Silvers[16] emphasize the following characteristics of alcohol hallucinosis: onset during withdrawal period; more frequent and free-running quality of hallucinosis; noises, music, and unintelligible voices; source of the hallucination outside the alcoholic's body and spatially localized; willingness to discuss the hallucinations; better insight; frequency independent of emotional state; and the tendency

Table 10–6. DIFFERENTIAL DIAGNOSIS OF ALCOHOL-INDUCED PSYCHOSES AND IDIOPATHIC PSYCHOSES

	Alcohol-induced Psychoses	Idiopathic Psychoses
Age of onset	40–50 years	Begins only infrequently after age 45 years
Type of onset	Usually acute	The majority begin insidiously over months or years
Duration of illness	Usually 1–3 months	Chronic
Premorbid personality	Various	May show certain personality traits, e.g., shy, aloof, withdrawn
Alcohol dependence	For many years	Not stated
Family history of alcoholism	Increased	Not stated
Family history of schizophrenia	No evidence of a positive family history of schizophrenia	Increased prevalence among close relatives
Hallucinations and delusions	Predominantly auditory, but visual and tactile frequently occur	Auditory hallucinations most common
Thought process	Unimpaired	Impaired
Affect	Anxious, depressed, perplexed but appropriate	Inappropriate
Intellectual function	May have subclinical or clinical findings consistent with alcoholism	Not compromised

to hallucinate in visual and auditory modalities simultaneously.

COCAINE AND AMPHETAMINE

In contradistinction to alcohol, induction of psychotic symptoms with cocaine and other stimulants is usually related to intoxication states, and delusions are more common than hallucinosis. Persecutory delusions often develop shortly after use and occasionally may be associated with hallucinations. In addition to these psychotic symptoms, repetitive compulsive behavior may occur.[17]

In a study[18] of 50 cocaine-dependent men, none of whom had other axis I diagnoses, 34 (68%) reported paranoid episodes limited to their periods of cocaine use. The paranoia did not extend beyond the "crash" or hypersomnolent phase of early abstinence. It developed after an average of 3 years use. These subjects did not differ significantly from those not reporting paranoia with respect to use characteristics such as route of administration, lifetime duration of use, cumulative exposure to cocaine, amount of cocaine consumed in the month of admission, or concurrent use of other drugs. These findings suggest that development of paranoia is not simply a result of exceeding a threshold of use and that affected individuals may be predisposed to this drug-induced state.

Another study,[19] which involved a 6-year follow-up of 51 addicted individuals, suggested that those who persistently used stimulants were likely to develop chronic psychotic disorders, mainly paranoid types that were not present at baseline. In this study, no changes in intellectual function (IQ) were observed despite the appearance of psychotic symptoms.

Pure hallucinations (delusional-independent) are reported by only a minority of stimulant users, with 15% relating histories of visual hallucinations, 13% tactile, 7% olfactory (usually of an unpleasant nature), 4% auditory, and 4% gustatory in one series.[17]

CANNABIS

High doses of marijuana may cause auditory and visual illusions or less commonly persecutory delusions, sometimes accompanied by unformed or complex hallucinations. At these high doses, users also often experience symptoms of anxiety and panic, emotional lability, and depersonalization.

PHENCYCLIDINE AND OTHER HALLUCINOGENS

Acute effects of phencyclidine (PCP) are roughly dose dependent. In low doses, PCP functions primarily as a depressant, producing mild intoxication with accompanying analgesia. Sensory distortions and altered body image are more frequent than are true hallucinations.

At higher doses, frank psychosis may occur, resembling catatonia or paranoid schizophrenia with persecutory auditory hallucinations. In addition, patients may show emotional lability including hostility and violent outbursts. The degree and persistence of the psychosis are related to the amount of drug ingested and may last from 24 hours to 1 month. An early, intermediate, and late phase are described. Agitation, hyperactivity, and paranoia initially predominate; during the intermediate phase, some control over behavior is obtained, although patients may still exhibit paranoid delusions. In the late phase, psychotic symptoms gradually resolve.

Chronic PCP use is sometimes accompanied by a chronic psychosis, which persists even when patients are drug free. It appears that the drug is capable of producing both acute and chronic psychosis in otherwise normal individuals.

In one study examining psychiatrically hospitalized PCP addicts,[20] 94% reported histories of feelings of unreality associated with drug use in the past, 75% reported various levels of paranoia, and 62% related a history of hallucinations.[12, 21]

Other hallucinogens (e.g., LSD, mescaline) may induce perceptual distortions, but frank hallucinations are not common. These drugs uncommonly produce psychotic symptoms, depending on the premorbid personality and the setting in which the drug is taken. In some patients, low-level perceptual symptoms such as *trailing*, a form of visual afterimage, may persist beyond the acute intoxication.

OPIATES

Unlike most other drugs, the opiates rarely produce psychotic symptoms during intoxication and actually exhibit antipsychotic properties. In fact, methadone has been used with some time-limited benefit in a well-controlled trial with refractory schizophrenic patients.[21]

Opiate withdrawal is associated with hyperadrenergic features, but psychosis is not a typical feature of this syndrome. However, Levinson and colleagues[22] reported on four cases of methadone withdrawal-related psychosis. The onset of psychosis followed methadone reduction in all cases, and none of these patients manifested typical symptoms of opiate withdrawal while experiencing psychotic symptoms. Others have also described psychosis associated with opiate withdrawal.[23-25]

Substance-Induced Mood Disorder

ALCOHOL

Alcohol may induce mood disturbance in either the intoxication or withdrawal state. Be-

cause alcohol is a CNS depressant, it follows that alcohol may produce intoxication state–related emotional and mood alterations. The subjective effects of alcohol are mediated by pharmacological action on brain neurotransmitters and their receptor sites. Specifically, alcohol enhances the neuronal activity of gamma-aminobutyric acid (GABA), a brain neurotransmitter, which counters the excitatory effects of norepinephrine. Increased flow of chloride ions across the GABA/benzodiazepine receptor membrane results in the membrane hyperpolarization that is thought to underlie the anxiolytic activity of alcohol, the benzodiazepines, and other CNS depressants.[26] A similar mechanism may be involved in the depressogenic effects induced by alcohol abuse and intoxication, although the precise pathophysiology is not well understood.

Alcohol withdrawal-induced depression is commonly encountered and may be clinically indistinguishable from the idiopathic depressive disorders. This depression probably results from alterations in brain chemistry after cessation from chronic exposure to alcohol, but the exact mechanism is unclear.

COCAINE AND PSYCHOSTIMULANTS

Cocaine and stimulant agents may induce an acute manic syndrome during the state of acute intoxication. The acute euphorigenic effects of these agents are attributable to their effects on brain catecholamines, specifically norepinephrine and dopamine, as well as serotonin.[27] Cocaine both facilitates the release of these catecholamines from presynaptic neurons and inhibits neuronal uptake and degradation. These actions are thought to constitute the neurobiological mechanism by which stimulant drugs produce euphoria, hyperactivity, and other reinforcing effects after acute administration.[26]

In contrast, chronic stimulant use leads to depletion of catecholamines from central presynaptic neurons, with a corresponding increase in the sensitivity of both noradrenergic and dopaminergic postsynaptic receptors. Chronic use has also been demonstrated to deplete intracellular stores of 5-hydroxytryptamine (serotonin) from presynaptic neurons and to block the neuronal uptake of tryptophan, an amino acid precursor important in serotonin synthesis. Collectively, these changes in neurotransmitter homeostasis are thought to have a role in the pathogenesis of the depression that accompanies stimulant withdrawal.

OPIATES

Opiates generally induce mood disturbance in the intoxication state, and chronic administration of opiates has been found to reduce noradrenergic tone in the CNS. It has been hypothesized that opiate-induced depression is a result of alterations in endorphin, noradrenergic, and adrenocorticotropic hormone/cortisol systems in the brain.[21]

Mood disturbance has also been documented as part of the withdrawal from opiates. Dakis and Gold[28] found a significantly higher prevalence of what they called "organic affective disorder" (depression) in patients withdrawn from methadone than in patients withdrawn from heroin (60% vs. 25%). They postulated that the longer-acting methadone had induced changes in brain neurophysiology that contributed to the depression in these patients and that these alterations took longer to reverse themselves once patients were detoxified.

Substance-Induced Anxiety Disorder

ALCOHOL

Because alcohol has depressive and anxiolytic properties, acute intoxication rarely involves acute anxiety or panic. However, acute alcohol withdrawal, as a hyperadrenergic state, may induce an anxiety disorder. Various degrees of subclinical anxiety ranging from panic to generalized anxiety can last for 3 to 12 months after cessation of drinking.

COCAINE AND PSYCHOSTIMULANTS

Cocaine and other psychostimulants may produce manifestations of anxiety, most commonly during the intoxication state. More commonly used drugs such as caffeine (intoxication) and nicotine (withdrawal) may also produce anxiety symptoms.

OPIATES

Opiate withdrawal actually may share neurochemical characteristics with panic disorder.[21] Protracted anxiety during methadone withdrawal may last several weeks or months owing to prolonged neuroreceptor alterations.

CANNABIS

Marijuana-induced anxiety usually occurs at high doses. The clinical picture typically is an exaggeration of the usual marijuana effects including anxiety, the fear of losing control or going crazy, depersonalization, and derealization. These symptoms can be experienced by individuals with no preexisting psychopathology as well as those who have a history of erratic or maladaptive behavior. These episodes usually occur in individuals with preexisting anxiety about drug use, especially novice users, or in experienced users who have taken more than their usual dose.

PHENCYCLIDINE AND OTHER HALLUCINOGENS

PCP and hallucinogens may acutely produce anxiety and panic, depending on the individual, dose, and setting. In some patients, low-level symptoms such as depersonalization and derealization may persist beyond the acute intoxication.

Substance-Induced Personality Syndrome

Chronic drug and alcohol abuse may create personality changes owing to the pharmacological properties and effects on brain function and the associated psychological sequelae of compromised coping, defenses, and socialization. As a result, substance abusers may develop feelings of isolation, an impaired sense of reality, impulsivity, and poor relationship ability. Preexisting personality disorders exhibiting such features must be considered in the differential, particularly borderline and antisocial, because these personality disorders have high rates of substance dependence.[27] However, it must not be assumed that addiction patients, because of their behavior, are character disordered independent of the biopsychosocial influences of the addiction. Dulit and colleagues[29] examined the prevalence of substance abuse in 137 patients given a diagnosis of borderline personality disorder. When substance abuse was not part of the diagnostic criteria, 32 (23%) of the patients no longer met criteria for borderline personality disorder. In this subgroup, symptoms were less severe and the course of the illness was more favorable than for the other group. This work adds weight to the possibility that drug abuse was an important factor in the development and diagnosis of the personality disorders observed in these patients.

Vaillant[30, 31] has discussed the concept of regression (neurobiopsychological) in addicts with substance-induced CNS impairment. These patients may revert to more primitive coping styles and defense mechanisms. In one study,[32] he found that abstinent substance abusers appeared to abandon the lifestyles of acting out and passive-aggressive behavior in favor of the hypothetically more mature defense patterns of isolation, dissociation, altruism, and reaction formation.

ALCOHOL

The later course of alcoholism is frequently marked by personality alterations that persist even during periods of sobriety. Although psychosocial vicissitudes are clearly involved, specific subclinical cognitive alterations characteristic of frontal lobe damage have been demonstrated in many alcoholics. Histological and radiographic evidence also suggests that the chronic toxic effects of alcohol seriously affect the frontal lobe structure and function first.[33] This may be extended to include, other than basic cognition, those aspects of personality structure that are supported by frontal lobe function, including higher-level cognition such as insight, reasoning, judgment, emotional and impulse control, anticipation and planning, and goal orientation.

Alcohol is also known to affect limbic system structures[33, 34] (temporal lobes, hippocampus, mamillary bodies, and so on). These areas are involved in motivation, emotions, memory, and sensory processing. It follows that damage to these areas by alcohol may also temporarily or permanently influence personality traits.

Chronic alcohol abuse may induce a range of CNS pathology, with chronic apathy as one manifestation of personality alteration.[34] This is understandable in terms of the findings of frontal and limbic system pathology. In the chronic stage of Wernicke-Korsakoff syndrome, in which damage occurs in frontal cortical areas and subcortical limbic areas, the majority of patients exhibit a placid and apathetic personality.[35] Granted that this is primarily a cognitive impairment syndrome, but it demonstrates how alcohol may, in addition, affect personality.

CANNABIS

The so-called amotivational syndrome associated with chronic cannabis use has been described in the Middle East, the Orient, and the United States.[21, 27] This syndrome is characterized by apathy and a diminished interest in activities and goals. The impact of the drug's pharmacology on motivation and performance varies according to individual personality patterns and the social milieu. Controversy exists about the importance of preexisting psychopathology in patients such as those with preexisting passive/dependent personality traits. In some users, cannabis clearly causes decreased motivation and worsening of performance on complex tasks. However, this may be related to altered concentration, impaired short-term memory, and decreased energy levels from the residual effects of marijuana.

PHENCYCLIDINE AND OTHER HALLUCINOGENS

Chronic personality changes with a shift in attitudes and evidence of magical thinking may occur after the use of hallucinogens.[21] Hallucinogenic drugs interact with the brain and personality in various nonspecific ways that may particularly impair developing adolescents.

Hallucinogen Persisting Perception Disorder

Only a small proportion of hallucinogen and cannabis users experience flashbacks in which the original drug experience is recreated with perceptual (time) and reality distortion.[21, 27] These may be pleasant or distressing and may occur spontaneously a number of weeks or months after the original drug experience. Flashbacks are usually brief events, lasting seconds to hours, often precipitated by stress, use of other drugs, or environmental stimuli that are reminiscent of the earlier original hallucinogenic experience.

The course of flashbacks is to decrease in intensity, frequency, and duration over time. In patients who experience flashbacks for more than a year after the original experience, an addiction-independent psychiatric disorder should be considered.

Conclusion

The most common substance-induced psychiatric syndromes have been presented and discussed. These disorders in general are intrinsically difficult to study methodologically because samples are small and based on random occurrence with naturalistic, uncontrolled conditions before presentation and evaluation. In addition, there are population sample difficulties: the use of multiple substances, preexistent axis I and II psychiatric disorders, preexistent brain pathology, self-report reliabilities, and variance in clinical assessment instruments and measures.

The study of these syndromes will continue to occur within the clinical context of assessment, diagnosis, and treatment. Assessments must accurately and reliably examine relevant historical data and current clinical findings in terms of the addiction and psychiatric symptoms. In general, these disorders are time limited and self-remitting with addictions treatment of intoxication and withdrawal and the establishment of sobriety. However, the differential diagnosis must entertain the existence of addiction-independent, idiopathic psychiatric disorders. Recognition and identification of such dual diagnosis patients must be a diagnostic priority because of their increased morbidity and the need for specialized treatment.

ACKNOWLEDGMENTS

The author would like to thank Gwendolyn Armster for assistance in manuscript preparation.

REFERENCES

1. American Psychiatric Association: Diagnostic and Statistical Manual of Mental Disorders, 4th ed. Washington, DC, American Psychiatric Association, 1994.
2. Schuckit MA, Monteiro MG: Alcoholism, anxiety and depression. Br J Addict 83:1373–1380, 1988.
3. Kulick AR, Ahmed I: Substance-induced organic mental disorders. Gen Hosp Psychiatry 8:168–172, 1986.
4. Monroe RR: Limbic ictus and atypical psychosis. J Nerv Ment Dis 170(12):711–716, 1982.
5. Post R, Kopanda R: Cocaine, kindling and psychosis. Am J Psychiatry 133:6, 1975.
6. Ballenger JC, Post RM: Kindling as a model for alcohol withdrawal syndromes. Br J Psychiatry 133:1–14, 1978.
7. Weiss RD, Mirin SM: The dual diagnosis alcoholic: Evaluation and treatment. Psychiatr Ann 19(5):261–265, 1989.
8. Reigier DA, Farmer ME, Rae DS, et al: Comorbidity of mental disorders with alcohol and other drug abuse: Results from the Epidemiologic Catchment Area (ECA) study. JAMA 264:2511–2518, 1990.
9. Weiss RD, Mirin SM, Frances RJ: The myth of the typical dual diagnosis patient. Hosp Community Psychiatry 43(2):107–108, 1992.
10. Lehman AF, Meyers CP, Corty E: Assessment and classification of patients with psychiatric and substance abuse syndromes. Hosp Community Psychiatry 40(10):1019–1025, 1989.
11. McKenna C, Ross C: Diagnostic conundrums in substance abusers with psychiatric symptoms: Variables suggestive of dual diagnosis. Am J Drug Alcohol Abuse 20(4):397–412, 1994.
12. Schuckit MA: The history of psychotic symptoms in alcoholics. J Clin Psychiatry 43(2):53–57, 1982.
13. Surawicz FG: Alcoholic hallucinosis: A missed diagnosis—differential diagnosis and management. Can J Psychiatry 25(1):57–63, 1980.
14. Strub RL, Black FW: Organic Brain Syndromes: An Introduction to Neurobehavioral Disorders. Philadelphia, FA Davis, 1981.
15. Cutting J: Hearing voices: May be normal but happens most commonly in schizophrenia and alcoholic hallucinosis. Br Med J 298(6676):769–770, 1989.
16. Albert M, Silvers KN: Perceptual characteristics distinguishing auditory hallucinations in schizophrenia and acute alcoholic psychoses. Am J Psychiatry 127(3):74–78, 1970.
17. Schuckit MA: Drug and Alcohol Abuse: A Clinical Guide to Diagnosis and Treatment. New York, Plenum, 1989.
18. Satel SL, Edell WS: Cocaine-induced paranoia and psychosis proneness. Am J Psychiatry 148:12, 1991.
19. Weinrieb RM, O'Brien CP: Persistent cognitive deficits attributed to substance abuse. Neurol Clin 11(3):663–691, 1993.
20. Khajawall AM: Characteristics of chronic phencyclidine abusers. Am J Drug Alcohol Abuse 8:301–310, 1981.
21. Lowinson JH, Ruiz P, Millman RB, Langrod JG: Substance Abuse: A Comprehensive Textbook. Baltimore, Williams & Wilkins, 1992.
22. Levinson I, Galynker II, Rosenthal RN: Methadone withdrawal psychosis. J Clin Psychiatry 56:73–76, 1995.
23. Fishbain DA, Goldberg M, Rosomoff RS, et al: Atypical withdrawal syndrome (organic delusional syndrome) secondary to oxycodone detoxification (letter). J Clin Psychopharmacol 8:441–442, 1988.
24. Harris B, Harper M: Psychosis after dextropropoxyphene (letter). Lancet 2:743, 1979.
25. Fruensgaard K, Vaaaf UH: Withdrawal psychosis following dextropropoxyphene. Ugeskr Laeger 137:631–632, 1975.
26. Group for the Advancement of Psychiatry Committee on Alcoholism and Addictions: Substance abuse disorders: A psychiatric priority. Am J Psychiatry 148(10):1291–1300, 1991.
27. Francis RJ, Miller SI (eds): Substance abuse and mental illness. In Clinical Textbook of Addictive Disorders. New York, Guilford Press, 1991.
28. Dakis CA, Gold MS: Depression in opiate addicts. In Mirin SM (ed): Substance Abuse and Psychopathology. Washington DC, American Psychiatric Association, 1984.
29. Dulit RA, Fyer MR, Haas GL, et al: Substance use in borderline personality disorder. Psychiatry 147:1002–1004, 1990.
30. Vaillant GE: Adaptation to Life. Boston, Little, Brown & Company, 1977.
31. Vaillant GE: Ego Mechanisms of Defense: A Guide for Clinicians and Researchers. Washington, DC, American Psychiatric Association, 1992.
32. Vaillant GE: A twelve-year follow-up of New York narcotic addicts, IV: Some characteristics and determinants of abstinence. Am J Psychiatry 123:573–584, 1966.
33. Parson OA, Nixon SJ: Neurobehavioral sequelae of alcoholism. Neurol Clin 11(1):205–217, 1993.
34. Adams RD, Victor M: Principles of Neurology. New York, McGraw-Hill, 1985.
35. Victor M, Adams RD, Collins GH: The Wernicke-Korsakoff Syndrome and Related Neurologic Disorders Due to Alcoholism and Malnutrition. Philadelphia, FA Davis, 1989.

Differential Diagnosis of Substance Abuse and Dependence

Dennis Beedle, MD

Social norms are shifting, and concern about substance disorders is increasing. Addictive substances are increasingly thought of as primary pathogens, rather than the abuse of substances being indicative of other psychopathology or as part of normal adolescent development.[1] Substance abuse and dependence are the primary issues related to a wide variety of behavioral, medical, and family problems. Increased cooperation and sharing of knowledge between the addiction field and psychiatry have led to greater appreciation and improved treatment of comorbid addictive and psychiatric illnesses. The increase in consumer-based self-help in psychiatry follows in the footsteps of 12-step programs. The similarities between the nature of chronic mental illness and addictions have been noted.[2]

The direct and indirect costs of substance abuse and dependence are enormous.[3] Appreciation of this has made earlier diagnosis of these problems very important, because treatment efforts that change behaviors before an individual is disabled may reduce the direct and indirect costs to individuals, families, businesses, and all levels of government.

Substance abuse disorders and addictions present with various medical, interpersonal, and social dysfunctions. The treatment of addictions has evolved from a self-help basis as developed in the 12-step program of Alcoholics Anonymous (AA). From the perspective of AA, psychiatric treatment and evaluation were viewed, at best, as adjunctive to the process of recovery. At worst, it was believed that psychiatric care could interfere with the process of recovery, and the long-term prescription of habituating psychotropics and poor understanding of the addictive illnesses by psychiatrists supported that perception.[4]

Identification of addiction now occurs in various settings and levels of care. The setting in which an addiction first presents can have an impact on the likelihood of receiving proper diagnosis and treatment interventions. Only widespread educational efforts will allow for early diagnosis and intervention. In some settings, the appropriate treatment strategies are not yet clearly developed, allowing the opportunity for innovative program development.

The Diagnostic Setting

The diagnosis of addiction was traditionally made in specialty inpatient units that dealt exclusively with addictive disorders. Patients would be admitted because of pressure from family and employers after the addiction had caused overwhelming dysfunction of the individual at home and work. The primary focus of these units was alcoholism. The length of stay was a standard 30 days, based on the maximum benefit period provided by insurance and the belief that relapse rates could be reduced by prolonging the period of abstinence before discharge. These units began to have a broader addictive focus and more individualized treatment length. Despite these changes, many have closed because of major reductions in insurance coverage for inpatient addictions treatment and studies that failed to show significant benefit from long-term inpatient treatment of addictive disorders.[5, 6]

Better understanding of the nature of the addictive process as a chronic illness with the need for intermittent interventions has led to the development of services that provide different levels of care depending on the acuity of need of a patient's illness. Patients are gradually moved to less intense levels of care, with the expectation that they will continue a lifelong involvement in an appropriate 12-step program.[7]

Cost containment has led to the shift of providing addictions treatment on an outpatient basis. A group of addicted patients are not well served by the unlocked inpatient addiction unit and are even less well served by outpatient-oriented services. The result is that severely addicted patients increasingly find themselves hospitalized in general psychiatric units. These units usually lack the knowledge and motivation to successfully initiate treatment for these patients, and referral to inpatient addictions treatment programs is no longer an option owing to insurance limitations.

In the past, when and if the diagnosis of addiction was made on a traditional psychiatric unit, the patient was referred to treatment at an addiction program. Addicted patients were sometimes thought of as self-medicating for a primary psychiatric disorder.[8] This thinking justified focusing efforts on the psychiatric disorder with the expectation that the substance abuse and dependence would normalize if the primary problem were treated and brought under better control. Formal diagnosis of the addictive or abuse disorder might result in psychiatric treatment not being reimbursed or provided. Psychiatric units and staff generally lacked the training and skills to make the diagnosis of substance dependence. Although the disease model was acknowledged, the reality commonly was that addicted patients were primarily thought of as manipulating themselves into psychiatric units for secondary gains.

Increased understanding of the comorbidity of addictions and other mental illnesses has led to active efforts to treat dually diagnosed patients.[2] The belief persists that primarily addicted patients are manipulating themselves onto psychiatric units rather than suffering from a disorder that often presents with risk of harm to themselves or others. It is clear that addictive disorders, including alcoholism, are significant causes of suicide attempts and completed suicides.[9, 10] They also represent a significant source of potential and actual violence toward others.[11] It is difficult to imagine these patients being effectively or safely treated in an unlocked setting. The reality is that incarceration after criminal activity or involuntary hospitalization is the only way that some addicts stop active use of the addictive substance. However, substance use may continue in both psychiatric hospitals and jails.[12] Despite widespread belief to the contrary, patients coerced into treatment do not differ significantly in long-term outcome from patients seeking treatment voluntarily.[13]

Efforts have recently been made to provide accurate and nonprejudicial diagnosis and treatment of addictions and substance abuse issues on psychiatric units. This effort is furthered by managed care companies that reimburse care based on intensity of care required rather than diagnosis. These patients have generally been hospitalized on locked psychiatric units because safety could not be maintained on an unlocked addiction unit. Stabilization of seriously suicidal or homicidal patients is inappropriate in an unlocked setting. Completed suicides do occur on detoxification units, and a patient with suicidal ideation must often be cleared by a psychiatrist before admission to an addictions program.

Medical and surgical service personnel often are able to diagnose addictions but lack knowledge about the natural history and treatment of addictive disorders. Significant prejudicial treatment and blaming of the patient or family have led some patients and families to feel that these issues are best not revealed to a physician. Compounding these problems is that addictive illness has not been routinely studied as a disease process as part of the standard medical school curriculum.[14]

Managed care companies have increasingly demanded that primary care physicians manage detoxification through medical services. The cost effectiveness as compared with specialized care is unknown. The traditional medical service does not provide addictions services that begin the behavioral aspect of treatment while patients are hospitalized. Medical and surgical services are currently best served by a consulting model of addiction services that parallels the traditional psychiatric consulting model.[15] The process of education can be both an informal and formal one. Over time, increased efforts to include addictions training in undergraduate medical education will increase the ability of all physicians to recognize and effectively intervene in addictive disorders.

Patients with addictions issues may present to outpatient psychiatric services with chief complaints related to interpersonal, academic, or work-related issues. In the past, the diagnosis may not have been made, owing to theories of self-medication, lack of knowledge about the diagnosis, and the tendency not to obtain a collateral history. As chemical dependence services have moved to outpatient settings, an understanding of the need for a focus on addictive illness in outpatient psychiatric services has increased.[16]

Substance abuse is rampant among college-age adults. These abuse issues have been normalized as part of the rite of passage of young adulthood. Only recently have questions been raised about the wisdom of not addressing these issues as health-related problems. Many addicted patients are clearly able to be identified retrospectively, with the onset of their addictions occurring during college or earlier in high school.[17] Student counseling centers have not traditionally examined the relationship between substance abuse and students presenting with interpersonal, social, and school performance problems.[18]

In systems where patients are referred prescreened with a probable diagnosis of addiction, confirmation of the diagnosis and screening for psychiatric and medical comorbidity are needed. A patient may occasionally be believed to have an addiction, which is later found not to be the cause of the presenting problems. Underrecognition of addictions remains the far more frequent problem.

Frontline screening and tentative diagnosis are made by employee assistance plans. These plans increasingly are the gatekeepers for both psychiatric and chemical dependence services. Employee assistance plans may provide treatment for patients with both psychiatric problems and chemical dependence on a short-term basis and refer longer-term or more impaired clients to other providers.

Primary physicians are the initial providers of medical services and the gatekeepers for specialty services. Accurate diagnosis and initial treatment strategies are difficult, given the short amount of time that most systems allow primary physicians to see patients and the inherent resistance of patients to reveal the problems related to substance use. These problems may not be recognized until relatively advanced medical complications occur.

The differential diagnosis of substance abuse and dependence is complicated by the wide variety of settings in which these disorders first present. The tendency for mental health professionals and patients to rationalize use and abuse of addictive substances contributes to the difficulty of the diagnostic process.

Diagnosis

DSM-IV uses the concept of substance-related disorders and describes use and induced disorders for each of the major categories of addictive substances. Use disorders are divided into dependence and abuse disorders. Dependence may be further specified by noting the presence or absence of physiological dependence.[19]

Use disorders are described for alcohol, amphetamine, cannabis, cocaine, hallucinogen, inhalant, nicotine, opioid, phencyclidine, sedative-hypnotic or anxiolytic, and polysubstance or unknown substance disorders. Induced disorders include intoxication, withdrawal, intoxication delirium, withdrawal delirium, persisting dementia, persisting amnestic disorder, psychotic disorder, mood disorder, anxiety disorder, sexual dysfunction, sleep disorder, and persisting perception disorder.

Substance dependence is diagnosed when three of the following criteria are noted in a 12-month period: (1) tolerance; (2) withdrawal or use of the substance to avoid withdrawal; (3) compulsive use; (4) unsuccessful effort to decrease or discontinue use; (5) major focus of time and life; (6) social, occupational, or recreational activities given up; and (7) continued use despite recognized psychological or physical problems related to or worsened by continued use.

Substance abuse is diagnosed when one or more of the following criteria are met and criteria for dependence are not met: (1) recurrent substance use leading to failure to fulfill major role obligations at work, school, or home; (2) use that puts the individual in physical danger; (3) legal problems related to use; and (4) adverse social and interpersonal consequences.

The 12-step program model does not explicitly diagnose its members but clearly believes in the disease model. Fundamental concepts used by AA and other 12-step programs overlap with DSM-IV and have influenced its development. For instance, DSM-IV criteria of loss of control over drinking despite efforts to cut back or stop, as well as inability to stop or to modify addictive use despite dire consequences, are summarized in the first step of the 12-step program: "We admitted we were powerless over alcohol and that our lives had become unmanageable."[20]

Differential Diagnosis

Acute and chronic toxicity of addictive substances often mimics and overlaps with other primary psychiatric disorders. Therefore, included in the differential diagnosis are affective disorders, psychotic disorders, personality disorders, and anxiety disorders. The adolescent age group includes the foregoing, plus conduct disorder, poor school performance, truancy, pregnancy, and criminal involvement. In children affected by neglect or abuse, addiction in the caregiver should be considered and is likely.

Adequate identification of patients with comorbid psychiatric and addictive disorders requires careful history taking, including a collateral history from family members, significant others, courts, schools, and other professionals involved with the patient. Prior hospital and clinic records may also reveal history supportive of an addictive disorder.[21] Patients who resist efforts to obtain a collateral history should raise suspicions about an overt addiction history that the patient is reluctant to acknowledge but others who know the patient could readily provide. Clinicians must recognize that patients and some families deny, minimize, distort, and lie about substance use disorders. Vague or incomplete responses require an examiner to be concrete in terms of questions related to the substance use and the relationship with dysfunctions in a patient's life. Urine toxicology screening should be routinely ordered as part of the workup in outpatient and inpatient settings. This is especially important when patients are presenting in crisis.[22] When results of the screening are positive, a high degree of suspicion should be raised about an addiction disorder.

When a patient presents with a depressive syndrome and evidence exists that the patient has active substance use, a minimum 72-hour delay before starting antidepressant treatment is indicated to allow for improvement in organic mood disorders. This is especially indicated when urine toxicology is positive for drugs associated with organic mood disorders. Cocaine, alcohol, and psychostimulants all cause depressive syndromes that may rapidly resolve without specific pharmacological interventions. For patients with alcoholism, a 2-week delay is preferable before starting antidepressant medication treatment. Rapidly introducing antidepressant treatment may confuse the diagnostic issues, reinforce addicts' belief that their drug or alcohol use is not the cause of the mood disorder, and reinforce a "better living through chemistry attitude," which undermines the importance of abstinence in later treatment efforts.

Psychotic presentations usually require immediate pharmacological intervention. Treatment should be targeted toward symptoms and syndromes. Rapid and complete resolution of psychotic symptoms should heighten suspicion about the presence of a primary addictive disorder. Medication treatment may be discontinued in approximately 4 weeks if the patient remains abstinent. Return of the psychotic symptoms while the patient is abstinent, as confirmed by urine toxicology screening and collateral history, suggests the likelihood of a true dual diagnosis. Certain psychotic disorders linked to alcoholism and drug dependence may be persistent and result in long-term psychiatric symptoms. These organic disorders qualify patients for inclusion in the category of dual diagnosis, and they most likely will not fare well in a primary addiction treatment program.

The diagnosis of personality disorder is difficult to establish in patients with active substance abuse or dependence. If it is possible to examine a patient's life and relationships before the substance abuse began, it may be possible to identify preexisting character pathology. Definitive diagnosis of character pathology is best undertaken after several months of sobriety. Occasionally, a patient's character disorder diagnosis significantly interferes with the process of recovery and involvement in addictions treatment. Antisocial, narcissistic, borderline, and paranoid patients are particularly likely to have difficulty with the large group format of 12-step programs.[23]

The 12-step approach acknowledges and focuses on the issue of character defects. The fourth step, which consists of taking a fearless moral inventory, is a particularly difficult step for severely disordered patients. These patients may benefit from individual treatment with a therapist knowledgeable about addictive disorders. The more common presentation is for a patient to present to individual therapy in a state of crisis related to psychiatric symptoms or interpersonal dysfunction and for the addictive issues to become evident only after treatment is under way. Individual treatment may need to precede the referral to addictions treatment and 12-step involvement. The issue of regression is an important one for the treatment of patients with addictions. Patients are often capable of functioning at a higher level when sober but become overwhelmed by affects, especially anger and sadness, while under the influence. This regression is compounded by the organic cognitive and personality changes that accompany long-standing addiction and acute intoxication.

The complaint of anxiety and panic is frequently expressed by patients with addictive disorders, especially alcoholism.[24] These patients may be prescribed benzodiazipines, which generally do not relieve the complaints. They commonly begin to complain about the ineffectiveness of the treatment yet demand further increase in the dose. Abuse of and dependence on other addictive substances continues, and the prescribing physician is placed in a difficult position because the patient feels that the prescribed medications are ineffective and that self-medication therefore is the only option. Another sign of probable addiction is simultaneous prescription of other medications and hypnotics by other physicians that the patient does not reveal to the physiatrist or prescribing physician. The diagnosis of an independent anxiety disorder requires a sustained period of abstinence and recovery of at least three months. The use of a nonbenzodiazepine psychotropic may be helpful, but behavioral therapies and interventions are a better first-line treatment. Patients often express a strong preference for pharmacological interventions, even if other pharmacological agents have been ineffective or harmful.

Addicted patients may present in an acutely delirious condition. The classical presentation of delirium tremens is generally recognized and is widely taught because of the high mortality rate if not properly diagnosed and treated. Other causes of delirium are acute intoxication and chronic conditions such as end-stage liver disease. Head injury is a common complication of addiction, and due diligence is required not to attribute all delirious presentations to secondary to delirium tremens.

The most problematic presentation of addiction is dementia.[25] This is most often encountered in advanced cases of alcoholism and in cocaine addiction. Avoidance of further substance use is essential to prevent further cognitive decline but is difficult even in advanced cases, because procuring and use of the substance is an overlearned behavior for most of these patients, who, despite significant cognitive declines and limitations, are still able to procure and use their substance of choice.

Addictions commonly present in primary care as sleep disorders or mood disorders. They may also present as chronic pain disorders, especially when a physician is enlisted to prescribe hypnotics, sedatives, and narcotics. Associated medical problems that addicted patients may seek help for include gastritis, hepatitis, human immunodeficiency virus infection, sexually transmitted diseases, cerebrovascular accidents, and traumatic injuries. These presenting problems may be the primary complaint of a patient but may be secondary to long-standing substance dependence. Careful focus on addictive issues in history taking and collateral history may reveal underlying addictive illness.

Family and marital dysfunction may be the presenting problem but may not be identified by the family or couple as an issue, especially if several family members are involved or if both members of the couple are addicted. Child abuse or neglect may be the primary presentation of addiction in parents or caregivers. A multitude of marital and child dysfunctions can be the presenting problem for a addicted spouse or child.

Summary

The differential diagnosis for substance abuse and dependence is a difficult but important skill for all physicians. Given the high prevalence of substance abuse and dependence in our society, physicians, therapists, counselors, and educators in a wide number of disciplines and settings must be aware of the high potential for patients, coworkers, clients, and students to be afflicted with chemical dependence or abuse problems. Addiction presents with diverse psychiatric symptoms and syndromes. Early recognition requires sensitivity and alertness from a wide variety of professionals, because early difficulties may first present at school, work, primary care, the court system, or a social agency.

Acknowledgment and understanding of the serious potential for violence and suicide among addictive patients and the growing understanding of the neurobiological basis of addiction will lead to integrated treatment programs in which addiction is seen and treated as a mental illness with a specific etiology, natural history, and treatment strategies.

REFERENCES

1. Baily GW: Current perspectives on substance abuse in youth. J Am Acad Child Adolesc Psychiatry 28(2):151–162, 1989.
2. Minkoff K: An integrated treatment model for dual diagnosis of psychosis and addiction. Hosp Community Psychiatry 40:1031–1036, 1989.
3. Rice DP, Kleman S, Miller LS: Estimates of economic costs of alcohol and drug abuse and mental illness, 1985 and 1988. Public Health Rep 106(3):280–292, 1991.
4. Decker KP, Ries RK: Differential diagnosis and psychopharmacology of dual disorders. Psychiatr Clin North Am 16(4):703–718, 1993.
5. McCrady BS, Longabaugh EF, Beattie M, et al: Cost effectiveness of alcoholism treatment in partial hospital versus inpatient settings after brief inpatient treatment 12-month outcomes. J Consult Clin Psychol 54(5):708–713, 1986.
6. Annis HM: Is inpatient rehabilitation of the alcoholic cost effective con position? National Association on Drug Abuse Problems scientific approach 1984. Adv Alcohol Subst Abuse 5(1–2):175–190, 1985–1986.
7. Hoffmann NG, Miller NS: Treatment outcome for abstinence based program. Psychiatr Ann 22(8):402–408, 1992.
8. Khantzian EJ: The self-medication hypothesis of addiction disorders from heroin and cocaine dependence. Am J Psychiatry 142:1259–1264, 1985.
9. Miller NS, Mahler JC, Gold MS: Suicide risks associated with drug and alcohol dependence. J Addict Dis 10(3):49–61, 1992.
10. Murphy GE: Suicide and substance abuse. Arch Gen Psychiatry 45:593–594, 1988.
11. Weisz JR, Martin SL, Walter BR, et al: Differential prediction of young adult arrest for property and personal crimes: Findings of a cohort follow-up study of violent boys from North Carolina's Willie M Program. J Child Psychol Psychiatry 32(5):783–792, 1991.
12. Sobell LC, Sobell MB, Maisto SA, et al: Alcohol and drug use by alcohol and drug abusers when incarcerated: Clinical and research implications. Addict Behav 8:88–92, 1983.
13. Watson CG, Brown K, Tilleskjor C, et al: The comparative recidivism rates of voluntary and coerced-admission male alcoholics. J Clin Psychol 44(4):573–581, 1988.
14. Goldsmith RJ, Miller NS: Training psychiatric residents in the addictions. Psychiatr Ann 24(8):432–439, 1994.
15. Spelman J: Interventions for hospitalized addicted patients through psychiatric consultation. Psychiatr Ann 24(8):424–426, 1994.
16. Silverman DC, O'Neill SF, Cleary PD, et al: Recognition of alcohol abuse in psychiatric outpatients and its effect on treatment. Hosp Community Psychiatry 40:644–646, 1992.
17. Helzer J, Burnam A: Epidemiology of alcohol addiction: United States. In Miller NS, ed: Comprehensive Handbook of Drug and Alcohol Addiction. New York, Marcel Dekker, 1991, pp 9–38.
18. Frances RJ, Bucky S, Alexopoulos GS: Outcome study of familial and non-familial alcoholism. Am J Psychiatry 141:1469–1471, 1984.
19. American Psychiatric Association: Diagnostic and Statistical Manual of Mental Disorders, 4th ed. Washington, DC, American Psychiatric Association, 1994.
20. Alcoholic Anonymous, 3rd ed. New York, World Services, 1976.
21. Anthenelli RM: The initial evaluation of the dual diagnosis patient. Psychiatr Ann 24(8):407–411, 1994.
22. Sanguineti VR, Brooks MO: Factors related to emergency commitment of chronic mentally ill patients who are substance abusers. Hosp Community Psychiatry 43:237–241, 1992.
23. Blume SB: Dual diagnosis: Psychoactive substance dependence and the personality disorders. J Psychoactive Drugs 21(2):139–144, 1989.
24. Schuckit MA, Hesselbrock V: Alcohol dependence and anxiety disorders: What is the relationship? Am J Psychiatry 151(12):1723–1734, 1994.
25. Cummings JL: Dementia syndromes: Neurobehavioral and neuropsychiatric features. J Clin Psychiatry 48(Suppl 5):3–8, 1987.

A Basic Clinical Approach to Diagnosis in Patients with Comorbid Psychiatric and Substance Use Disorders

Robert M. Anthenelli, MD

Mental health workers have started to pay more attention to the role of substance use disorders in many psychiatric complaints. Within the past half decade, two major epidemiological surveys[1, 2] have documented high rates of comorbid psychiatric and addictive disorders ranging from 15% to 40%. In addition, the Diagnostic and Statistical Manual of Mental Disorders, 4th edition (DSM-IV), now contains specific *substance-induced* psychiatric disorders in each of the major categories of mental illness.[3] Similarly, thanks to the concerted efforts of groups such as the Committee on Alcoholism and the Addictions[4] and the Committee on Training and Education in Addiction Psychiatry, the American Psychiatric Association has issued an official action statement acknowledging what workers in the field have long known: "The prevalence of substance abuse and dependence among general psychiatric patients is one of the major health problems confronting the mental health field today."[5] Taken together, these developments are signs that psychiatry is committed to becoming more active in addressing the special needs of patients with comorbid psychiatric and substance use problems.

This clinically oriented chapter presents some general guidelines useful in the assessment and diagnosis of patients who have some combination of a psychiatric and substance use problem. For heuristic purposes, this practical approach to assessment and diagnosis is then applied in three clinical case scenarios: (1) antisocial behavior, (2) psychosis, and (3) mood disturbance. The case examples have been designed to illustrate the major principles outlined next.

A Basic Approach to Diagnosis

Figure 12–1 illustrates a basic approach to diagnosis in individuals presenting with some combination of psychiatric and possible substance use problems. The following sections explain the rationale behind each step in this decision-making process.

PROBE FOR ALCOHOL AND DRUG PROBLEMS WHEN EVALUATING ALL PSYCHIATRIC COMPLAINTS

Analyzing data from the Epidemiologic Catchment Area study, Helzer and Przybeck

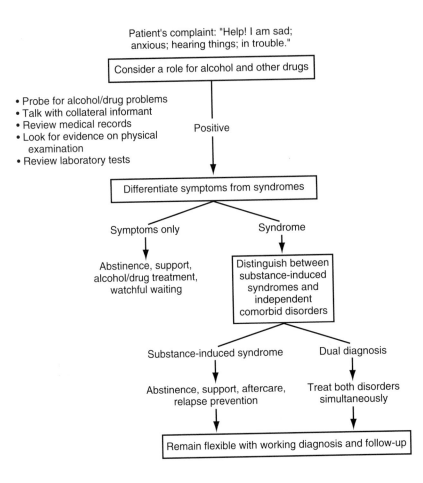

Patient's complaint: "Help! I am sad; anxious; hearing things; in trouble."

Consider a role for alcohol and other drugs

- Probe for alcohol/drug problems
- Talk with collateral informant
- Review medical records
- Look for evidence on physical examination
- Review laboratory tests

Positive

Differentiate symptoms from syndromes

Symptoms only

Abstinence, support, alcohol/drug treatment, watchful waiting

Syndrome

Distinguish between substance-induced syndromes and independent comorbid disorders

Substance-induced syndrome

Abstinence, support, aftercare, relapse prevention

Dual diagnosis

Treat both disorders simultaneously

Remain flexible with working diagnosis and follow-up

Figure 12–1. Initial assessment of patients presenting with psychiatric and possible substance use problems.

showed that the co-occurrence of psychological and alcohol problems is more likely to lead an individual to seek help at a clinic.[6] This principle contributes, in part, to the high rates of comorbidity found in clinical populations. For example, in a sample of substance abusers seeking treatment, Ross and colleagues found lifetime rates of psychiatric conditions to be as high as 80%, with almost two thirds of the patients currently fulfilling DSM-III-R criteria for some additional psychiatric diagnosis.[7]

Although patients with two or more problems are more likely to visit mental healthcare providers and use services, they seldom volunteer information about their alcohol and drug use patterns when they present their psychiatric complaints.[6] Unless asked directly about their use of alcohol and other drugs, patients' denial and minimization of their substance-related problems keep this important information buried, making assessment and diagnosis difficult.[8] In addition to patients' denial of their drug problems, certain drugs (e.g., central nervous system [CNS] depressants such as alcohol) impair memory and make history taking less reliable.[9] Therefore, when assessing patients with possible substance use problems, clinicians should gather information from several resources.[8, 10]

After obtaining a patient's permission, the history should be obtained from both the patient and a collateral informant (usually a relative or close friend).[8, 10] Such a collateral informant interview serves several purposes. First, by establishing how patterns of alcohol and drug use relate to psychological symptoms and their time course, a clinician obtains additional information to be used in the longitudinal evaluation of psychiatric and substance use problems described later. Second, by defining the role of substance use in a patient's psychological complaints, the clinician is starting to confront some of the patient's denial, the defense mechanism that helps keep these associations out of mind.[8, 11] Third, by knowing that a clinician will be talking to a family member, patients might be more likely to offer more accurate information. Fourth, patients observe that the clinician is interested enough in their case to contact family members, helping to establish the therapeutic alliance. Finally, by involving family members early in the course of treatment, the physician begins laying the groundwork toward establishing a network that will become an important part of the patient's recovery program.[12]

Medical records are another potentially rich source of information.[8] This review of the medical record should look for evidence of previous psychiatric contacts or laboratory results (e.g., positive urine toxicology screens, elevations in markers of heavy drinking such as gamma-glutamyltransferse [GGT], mean corpuscular volume, and so forth) that might further implicate a role for alcohol or other drugs in the patient's psychiatric problems.[13] For instance, previous documentation of repeated admissions for brief psychotic episodes in a patient whose urine toxicology screens were also positive for methamphetamine would raise the clinician's level of suspicion that drugs are likely an important causative factor in the patient's new complaints.

Laboratory tests including chemistry profiles and liver panels, complete blood count, and urine or blood toxicology screens should be performed to search for evidence of alcohol or drug use that might aid assessment.[13, 14] Because most drugs of abuse have short half-lives and cannot be detected in blood or urine more than 24 hours after the drug was last used, it is important to obtain the toxicology screens at the time of the initial presentation of psychiatric complaints.[15] These results might also provide indirect evidence of tolerance to alcohol or drugs if the clinician documents relatively normal cognitive, behavioral, and psychomotor performance in the presence of very high blood alcohol or drug concentrations that would usually render most individuals markedly impaired.[13] Subsequent laboratory testing might also need to include other diagnostic procedures (e.g., brain imaging studies and so forth) to rule out indirect alcohol- and drug-related organic causes of the psychiatric complaints. For example, alcoholics suffering head trauma might present with subdural hematomas or other traumatic brain injuries causing psychiatric symptoms and signs.

Finally, all patients should undergo a complete physical examination.[8] Attention should be paid to physical manifestations of heavy alcohol and other drug use such as injected sclerae, enlarged tender liver, or needle track marks. The combination of positive results on laboratory testing and physical examination points strongly to a diagnosis of substance abuse or dependence. This information can be used later on when the physician presents his or her diagnosis to the patient and starts to confront the denial associated with the addiction.

HEAVY ALCOHOL OR OTHER DRUG USE CAUSES PSYCHIATRIC SYMPTOMS AND SIGNS

Alcohol and other drugs of abuse cross the blood-brain barrier and produce changes in mood, perception, psychovegetative state, and behavior.[8, 16] These agents produce their mind-altering and reinforcing effects by causing changes in the same neurotransmitter and receptor systems associated with most major psychiatric disease states.[17] Partly as a result of these direct CNS effects, heavy alcohol or other drug use causes psychiatric symptoms and signs and mimics most major psychiatric disorders. These changes occur in various contexts, and during the initial assessment the clinician should determine when in the patient's drinking and drug use cycle (i.e., intoxication, acute withdrawal, protracted withdrawal, stable abstinence) these complaints are occurring.[8]

Using psychosis as an example, heavy, prolonged *intoxication* with a CNS stimulant drug such as cocaine frequently leads to persecutory delusions and auditory hallucinations that, if viewed only cross-sectionally, can resemble a psychotic disorder. A similar clinical picture is seen in some cases of depressant *withdrawal*, which may or may not be accompanied by delirium. In both of these instances, the psychosis is likely a result of acute pharmacological effects of the drugs on brain functioning as well as more chronic changes associated with recurrent alcohol and drug use. Therefore, clinicians need to probe for alcohol and drug problems and determine in which context the psychiatric symptoms and signs have developed.

DIFFERENTIATE ALCOHOL- AND DRUG-RELATED SYMPTOMS FROM SYNDROMIC MENTAL DISORDERS

Because of the propensity for heavy alcohol and drug use to cause psychological disturbances, when patients come to the clinic for help with co-occurring psychiatric and substance use problems, two *independent* diagnoses are not necessarily implicated. The preferred definition of *diagnosis* used here refers to a constellation of symptoms and signs, or syndrome, with a generally predictable course and duration of illness as outlined by DSM-IV.

Thus, it is the clinician's job to synthesize the data obtained from the multiple resources cited earlier and to put together a working diagnosis. It can be helpful to differentiate between substance-related symptoms and signs and substance-induced syndromes. The latter designation is now being used in DSM-IV to designate symptoms that "are in excess of those usually associated with the intoxication or withdrawal syndrome" and that "are sufficiently severe to warrant independent clinical attention."[3]

Although heavy, prolonged use of alcohol and other drugs can produce psychiatric symptoms or, at times, more severe and protracted substance-induced psychiatric syndromes, these substance-related conditions are likely to improve markedly with abstinence, unlike the major independent psychiatric disorders they mimic.[8, 16] Perhaps the best empirical evidence documenting that alcohol-induced psychiatric conditions generally abate with conservative treatment within 2 to 4 weeks can be garnered from studies assessing depression and anxiety in recently abstinent alcoholics. Studies by Brown and Schuckit[18, 19] and others[20] have demonstrated that the course of these alcohol-induced psychiatric syndromes differs from frank independent major psychiatric disorders and that symptoms are not diagnoses.

In summary, alcohol and other drugs of abuse can cause signs and symptoms of depression, anxiety, psychosis, and antisocial behavior in the context of intoxication or withdrawal. At times, these symptoms and signs cluster, last for weeks despite abstinence, and mimic frank psychiatric disorders (i.e., are substance-induced syndromes). These substance-related conditions usually disappear after days to weeks of abstinence. Prematurely labeling them as major depression, panic disorder, schizophrenia, or antisocial personality disorder (APD) can lead to misdiagnosis and inattention to a patient's principal problem with alcohol and other drugs.[8]

DISTINGUISH SUBSTANCE-INDUCED SYNDROMES VERSUS INDEPENDENT COMORBID DISORDERS

Making proper diagnosis more difficult is evidence demonstrating that individuals with APD, schizophrenia, and bipolar disorder have an increased risk of developing alcoholism or other drug abuse.[1, 8] Thus, even after determining that a patient's constellation of symptoms and signs has reached syndromic levels and warrants a label of a substance-induced mood,

anxiety, or psychotic disorder, the possibility remains that the patient has an independent comorbid disorder that might also require treatment. I reserve the dual-diagnosis label for these patients, although there remains controversy about how to treat individuals with more persistent substance-related conditions.[8]

When the symptoms and signs persist long enough and are severe enough to consider the possibility of two independent diagnoses, the approach used in San Diego is to start by determining independent versus substance-induced diagnoses based on the chronology of development of symptom clusters. Using this technique, substance-induced disorders are those conditions in which symptoms and signs cluster in the setting of heavy alcohol or other drug use or withdrawal. For example, patients exhibiting psychiatric symptoms and signs only in the setting of recurrent use of alcohol and after they have developed repeated severe life problems because of its recurrent use (i.e., meet criteria for alcohol abuse or dependence) are likely to have a substance-induced psychiatric condition. In contrast, patients exhibiting symptoms and signs of a psychiatric condition such as bipolar disorder in the absence of problematic use of alcohol and other substances will most likely follow the course typified by bipolar disorder with episodic mood shifts requiring treatment with mood stabilizers.[8, 16, 21]

If it is determined that a patient probably does have two or more diagnoses, then one useful technique is to try to establish a time line of the patient's comorbid conditions.[8, 10, 16] This reconstruction of the clinical history allows one to disentangle the chronological course of the disorder and helps establish substance-induced versus independent diagnoses. Collateral information from outside informants and the data obtained from the review of the medical records are very useful in determining this longitudinal history. Rather than focusing on the age when the patient first imbibed or the time he or she first become intoxicated, instead, the age at which the patient first met criteria for alcohol dependence or drug abuse is noted. This can be approximated by determining when patients developed alcohol or drug problems that interfered in their lives in a major way and affected their ability to function. Probing is typically begun in four areas: (1) legal, (2) social relationships, (3) occupational, and (4) medical.[8, 22] Thus, the onset of alcoholism is denoted by determining the first time that alcohol or drug use actually interfered in two or more of these major domains or the first time an individual received treatment for alcoholism or drug abuse. Further questioning should include whether the patient ever developed *tolerance* to the effects of alcohol and/or other drugs or suffered from signs and symptoms of *withdrawal* when he or she stopped using the substance. At the same time, psychiatric symptoms and signs are reviewed across the life span. Recollection of the chronology of appearance of these problems is improved by framing the interview around important landmarks in time (e.g., the year the patient enlisted in the military, his or her graduation date, military discharge date, and so forth) and by the collateral information obtained. This method not only ensures the most accurate chronological reconstruction of a patient's problems but also, on a therapeutic basis, helps patients see the relationship between their substance abuse and psychological problems and begins to confront some of the denial mechanisms that tend to keep these associations out of mind.[8, 16]

Throughout this chronological history, it is important to probe for any periods of stable abstinence that a patient may have had, noting how this period of sobriety affected the patient's psychiatric problems. Somewhat conservatively, I probe for periods of abstinence of about 3 months' duration because it is common for some mood, psychovegetative, perceptual, and behavioral symptoms and signs to persist in a protracted manner in some alcoholics and drug abusers.[3, 16] By using this time line approach, it is generally possible to arrive at a preliminary working diagnosis that helps to predict the most likely course of the disorder and to begin putting together a treatment plan.[8, 16]

It is important to remain flexible with this working diagnosis and to continue to monitor patients over time.[8, 10] Like most initial psychiatric assessments, this basic approach is hardly foolproof. It is important to monitor a patient's course even if improvement occurs with abstinence and supportive treatment alone during the first weeks of sobriety. Empirical data show a resolution of most major symptoms and signs within the first 4 weeks of abstinence.[19, 20, 23] Therefore, a 2- to 4-week observation period is usually advised before considering the use of any psychotropic medications.

Practical Applications

The following sections demonstrate how this basic approach can be used in assessing the three most prevalent co-occurring clinical scenarios: (1) APD versus substance-induced antisocial behavior, (2) schizophrenia versus substance-induced psychotic disorder, and (3) independent versus substance-induced mood disorder. These comorbid conditions are addressed in detail in other chapters of this textbook and are only briefly discussed here to illustrate the diagnostic decision-making process.

ANTISOCIAL PERSONALITY DISORDER

The mental disorder that is most frequently associated with alcoholism and other substance use disorders is APD.[1, 2] Alcoholics with APD appear to have a more severe course and worse prognosis for their illness than alcoholics without comorbid APD, including having more psychiatric symptoms.[21, 24] Making the diagnosis requires establishing a pattern of antisocial and irresponsible behaviors starting in childhood or early adolescence that predates the onset of alcohol or other drug dependence.[3, 25] Antisocial behavior occurring later in adolescence or adulthood after the onset of multiple alcohol- and drug-related problems is better described as early onset substance dependence with adult antisocial behavior, which might have different treatment implications.[21, 26]

CASE EXAMPLE 1

A 27-year-old man was brought to the emergency room in handcuffs by the police after being arrested and charged with domestic violence. On questioning by the psychiatrist on call, the patient denies any recollection of spousal abuse. He states that he "doesn't remember anything" because he was "in an alcoholic blackout."

The psychiatrist on call obtained a urine toxicology screen that was positive for Δ9-tetrahydrocannabinol (the active ingredient in marijuana), ethanol, and amphetamine. Notably, the patient denies any drug use other than alcohol and states that such would be in violation of his parole.

The childhood developmental history section of the interview is remarkable for a history of truancy starting at age 11 years and frequent fights with peers. The patient admits to shooting birds, squirrels, and cats with pellet guns and states that he was sent to reform school at age 13 after being found guilty of shoplifting. The pattern of violating the rights of others and committing antisocial acts persists into adulthood, as marked by the patient's being jailed repeatedly for assorted crimes including previous spousal abuse charges.

The patient states that he started using alcohol and other drugs at age 13 and that he had his first alcohol-related public intoxication charge at age 16 years. He was expelled from school for being intoxicated in class at age 16, and he was fired from a part-time job at the same age also for being intoxicated. He had his first inpatient alcohol and drug treatment program at age 21 after his dishonorable discharge from the military.

In this instance, the clinician is comfortable making a diagnosis of APD with comorbid alcohol dependence because the pattern of irresponsible and antisocial behaviors developed *before* the onset of alcohol dependence. The use of the urine toxicology screen and medical record to uncover covert drug use and a previous history of spousal abuse charges, respectively, provided important diagnostic information.

The alternative clinical presentation (i.e., early onset alcohol dependence with adult antisocial behavior) would have been marked by the patient's not fulfilling criteria for conduct disorder before the onset of the multiple life problems related to alcohol. It remains unclear, however, how individuals who have early onset of alcohol and drug dependence and who do not fulfill criteria for the APD differ from frank APD alcoholics.[25, 27] Regardless of this nosological distinction, both forms of this early-onset alcoholism appear to be associated with a more severe course of alcohol-related problems.

SCHIZOPHRENIC SPECTRUM DISORDERS VERSUS SUBSTANCE-INDUCED PSYCHOTIC DISORDER

Because alcohol and other drugs can produce symptoms and signs of psychosis in various settings, clinicians frequently face situations in which individuals presenting with psychosis have been using drugs or alcohol. Although in many instances the substance-induced psychotic symptoms and signs are likely to diminish with abstinence and supportive treatment over several weeks, the strong association between schizophrenia and comorbid substance use disorders bears consideration.[1, 28] In order to disentangle the role of alcohol and drugs in patients presenting with psychosis, a clinician must assess the quality, duration, and severity of the psychotic symptoms and signs in relation to alcohol and drug use. Individuals who continue to manifest active and residual signs and symptoms of schizophrenia that meet the DSM-IV diagnostic criteria for this disorder during periods of abstinence most likely have an independent schizophrenic spectrum disorder in addition to their alcohol or drug dependence. It is also important to rule out the possibility of a mood disorder with psychotic features in making this differential diagnosis.

CASE EXAMPLE 2

A 22-year-old man is brought to the emergency room by his dormitory advisor for evaluation of bizarre behavior. The advisor states that for the past week the patient has been staying in his room, skipping classes, and missing meals. At times he paces the room and appears to be in a conversation with someone; however, the room is empty. He has told his dormitory advisor that "(his) chemistry professor, dean of the university, and roommate," are involved in a plot against him to "flunk (him) out of school." He believes this conspiracy is being masterminded by the CIA. The dormitory advisor learned from the patient's roommate that he has been using crystal methamphetamine to stay awake later and study, and a urine toxicology screen performed in the emergency room later confirms this.

The clinician admits the patient to the locked psychiatric ward for observation. After obtaining the patient's permission, he speaks with the patient's parents, who state that their son has always been an outgoing overachiever with many friends. The parents became concerned, however, about their son's drug use, which started during his senior year of high school. He was kicked off the baseball team for using drugs and had an alcohol-related motor vehicle accident later that same year.

Given this information about the patient's drug use antedating any psychiatric symptoms, the clinician chooses a conservative course and observes the patient in the hospital while prescribing only low doses of neuroleptic medications as needed for severe agitation. During the first few weeks of hospitalization, the patient's psychotic symptoms and signs gradually improve. By discharge, he no longer complains of any persecutory delusions and the voices he was experiencing have all but disappeared.

Treatment focuses on his problems with alcohol and methamphetamine, and he begins attending meetings in the hospital's alcohol and drug treatment program, where he goes after discharge.

In this case scenario, the diagnosis of a substance-induced psychotic disorder is obvious because the psychotic symptoms and signs resolve after cessation of stimulant drug use. However, had the psychotic symptoms and signs persisted for months despite abstinence from drugs and had there been evidence of other residual symptoms and signs of schizophrenia in this young man (i.e., deterioration of social functioning, negative symptoms and signs, and so forth), then a diagnosis of schizophrenia would have been more seriously entertained. In either event, the clinician needs to remain flexible with the working diagnosis and to provide follow-up evaluation.

INDEPENDENT VERSUS SUBSTANCE-INDUCED MOOD DISORDER

About one third of patients with mood disorders also fulfill criteria for substance abuse or dependence at some time in their lives.[1, 6] The strength of the association between the substance use and mood disorders is due primarily to the fact that many patients with bipolar disorder abuse alcohol and other drugs.[29, 30] More than 50% of individuals with bipolar disorder develop alcohol or other drug abuse or dependence at some time in their lives.[1] Because alcohol is a brain depressant and because symptoms and signs of depression also occur during stimulant withdrawal, clinicians must frequently evaluate patients complaining of depression when substance abuse looms in the clinical picture.

CASE EXAMPLE 3

A 52-year-old man presents in the clinic complaining of hopelessness and suicidal ideation. The physician detects the faint smell of alcohol on the man's breath, but the patient denies being alcoholic.

Recognizing that this an emergency situation and that there is an increased prevalence of suicides in alcoholics,[31] the clinician admits the patient to the acute psychiatric ward for an evaluation. The psychiatrist obtains the patient's permission to speak with his daughter. Despite the patient's denial of alcoholism, this collateral informant interview corroborates the physician's suspicion that the man has long-standing problems with alcohol that date back to his mid-20s. Physical examination findings of an enlarged liver and spider telangiectases support the diagnosis, as do laboratory tests showing an elevated GGT level and mild macrocytic anemia. Review of the patient's medical record shows a previous hospitalization for suicidal ideation and depression 2 years earlier, after the patient's wife died.

The psychiatrist relies on three pieces of information when formulating a working diagnosis of probable substance-induced mood disorder with depressive features.

First, the patient states that his depression started 3 days before admission after he was asked to leave his sister's home for being disruptive. This triggered a more intense drinking binge that ended hours before his arrival in the emergency room. Although he complains of difficulty sleeping and concentrating during the past 2 weeks, he admits he had been drinking on and off during that period. However, he denies anhedonia, suicidal ideation, or impairment in his ability to function during that period.

Second, the medical record indicates that the patient's other bout of depression and suicidal ideation improved with abstinence and supportive and group psychotherapy during his previous hospitalization. After 2 weeks, he was transferred to the hospital's alcoholic treatment unit, where he learned some of the principles that led to his longest abstinence of 18 months.

Third, both the patient and his daughter said that during this period of lengthy abstinence, the patient showed gradual, continued improvement in his mood. He worked an active 12-step program of sobriety and returned to his job as an office manager.

During the 2 weeks of hospitalization, the patient's suicidal ideation disappeared and his mood gradually improved. He was transferred to the open unit and participated more actively in support groups. His denial of his alcoholism waned with persistent gentle confrontation by his counselors, and he began attending the hospital's 12-step program.

Three weeks after admission, he continued to exhibit improvement in his mood but still complained of some difficulty sleeping. The patient felt reassured by the psychiatrist's explanation that the sleep disturbance was likely a remnant of his heavy drinking that should continue to improve with prolonged abstinence. However, the psychiatrist scheduled follow-up appointments with the patient to continue monitoring his mood and sleep patterns.

In summary, initial assessment of patients presenting with both psychiatric and substance abuse problems is challenging. It depends on (1) the clinician's awareness that alcoholism and drug dependence are relatively common disorders that frequently go hand in hand with psychiatric symptoms, (2) careful probing of multiple resources to establish diagnoses, (3) a longitudinal evaluation of the relationship between psychiatric complaints and substance-related problems, and (4) follow-up and flexibility with the initial working diagnosis. With practice, following this decision-making process can lead to better diagnosis in this challenging patient population.

ACKNOWLEDGMENTS

The author would like to thank Marc A. Schuckit, M.D., for his guidance and original contributions to some of the ideas expressed in this chapter.

This chapter was adapted in part from articles by the author (see references 8 and 16).

This work was supported by NIAAA Grant #09735, a VA Research Advisory Group Grant, and the Veterans Affairs Research Service.

REFERENCES

1. Regier DA, Farmer ME, Rae DS, et al: Comorbidity of mental disorders with alcohol and other drug abuse—results from the Epidemiologic Catchment Area (ECA) study. JAMA 264:2511–2518, 1990.
2. Kessler RC, McGonagle KA, Zhao S, et al: Lifetime and 12-month prevalence of DSM-III-R psychiatric disorders in the United States: Results from the National Comorbidity Survey. Arch Gen Psychiatry 51:8–19, 1994.
3. American Psychiatric Association: Diagnostic and Statistical Manual of Mental Disorders, 4th ed. Washington, DC, American Psychiatric Association, 1994, pp 190–194.
4. Khantzian EJ, Bean-Bayog M, Blumenthal S, et al: Substance abuse disorders: A psychiatric priority. Am J Psychiatry 148(10):1291–1300, 1991.
5. Committee on Training and Education in Addiction Psychiatry: Position statement on the need for improved training for treatment of patients with combined substance use and other psychiatric disorders. Am J Psychiatry 151:795–796, 1994.
6. Helzer JE, Przybeck TR: The co-occurrence of alcoholism with other psychiatric disorders in the general population and its impact on treatment. J Stud Alcohol 49:219–224, 1988.
7. Ross HE, Glaser FB, Germanson T: The prevalence of psychiatric disorders in patients with alcohol and other drug problems. Arch Gen Psychiatry 45:1023–1031, 1988.
8. Anthenelli RM: The initial evaluation of the dual diagnosis patient. Psychiatric Ann 24:407–411, 1994.
9. Anthenelli RM, Schuckit MA: Alcohol and cerebral depressants. In Glass IB (ed): The International Handbook of Addiction Behavior. London, Routledge, 1991, pp 57–63.
10. Schuckit MA: Evaluating the dual diagnosis patient. Drug Abuse & Alcoholism Newsletter 17(10):1–4, 1988.
11. Vaillant GE: Theoretical hierarchy of adaptive ego mechanisms. Arch Gen Psychiatry 24:112–118, 1971.
12. Galanter M: Appendix—the rules of network therapy summarized: Network Therapy for Alcohol and Drug Abuse: A New Approach in Practice. New York, Basic Books, 1993, pp 195–199.
13. Schuckit MA, Irwin M: Diagnosis of alcoholism. Med Clin North Am 72(5):1133–1153, 1988.
14. Irwin M, Baird S, Smith TL, Schuckit MA: Use of laboratory tests to monitor heavy drinking by alcoholic men discharged from a treatment program. Am J Psychiatry 145(5):595–599, 1988.
15. Mullen J, Bracha HS: Toxicology screening: How to assure accurate results. Postgrad Med 84(5):141–148, 1988.
16. Anthenelli RM, Schuckit MA: Affective and anxiety disorders and alcohol and drug dependence: Diagnosis and treatment. J Addict Dis 12:73–87, 1993.
17. Koob GF, Bloom FE: Cellular and molecular mechanisms of drug dependence. Science 242:715–723, 1988.
18. Brown SA, Schuckit MA: Changes in depression among abstinent alcoholics. J Stud Alcohol 49(5):412–417, 1988.
19. Schuckit MA, Irwin M, Brown SA: The history of anxiety symptoms among 171 primary alcoholics. J Stud Alcohol 51(1):34–41, 1990.
20. Weingold JP, Lachin JM, Bell H, Coxe RC: Depression as a symptom of alcoholism: Search for a phenomenon. J Abnorm Psychol 73:195–197, 1968.
21. Schuckit MA: The clinical implications of primary diagnostic groups among alcoholics. Arch Gen Psychiatry 42:1043–1049, 1985.
22. Schuckit MA: Drug and Alcohol Abuse: A Clinical Guide to Diagnosis and Treatment, 3rd ed. New York, Plenum, 1989.
23. Brown SA, Inaba RK, Gillin JC, et al: Alcoholism and affective disorder: Clinical course of depressive symptoms. Am J Psychiatry 152(1):45–52, 1995.
24. Hesselbrock MN, Meyer RE, Keener JJ: Psychopathology in hospitalized alcoholics. Arch Gen Psychiatry 42:1050–1055, 1985.
25. Anthenelli RM, Smith TL, Irwin MR, Schuckit MA: A comparative study of criteria for subgrouping alcoholics: The primary/secondary diagnostic scheme versus variations of the type 1/type 2 criteria. Am J Psychiatry 151(10):1468–1474, 1994.
26. von Knorring L, Palm U, Anderson H-E: Relationship between treatment outcome and subtype of alcoholism in men. J Stud Alcohol 46(5):388–391, 1985.
27. Gerstley LJ, Alterman AI, McLellan AT, Woody GE: Antisocial personality disorder in patients with substance abuse disorders: A problematic diagnosis? Am J Psychiatry 147:173–178, 1990.
28. Mueser KT, Bellack AS, Blanchard JJ: Comorbidity of schizophrenia and substance abuse: Implications for treatment. J Consult Clin Psychol 60(6):845–856, 1992.
29. Brady KT, Lydiard RB: Bipolar affective disorder and substance abuse. J Clin Psychopharmacol 12:17s–22s, 1992.
30. Schuckit MA: Genetic and clinical implications of alcoholism and affective disorder. Am J Psychiatry 143(2):140–147, 1986.
31. Murphy GE: Suicide and substance abuse. Arch Gen Psychiatry 45:593–594, 1988.

The Medical Basis of Addictive Disorders

Wilson M. Compton, III, MD •
Samuel B. Guze, MD

The Merriam-Webster dictionary defines disease as "an impairment of the normal state of the living animal or plant body or of any of its components that interrupts or modifies the performance of the vital functions, being a response to environmental factors (as malnutrition, industrial hazards, or climate), to specific infective agents (as worms, bacteria, or viruses), to inherent defects of the organism (as various genetic anomalies), or to combinations of these factors."[1] It is clear that this definition of disease can be applied to alcoholism and other addictions, but the ways in which these conditions fit this disease model bear scrutiny—and that is the main topic of this chapter. Consideration of whether alcoholism and other addictions fit the definition of disease is more than an abstract issue; accepting and validating the disease model (and thus the medical model) has critical implications for the ways in which the medical community and the public approach substance dependence. This chapter reviews the evidence for the applicability of the disease (and medical) model to alcoholism and other addictions. Thus, the main question addressed in this chapter is, What is the evidence for addictions being valid diseases?

The validity of any diagnostic category depends on many different factors. For most of medicine, classification ultimately depends on pathological evaluation and a thorough under-standing of pathophysiology and etiology. In psychiatry (including addiction psychiatry), the limited understanding of the underlying brain pathophysiology and etiology means that somewhat indirect measures must be used to support the validity of disease conditions. Robins and Guze described five phases for validating a psychiatric diagnosis in their seminal 1970 paper.[2] These phases are (1) clinical description, (2) laboratory studies, (3) delimitation from other disorders, (4) follow-up study, and (5) family study. Cloninger further described these phases in terms of standard psychometric nomenclature in that clinical description is a form of content validity, laboratory study is a form of concurrent validity, delimitation from other disorders is a form of discriminative validity, follow-up study is a form of predictive validity, and family study is a form of criterion-related validity.[3] This chapter includes a review of some of the data that allow us to believe in the validity of alcoholism and other addictions. The conclusion is a discussion about some of the major questions that confront clinicians and researchers interested in the validity of these disorders.

History and Clinical Description

Alcoholism as a term originated in the mid-nineteenth century, but descriptions of problems due to alcohol consumption date from antiquity.[4-6] The first writings to describe alcoholism as a disease were in the early nineteenth century,[7] and by the end of that century several facilities had been established for the treatment of alcoholics. In fact, the *Journal of Inebriety* was started in 1876 based on the explicit idea that drunkenness was a mental disease.[8] In the modern era, perhaps the best-known descriptions of alcoholism as a disease were written by Jellinek.[9, 10] Jellinek's writings helped to convince the medical community about the usefulness of the disease model of alcoholism. He described the symptoms and signs of alcoholism and emphasized the chronic progressive course of the syndrome. His detailed analyses of the differences between men and women in symptoms and course remain a major contribution to the clinical understanding of these difficult conditions.

Since Jellinek's time, several researchers have had key roles in the acceptance of alcoholism as a disease. A major contribution came from the highly structured and clearly operationalized diagnostic systems first developed 25 years ago. Feighner and colleagues' psychiatric diagnostic criteria of Washington University[11] were the first of these systems and included criteria for alcoholism. These criteria served as the foundation for other modern U.S. diagnostic systems (i.e., the Research Diagnostic Criteria[12] and the American Psychiatric Association's *Diagnostic and Statistical Manual of Mental Disorders*, third edition, third edition-revised, and fourth edition[13-15] [DSM-III, DSM-III-R, and DSM-IV]). The inclusion of alcoholism as a separate category in all of these nomenclatures is evidence of the recognition of its relevance to psychiatry.

In the mid-1970s, Edwards and colleagues described the dependence syndrome, which emphasized symptoms of loss of control over substance use in addition to tolerance and withdrawal.[16] This approach to the diagnosis of alcoholism was adopted in DSM-III-R, DSM-IV, and the International Classification of Diseases, tenth edition (ICD-10),[17] although the precise criteria vary between each of these systems. The approach has been applied as well to other substance dependence syndromes, and thus a single set of criteria is used for all addictive syndromes in DSM-IV and ICD-10. What can be learned from these writings is that the specific diagnostic criteria for alcoholism and other substance dependence may not be completely agreed on, but the overall acceptance of these conditions as diseases is well established.

Genetics of Alcoholism and Other Addictions

Family, twin, and adoption studies have provided evidence for a genetic component of alcoholism. Virtually all family studies have shown much higher than expected rates of alcoholism among the relatives of alcoholics.[18, 19] Of course, familial clustering does not prove a *genetic* component of the inheritance of alcoholism. For such evidence, we look to adoption studies and twin studies. Adoption studies have generally shown that alcoholism in offspring is predicted by alcoholism among biological but not adoptive relatives.[20-23] One study showed some evidence that drug misuse also was associated with alcoholism in biological relatives,[24] and one study showed a tendency for antisocial behavior to be inherited by a subgroup of adoptees of alcoholics,[25] but otherwise, no other psychiatric conditions were consistently found to coexist with alcoholism.

Twin studies have consistently shown an excess of alcoholism in the co-twins of monozygotic (MZ) twins compared with dizygotic (DZ) twins.[26, 27] Most recently, twin studies from Minnesota[28] and Virginia[29] have improved our knowledge about the inheritance of alcoholism and showed that MZ twins had higher concordance than DZ twins among both male and female twin pairs. These studies, from the general family studies to the most specific twin projects, clearly indicate a genetic predisposition to alcoholism.

A major project supported by the National Institute on Alcoholism and Alcohol Abuse (NIAAA) is currently under way to determine the genetic basis for alcoholism through the molecular genetic study of high-risk families.[30] This project is based on the long-standing observation that alcoholism clusters in families and has a strong genetic component. Thus, acceptance of the familial/genetic nature of alcoholism has led to a study that may be able to uncover a specific cause of these devastating conditions.

For other addictions, less work in the area of genetic/family study has been completed. This is partly because of the complications in studying illicit substance use across generations when the exposure to substances in the social environment has changed dramatically during the past decades. Because the exposure to various substances has changed so much over time, specific study of parental rates of illicit substance dependence may be confounded by differential environments. This problem may be solved by the sibling-pair method of genetic studies or by the twin methods. In fact, one twin study has demonstrated preliminary evidence for the heritability of drug dependence.[31] Nevertheless, the family/twin/adoption study of illicit substance dependence has lagged significantly behind the alcoholism projects.

Epidemiology of Addiction

Understanding the rates of alcoholism and substance dependence among different groups gives an important glimpse of the places where prevention is most needed. Furthermore, the consistency of these studies gives some indirect support to the validity of the conditions themselves. Although the rates of alcoholism and illicit substance dependence vary across studies (perhaps based on different samples, diagnostic instruments, and different diagnostic criteria), the association with certain risk factors remains consistent. For example, in a large number of epidemiological samples[32–34] using the National Institute of Mental Health (NIMH) Diagnostic Interview Schedule (DIS)[35] and in the more recent National Comorbidity Survey,[36] strong associations have been found between male gender and substance dependence and between antisocial personality disorder and substance dependence. The consistency of these findings lends credence to the validity of the underlying addictive conditions in that they are not randomly distributed in the population but take on certain predictable forms.

As described by Helzer and Canino, cross-cultural similarity is also supportive of the validity of psychiatric conditions.[37] The argument is that if similar symptoms are found in widely divergent cultural settings, this is indirect (but strong) evidence for a common underlying condition. Helzer and colleagues have followed their theoretical paper with a contribution describing alcoholism in North America and Asia.[32] The researchers found a remarkably similar presentation of symptoms of alcoholics across the sites, which included Puerto Rico, St. Louis, Edmonton, Seoul, and Taiwan. At present, a large study being conducted by the World Health Organization is examining the reliability and validity of alcohol and drug use disorders at 12 sites internationally, a study that should allow further examination of the consistency of the addictive syndromes across a wide variety of cultural settings.[38]

Animal Studies

Some of the strongest evidence for addictive diseases as valid entities comes from the animal and behavioral models of addiction. Because these studies have begun to unravel the underlying brain mechanisms of reward and reinforcement (which are key components of addiction), they may provide evidence about the etiology of addictive behavior. The circuitry and neurochemistry of the brain reward system are described in other chapters and primarily involve the mesolimbic and mesocortical dopamine pathways.[39] Investigation of the brain mechanisms of reward is based on demonstration of the ability to addict animals to various illicit substances and has provided some of the strongest evidence of the external validity of addiction.[39, 40] No longer can simple morality be invoked to explain addictive behavior. Furthermore, as major strides have been made to unravel the brain reward systems, these studies have allowed us to begin to integrate basic science and clinical medicine in a way that has not been possible in other areas of psychiatry. Thus, the validity of addiction as specific entities may even be better established than other psychiatric conditions.

Treatment Response

Treatment response is sometimes considered a validation of a diagnostic category in that a predictable response to treatment represents indirect evidence for the reasonableness of a classification. In substance dependence, the main treatments have been behaviorally based and thus do not directly support hypotheses about the medical nature of alcoholism and other addictions. However, the demonstrated efficacy of naltrexone in the treatment of alcoholism[41, 42] supports the validity of the disease model in that as a mu opiate receptor blocker, naltrexone is a treatment regimen with theoretically based ties to the brain reward mechanisms. For the purposes of this chapter, the main point is not the specific theoretical mechanisms of action of naltrexone (these are described elsewhere) but how a specific diagnosis with a specific treatment leads to a predictable result. This is expected with the medical model of alcoholism and helps to support both the validity and the usefulness of the model.

Natural History

The course of alcoholism and other addictions has been described by many different investigators from retrospective analysis, but only a few have examined these conditions prospectively—most of these have primarily focused on alcoholism, not on other substances. Published longitudinal studies have included (among others) samples from various settings: prisons,[43] outpatients,[44–46] inpatients,[47] and college students.[48] Despite different samples, different definitions of alcoholism/addiction, and different lengths of follow-up, several important characteristics emerge from these studies: A small but significant percentage of addicts undergo remission each year, no matter what the source of the sample. Return to controlled substance use (mostly shown for drinking) seems to be rare and primarily limited to mild cases at baseline. The onset of addiction is generally insidious, and the course and symptoms vary between men and women.[10, 49–51] Women seem to begin substance use at a later age, have more varied courses, and may have a more rapid progression of symptoms. In general, alcoholism and other addictions fit the pattern of chronic, relapsing disorders. Periods of remission may last for varying times, and outcome can be expected to include relapse in the majority of cases.

Applying the Medical Model to Addiction Psychiatry

The epitome of the medical approach to any disorder is to diagnose the illness, plan treatment, and predict outcome. Applying the medical model to addiction psychiatry implies that the "concepts, strategies, and jargon of general medicine are applied to psychiatric disorders: diagnosis, differential diagnosis, etiology, pathogenesis, treatment, natural history, epidemiology, complications, and so on."[52] In addictions, the medical model is used because it may give the greatest chance to discern new ways to prevent morbidity (i.e., primary, secondary, or tertiary prevention) just as it has in other branches of medicine. The medical model is a skeptical approach in that clear, scientifically plausible evidence is needed for a theory to be accepted. On the other hand, like all other medical specialties, evidence about treatment does not necessarily have to go hand in hand with knowledge of pathophysiology, and novel approaches are always acceptable if based on available evidence. Differential diagnosis is a key component in the medical approach because it forces a clinician to weigh the possible explanations for a given patient's symptoms/signs and is based on a general understanding that variability of presentation is usual for virtually all illnesses (at least to some degree).

Despite the popularity and the success of the medical model, this approach to addiction psychiatry has several competitors in the literature. Most prominent are the moral models, the psychodynamic (or psychoanalytical) models, the sociocultural models, the behavioral models, and that recent hybrid particularly promulgated by the American Psychiatric Association the biopsychosocial models. The plural *models* is used for these discussions to acknowledge that each of the mentioned categories has several (at least) markedly different constructs within the general category. The medical model differs from the other models in many important ways. The most fundamental difference is that each of the other models seeks to explain addiction in terms of various external factors and neglects the primary organ of addiction, the brain/mind. The medical model is without a priori theory but does consider brain mechanisms to be a priority. Because it can encompass the other models to the extent that they are backed up by scientific evidence, the medical model can be considered one of the most liberal models. Practitioners are constrained only by practical application of theory to clinical situations. All the other models require strict adherence to particular theoretical perspectives.

Moral models of addictive conditions were well represented in the temperance movement, in which alcoholics were considered lost souls who needed redemption. Excessive drinking was considered a kind of moral weakness. Alcoholics and drug addicts were thought of as having character defects that they brought upon themselves through personal weakness.

Psychodynamic models have offered comprehensive explanations of all human behavior, including normal behaviors and pathological conditions. Most psychodynamic theories developed from the notion that unconscious memories and experiences from childhood and infancy are expressed indirectly through dreams, slips of the tongue, and psychiatric symptoms. The underlying assumptions have been called *psychological determinism*, in which all behavior is a result of psychological causes.[53, 54] A second and related assumption is that a symptom must have some underlying meaning for a patient. In this way, symptoms are considered to be windows into the unconscious rather than to have some external validity of their own. Psychodynamic models encounter difficulties when they ignore evidence from genetics, physiology, and epidemiology because they do not fit into the preconceived causal framework. It is also a problem that psychodynamic theories are essentially untestable because they provide no dependable ways to correct for suggestion, bias, and circularity of argument.[55] Being essentially untestable (and also impossible to *dis*prove), these models violate a fundamental scientific principle that only testable hypotheses are worthy of investigation.

The sociocultural models in their extreme form also seek to explain psychiatric symptoms and conditions as being caused by external factors.[56, 57] The limitations of these theoretical positions have been discussed in the literature.[58] Sociocultural models are useful in part because (unlike psychodynamic models) they are often testable. Furthermore, most would agree that social and cultural factors have been shown to be important in various illnesses, not just psychiatric.[59] The medical model does not eliminate social and cultural factors from the understanding of disease processes but does not ascribe to social and cultural factors alone a causative role. To do so would ignore much evidence from genetics, physiology, and epidemiology that the brain is also important in the expression of alcoholism and other addictions.

Similar to sociocultural models, behavioral models of psychopathology have many appealing aspects, particularly in that behavioral treatments have been shown to be quite helpful in treating certain psychiatric conditions, especially addictive disorders.[60] Behavioral theory has been particularly useful in describing certain human behaviors in terms of experimental paradigms. The limitation is that not all addiction psychiatry can be explained in terms of behaviorism. The brain as the organ of addiction is particularly ignored in behavioral models in which responses may be considered solely due to environmental factors.[61]

Finally, the last alternative model, the biopsychosocial, seems appealing in that all other models are given equal weight. In many ways, all medical specialties could be considered as having a biological component, a psychological component, and a sociocultural component. What is missing from this model is the usual respect for the organ system involved—the brain. In other branches of medicine, the spe-

cific organ system would take priority for a physician. The medical model when applied to addiction psychiatry would imply the same priorities: The brain and how brain mechanisms are related to functional impairment would be considered the first goal of the medical model. Psychological and sociocultural factors remain important and in certain cases are of primary interest, but they do not supplant study of the brain as the organ of addiction.

Models other than the medical model may have meaning outside of science and medicine, but they are not useful in planning treatment to help someone overcome the difficulties inherent in the behaviors associated with alcoholism and other substance use disorders. This does *not* mean that social, cultural factors are unimportant. They may be influential intervening variables. The value of the medical model is that it allows a rational approach to a complex set of behaviors and situations that are agreed on by the health establishment and the public. With this approach, a scientific exploration of etiology and treatment is promoted so that the focus is on the brain as the substrate for predisposition to addiction and as the organ system affected by various substances. The implications of accepting this model are a hope and expectation that a medical approach to addiction (in contrast to other approaches) will lead to the most progress in understanding and improving treatment of these devastating and common brain/mind illnesses, just as the medical model has led to great progress in treating diseases of other major organ systems (such as the heart, lungs, or endocrine systems).

In addition to the potential effect of the medical model on clinical practice and research, the implications for patients and families are profound. This approach means that patients and families can dispense with at least some of the guilt about behavior related to alcoholism and other addictions. They can understand that they do not have control over the conditions but have a disease. Just as they would not feel personally responsible for getting colon cancer, they can learn to feel less guilty about their addiction and more hopeful about treatment.

Future Work

Much has been learned about the validity of addictive disorders, and the medical model of addiction has achieved a high level of acceptance, yet much work remains. In the area of validity of alcoholism and other addictions, many questions remain to be answered. Some of this work is outlined next.

The *first* question is whether a set of true diagnostic criteria could be developed. Given the recent revisions of the DSM and ICD nomenclatures, this has been an extremely relevant question with which both American and international colleagues have wrestled. The DSM-IV and ICD-10 substance disorders committees defined overlapping but distinct criteria for substance dependence, and the criteria for DSM-IV abuse and ICD-10 harmful use are markedly different. These discrepancies persisted in the presence of efforts by both committees to coordinate results. Thus, even with the best intentions, it has been difficult for experts to agree on criteria. Nevertheless, much can be learned from diagnostic criteria. Perhaps by using newer psychometric methods to examine the underlying factor structure of addictive symptoms, we will be able to learn more about the most applicable criteria and about the underlying conditions.[62] Such factor analysis has been applied by Muthen and colleagues to alcoholism, and a two-factor solution emerged.[63] Using these techniques for other addictions is one way to make a scientific study of diagnostic groupings. Despite some optimism, *all* diagnostic systems should be considered working models that are designed to "facilitate communication, understanding, and treatment."[64] Diagnostic systems should not remain static but must change and respond to new evidence until such time as the pathogenesis is completely understood and direct symptoms can be separated from the ancillary (nonspecific) phenomena.

Second, can valid subtypes of alcoholism and other addictions be elucidated? Jellinek's alpha, beta, gamma, delta, and epsilon groups[10]; Cloninger's type I and II alcoholism[65]; and Babor's type A and B[66] represent a few of the better-known typologies. In fact, this area has been critically summarized by Bohn and Meyer.[60] The utility of these subtypes for treatment planning and prognostication remains to be proved, but the heterogeneity of alcoholism symptom profiles is clear. The identification of valid, reliably determined subtypes remains appealing to researchers and clinicians. For addictions other than alcohol, identifying subtypes has not been accomplished, and the field is ripe for exploration.

Third, are alcoholism and other drug abuse syndromes the same disorders with different substance exposure? Are these separate illnesses with certain commonalities? Many stud-ies have shown that alcoholism and other addictions frequently overlap in patients and families.[67, 68] Assuming that both alcoholism and other drug addictions are heritable, these conditions may represent a single transmitted trait or each individual substance may have its own inheritance.[69] Early evidence has shown a tendency for respondents with both alcoholism and another addiction to have higher rates of alcoholism among their relatives compared with relatives of respondents with the other addiction alone.[34, 70–72] More specific evidence about the separation of alcoholism and other addictions is lacking.

Fourth, what are the overlaps between substance dependence and other disorders? How can we understand the meaning of the overlap? Is it nonspecific—as in the stress model of affective disorders? Are psychiatric symptoms seen in those with substance dependence an epiphenomenon of the dependence? Or is there some specific etiological relationship between substance dependence and other psychiatric problems? The comorbidity of substance use disorders and other psychiatric conditions has been shown in both treatment and general population samples,[34] but the reasons for this overlap remain to be studied.

Conclusions

This chapter summarizes some of the evidence that alcoholism and other addictions are diseases. Because acceptance of addictions as diseases is central to the medical model of alcoholism and other addictions, this chapter also describes the rationale for acceptance of the medical model. Support for this model comes from various sources: clinical description, longitudinal studies, epidemiology, laboratory and animal studies, family and other genetic studies, and treatment response. The implications of the medical model are profound for research and treatment, but much work is left to be completed because the underlying pathophysiology of addiction is yet to be determined.

REFERENCES

1. Webster's Third New International Dictionary. New York, G & C Merriam, 1966.
2. Robins E, Guze SB: Establishment of diagnostic validity in psychiatric illness: Its application to schizophrenia. Am J Psychiatry 126:107–111, 1970.
3. Cloninger CR: Establishment of diagnostic validity in psychiatric illness: Robins and Guze's method revisited. In Robins LN, Barrett JE (eds): The Validity of Psychiatric Diagnosis. New York, Raven Press, 1989.

4. Babor T: Alcohol: Customs and Rituals. London, Burke, 1988.
5. Keller M: On defining alcoholism: With comment on some other relevant words. In Gomberg EL, White HR, Carpenter SA (eds): Alcohol, Science and Society Revisited. Ann Arbor, University of Michigan Press, 1982.
6. Rouche B: Alcohol. New York, Grove Press, 1960.
7. Rush B: An Inquiry into the Effects of Ardent Spirits upon the Human Body and Mind, 6th ed. New York, 1811.
8. Goodwin D, Guze SB. Psychiatric Diagnosis, 4th ed. New York, Oxford University Press, 1989, p 172.
9. Jellinek EM: Phases of alcohol addiction. Q J Stud Alcohol 13:673–684, 1952.
10. Jellinek EM: The Disease Concept of Alcoholism. New Haven, College and University Press, 1960.
11. Feighner JP, Robins E, Guze SB, et al: Diagnostic criteria for use in psychiatric research. Arch Gen Psychiatry 26:57–63, 1972.
12. Spitzer RL, Endicott J, Robins E: Research diagnostic criteria: Rationale and reliability. Arch Gen Psychiatry 35:773–789, 1978.
13. American Psychiatric Association: Diagnostic and Statistical Manual of Mental Disorders, 3rd ed. Washington, DC, American Psychiatric Association, 1980.
14. American Psychiatric Association: Diagnostic and Statistical Manual of Mental Disorders, 3rd ed, revised. Washington, DC, American Psychiatric Association, 1987.
15. American Psychiatric Association: Diagnostic and Statistical Manual of Mental Disorders, 4th ed. Washington, DC, American Psychiatric Association, 1994.
16. Edwards G, Gross MM, Keller M, et al: Alcohol-Related Disabilities. Geneva, World Health Organization, 1977.
17. World Health Organization: The ICD-10 Classification of Mental and Behavioural Disorders. Geneva, World Health Organization, 1992.
18. Cotton NS: The familial incidence of alcoholism: A review. J Stud Alcohol 40:89–116, 1979.
19. Goodwin DW: Alcoholism and genetics: The sins of the fathers. Arch Gen Psychiatry 42:171–174, 1985.
20. Goodwin DW, Schulsinger F, Hermansen L, et al: Alcohol problems in adoptees raised apart from alcoholic biological parents. Arch Gen Psychiatry 28:238–243, 1973.
21. Bohman M: Genetic aspects of alcoholism and criminality. Arch Gen Psychiatry 35:269–276, 1978.
22. Bohman M, Sigvardsson S, Cloninger CR: Maternal inheritance of alcohol abuse: Cross-fostering analysis of adopted women. Arch Gen Psychiatry 38:965–969, 1981.
23. Cadoret RJ, Cain CA, Grove WM: Development of alcoholism in adoptees raised apart from alcoholic biologic relatives. Arch Gen Psychiatry 37:561–563, 1979.
24. Cadoret RJ, Troughton E, O'Gorman TW: Genetic and environmental factors in alcohol abuse and antisocial personality. J Stud Alcohol 48:1–8, 1987.
25. Cloninger CR, Bohman M, Sigvardsson S: Inheritance of alcohol abuse: Cross-fostering analysis of adopted men. Arch Gen Psychiatry 38:861–868, 1981.
26. Kaij L: Studies on the Etiology and Sequels of Abuse of Alcohol. Lund, University of Lund, 1960.
27. Hrubec Z, Omenn GS: Evidence of genetic predisposition to alcoholic cirrhosis and psychosis: Twin concordances for alcoholism and its biological end points by zygosity among male veterans. Alcohol Clin Exp Res 5:207–215, 1981.
28. Pickens RW, Svikis DS, McGue M, et al: Heterogeneity in the inheritance of alcoholism. Arch Gen Psychiatry 48:19–28, 1991.
29. Kendler KS, Heath AC, Neale MC, et al: A population-based twin study of alcoholism in women. JAMA 268:1877–1882, 1992.
30. Reich T: Personal communication, St. Louis, 1995.
31. Grove WM, Eckert ED, Heston L, et al: Heritability of substance abuse and antisocial personality of monozygotic twins reared apart. Biol Psychiatry 27:1293–1304, 1990.
32. Helzer JE, Canino GJ, Hwu HG, et al: Alcoholism: North American and Asia. Arch Gen Psychiatry 47:313–319, 1990.
33. Robins LN, Regier DA (eds): Psychiatric Disorders in America. New York, Free Press, 1991.
34. Regier DA, Farmer ME, Rae DS, et al: Comorbidity of mental disorders with alcohol and other drug abuse. JAMA 264:2511–2518, 1990.
35. Robins LN, Helzer JE, Croughan J, et al: NIMH Diagnostic Interview Schedule: Version III. Rockville, MD, National Institute of Mental Health, 1981.
36. Kessler RC, McGonagle KA, Zhao S, et al: Lifetime and 12-month prevalence of DSM-III-R psychiatric disorders in the United States. Arch Gen Psychiatry 51:8–19, 1994.
37. Helzer JE, Canino G: The implications of cross-national research for diagnostic validity. In Robins LN, Barrett JE (eds): The Validity of Psychiatric Diagnosis. New York, Raven Press, 1989.
38. World Health Organization: Reliability and Validity Study. Geneva, World Health Organization, Mental Health Division, 1995.
39. Liebman JM, Cooper SJ (eds): The Neuropharmacological Basis of Reward. Oxford, Oxford University Press, 1989.
40. Spragg SDS: Morphine addiction in chimpanzees. Comprehensive Psychological Monographs 15:1–132, 1940.
41. O'Malley SS, Jaffe AJ, Chang G, et al: Naltrexone and coping skills therapy for alcohol dependence. Arch Gen Psychiatry 49:881–887, 1992.
42. Volpicelli JR, Alterman AI, Hayachida M, O'Brien CP: Naltrexone in the treatment of alcohol dependence. Arch Gen Psychiatry 49:876–880, 1992.
43. Goodwin DW, Crane JB, Guze SB: Felons who drink: An 8-year follow-up. Q J Stud Alcohol 32:136–147, 1971.
44. Hyman MM. Alcoholics 15 years later. Ann N Y Acad Sci 273:613–623, 1976.
45. Vaillant GE: A 20-year follow-up of New York narcotic addicts. Arch Gen Psychiatry 19:237–241, 1973.
46. Anglin MD, Hser Y, Booth MW: Sex differences in addict careers. Am J Drug Alcohol Abuse 13:253–280, 1994.
47. Helzer JE, Robins LN, Taylor JR, et al: The extent of long-term moderate drinking among alcoholics discharged from medical and psychiatric treatment facilities. N Engl J Med 312:1678–1682, 1985.
48. Vaillant GE: The Natural History of Alcoholism: Causes, Patterns, and Paths to Recovery. Cambridge, Harvard University Press, 1983.
49. Pemberton DA: A comparison of the outcome of treatment in female and male alcoholics. Br J Psychiatry 113:367–373, 1967.
50. Cloninger CR, Bohman M, Sigvardsson S: Inheritance of alcohol abuse: Crossfostering analysis of adopted men. Arch Gen Psychiatry 36:861–868, 1981.
51. Schuckit MA: Drug and Alcohol Abuse. New York, Plenum, 1989.
52. Guze SB: Why Psychiatry Is a Branch of Medicine. New York, Oxford University Press, 1992, p 4.

53. Gabbard GO: Psychodynamic Psychiatry in Clinical Practice. Washington, DC, American Psychiatric Association, 1990.
54. Sulloway FJ: Freud, Biologist of the Mind. New York, Basic Books, 1979.
55. Spence DP: The Freudian Metaphor. New York, WW Norton & Co, 1987.
56. Dunham HW: Community and Schizophrenia. Detroit, Wayne State University Press, 1965.
57. Brown GW, Harris T: Social Origins of Depression. London, Tavistock Publications, 1978.
58. Tennant C, Bebbington P: The social causation of depression: A critique of the work of Brown and his colleagues. Psychol Med 8:565–575, 1978.
59. Feinstein AR: Clinical Epidemiology. Philadelphia, WB Saunders, 1985.
60. Bohn MJ, Meyer RE: Typologies of addiction. In Galanter M, Kleber HD (eds): The American Psychiatric Press Textbook of Substance Abuse Treatment. Washington, DC, American Psychiatric Associations, 1994.
61. Skinner BF: Cumulative Record. New York, Appleton-Century-Crofts, 1959.
62. Muthen B: Latent variable modeling in epidemiology. Alcohol Health Res World 16:286–292, 1992.
63. Muthen B, Grant B, Hasin D: The dimensionality of alcohol abuse and dependence: Factor analysis of DSM-III-R and proposed DSM-IV criteria in the 1988 National Health Interview Survey. Addiction 88:1079–1090, 1993.
64. Guze SB: Discussion of C. Robert Honinger's paper. In Robins LN, Barrett JE (eds): The Validity of Psychiatric Diagnosis. New York, Raven Press, 1989, p 16.
65. Cloninger CR: Neurogenetic adaptive mechanisms in alcoholism. Science 236:410–416, 1987.
66. Babor TF, Hofman M, DesBoca FK, et al: Types of alcoholics, I: Evidence for an empirically derived typology based on indicators of vulnerability and severity. Arch Gen Psychiatry 49:599–608, 1992.
67. Croughan JL: The contribution of family studies to understanding drug abuse. In Robins LN (ed): Studying Drug Abuse. New Brunswick, Rutgers University Press, 1985.
68. Rounsaville BJ, Kosten TR, Weissman MM, et al: Psychiatric disorders in the relatives of probands with opioid addiction. Arch Gen Psychiatry 48:33–43, 1991.
69. Pickens RW, Svikis DS: Genetic vulnerability to drug abuse. In Pickens RW, Svikis DS (eds): Biological Vulnerability to Drug Abuse, NIDA Research Monograph 89. Rockville, MD, US Dept of Health and Human Services, 1988.
70. Hill SH, Cloninger CR, Ayre FR: Independent familial transmission of alcoholism and opiate abuse. Alcohol Clin Exp Res 1:335–342, 1977.
71. Handelsman L, Branchey MH, Buydens-Branchey L, et al: Morbidity risk for alcoholism and drug abuse in relatives of cocaine addicts. Am J Drug Alcohol Abuse 19:347–357, 1993.
72. Compton WM, Cottler LB: Family history of substance abuse in cocaine abusers. In Harris L (ed): Problems of Drug Dependence 1994, NIDA Research Monograph. Rockville, MD, 1995.

Addiction and Psychiatric Settings

Mark C. Wallen, MD

Since their inception, addiction and psychiatric treatment programs have been involved with patients with coexisting psychiatric and addictive disorders. Unfortunately, most of these patients are never diagnosed with a second major illness, commonly resulting in poor treatment results for the initial problem diagnosed. Even if a coexisting problem is recognized to a degree, it often is relegated to a secondary status. As a result, many of these individuals are shuttled back and forth between psychiatric and addiction treatment settings, depending on which of their symptoms predominate at any one time.[1] The end result of this type of care is multiple exacerbations of psychiatric symptoms and addiction relapses.

Concordance rates for coexisting psychiatric and addictive disorders have been highly variable, controversial, and at times contradictory, resulting in difficulties in formulating appropriate clinical treatment approaches to meet the complicated needs of patients who truly have a dual diagnosis. In order to formulate effective treatment approaches, clinicians first need to assess patients comprehensively to establish at least working diagnoses of both problems and then need to provide the long-term simultaneous treatment of both disorders that is required in order to be successful.

To address this topic adequately, a number of critical issues need to be examined and reviewed. Clinicians need to be aware of the results of epidemiological studies that have been reported, including the limitations associated with drawing valid conclusions from the available data. Clinicians also need to be aware of the treatment concepts and approaches inherent in the addiction and psychiatric fields that have impeded the development of effective treatment approaches for patients with a dual diagnosis. Finally, clinicians need to be cognizant of treatment models and treatment approaches that have been shown to be helpful in meeting the complex treatment needs of these patients.

Epidemiology

The prevalence of comorbid psychiatric and addictive disorders has historically been viewed as being quite high. Overall, however, concordance rates have been extremely variable, in the range of 15% to 75%.[2-6] Results of the Epidemiologic Catchment Area Study, as reported by Reiger and colleagues,[7] found lifetime prevalence rates of 29% for an addictive disorder in those patients with mental disorders, an increase of odds ratio of 2.7 over those without mental disorders. Among those with an alcohol disorder, 37% had a comorbid mental disorder. In patients with an addictive disorder other than alcoholism, 53% were found to have a mental disorder. Comorbidity rates

135

in mental health and addiction treatment settings were double those in the overall population, thus reinforcing the additive effect on illness severity of comorbid disorders.

Miller and Fine reported on a comprehensive analysis of studies of the comorbidity of psychiatric and addictive disorders during the past four decades. They concluded that the wide disparity of concordance rates was due to a number of factors, including the populations sampled, methodology of the study, perspective of the examiner, longitudinal perspectives, and treatment interventions.[8] As a result of all these factors, they further concluded that the prevalence rates for psychiatric symptoms generated by alcohol or drug use and addiction are much greater than those for concomitant independent psychiatric disorders in the addiction population; prevalence rates for the comorbidity of addictive disorders in psychiatric populations are no greater than those for the general population, except for schizophrenia and antisocial personality disorder; and prevalence rates for comorbid psychiatric disorders in addiction settings reflect inflated rates for comorbidity.

An extensive review of epidemiological studies was presented in previous chapters. One must be extremely cautious in interpreting the results of these studies as a result of the factors noted earlier. Many studies have not taken into consideration the wide array of psychiatric symptoms produced by addictive substance use and withdrawal, resulting in inflated diagnoses of psychiatric disorders. A tendency also has been to assume that treatment of psychiatric symptoms will result in lowered morbidity and mortality due to the addictive disorders, a theory that arises from the assumption that the addictive disorders are caused by the psychiatric disorder or are secondary to it. This assumption is inconsistent with our current view of addictive disorders being chronic primary illnesses. One unfortunate result of this, however, has been not to diagnose coexisting addictive disorders, resulting in the lack of the provision of the addiction treatment services needed to reduce the secondary psychiatric morbidity and mortality associated with addictive disorders.

Systems Impediments

Sensible treatment of individuals with coexisting psychiatric and addictive disorders requires blending of elements from both psychiatric and addictions treatment methods. In order to understand the difficulties associated with the development of treatment models for dually diagnosed patients, one must first realize how the mental health and addiction fields have differed in their philosophies and treatment approaches and have generally lacked understanding of each other. The two fields have historically not worked well together and at times have even been adversarial in their relationships.[9]

Psychiatric treatment is usually provided by licensed and degreed professionals including psychologists, social workers, and nursing staff under the general direction of psychiatrists. All of these disciplines receive minimal education related to addictive disorders during their professional training. Many of these individuals are victims of the common bias and prejudices in society today regarding addicts, including the perspective that these disorders are self-inflicted and due to immoral behaviors or simply a lack of willpower. As a result, many of these clinicians develop extremely negative countertransference feelings for addicted patients, often maintaining a view that addiction is not a treatable illness. Treatment tends to be centered around psychiatric differential diagnosis, including a focus on the use of psychotropic medications and uncovering psychotherapies. Although insight-oriented psychotherapy may be very useful in treating many types of psychiatric disorders, it also results, as part of the treatment process, in increased anxiety and other dysphoric feelings, which addicted patients commonly deal with by increasing substance use. This approach to treating patients with coexisting addictive disorders often causes these individuals to drop out of treatment as a result of their increased substance use. Treatment also often tends to be nondirective in focus, with patients encouraged to increase their autonomy. Although almost all clinicians in the mental health field have heard of the 12-step programs of Alcoholics, Cocaine, and Narcotics Anonymous, they tend to have many misperceptions and misbeliefs about these programs. They tend to believe that these programs are unscientific because they are peer-led support groups. They also tend to view these programs as being religious in nature because of the reference to God in the 12 steps and the use of the term *spirituality* as a major component of addictive disorders.

Current chemical dependence treatment has evolved since the formulation of the 12-step program of Alcoholics Anonymous (AA) in 1935. Treatment is often provided by non–degree-holding certified addiction counselors who are not formally licensed in most states. A majority of treatment staff are also recovering individuals themselves. Treatment tends to be centered around the philosophies of the 12-step programs, focusing on behavioral changes and peer feedback along with attendance at 12-step program meetings. Treatment tends to encourage patients to give up control and to adhere to a direct and often dogmatic treatment approach. Until fairly recently, treatment centered around a relatively fixed inpatient length of stay (usually 28 days) followed by some minimal outpatient treatment, with a major emphasis on continuing to attend 12-step program meetings. Addiction counselors receive minimal to no education or training regarding psychiatric disorders. These clinicians tend to have many of the biases and prejudices that people in general society today have about psychiatric disorders and often view these illnesses as untreatable. An emphasis of treatment is placed on patients' assuming personal responsibility for their recovery and on "living the program" (12-step programs) on a daily basis. Treatment is often highly confrontational in nature because of the denial most of these patients present with. This approach, although effective in dealing with individuals with chemical addiction problems only, often results in elicitation of anxiety, which could have the effect of worsening psychiatric symptoms in a person with a coexisting psychiatric disorder. As a result, patients have at times decompensated psychiatrically and then have to be referred for intensive psychiatric treatment. Individuals who are involved with the 12-step programs are often advised to avoid any mood- or mind-altering substances. Many addiction counselors thus have the perspective that patients should avoid the use of psychotropic medications, because they lack an understanding of what these medications actually do. Unfortunately, this perspective has also been reinforced in the past by physicians' and psychiatrists' prescribing addicting medications for the treatment of psychiatric symptoms resulting from patients' substance use or withdrawal. These prescription practices have also led to a general negative view of physician/psychiatrist involvement in the treatment of addicted patients. More mental health professionals, including psychiatrists, are becoming involved in addiction treatment. Many of these individuals are themselves recovering and also unfortunately develop many of the misbeliefs and misperceptions previously noted, once they have been involved in their own treatment and have become involved in 12-step programs.

During the past several years, each field has become increasingly aware of the existence of patients with problems in the other field. This has led to each field's attempting to address the other problem in a somewhat simplistic fashion. Psychiatric settings have commonly attempted to address substance abuse and addiction problems by hiring certified addiction counselors to become part of their treatment approach. Unfortunately, addiction counselors often attempt to approach treatment from a traditional perspective as noted earlier, and this plan commonly does not work well and may even worsen the patient's psychiatric symptoms. Similarly, in the addiction field, attempts have been made to include psychiatric staff to help deal with patients with coexisting psychiatric disorders. If a psychiatrist has no training in treatment or understanding of addiction and of dealing with dually diagnosed patients, problems can arise if addicting medications are prescribed or if an attempt is made to involve the patient in intensive, inside-oriented psychotherapy.

These attempts by each field to address the other's problem has often resulted in reinforcement of the negative perspective each field has for the other and impedes the process of psychiatric staff and addiction treatment staff working together to formulate effective treatment approaches to deal with patients' coexisting problems.

Treatment Model Overview

Various conceptual models have been formulated and used to address the treatment needs of dually diagnosed patients. From a general systems perspective, these programs may be viewed as being serial, parallel, or integrated in nature.[10] In serial treatment, a patient is treated first in one setting (either psychiatric or addiction) and then in the other. This approach, which has commonly been used in the past, tends to maintain and reinforce the separateness between the two systems, including all of the impediments to effective treatment noted previously. In parallel treatment, patients are involved simultaneously in treatment for both problems but at different locations. Common examples include patients who are admitted to a hospital psychiatric inpatient treatment unit and who also attend treatment components in the hospital's addiction treatment unit or patients who attend two separate outpatient programs in the community. Although this approach is an improvement over the serial model, because patients at least are introduced to the concept that they need treatment for both problems and clinicians in each field may be led to become more aware of the other, it tends to be inefficient, expensive, and often quite stressful to patients. Again, the impediments to effective treatment in each system noted previously may also cause patients to receive conflicting messages about their treatment, causing confusion and misunderstanding and resulting in a tendency for patients to focus their attention on treatment for one of their problems to the detriment of the other. Although this is not the most effective treatment approach to deal with the treatment needs of dually diagnosed patients, many patients are left with no choice but to be involved in treatment in this manner because of insurance coverage constraints, state agency and bureaucratic turfdom issues, and the lack of the availability of more effective treatment programs.

In integrated treatment models, patients receive simultaneous treatment for both their psychiatric and addiction problems in the same setting. This is the most efficacious way to provide treatment for dually diagnosed patients. In such programs, treatment components from both fields are integrated with each other to provide a treatment approach to address the multiple needs of the dually diagnosed patient population. The initial development of these programs was focused on integrating features of one model of treatment, such as the addiction treatment model, into an established psychiatric treatment program. Subsequent to this, programs were specifically formulated right from the beginning for dually diagnosed patients. Regardless of their mode of formulation, a number of programs, both inpatient and outpatient, have begun to focus, promote, and advertise themselves as being specifically for dually diagnosed patients.

Osher and Kofoed outlined a conceptual model of integrated treatment for dually diagnosed patients that includes four treatment phases: engagement, persuasion, active treatment, and relapse prevention.[11] Specific treatment components consisted of milieu therapy, case management, psychopharmacology, detoxification, toxicologic screening, family involvement, and self-help groups. Lehman and colleagues outlined an integrated treatment model that consists of two general phases of treatment: (1) acute treatment and stabilization and (2) maintenance and rehabilitation.[12]

Rosenthal and associates reported on a model of integrated services for outpatient treatment of patients with comorbid schizophrenia and addictive disorders. It was based on weekly group therapy[13] and focused on establishing a sense of group identity, educating patients about both problems, appropriately controlling psychotic symptoms with antipsychotic medications, encouraging attendance at 12-step program meetings, and improving peer communication skills. A hybrid model of addiction involving integrated treatment provided in a parallel fashion was reported by Minkoff, developed for treatment within a general hospital psychiatric unit.[14] This model included four treatment phases: acute stabilization, engagement, prolonged stabilization, and rehabilitation.

Most all integrated treatment models emphasize the need for comprehensive assessment and concurrent treatment of both problems based on individualized patient needs. It is important to keep in mind that the dually diagnosed patient population is not a homogeneous group and that treatment needs can vary considerably depending on the type and severity of the psychiatric and addictive disorders being treated. Treatment services for well-stabilized patients with coexisting addictive and affective disorders may differ from treatment approaches needed for individuals with coexisting addictive disorders and chronic thought disorders. Regardless of this, however, the key point involves integration of both mental health and addiction services. The mental health services should include crisis management and stabilization, medication management, psychotherapy, education and vocational programming, and case management. Addiction services should include addiction education seminars, group therapy, 12-step program involvement, and relapse prevention. Family support and education are required for both problems, as is focusing on the development of appropriate social networks and constructive use of leisure time. Patients also require education about how both problems affect each other and the need to continue in long-term, simultaneous treatment for both of them. A major overall focus of treatment, therefore, needs to be placed on helping patients develop an identification as having a dual diagnosis with two coexisting treatable disorders.

Treatment Approaches

From a general systems perspective, the ideal way to provide treatment for dually diagnosed patients is to refer all of them to clinicians who, by virtue of education, training, and experience, are believed to be experts in both fields. Such clinicians do actually exist—for example, psychiatrists who have experience and training in addiction or who are certified in addiction psychiatry. Unfortunately, however, not enough of these clinicians are available to adequately assess and provide treatment for all dually diagnosed patients. A more practical alternative is to have individuals from each field obtain additional training in the other field along with training in the integration of treatment for dually diagnosed patients. These individuals could then work together under the direction and supervision of individuals who are experts in both fields. This could be accomplished in either psychiatric or addiction treatment settings and in dual-diagnosis programs. The most critical issue is that all of these treatment professionals have common philosophies and concepts regarding the treatment of individuals with two primary disorders that are related to but not caused by each other. Treatment needs to center around integrating components from both fields to provide a comprehensive multidisciplinary treatment approach to meet the complex needs of patients with a dual diagnosis.

Regardless of the initial setting, the first component of treatment is completion of a comprehensive assessment to evaluate patients for the presence of addictive and psychiatric disorders. A substance use history needs to be completed, including the following components: substances used, age of onset, amount and pattern of substance use, signs of tolerance and withdrawal, addiction-related complications, prior treatment, family history of addiciton, and prior involvement with 12-step programs. It is important to ask questions about the use of all of the different categories of abusable substances including alcohol, illicit drugs, and prescription medications. An initial urine drug screen should be completed, although it is important to keep in mind that a negative urine drug screen does not rule out substance use, abuse, or addiction. A comprehensive physical examination should be completed with a focus on looking for clinical signs of substance use/withdrawal (i.e., tremulousness, diaphoresis, abnormal pupil size, needle tracks, and so forth). A comprehensive psychiatric evaluation should be completed by a psychiatrist who is knowledgeable about addiction in order to assess for the presence of a psychiatric disorder. As a result of the wide variety of psychiatric symptoms that can be caused by addiction,

it may be extremely difficult to accurately diagnose a coexisting separate psychiatric disorder until a patient has been free from the use of addicting chemicals for a significant period. Certain factors, however, do increase the probability that a person has a coexisting psychiatric disorder. They include a history of symptoms consistent with a psychiatric disorder before substance use or during a period of significant total abstinence (at least 2 to 3 months) and a family history of psychiatric illnesses not associated with substance use or addiction.

Once a dual diagnosis is established, patients need to become involved in a treatment regimen that integrates their psychiatric and addiction treatment needs. Clinicians need to provide a therapeutic milieu within which patients feel comfortable in dealing with both of their problems. Clinicians need to provide patients with considerable structure, direction, and support. Clinicians need to be aware of the emergence of negative countertransferance feelings that these patients often elicit. These feelings need to be identified and handled appropriately. Similarly, patients also develop transference feelings toward treating clinicians; these need to be identified and dealt with as part of the treatment process. It is important to keep in mind that patients often enter into treatment with various degrees of denial regarding both their addiction and psychiatric disorders. Although confrontation is necessary to deal with this issue, clinicians need to be aware that intense confrontation can result in worsening of psychiatric symptoms or increasing the risk for relapse to substance use.

Treatment planning should be provided in a highly individualized manner based on the clinical state of the patient. Although the treatment program may have a wide variety of treatment components, it may not be clinically appropriate for every patient to be involved in all of the treatment components right from the beginning of treatment. Dually diagnosed patients often fare poorly in this lockstep approach. Patients should be slowly assimilated into treatment program components as they appear capable of participating in them.

Psychotherapy and counseling should be recovery oriented with a focus on immediate issues that patients need to address at once in order to maintain their recovery. A focus on highly charged emotional issues from the past can result in patients' feeling overwhelmed, resulting in a worsening of their psychiatric symptoms or putting them at risk for relapse. Similarly, individuals who might be identified as adult children of alcoholics or addicts should also delay focusing on issues resulting from addiction in their family of origin until they have been able to maintain a period of recovery and psychiatric stability. Uncovering or insight-oriented psychotherapy should therefore be avoided for most patients.

Patients requiring psychotropic medications for treatment of their psychiatric disorder should be maintained on these medications and continually monitored by a psychiatrist. Potentially addicting medication, such as benzodiazepines and other sedative-hypnotic medications, should be avoided. Patients should be made aware of the fact, however, that if they attend 12-step program meetings, they may be told by well-intentioned but misinformed 12-step program members that they should not take the medication because they are not sober/straight if they are taking it. This problem can be addressed by making patients aware that AA has produced a pamphlet entitled *The AA Member—Medication and Other Drugs*, which clearly states AA's official position that patients should take other medications that are appropriately prescribed for medical or psychiatric problems.[15] This pamphlet can be obtained by ordering it through the local AA Intergroup, whose phone number can be obtained from the local phone directory.

Educational seminars can be a very useful treatment component. They should focus on addressing multiple addiction–related topics as well as educating patients about their psychiatric illnesses. It is also helpful to include information about how psychiatric disorders and addiction are related to each other so that patients can develop a better idea of what it actually means to have two disorders that require long-term treatment. These seminars can help patients formulate an identification as having a dual diagnosis.

Patients should become involved in the 12-step programs of AA and Narcotics and Cocaine Anonymous. These peer self-help support groups can help provide a social network for patients to help them maintain their recovery from addiction. As noted previously, patients who are on medications have often been advised by 12-step program members not to take them. As a result of this, specialized 12-step programs for patients with dual problems have been established. They include AA meetings for psychiatrically recovering patients as well as meetings that have been identified as "double-trouble" meetings. In some areas of the country, these programs have become highly developed. In the Philadelphia area, for example, the double-trouble groups have formulated an intergroup association and have established themselves as a totally autonomous 12-step program with their own 12 steps and 12 traditions. By attending these types of meetings, patients can feel comfortable talking about being on medications and need not be fearful that they will be told to stop them.

As part of the treatment program, patients need to begin to identify cues or triggers for substance use. These have been commonly referred to in the addiction field as the people, places, and things that have been associated with the patient's pattern of substance use in the past. Patients need to formulate plans to deal with these situations effectively in the future. One way in which this can be addressed is through role-playing situations. By using role-playing techniques, patients can be helped to develop the skills necessary to turn down the use of addicting chemicals when they are urged to do so by others.

A focus on leisure-time education and other types of adjunctive therapy should be included as part of the treatment program. Social skills training, relaxation training, assertiveness training, communication skills training, and art and music therapies all are related aspects. Vocational training should be considered for individuals with poor work histories or poor job skills. Individuals who have dropped out or have been suspended from school can be helped to formulate a plan to obtain their general equivalency diploma.

Family involvement also is a very important treatment program component, when clinically appropriate. Family members are often also victimized by the two disorders afflicting the patient. They need to develop an awareness and understanding of how the disorders have affected their loved one and themselves. Family assessments and family counseling should be available. It is also helpful to involve family members in an educational program to teach them about addiction and psychiatric illnesses. Many family members find it useful to become involved in the associated 12-step programs of Al-Anon and Naranon to help them deal with the effects of addiction on themselves. Involvement in Families Anonymous meetings and mental health support groups in the community can also be helpful for many family members.

Before movement from one level of care to another (i.e., inpatient to outpatient), it is helpful for patients to formulate a comprehensive continuing care plan as well as a relapse prevention plan. The continuing care plan should include the treatment components that the patient will be involved in at the next level of care. It should be comprehensive in nature to address on an ongoing basis both of the patient's problems. Attendance at 12-step program meetings is also very important and should be part of the continuing care plan. Patients should also formulate a relapse prevention plan that should include strategies for how they will avoid returning to substance use in the future. It is very helpful for patients to write this plan down in a summary fashion and carry it with them at all times. It can then be used should they find themselves in high-risk situations or in circumstances where they begin to develop intense cravings to use once again.

Dually diagnosed patients being treated in outpatient settings may not be able to achieve immediate abstinence after initiation of treatment. Clinicians may find themselves in the uncomfortable position of having to reinforce continued substance use, albeit at a reduced amount or frequency. This can be addressed by reframing the issue so that patients perceive their reduced use as progress made toward the long-term goal of total abstinence. By presenting the issue in this manner, clinicians can avoid directly reinforcing substance use.

The following case history exemplifies how all of these treatment approaches can be used in the treatment of patients with a dual diagnosis.

CASE HISTORY

Ms. Jane Doe is a single 31-year old unemployed woman who was referred for dual-diagnosis treatment by her local community mental health center. She presented with a 7-year history of progressive alcohol consumption and a 3-year history of crack cocaine smoking. Most recently she had been smoking crack cocaine on an almost every-other-day basis and consuming up to a fifth of hard liquor on an almost daily basis. At the age of 18 years, she had been hospitalized for the first time because of an acute psychotic episode. Before that time, she had not been involved with any type of substance abuse. She was diagnosed at that time as suffering from paranoid schizophrenia. Since then she has been hospitalized on two additional occasions for similar problems, with one episode occurring after she had been admitted to a detoxification unit, where

her psychotropic medication had been discontinued. She had been attending the local community mental health center on an outpatient basis and was being treated with Haldol and Symmetrel. Compliance with medication was poor, and her schizophrenic symptoms appeared to worsen when she smoked cocaine or drank alcohol. Her relationship with her parents, with whom she had been residing, had been deteriorating because she had been taking things from the household and selling them to obtain money to purchase cocaine. She had some brief odd jobs in the past but commonly would be terminated because of poor attendance. Approximately 2 weeks before admission, she had been arrested for possession of cocaine. Because of all of these difficulties, her parents had threatened to throw her out of the household. Her psychiatric symptoms began to worsen, and she was finally referred by her therapist at the local community mental health center to the newly established dual-diagnosis treatment program at a local psychiatric hospital.

Physical examination at the time of admission revealed evidence of mild hepatomegaly thought to be secondary to her alcohol use and chronic bronchitis believed to be secondary to her smoking of freebase cocaine. She initially was detoxified from her alcohol dependence with tapering doses of benzodiazepines. She resumed taking Haldol and Symmetrel, which appeared to be quite effective in reducing her paranoid delusional thinking and auditory hallucinations. After she was completely detoxified and her acute psychiatric problem was stabilized, a staff psychiatrist who was certified in addiction psychiatry performed a comprehensive psychiatric assessment. A diagnosis of schizophrenia, chronic paranoid type, along with cocaine and alcohol dependencies was made. She was informed of these diagnoses, and it was recommended to her that she continue in treatment in the dual-diagnosis program. She reluctantly agreed to do so.

Initially, Ms. Doe appeared to be anxious, guarded, and suspicious. She did not, however, display any evidence of gross delusions or hallucinations. As part of her treatment plan, she was seen by the staff psychiatrist at least three times per week for monitoring of her mental status and adjustment of her medication. During the first 3 days of treatment, she was seen in individual sessions by the therapy staff because it was thought that she was not ready for immediate involvement in group therapy sessions. She subsequently was able to attend group therapy sessions, and although somewhat fearful and apprehensive, she did fairly well with appropriate support and guidance from the group therapist. During individual counseling sessions, she was able to identify specific problems resulting from her addiction, was able to identify some of the deleterious effects her use of cocaine and alcohol had on her thinking and behavior, and was able to develop an awareness of the need for the continued use of psychotropic medication. She was involved in leisure-time education and other adjunctive therapies, with an emphasis placed on assertiveness training, relaxation training, and social skills development. She expressed an interest in obtaining her general equivalency diploma and, with her therapist's help, was able to formulate a plan to obtain it by attending night courses at a local community college after discharge. She also attended AA, Cocaine Anonymous, and double-trouble meetings held at the treatment center. She initially appeared to be somewhat apprehensive at these meetings, but she later felt more comfortable and was even able to speak briefly at one of the meetings.

A family session was completed with Ms. Doe and her parents. They initially appeared quite distraught and were not really sure whether their daughter was "crazy" or whether she was just an alcoholic and an addict. Her parents, with Ms. Doe present, were informed of their daughter's dual diagnoses and received some educational information about both problems. They were quite supportive of their daughter's involvement in treatment and were willing to become involved in family counseling sessions after her discharge. They also agreed to attend Al-Anon meetings and support groups for families of the mentally ill, and they were referred to such programs in their community.

Ms. Doe subsequently worked with her therapist to formulate an aftercare plan. She was agreeable to becoming involved in the dual-diagnosis outpatient program, which was an extension of the inpatient program. She agreed to see a psychiatrist there for medication monitoring. Arrangements were made for her to attend the dual-diagnosis partial hospitalization day treatment program 3 days per week. Because of her interest in returning to work, arrangements were

made for her to attend a program at the local bureau of vocational rehabilitation the other 2 days per week. She agreed to see a therapist in the outpatient dual-diagnosis program who was skilled and experienced in working with dually diagnosed patients. She also agreed to attend at least one AA or Cocaine Anonymous meeting weekly as well as one double-trouble meeting weekly. Specific meetings were identified for her to attend, and she wrote these down in her aftercare workbook for future reference. She also completed a comprehensive relapse prevention plan that she kept with her in her pocketbook on an ongoing basis.

At the time of discharge, Ms. Doe's psychiatric symptoms were well controlled using Haldol and Symmetrel. She stated that for the first time in her life she felt that she finally had some understanding of what was happening to her as a result of both her psychiatric and addictive disorders.

Conclusion

The treatment of patients with a dual diagnosis poses many challenges for clinicians in the mental health and addiction fields. It is hoped that further research will validate that the treatment models and approaches presented result in decreased overall morbidity and mortality for patients with coexisting addictive and psychiatric disorders. It is critical that psychiatrists knowledgeable about and experienced in addictive disorders assume a leadership role in developing and administering programs, conducting research, and advocating for the complex needs of patients with a dual diagnosis.

REFERENCES

1. Wallen MC, Weiner HD: The dually diagnosed patient in an inpatient chemical dependency treatment program. Alcoholism Treatment Quarterly 5(1/2):197–218, 1988.
2. Halikas JA, Crosby RD, Pearson VL, et al: Psychiatric comorbidity in treatment-seeking cocaine abusers. American Journal on Addictions 3:25–35, 1994.
3. Barbee JG, Clark PD, Crapanzano MS, et al: Alcohol and substance abuse among schizophrenic patients presenting to an emergency psychiatric service. J Nerv Ment Dis 177(7):400–407, 1989.
4. Miller F, Busch F, Tanenbaum J: Drug abuse in schizophrenia and bipolar disorder. Am J Drug Alcohol Abuse 15(3):291–295, 1989.
5. Rounsaville B: Psychiatric co-morbidity in alcoholics. Substance Abuse 11(4):186–191, 1990.
6. Lydiard RB, Brady K, Ballenger JC, et al: Anxiety and

mood disorders in hospitalized alcohol individuals. American Journal on Addictions 1(4):325–331, 1992.

7. Reiger DA, Farmer ME, Rae DS, et al: Comorbidity of mental disorders with alcohol and other drug abuse: Results from the Epidemiologic Catchment Area (ECA) Study. JAMA 264:2511–2518, 1990.

8. Miller NS, Fine J: Current epidemiology of comorbidity of psychiatric and addictive disorders. Psychiatr Clin North Am 16(1):1–10, 1993.

9. Wallen MC, Weiner HD: Impediments to effective treatment of the dually diagnosed patient. J Psychoactive Drugs 21(2):161–168, 1989.

10. Ries R: Clinical treatment matching models for dually diagnosed patients. Psychiatr Clin North Am 16(1):167–175, 1993.

11. Osher F, Kofoed L: Treatment of patients with psychiatric and psychoactive substance abuse disor-ders. Hosp Community Psychiatry 40(10):1025–1029, 1989.

12. Lehman A, Myers C, Corty E: Assessment and classification of patients with psychiatric and substance abuse syndromes. Hosp Community Psychiatry 40(10):1019–1024, 1989.

13. Rosenthal RN, Hellerstein DJ, Miner CR: A model of integrated services for outpatient treatment of patients with comorbid schizophrenia and addictive disorders. American Journal on Addictions 1(4):339–348, 1992.

14. Minkoff K: An integrated treatment model for dual diagnosis of psychosis and addiction. Hosp Community Psychiatry 40(10):1031–1036, 1989.

15. Alcoholics Anonymous: The AA Member—Medication and Other Drugs. New York, Alcoholics Anonymous World Services, 1984.

15

Medical Disorders in Addicted Patients

Michael D. Stein, MD

Since the advent of the epidemic of human immunodeficiency virus (HIV) infection in the early 1980s, the medical care of illicit drug users has become central to national and local public health planning. Drug users are at high risk of acquiring and transmitting HIV to their social network via needle sharing, trading sex for drugs, sexual relations with steady partners, and perinatally. The association between alcohol abuse and high-risk behaviors for contracting acquired immunodeficiency syndrome (AIDS) has more recently been demonstrated by the finding of a substantial prevalence of HIV infection among clients in alcohol treatment programs.[1]

Before HIV disease, life-threatening events were not new to populations of drug and alcohol abusers.[2, 3] Indeed, injection drug addicts have been found to die at seven times the rate of comparable age groups in the general population.[4] Population studies have shown that heavy drinkers have an increased risk of death due to cirrhosis, motor vehicle accidents, suicide, homicide, certain malignancies, and hemorrhagic cerebrovascular disease.[5] Behaviors and environment often dictate health, and a disproportionate share of addicts still reside in high-risk neighborhoods; that they die drug-related and violence-related deaths comes as no surprise.

Although HIV disease has focused attention on *injection* drug use, other routes of drug administration may lead to equally pernicious medical complications. This chapter is divided into four parts. Discussed first are the complications of alcohol, the most commonly abused substance in the United States. The second section discusses the complications of injected drug use, focusing on those illnesses that are specifically due to needle use. Most of this literature derives from series of opiate abusers. The third part discusses the complications of cocaine use. Cocaine has toxicities apart from its route of administration, and these are highlighted. The final part discusses the complications of HIV disease that have been described in persons who use illicit drugs. Because the complications that bring persons into medical care are mostly due to alcohol, opiate, and cocaine abuse, these three drugs are the focus of this chapter, and discussions of other classes of drugs are not included. Discussion of the psychological and social complications of drug use are found elsewhere in this book.

The spectrum of disease related to drugs of abuse is broad and often insidious. Healthcare providers must actively consider drug use when taking patients' histories, performing physical examinations, and considering differential diagnoses in order to identify drug users before serious complications occur.[6] Preventive healthcare requires early identification of those at risk for drug use complications. When drug-related complications occur, providers may have a special opportunity to direct particularly receptive patients into drug treatment.[7]

The literature concerning the range of medical complications due to alcohol, opiates, and cocaine is based on case series and individual case reports. No large surveys documenting the natural history of the complications of opiates or cocaine use exist. Therefore, it is difficult to assess the precise toxicity of drugs of abuse because most reports do not and cannot report standard doses, because patient-reported histories are often unreliable, and because concomitant multidrug use is common among chemically dependent persons.

Alcohol

Although there is continued disagreement about risk levels of alcohol consumption for individuals, once a medical complication of alcohol use has occurred, it may serve as an aid in breaking though patients' denial of their problem drinking. Higher than expected rates of care seeking for digestive disorders and traumatic injuries are associated with heavy alcohol use across broad populations of patients, although many other health problems have been described among heavy users.[8] Population studies have shown that heavy drinkers have an increased risk of death due to cirrhosis, motor vehicle accidents, suicide, homicide, particular malignancies, and cerebrovascular disease.[5, 9] The importance of controlling for cigarette smoking, a strong correlate of alcohol use and a predictor of death due to several of these causes, is well known.[10] Nonetheless, the risk of death among heavy drinkers is at least 50% higher than the risk among light drinkers, and this risk is increased more for women than men.[11] Alcoholic men who achieve stable abstinence return to age-, sex-, and race-matched mortality experience.[12]

There is generally a direct relationship between alcohol consumption level or duration of use and clinical problems. It has been noted that women have higher blood levels than

Table 15–2. PHYSICAL FINDINGS AMONG HEAVY ALCOHOL USERS

Spider angiomata	Tachycardia
Palmar erythema	Hypertension
Gynecomastia	Dupuytren's contracture
Parotid gland enlargement	Proximal myopathy
Polyneuropathy	Periorbital edema
Hepatomegaly	Jaundice
Splenomegaly	Heme-positive stool

men, given an equivalent dose of alcohol,[13] most likely because of smaller size and less first-pass gastric metabolism.

Chronic heavy alcohol use is associated with protean medical complications. A wide range of symptoms (Table 15–1), physical findings (Table 15–2), and laboratory abnormalities (Table 15–3) have been described. Many of the disorders described next can be halted or reversed by cessation of alcohol intake. The most common disorders associated with alcohol use are described, concentrating on clinical findings but also touching on treatments and prognosis.

GASTROINTESTINAL

The most common complaints related to alcohol use are gastrointestinal: pain, bloating, nausea, and vomiting.[14] Alcohol slows gastric emptying, stimulates gastric secretions, and injures gastric mucosa. Although symptoms often subside with the cessation of intake, for even moderate drinkers the risk of gastritis and ulcers is not trivial. Heavy chronic drinking is associated with acute and chronic pancreatitis, which must be differentiated from gastritis and ulcer for those patients with abdominal symptoms.

Right upper quadrant pain is a frequent presentation of liver disease and often occurs in persons consuming modest quantities of alcohol (20 to 40 g/day). It may signify fatty liver (the most common histological abnormality on biopsy), hepatitis, cholestasis, or portal hypertension. Alcoholic hepatitis may be asymptom-

Table 15–1. MEDICAL SIGNS AND SYMPTOMS OF ALCOHOL ABUSE

Nausea	Abdominal pain
Vomiting	Weight loss
Anorexia	Muscle weakness
Diarrhea	Dizziness
Tremor	Confusion
Myalgia	Headache

Table 15–3. LABORATORY ABNORMALITIES DUE TO ALCOHOL ABUSE

Hyponatremia	Thrombocytopenia
Hypokalemia	Hypophosphatemia
Hypomagnesemia	Transaminitis
Hyperamylasemia	Anemia
Hyperbilirubinemia	Leukopenia
Prolonged prothrombin time	

atic or florid and life threatening, usually developing over weeks and accompanied by vomiting, weight loss, and sometimes jaundice. In mild cases, the course is benign, but a significant number of persons worsen despite abstinence and nutritional care. The clinical, biochemical, and histological consequences of hepatic injury may occur separately or in combination, although there is a poor correlation between clinical syndromes and pathological abnormalities.

Early diagnosis of alcohol-related liver complications is important because both fatty liver and alcohol hepatitis are reversible but cirrhosis is not. Cirrhosis occurs in 10% to 20% of chronic heavy alcohol users (120 to 180 g/day for more than 15 years) but is discovered in only 25% of patients antemortem. Women may have a greater susceptibility to cirrhosis.[15] Non–alcohol-related liver disease must be considered even among heavy alcohol users.

CARDIOVASCULAR

Chronic alcohol abuse can be associated with various cardiovascular disorders including hypertension, stroke, heart failure, and sudden death. Alcoholic cardiomyopathy is often subclinical. Clinical decompensation typically occurs in persons who have ingested at least 80 g/day for at least 10 years.[16] If diagnosed early, alcoholic cardiomyopathy responds to cessation of alcohol intake.

Cardiac arrhythmias, mostly atrial, can occur during intoxication, withdrawal, and even moderate intake in persons without cardiomyopathy. Atrial fibrillation is the most common presenting rhythm, and electrolyte levels are usually normal.[17] Cardioversion is often required to return patients to sinus rhythm. An increased risk of sudden cardiac death in persons who abuse alcohol but who do not have known heart disease has been noted in cohort studies and case-control series.[18]

Epidemiological studies have also found a positive association between the amount of alcohol consumed and cerebrovascular accidents including subarachnoid hemorrhage and stroke.[5] This increased risk may be mediated by alcohol-induced hypertension.[19] Primary care providers should consider alcohol consumption as a potential cause of hypertension, because 5% to 10% of hypertensive cases are thought to be due to alcohol intake. Certainly, response to antihypertensive agents is lessened by active alcohol use. For heavy drinkers (six or more drinks per day), the prevalence of hypertension is double that of abstinent individuals.[20]

HEMATOLOGICAL

The hematological disorders related to alcohol result from the direct effects of ethanol, those resulting from secondary nutritional deficiencies, and those due to hepatic disease.[21] A spectrum of hematological problems involving red blood cells, white blood cells, platelets, and other hemostatic factors has been described, because the production of erythrocytes, white blood cells, and platelets can be suppressed by alcohol. In severe alcoholism, anemia with macrocytosis is a frequent finding. In alcohol users without marked liver disease, folate deficiency, reticulocytosis, and macrocytosis predominate, often without anemia. As many as 75% of heavy alcohol users may have bone marrow hypofunction, and half of these cases are related to folate deficiency, which may be due to poor intake, decreased capacity to store folate, and impaired jejunal folate absorption. Anemia in heavy alcohol users is due to multiple causes including iron deficiency (from gastrointestinal bleeding), decreased red blood cell survival, defects of marrow production, and nutritional deficiencies.[21]

Persistent leukopenia and thrombocytopenia are markers of long-term alcoholism. A minority of alcoholics have neutropenia, although this may be more common among those with infections. Thrombocytopenia, which may be present in as many as 25% of acutely intoxicated patients, is likely due to both decreased production and survival of platelets; return to normal platelet counts occurs after 2 to 4 weeks of abstinence. Results of coagulation studies do not change after acute alcohol ingestion; fibinolytic and coagulation factor changes occur only with chronic alcohol intake.

GYNECOLOGICAL

Numerous gynecological and obstetrical complications are associated with heavy alcohol consumption. Specifically, amenorrhea, dysfunctional uterine bleeding, dysmennorhea, infertility, and premenstrual syndrome have been described. The obstetrical complications of alcohol consumption include spontaneous abortion, stillbirth, premature labor, and low-birth-weight infants. It is estimated that one third of babies born to women drinking more than six alcoholic beverages per day during pregnancy have fetal alcohol syndrome.[22]

METABOLIC

The metabolic disturbances due to acute alcohol intoxication are complex. Metabolic acidosis due to vomiting and dehydration, respiratory alkalosis due to withdrawal, sepsis or pain, and metabolic ketoacidosis all may be superimposed.[23] Electrolyte disturbances including hypokalemia, hyponatremia, hypomagnesemia, and hypophosphatemia are not uncommon, particularly when persons with chronic alcohol abuse and malnutrition start binge drinking.

CENTRAL NERVOUS SYSTEM

Neurological disorders constitute a large, diverse, and devastating subset of medical complications of alcoholism.[24] Complications involve every level of the nervous system and may be caused by a combination of direct neurotoxic effects, nutritional factors, and genetics. Alcohol intoxication (with blood levels reflecting levels in the brain) first affects vestibular and cerebellar functions, causing nystagmus, dysarthria, and ataxia; further intake may lead to mild confusion, stupor, respiratory suppression, and coma. Comatose alcoholic patients pose an array of diagnostic possibilities including mixed-drug overdose, head trauma, electrolyte disturbances, meningitis, and ketoacidosis. Although intoxication is legally defined in most places as 100 mg/dl, levels as low as 47 mg/dl are associated with increased risk of motor vehicle accidents.[25] Chronic tolerance (thought to be due to adaptive changes in membrane lipids, neuromodulators, neurotransmitter receptors, ion channels, and G-proteins) permits alcoholic patients to remain sober despite extremely high ethanol concentrations.

Heavy alcohol intake for short periods or lower level ingestion for prolonged period leads to physical dependence. Cessation of drinking or reduction in intake in physically dependent persons may lead to a withdrawal syndrome.[25] This syndrome is characterized by autonomic hyperactivity, nausea and vomiting, insomnia, tremor, agitation, and perceptual disturbance that includes visual or auditory illusions. Symptoms begin within hours of withdrawal onset, peak at 24 to 36 hours, and may be suppressed by resumption of drinking, beta-adrenergic receptor blockade, or alpha-2-adrenergic blockade.

A minority of persons (20% to 30%) undergoing withdrawal have generalized tonic-clonic seizures early in withdrawal. For patients who have seizures *after* the first 24 hours of withdrawal, who have focal neurological deficits, or who have signs of head trauma, brain imaging is required to evaluate for a treatable abnormality such as a subdural hematoma.

The most serious and delayed (day 2 to 4) manifestation of withdrawal is delirium tremens. Approximately 5% of those hospitalized for withdrawal develop delirium tremens, which is characterized by profound confusion and agitation and severe autonomic hyperactivity including tachycardia and fever. Frequently precipitated by other illnesses (pancreatitis, trauma), delirium tremens resolves in 80% of cases within 72 hours, but 5% of patients may die. These outcomes have not changed significantly during the past two decades despite the widespread use of benzodiazepines to limit the discomfort of withdrawal.

Wernicke's encephalopathy, caused by thiamine deficiency, classically includes the triad of encephalopathy, ophthalmoplegia (nystagmus, lateral rectus palsies), and ataxia. Although only a third of patients with acute Wernicke's encephalopathy have all three signs, a majority are profoundly disoriented.[24] Only a subset of thiamine-deficient alcoholics have Wernicke's encephalopathy, however; how thiamine deficiency leads to the characteristic brain lesions is unclear. With prompt repletion of thiamine (100 mg of thiamine per day for at least 5 days), ocular signs improve within hours and ataxia and cognitive signs within days, most likely representing biochemical improvement rather than a structural lesion's reversal. A majority of these patients are left with Korsakoff's syndrome, a disabling anterograde and retrograde memory disorder.

Many long-term heavy alcohol users have impaired performance on neuropsychological tests even when sober; this may be due to premorbid intellectual deficits, ethanol neurotoxicity, head trauma, and nutritional deficiencies.[24] Chronic cerebral degeneration may occur after 10 or more years of heavy use, although this condition does not correlate with daily or lifetime consumption patterns, and the cause remains unknown.[24] It is usually of subacute onset, and gait ataxia is the prominent symptom.

Alcoholic patients also have a high incidence of peripheral nerve disorders, most commonly polyneuropathies thought to be due to thiamine deficiency and other B vitamin deficits. Gradually progressive, the clinical findings are usually symmetrical and distal including numbness, paresthesias, cramps, weakness, and loss of tendon reflexes. Improved nutrition and abstinence often result in improvement.

Alcoholic myopathy may present acutely or more slowly. The acute form, which is rare, develops over hours (often during a binge) and is characterized by weakness, tenderness, and swelling of the affected muscle. It most often involves proximal muscles. Serum creatinine kinase levels are elevated, myoglobinuria is noted, and necrosis of muscle fibers is found on biopsy. Chronic myopathy is more common. The major findings are muscle weakness and atrophy affecting the hip and shoulder groups. Cessation of drinking leads to improvement in most patients.

TRAUMA

The degree of alcohol intake is related to the risk of traumatic death.[26] Younger drinkers are known to be more likely to be involved in alcohol-related accidental deaths than older persons.[11] Alcohol is also associated with non-fatal injury, and minor trauma may be a clue to excessive drinking. Alcohol and drug addiction are also major risk factors for suicide, as both cause and precipitant.[27]

DRUG INTERACTIONS

Alcohol interacts with hypnosedatives (antihistamines, barbiturates, benzodiazapines, phenothiazines, and opiates) to cause respiratory depression. With warfarin, alcohol can increase anticoagulant potency. With acetominophen, hepatotoxic metabolites cause liver necrosis. Alcohol may interact with tricyclic antidepressants to increase the risk of seizures and arrhythmias. Disulfiram-like reactions can occur with chlorpropamide, metronidazole, isoniazid, and some cephalosporins.

Injection Drug Use

Illicit drug use leads to approximately 20,000 deaths each year in the United States.[28] These deaths result from such causes as overdose, suicide, homicide, motor vehicle injuries, pneumonia, hepatitis, endocarditis, and HIV disease[29] (Table 15–4).

Before the advent of AIDS, medical epidemics penetrating this population included hepatitis and tetanus. In the 1950s, in New York City, 8.3% of deaths among addicts were due to tetanus. In the late 1960s, acute hepatitis was "the foremost cause of addicts' admissions to municipal hospitals."[2] During the past decade,

Table 15–4. MEDICAL COMPLICATIONS OF PARENTERAL DRUGS

Infectious	Noninfectious
Endocarditis	Nephrotic syndrome
Pneumonia	Glomerulonephritis
Cellulitis	Renal failure
Cutaneous abscess	Arrhythmia
Gas gangrene	Mycotic aneurysm
Infected false aneurysm	Talc granuloma
Osteomyelitis	Pulmonary edema
Septic arthritis	Pneumothorax
Sexually transmitted	Pneumomediastinum
diseases	Pulmonary fibrosis
Tuberculosis	Pulmonary hypertension
Tetanus	Motility disorders
Malaria	Constipation
Human immunodeficiency	Stroke
virus infection	Myositis
Epidural abscess	Overdose
Subdural abscess	Trauma
Brain abscess	Needle embolus
Hepatitis A, B, C, and D	Necrotizing angiitis
viruses	Amenorrhea
	Thrombocytopenia

novel infectious and noninfectious syndromes have been identified among injection drug users (IDUs).[30]

The drugs injected by addicts include heroin, cocaine, Demerol, Dilaudid, pentazocine, tripelennamine, and barbiturates.[2] These are used individually or mixed and before injection are usually liquefied then filtered through cotton into syringes. Opiates are sold in bags that arrive on the street with a wide range of purity. Users' lack of awareness of the exact dose injected may be one cause of overdoses. Even in the era of AIDS, drug overdoses remain the leading cause of death among IDUs.[31]

The possibilities of contamination between bag and bloodstream are both chemical and microbial. Quinine, used as a diluter, may produce anaerobic skin abscesses. Cotton, used as a filter, itself causes granulomatous pulmonary reactions.[2] An addict's skin flora is the likely source of infecting organisms, as demonstrated by the microbiology of soft tissue infections such as cellulitis and skin abscesses.[32] Skin flora may be expected to differ among institutions as well as according to individuals' injection sites. Beta-hemolytic streptococci and *Staphylococcus aureus* account for the majority of microbial causes, although anaerobes predominate in some series.[33, 34]

FEVER

Fever is a frequent reason for hospital admission among IDUs and can be a manifestation of both common and unusual medical conditions. The major concern in the evaluation of a febrile IDU is differentiating serious illness (such as endocarditis) from less serious illness that can be managed without hospitalization. Two studies have examined consecutive series of febrile IDUs.[35, 36] Although in a majority of cases the cause of fever is clinically apparent after a physical examination and initial testing (e.g., pneumonia, cellulitis), in roughly one third of cases the cause of fever is not apparent. Neither study could identify clinical or laboratory features that might assist clinicians in identifying serious illness in this group. Therefore, hospitalization is often recommended for febrile IDUs in order to ensure adherence to follow-up examinations and to initiate parenteral antibiotics for those who may have occult bacteremia. The differential diagnosis of fever in IDUs presenting to emergency departments is shown in Table 15–5.

ENDOCARDITIS

Injection drug use creates the endothelial valvular damage and platelet fibrin deposition thought necessary for bacterial endocarditis. Endocarditis is diagnosed by the presence of persistently positive blood cultures and cardiac valve involvement.[37] The incidence of bacterial endocarditis is estimated at 2 cases per 1000 addicts per year. An affinity between particular organisms and particular valves may exist.[38] S. aureus remains the most frequent isolate in endocarditis, and the tricuspid valve is the valve most frequently involved. Right-sided endocarditis generally has a favorable prognosis, with septic pulmonary emboli the major complication. Streptococcus, the next most common organism, may have a proclivity for left-sided valves, where systemic embolization more often leads to fatal outcomes. Echogenic vegetations are predictive of complications of endocarditis, and their appearance may persist after bacteriological cure. Clinical prediction of the infecting species is difficult, and directed antibiotic therapy remains of greatest importance.

PULMONARY

Dyspnea is another common IDU complaint that results from common diseases as well as syndromes unique to this population. For instance, talc granulomatosis is unique to those addicts who dilute their drug of choice with talc. Deposition of talc crystals in pulmonary arterioles leads to granuloma formation and chronic dyspnea.[39] Acute onset of shortness of breath suggests a toxic drug reaction. Bronchospasm has been reported after intravenous opiate use. Pulmonary edema from heroin use may also occur, although the proposed mechanisms remain speculative and include allergic reaction, opiate-induced histamine release, and a central nervous system effect.[2]

Pneumonia, with typical community-acquired organisms such as Hemophilus influenzae and Streptococcus pneumoniae, is common. Alcohol use, in addition to cigarettes and drug injection, increases the risk of aspiration. Consideration of opportunistic pulmonary infections is important even in the absence of documented HIV seropositivity.

The resurgence of tuberculosis in general and among IDUs in particular geographical areas has been alarming during the past 5 years. Latent tuberculosis has been found in as many as 25% of selected urban drug-using populations.[40] Alcohol has been associated with the reactivation of tuberculosis, partly because of malnutrition and poor compliance with antituberculous chemotherapy. The possibility of tuberculosis must be considered with any pulmonary infiltrate. Respiratory precautions, before definitive diagnosis, are appropriate for IDUs admitted to the hospital with abnormal findings on chest radiographs.

HEPATITIS

IDUs are at high risk for various forms of infectious and toxic hepatitis. Approximately two thirds of long-term injectors have serological evidence of hepatitis B virus and hepatitis C virus infection.[41, 42] Acute and chronic liver disease may be exacerbated by concomitant alcohol abuse. Outbreaks of delta hepatitis leading to fulminant liver failure have been described among drug injectors.[43] Clinically important cytomegalovirus or Epstein-Barr vi-

Table 15–5. DIFFERENTIAL DIAGNOSIS OF FEVER IN 370 INTRAVENOUS DRUG USERS

Diagnosis	Number	%
Pneumonia	96	26
Cellulitis	70	19
Endocarditis	30	8
Abscess	11	3
Other major or nontrivial illness	48	13
Minor or trivial illness	115	31

Adapted from O'Connor PG, Samet JH, Stein MD: Management of hospitalized intravenous drug users: Role of the internist. Am J Med 96:551–558, 1994.

rus hepatitis is very rare among addicts. The progression from chronic persistent to chronic active hepatitis may be more common in IDUs, perhaps because of continued viral exposure and higher viral load.[42] The majority of alcohol-using IDUs have histological evidence of chronic liver disease ranging from chronic persistent hepatitis to cirrhosis.

SEXUALLY TRANSMITTED DISEASES

Sexually transmitted infections have been associated with substance abuse owing to the exchange of sex for drugs and the finding that sexual impulsivity has been associated with psychoactive substance use, particularly cocaine and alcohol. Those infections that cause genital ulceration facilitate the transmission of HIV infection. The high false-positive rate of nontreponemal test results for syphilis in IDUs justifies the use of specific treponemal tests.[44] Recommending and distributing latex condoms may prevent infections.

RENAL DISEASE

Various chronic renal conditions have been reported among IDUs. Urinalysis commonly demonstrates mild to moderate proteinuria, as well as hematuria. Nephrotic syndrome (heroin nephropathy) is most often due to focal or diffuse glomerulosclerosis and may progress to end-stage renal disease.[45] Renal amyloidosis occurs in addicts who "skin pop" or have repeated skin ulceration or abscesses.[46]

WITHDRAWAL

For opiate users, hospitalization with any of the aforementioned complications puts them at risk for withdrawal. In patients with known or suspected substance abuse, a detailed substance use history and toxicological screening can help clinicians anticipate the development of withdrawal syndromes. Heroin withdrawal typically begins from 3 to 5 hours after the last heroin use.[47] Other opiates have different time courses of withdrawal, depending on their half-lives. Left untreated, heroin withdrawal typically peaks at 3 days and may last as long as 2 weeks. Unlike alcohol withdrawal, heroin withdrawal is not associated with either severe morbidity or mortality. Symptoms of withdrawal include piloerection, perspiration, lacrimation, nausea, myalgia, yawning, and restlessness (Table 15–6). Physical findings include tachycardia, hypertension, fever, and diarrhea. Mild withdrawal symptoms may be treated

Table 15–6. WITHDRAWAL SYNDROMES FOR OPIOIDS AND COCAINE

Opioid Withdrawal	
Vital signs	Tachycardia, hypertension
Central nervous system	Craving, restlessness, insomnia, muscle cramps, yawning
Eyes, nose	Lacrimation, rhinorrhea
Skin	Perspiration, piloerection
Gastrointestinal	Nausea, vomiting, diarrhea
Cocaine Withdrawal	
Crash	Depression, fatigue
Withdrawal	Anxiety, high craving
Extinction	Normalization of mood, episodic craving

effectively with clonidine, which suppresses those manifestations of autonomic nervous system dysfunction. Persons with moderate to severe withdrawal may require methadone, which can be tapered over 5 to 7 days.

Cocaine

During the past decade, with the escalation of cocaine use and the arrival of crack cocaine, the medical complications of cocaine use have been amplified (Table 15–7). Although many of the complications of cocaine use are due to

Table 15–7. COMPLICATIONS ASSOCIATED WITH COCAINE USE

Cardiac	Pulmonary
Chest pain	Pneumothorax
Myocardial infarction	Pneumomediastinum
Arrhythmias	"Crack lung"
Cardiomyopathy	Pulmonary edema
Myocarditis	Exacerbation of asthma
Endocrine	Pulmonary hemorrhage
Hyperprolactinemia	Psychiatric
Gastrointestinal	Anxiety
Intestinal ischemia	Depression
Gastroduodenal perforations	Paranoia
	Delirium
Head and neck	Psychosis
Dental enamel erosions	Suicide
Gingival ulceration	Overdose
Keratitis	Withdrawal
Corneal epithelial defects	
Chronic rhinitis	Renal
Perforated nasal septum	Rhabdomyolysis
Altered olfaction	
Optic neuropathy	Obstetrical
	Placental abruption
Neurological	Lower infant weight
Headaches	Prematurity
Seizures	Microcephaly
Cerebral hemorrhage	
Cerebral vasculitis	

needle puncture and are therefore similar to those described among opiate users, others are due to direct drug toxicity. The most common complaints that bring cocaine users to emergency rooms are cardiac (chest pain, palpitations) and neurological problems (seizures). Cocaine's toxicity is most likely due to its primary physiological effect, vasospasm.[48] Psychiatric symptoms, such as suicidal intent, are also a common presentation. Of note, however, is that no pathognomonic feature of cocaine abuse exists; therefore, those complications ascribed to cocaine can be determined only by a patient's history or toxicology studies.

CARDIAC

Cocaine use has been associated with sudden death.[49] Hypothesized mechanisms include arrhythmias (ventricular fibrillation, asystole), with or without cocaine-induced cardiomyopathy or myocardial ischemia. Angiographic studies of patients with cocaine-related myocardial infarctions have demonstrated both diseased and normal coronary vasculature. In those one third of persons who have normal coronary arteries, vasospasm, enhanced platelet aggregation, and increased myocardial oxygen demand due to cocaine-related tachycardia and hypertension may be the cause of infarction. The onset of ischemia may occur minutes to up to 36 hours after cocaine use. Silent ischemia has been documented in cocaine users undergoing withdrawal.

NEUROLOGICAL

The most common symptom reported by regular cocaine users is headaches. High levels of cocaine may lead to cerebral vasospasm and strokes, particularly with crack use.[50] Injection of cocaine has been associated with hemorrhagic stroke.[50] Long-term cocaine users may develop cerebral atrophy. Cerebral vasculitis has also been described.[51]

PULMONARY

Inhalation of cocaine commonly causes wheezing, and exacerbations of asthma have been described. Pain, hemoptysis, and diffuse alveolar infiltrates, known as *crack lung*, may be a hypersensitivity reaction to cocaine or an unknown cocaine diluter.[52] Smoking cocaine has been associated with pulmonary edema (possibly due to altered capillary permeability) and barotrauma leading to pneumothorax.[49]

The long-term effects of regular cocaine smoking remain unknown. Smoking of cocaine has also been found to be a risk factor for bacterial pneumonia.[47]

OTHER COMPLICATIONS

Acute renal failure as a result of rhabdomyolysis has been described. Most patients have mild or no neuromuscular symptoms with cocaine-associated rhabdomyolysis. In one series, one third of patients developed acute renal failure, and half of these patients died.[53] Aggressive supportive care is necessary, often including dialysis.

Intestinal ischemia has been reported after cocaine use. Otolaryngological complications include gingival ulceration, erosion of dental enamel, and perforated nasal septum.

The use of cocaine during pregnancy has been associated with an increased risk for low infant birth weights, prematurity, microcephaly, and placental abruption.[54]

Cocaine has also been associated with violent behavior. Forty percent of homicide victims in one study tested positive for cocaine.[55] In New York, 21% of suicide victims younger than 60 tested positive at autopsy.[56]

HIV Disease

Injection drug use has been established as an important risk factor for infection with HIV. The proportion of AIDS cases related to injection drug use has steadily increased and currently constitutes half of all cases among women. However, the natural history of HIV infection among drug users remains understudied. Two issues are in question. First, does HIV disease progress faster or slower among persons with a history of injection drug use or among those who are still using drugs than among those persons who have been infected with HIV via other behaviors? Second, are the clinical manifestations that characterize HIV disease different in drug users from those in other populations?

HIV DISEASE PROGRESSION

Two studies early in the HIV epidemic suggested that IDUs had a more rapid decline in CD4 lymphocyte count than that reported in homosexual men.[57, 58] However, these studies were limited by small cohort size and short duration of follow-up. Other studies have demonstrated depletion of CD4 lymphocytes among IDUs at rates no different from cohorts of gay men.[59] These studies also suggest that use or nonuse of drugs does not significantly affect CD4 cell count decline. Further, no relationship was found between the rate of change in CD4 cell counts and frequency of drug injection.[59] Studies with longer follow-up and better functional immunological assays are needed.

Fewer studies have attempted to describe the relationship between use of psychoactive drugs or alcohol and subsequent occurrence of AIDS in HIV-infected persons.[60] Research from a large cohort of gay men demonstrated that neither alcohol nor other classes of commonly used substances (cocaine, nitrites, phencyclidine, amphetamines, barbiturates) were important cofactors for the development of AIDS. Certainly drug and alcohol use may lead to those complications described in the earlier parts of this chapter, unrelated to HIV disease, or may influence behavior that leads to dissemination of HIV infection, but the immunological expression of HIV infection seems to be unchanged.

HIV DISEASE MANIFESTATIONS

The inverse correlation between CD4 cell counts and incidence of AIDS (as defined by the Centers for Disease Control's list of diagnoses) is noted in IDUs as in all other populations of persons infected with HIV.[61] Indeed, IDUs have a pattern of HIV-related disease that is largely similar to that in other populations with AIDS.[62] However, several distinctions are worthy of note.

IDUs were known to be at risk for bacterial pneumonia before the AIDS epidemic.[63] Several studies have documented a risk of bacterial pneumonia more than four times greater in seropositive drug users than in seronegative drug users.[64] S. pneumoniae and H. influenzae are again the most frequently found organisms, suggesting the importance of vaccination to prevent these infections early in the course of HIV infection. Higher rates of bacteremia are found in HIV-infected persons with pneumonia, although response to treatment is similar. Bacterial pneumonia itself may be associated with more rapid HIV disease progression.[63.]

HIV-associated tuberculosis has been related to injection drug use.[65] Extrapulmonary mycobacterial disease (meningitis, bone involvement) is not uncommon in drug users with advanced HIV infection, representing between 25% and 70% of cases.[66] The classical findings of upper lobe involvement and cavitation are in fact uncommon in patients with AIDS. Drug users with positive skin test results have a high risk of active tuberculosis, highlighting the importance of antituberculosis therapy.[67] Such therapy (isoniazid) must be monitored closely because of the high frequency of underlying liver disease. Once a diagnosis of active tuberculosis is made, four or five drug regimens are recommended, often with direct observation of patient compliance, to prevent the development of drug resistance, which is a growing problem.[68]

Because drug use has long been associated with sexually transmitted infection and because most women with AIDS in the United States have a history of injected drug use, women with human papillomavirus are at high risk for cervical dysplasia and cervical cancer. Regular surveillance with Papanicolaou smears in this group is important.[69] Studies have noted that HIV-positive persons have an increased risk of being chronic hepatitis B virus carriers.[70] These coinfected patients also have a greater replication of virus. Vaccination of HIV-positive persons who are hepatitis B seronegative is recommended.

Although cancer of the nasopharynx, larynx, and esophagus has a higher incidence in heavy drinkers and smokers, increased mortality due to solid malignancies is also observed in HIV-infected drug users.[31]

Recommendations for HIV treatments, including prophylaxis of opportunistic infections and antiretroviral therapy, should not be different for drug abusers.[71, 72] The importance of early medical intervention in this population has been amply demonstrated.[73]

Conclusion

Given the preceding review, it is obvious that differentiating the complications of parenteral drug use, HIV disease, and the toxicity from drugs such as alcohol or cocaine may be a difficult matter for clinicians. Nonspecific complaints such as weight loss, fatigue, diarrhea, or sweating may be due to a wide range of causes. The risk of coexisting morbidities is high. Thus, obtaining accurate and complete medical histories is of paramount importance. Once a diagnosis is made and a treatment plan initiated, drug abuse treatment and follow-up medical care often involve multiple health care providers. The integration of primary prevention plans with the reinforcement of drug abstinence requires time, commitment, and the coordination of services. This integration should be a priority for the individual patient and the clinician and for public health planning.

REFERENCES

1. Avins AL, Woods WJ, Lindan CP, et al: HIV infection and risk behaviors among heterosexuals in alcohol treatment programs. JAMA 27:515–518, 1994.
2. Stein MD: Medical complications of intravenous drug use. J Gen Intern Med 5:249–257, 1990.
3. Cherubin CE, Sapira JD: Medical complications of drug addiction and the medical assessment of the intravenous drug user: 25 years later. Ann Intern Med 119:1017–1028, 1993.
4. Joe GW, Simpson DD: Mortality rates among opioid addicts in a longitudinal study. Am J Public Health 77:347–348, 1987.
5. Klatsky AL, Armstrong MA, Friedman GD: Alcohol and mortality. Ann Intern Med 117:646–654, 1992.
6. Haverkos HW, Stein MD: Illicit drug use. Am Fam Physician (in press).
7. Gerstein DR, Lewin LS: Treating drug problems. N Engl J Med 323:844–848, 1990.
8. Putnam S: Alcoholism, morbidity and care-seeking; the inpatient and ambulatory service utilization and associated illness experience of alcoholics and matched controls in a health maintenance organization. Med Care 20:97–121, 1982.
9. Anda RH: Alcohol and fatal injuries among US adults: Findings from the NHANES I Epidemiologic Study. JAMA 260:2529–2532, 1988.
10. Friedman GD, Tekawa I, Klatsky AL, et al: Alcohol drinking and cigarette smoking: An exploration of the association in middle-aged men and women. Drug Alcohol Depend 27:283–290, 1991.
11. Andreasson S, Allebeck P, Romelsjo A: Alcohol and mortality among young men; longitudinal study of Swedish conscripts. Br Med J 296:1021–1025, 1988.
12. Bullock KD, Reed RJ, Grant I: Reduced mortality risk in alcoholics who achieve long-term abstinence. JAMA 267:668–672, 1992.
13. Frezza M, Dipadova C, Pozzato G, et al: High blood alcohol levels in women. N Engl J Med 322:95–99, 1990.
14. Geokas MC (ed): Symposium on ethyl alcohol and disease. Med Clin North Am 68:1–255, 1984.
15. Sherlock S: Liver disease in women. West J Med 149:683–686, 1988.
16. Burch GE, Gilles TD: Alcoholic cardiomyopathy: Concern of the disease and its treatment. Am J Med 50:141–145, 1971.
17. Engel TR, Luck JC: Effect of whisky on atrial vulnerability and "holiday" heart. J Am Coll Cardiol 1:816–818, 1983.
18. Regan TJ: Alcohol and the cardiovascular system. JAMA 264:377–381, 1990.
19. MacMahon SW, Norton RN: Alcohol and hypertension: Implications for prevention and treatment. Ann Intern Med 105:124–126, 1986.
20. Klatsky AL: The cardiovascular effects of alcohol. Alcohol Alcholol 22:117–124, 1987.
21. Herbert V (ed): Hematologic complications of alcoholism. Semin Hematol 17:83–176, 1980.
22. Cyr MG, Moulton AW: Substance abuse in women. Obstet Gynecol Clin North Am 17:905–923, 1990.
23. Wrenn KD, Slovis CM, Minion GE, Rutkowski R: The syndrome of alcoholic ketoacidosis. Am J Med 91:119–128, 1991.
24. Charness ME, Simon RP, Greenberg DA: Ethanol and the nervous system. N Engl J Med 321:442–452, 1989.
25. Zylman R: Accidents, alcohol and single-cause explanations: Lessons from the Grand Rapids Study. Q J Stud Alcohol S4:212–233, 1968.
26. Andaa RF, Williamson DF, Remington PL: Alcohol and fatal injuries among US adults. JAMA 260:2529–2532, 1988.
27. Miller NS, Giannini J, Gold MS: Suicide risk associated with drug and alcohol addiction. Cleve Clin J Med 59:535–538, 1992.
28. McGinnis JM, Foege WH: Actual causes of death in the United States. JAMA 270:2207–2212, 1993.
29. Ghodse AH, Sheehan M, Taylor C, et al: Deaths of drug addicts in the United Kingdom 1967–81. Br Med J 290:425–428, 1985.
30. Haverkos HW, Lange WR: Serious infections other than human immunodeficiency virus among intravenous drug abusers. J Infect Dis 5:894–902, 1990.
31. Perucci CA, Davoli M, Rapiti E, et al: Mortality of intravenous drug users in Rome: A cohort study. Am J Public Health 81:1307–1310, 1991.
32. Orangio GR, Della Latta P, Marino C, et al: Infection in parenteral drug abusers, further immunologic studies. Am J Surg 146:738–741, 1983.
33. Orangio GR, Pitlick SD, Della Latta P, et al: Soft tissue infections in parenteral drug abusers. Ann Surg 199:97–100, 1984.
34. Webb D, Thadepoli T: A skin and soft tissue polymicrobial infections from intravenous abuse of drugs. West J Med 130:200–204, 1979.
35. Samet JH, Shevitz SA, Fowle A, Singer DE: Hospitalization decision in febrile intravenous drug users. Am J Med 89:53–57, 1990.
36. Marantz PR, Linzer M, Feiner CJ, et al: Inability to predict diagnosis in drug abusers. Ann Intern Med 106:823–828, 1987.
37. Farber HW, Falls R, Glauser PL: Transient pulmonary hypertension from the intravenous injection of crushed suspended pentacozine tables. Chest 80:178–182, 1981.
38. Durack DT, Beeson PB: Experimental bacterial endocarditis: Colonization of a sterile vegetation. Br J Exp Pathol 53:44–49, 1972.
39. Scheld WM, Zak O, Vosbeck K, et al: Bacterial adhesion in the pathogenesis of infective endocarditis. Effect of subinhibitory antibiotic concentration on streptococcal adhesion in vitro and the development of endocarditis in rabbits. J Clin Invest 68:1381–1384, 1981.
40. Friedman LN, Sullivan GM, Bevilacqua RP, et al: Tuberculosis screening in alcoholics and drug addicts. Am Rev Respir Dis 136:1188–1192, 1987.
41. Donahue JG, Nelson KE, Munoz A, et al: Antibody to hepatitis C virus among cardiac surgery patients, homosexual men, and intravenous drug users in Baltimore, Maryland. Am J Epidemiol 134:1206–1211, 1991.
42. Seeff LB: Hepatitis in the drug abuser. Med Clin North Am 59:843–848, 1975.
43. Lettau LA, McCarthy JG, Smith MH, et al: Outbreak of severe hepatitis due to delta and hepatitis B viruses in parenteral drug abusers and their contacts. N Engl J Med 317:1256–1261, 1987.
44. Gourevitch MN, Selwyn PA, Davenny K, et al: Effects of HIV infection on the serologic manifestations and response to treatment of syphilis in intravenous drug users. Ann Intern Med 118:350–355, 1993.
45. Rao TKS, Nicastri AD, Friedman EA: Natural history of heroin associated nephropathy. N Engl J Med 290:19–23, 1974.
46. Neugarten J, Gallo GR, Buxbaum J, et al: Amyloidosis in subcutaneous heroin abusers. Am J Med 81:635–640, 1986.
47. O'Connor PG, Samet JH, Stein MD: Management of

hospitalized intravenous drug users: Role of the internist. Am J Med 96:551–558, 1994.

48. Rich JA, Singer DE: Cocaine-related symptoms in patients presenting to an urban emergency department. Ann Emerg Med 20:616–621, 1991.

49. Warner EA: Cocaine abuse. Ann Intern Med 119:226–235, 1993.

50. Levine SR, Brust JC, Futrell N, et al: Cerebrovascular complications of the use of the "crack" form of alkaloidal cocaine. N Engl J Med 323:699–704, 1990.

51. Fredericks RK, Lefkowitz DS, Challa VR, et al: Cerebral vasculitis associated with cocaine abuse. Stroke 22:1437–1439, 1991.

52. Forrester JM, Steele AW, Waldron JA, et al: Crack lung: An acute pulmonary syndrome with a spectrum of clinical and histopathologic findings. Annu Rev Respir Dis 142:462–467, 1990.

53. Welch RD, Todd K, Krause GS: Incidence of cocaine-associated rhabdomyolysis. Ann Emerg Med 20:154–157, 1991.

54. Volpe JJ: Effect of cocaine use on the fetus. N Engl J Med 327:399–407, 1992.

55. Hanzlick R, Gowitt GT: Cocaine metabolite detection in homicide victims. JAMA 265:760–761, 1991.

56. Marzuk PM, Tardiff K, Leon AC, et al: Prevalance of cocaine use among residents of New York City who committed suicide during a one-year period. Am J Psychiatry 149:371–375, 1992.

57. Desjarlais DC, Friedman SR, Mamor M, et al: Development of AIDS, HIV seroconversion, and potential cofactors for T4 cell loss in a cohort of intravenous drug users. AIDS 1:105–111, 1987.

58. Galli M, Lazzarin A, Saracco A, et al: Clinical and immunological aspects of HIV infection in drug addicts. Clin Immunol Immunopathol 150:S166–S176, 1989.

59. Margolick JB, Munoz A, Vlahov D, et al: Changes in T-lymphocyte subsets in intravenous drug users with HIV-1 infection. JAMA 267:1631–1636, 1992.

60. Kaslow RA, Blackwelder WC, Ostrow DG, et al: No evidence for a role of alcohol or other psychoactive drugs in accelerating immunodeficiency in HIV-1-positive individuals. JAMA 261:3424–3429, 1989.

61. 1993 Revised classification system for HIV infection and expanded surveillance case definition for AIDS among adolescents and adults. MMWR Morb Mortal Wkly Rep 41:1–19, 1992.

62. Fernandez-Cruz E, Desco M, Montes MG, et al: Immunological and serological markers predictive of progression to AIDS in a cohort of HIV-infected drug users. AIDS 4:987–994, 1990.

63. Selwyn PA, Alcabes P, Hartel D, et al: Clinical manifestations and predictors of disease progression in drug users with human immunodeficiency virus. N Engl J Med 327:1697–1703, 1992.

64. Farizo KM, Buehler JW, Chamberland ME, et al: Spectrum of disease in persons with human immunodeficiency virus infection in the United States. JAMA 267:1798–1805, 1992.

65. Selwyn PA, Hartel D, Lewis VA, et al: A prospective study of the risk of tuberculosis among intravenous drug users with HIV infections. N Engl J Med 320:545–550, 1989.

66. Barnes PR, Bloch AB, Davidson PT, et al: Tuberculosis in patients with human immunodeficiency virus infection. N Engl J Med 324:1644–1650, 1991.

67. Selwyn PA, Sckell BM, Alcabes P, et al: High risk of active tuberculosis in HIV-infected drug users with cutaneous anergy. JAMA 268:504–509, 1992.

68. Fischl MA, Uttamchandani RB, Daikos GL, et al: An outbreak of tuberculosis caused by multiple-drug-resistant tubercle bacilli among patients with HIV infection. Ann Intern Med 117:177–183, 1992.

69. Feingold AR, Vermund SH, Burk RD, et al: Cervical cytologic abnormalities and papilloma virus in women infected with human immunodeficiency virus. J AIDS 3:896–903, 1990.

70. Hadler SC, Judson FN, O'Malley PH, et al: Outcome of hepatitis B virus infection in homosexual men and its relation to prior human immunodeficiency virus infection. J Infect Dis 163:454–459, 1991.

71. Sande MA, Carpenter CCJ, Cobbs CG, et al: Antiretroviral therapy for adult HIV-infected patients. JAMA 270:2583–2589, 1993.

72. Gallant JE, Moore RD, Chaisson RE: Prophylaxis for opportunistic infections in patients with HIV infection. Ann Intern Med 120:932–944, 1994.

73. Jewett JF, Hecht FM: Preventive health care for adults with HIV infection. JAMA 269:1144–1153, 1993.

The Course of Alcoholism in Men and Women

Joseph A. Flaherty, MD •
Kathleen Kim, MD • Susan Adams, MA

The history of psychiatric nosology has always included lumpers and splitters—that is, those who seek parsimony through the natural aggregation of syndromes or disorders and those who highlight differences. Taking the latter to the extreme, of course, there are as many different syndromes and presentations of disorders as there are individual sufferers. Likewise, the course of a particular disorder or syndrome has many paths resulting in various methods for charting a modal course or courses. In the case of alcoholism, the historical and competing criteria as well as the wide variety of social, psychological, physiological, and legal "symptoms" of the illness magnify the difficulty of presenting a typical or modal course.

Other specific problems arise in plotting a clinical course with regard to alcoholism. First, it is conservatively estimated that fewer than 20% of people with alcoholism ever seek treatment, highlighting the limited utility of examining the clinical course in treated populations alone. Second, there are various ways of measuring or labeling alcoholism: heavy drinkers, problem drinkers, alcohol abusers, and alcohol-dependent individuals, all of whom may have different courses. Third is the issue of the temporal course of alcoholism in relationship to other psychiatric disorders (i.e., does problematic drinking occur before or after the onset of another psychiatric disorder?).

Although we are not at the point of being able to stage alcoholism, as in cancer or diabetes research, or to chart a modal course, it is useful to explore this possibility for several reasons. Some of these reasons have been summarized by Schuckit and colleagues.[1] First is the issue of prevention. In order to plan preventive strategies against the onset of alcohol problems, it would be useful to know what the general clinical course is for different populations for which these interventions are being planned. Second, treatment in general is best informed by having a basic idea of the course of alcoholism, bearing in mind the limitations of this method. Treatment decisions by both the clinician and the patient are usually determined by a cost-benefit analysis at each particular point in illness; this will be increasingly important as managed care gains a major role in authorizing treatment. Finally, the evaluation of treatment efficacy makes it essential to compare the effects of treatment with what might be described as the natural course without treatment.

Vaillant[2] argues strongly for prospective studies to clarify the course of alcoholism and to dispel long-standing myths. He cites diverse data to dispel the notion that alcoholism is the result of an unhappy childhood, family discord, or personality disorder.[3-5] He also provides compelling evidence that studies of treated populations (versus community samples) have contributed to a false sense of pessimism about treatment. Vaillant also concludes that only community-based follow-up can clarify the "cart and horse" relationship with coexisting conditions such as depression.

This chapter begins by examining some of the classical studies of the course of alcoholism and highlights key limitations. To a great extent, our knowledge of the natural course of alcoholism has been limited to work in the United States and other industrialized countries. This knowledge has been based primarily on the experiences of white men in treatment. We then move on to newer studies focusing on typology and clinical course. Finally, we address particular issues in the developing literature on gender differences.

Although it might be ideal to compare a natural course of alcoholism with the *clinical courses* with different types of interventions, this is more difficult than decades ago. The prevalence of Alcoholics Anonymous (AA) in the United States and internationally; the increasing use of employee assistance programs in the workplace; and the growing practice of primary care providers in screening, educating, or advising people with problem drinking have become so widespread that it is difficult to separate out a natural course in its purest form from courses of different treatments. The majority of studies reviewed have in common the longitudinal course of alcoholism with the identification of possible risk factors and include attempts at treatment as both predictor and outcome variables. Although this presents a more complex view of the course of alcoholism, as, for example, contrasted with studies comparing the efficacy of antidepressant drugs, it is more representative of the phenomenon of alcoholism in U.S. society, where the course varies markedly over time in symptoms, functional capacity, and treatment receptivity.

Classical Studies

There are few areas in medicine where the disease in question, with the possible exception of acquired immunodeficiency syndrome (AIDS), has provoked so much ethical, moral, sociopolitical, and religious debate as has alcoholism. To a great extent, the complexity and controversy of this debate are not merely due to social vectors but are inherent in the phenomenon of alcoholism itself. Alcoholism is a disorder that is markedly influenced by a complex set of environmental and biological factors. Jellinek's[6] work must be understood in the context of its time. In the postprohibition era, Jellinek may have been responding to various issues, including the psychotherapeutic view that regarded alcoholism as a symptomatic response to psychodynamic conflict, the need to legitimize alcoholism as a disease in order to promote treatment, and the growing importance of AA as both a treatment venue as well as a group of people who collectively held an astute awareness of warning signals in the everyday course of drinking behavior. To a significant degree, Jellinek tried to expand our understanding of the heterogeneity of drinking careers and to reconcile the many "types" of drinking behaviors ranging from binge drinking to going on and off the "water wagon." To this end, he devised a system of types of alcohol abuse: *Alpha* individuals had symptoms and behavior consistent with alcoholism but did not have physical dependence, *beta* individuals had medical symptoms but not physical dependence, *gamma* individuals had both symptoms and physical dependence, *delta* individuals had physical dependence but few symptoms, and *epsilon* individuals were the binge drinking type. Using his own observations as well as a questionnaire developed with AA, which was completed by 98 alcoholic men, he devised a useful cross-sectional classification and provided some insights into lifelong patterns. Perhaps most important toward the development of typologies of alcoholism, Jellinek described several concepts of continued importance:

1. There are marked changes in the types of symptoms and problems over the course of time.

2. There may be differences between physical dependence on alcohol and psychological dependence.

3. There are different psychological, psychiatric, and medical consequences of drinking.

4. There are pronounced effects of alcoholic behavior on a person's social and occupational functioning and the strong reactions from others.

The assumption that the course of alcoholism leads from one stage to the next as a progressive disease illness toward gamma alcoholism, which is a common inference from Jellinek's work, is analogous to Kubler-Ross' efforts in delineating stages of mourning. Both are useful attempts to chart modal phases in a complex process, both serve as more of a generalization than as the single common course, and both were presented without benefit of comprehensive longitudinal data that would show the extent to which individuals actually traverse these phases and in what sequence.

Lemere,[7] a contemporary of Jellinek, tried to chart the course of untreated alcoholism through interviews with family members of 500 deceased alcoholics. Although his study suffers the usual problems of retrospective surveys, compounded by the fact that the respondents were psychiatric patients themselves, it does provide one picture of the untreated course before the current era (when treatments and awareness are more common). Lemere stated that one fifth of the alcoholics achieved remission; of these alcoholics, approximately one half had become abstinent and one half had returned to "normal" or "controlled" asymptomatic drinking. In either case, this 20% seemed to fare reasonably well. Another 20% stopped drinking later in life because of severe illness rendering them too sick to continue drinking. A full 60% in Lemere's study continued to abuse alcohol until their death. Significantly, the average age of death was 52 for this group; 11% of the total sample committed suicide. In a smaller study using a follow-up design, Kendall and Staton[8] monitored 57 untreated alcoholics for an average of 7 years. Approximately 20% had died, and of the survivors, 20% achieved stable abstinence and another 11% had returned to social but controlled drinking.

Highlighting the dangers of generalizing from cross-sectional data, Drew[9] examined the first admissions for alcoholism in the Australian state of Victoria, with a population of three million people. Admission increased up to age 55, after which the admission of older alcoholics in the population steadily declined. Drew also noted that the peak in arrests for drunken driving occurred between ages 40 and 50. Based on his study and review of the literature, Drew concluded that alcoholism was a disease of younger people and that there was a strong decline in alcoholism after age 50. He further proposed, given the limits of available treatments at that time and the limited use of such services, that this decline in the older years was a process of spontaneous recovery. As Vaillant[2] suggested, Drew failed to address the alternative that alcoholism is not a self-limiting disease but a fatal one.

The Work of George Vaillant

Much of our current knowledge of the natural history of alcoholism comes from the work of George Vaillant summarized in *The Natural History of Alcoholism* in 1983 and in subsequent publications. Vaillant[2, 11, 12] described his own longitudinal study of the course of alcoholism and carefully summarized the existing literature. Vaillant[2] reviewed ten studies (each lasting 7 years or longer) representing both partially treated, treated, and untreated populations. Conclusions based on this review include the following:

1. It is not feasible to distinguish treated from untreated populations because treatment can reflect brief treatments, intense treatments with follow-up, and interventions associated only with the onset of medical disorders (as occurs with increasing age).

2. The length of the follow-up rather than the intensity of treatment is associated with a decline in the proportion of active alcoholics.

3. High abstinence rates in longitudinal studies may be an artifact related to morbidity. Vaillant reports, for example, that in Sundby's[13] follow-up study of up to 35 years, the abstinence rate was 64%. Vaillant points out that 62% of the original sample (including many of the most severe alcoholics) had died by the last report. Sundby estimated, however, that 48% of the sample had died sober, supporting the view that if alcoholics can survive their illness, they often recover.

4. Studies of young alcoholics show the highest return to asymptomatic drinking. For example, Goodwin and colleagues,[14] in their study of convicted felons with an average age of 27, report the highest rate of return to asymptomatic drinking (33%). Vaillant contrasted this study with Bratfos'[15] study in which no one returned to asymptomatic drinking and 87% remained alcoholic after 10 years. However, Bratfos' sample began as inpatients, and the great majority of his sample were middle-aged at the beginning of the study and were already estimated to be in the gamma stage of alcoholism.

5. Marriage seemed to be the most common reason to a return to asymptomatic drinking for young men in both Goodwin's study of felons as well as Vaillant's own study of the Core City men.

Vaillant's own work compares and contrasts two of the most comprehensive longitudinal samples. The Harvard Study of College Sophomores begun in 1938 (average age of 18) has now continued for more than 50 years. The Core City sample, also collected in Boston, was begun in 1940 with 500 boys (ages 11 to 16) selected from the conditions of inner city poverty and for the absence of serious sociopathy. It is beyond the scope of this review to present all the data or even all the conclusions from this notable body of work. Some important highlights are relevant, however. First, Vaillant reports that the progression from asymptomatic drinking to alcohol abuse to alcohol dependence occurred gradually over many years. In the college sample, this progression was even slower than in the Core City sample, with many of the college sample becoming alcohol dependent after 20 years of asymptomatic use. A key predictor in both the rapidity of onset of alcohol dependence as well as its severity is antisocial behavior and alcohol use in adolescence. Interesting, however, is the finding that a greater percentage of the Core City men than the Harvard men achieved stable remission. Perhaps most interesting in Vaillant's further follow-up of these samples[11] are two phenomena that begin to emerge at age 50: Alcoholics have a much higher mortality than nonalcoholics, and both abstinence rates and returns to asymptomatic drinking increase among survivors in later years.

Typologies and the Life Course of Alcoholism

Both clinical studies and anecdotal clinical experience have led to the conclusion that even if alcoholism deserves a single disease label, it also represents a heterogeneous group of individuals distinguished by clinical course, the presence and absence of other psychiatric disorders, and background characteristics. This understanding has led to an examination of risk factors such as family history or antisocial personality that might predict prognosis. The natural evolution of studies of risk factors has led to the development of typologies that, like diagnoses themselves, may have treatment implications and predictive validity—that is, a priori groupings hold "true" in longitudinal studies of phenomenology, response to treatment, or outcomes. The corollary is to avoid a similar tautological trap set by Kraeplin. He suggested that because schizophrenics have a progressively downhill course, patients with psychosis who have a downhill course are by definition schizophrenic.

Attempts at looking at a single domain, although shedding some light on the effects of that domain on the course of alcoholism, have in general failed to lead to development of a typology. These attempts include the presence or absence of a family history (usually presumed to be a proxy for a genetic diathesis), primary or secondary antisocial personality disorder (usually determined by the antecedent presence of a specific psychiatric disorder such as depression or schizophrenia), and gender. Jellinek's early gamma-delta distinction was multidimensional in its attempt to include at least three defining characteristics: (1) etiology, (2) the process of dependence, and (3) the consequences caused by drinking.

A number of multidimensional typologies have in recent years been derived from either cluster analyses or from empirical or theoretical bases. Morey and Skinner[16] used cluster analyses developed from a questionnaire, and they identified three types of drinkers. *Early-stage problem drinkers* showed strong evidence of problem drinking behavior but not alcohol dependence. *Affiliative drinkers* were more socially oriented, drank daily, and demonstrated a moderate degree of alcohol dependence. *Schizoid drinkers* were more socially isolated, drank in binges, and reported the most severe symptoms of alcoholism.

Zucker[17] used a developmental model to formulate four types of alcoholism. *Antisocial alcoholism* is presumed to have a genetic basis and a poor prognosis; it is characterized by early onset of alcohol problems and antisocial behavior. *Cumulative alcoholism* is believed to be primary and antecedent to other psychiatric disorders; it is characterized by progressive use of alcohol, is endorsed by cultural drinking patterns, and leads to alcohol dependence. *Negative affect alcoholism* is considered to occur primarily in women and is characterized by the use of alcohol for mood regulation and to enhance social relationships. Finally, *developmentally limited alcoholism* characterizes those individuals who have frequent heavy drinking or binges and whose drinking tends to remit with the assumption of adult career and family roles.

Based on work with adoption studies and using a genetic and neurobiological learning model, Cloninger[18] distinguished two genetic subtypes that he terms type I and type II. *Type I (milieu-limited)* alcoholics have a later age of onset of alcohol problems, show psychological more than physical dependence, and experience guilt about their alcohol use. *Type II (male-limited)* alcoholics manifest alcohol problems at an early age, are socially disruptive when drinking, and have dependence manifested by alcohol-seeking behavior. Babor and his colleagues[19, 20] have summarized some of these typologies by saying that "one type of alcoholic is characterized by later onset, slower course, fewer complications, less psychological impairment and better prognosis. Another type is characterized by early onset, a more rapid course, more severe symptoms, greater psychological vulnerability and poor prognosis."

Babor and his colleagues[19, 20] have provided a rigorous attempt at a typology by the use of an empirical clustering technique applied to 321 alcoholic men and women who were volunteers from three residential treatment centers. These individuals were observed for 3 years with a 74% follow-up rate. Subtypes were based on these categories of characteristics: Premorbid factors included (1) family history, childhood disorders, and the age of onset of problem drinking; (2) the use of alcohol and other substances, including the amount of alcohol consumed, the severity of the dependence, benzodiazepine use, and concurrent polydrug use; (3) chronicity and consequences including physical conditions and consequences, social consequences, and years of heavy drinking; and (4) psychiatric symptoms including those of depression, antisocial personality, and anxiety. Sequestering technique differentiated two clear types. Type A was characterized by fewer childhood risk factors, a later age of onset, fewer alcohol-related physical and social consequences, less psychopathological dysfunction, and less distress in the areas of work and family. Type B was characterized by early childhood and familiar risk factors, an earlier age of onset, greater dependence, greater use of other substances, more serious consequences, and more comorbidity with other psychiatric disorders (construct validity). In testing the discriminant validity of this classification, type A and type B were contrasted in terms of personality variables, drinking history, alcohol-related consequences, and clinical ratings. Type B alcoholics were significantly more experimental (versus conservative) in their drinking behavior, were less controlled, and had more tension than their type A counterparts. Type B alcoholics also reported more symptoms of childhood aggression and a greater number of treatment episodes for alcohol dependence.[19, 20]

The 1- and 3-year outcome data were used as a measure of predictive validity. A measure of global outcome was made up of various outcome variables including distress, social problems, concurrent drug use, pathological drinking, and relapses or "slips." Type B alcoholics indicated more problem drinking at 1 and 3 years; 64% of the type B alcoholic men had suffered a relapse at 1 year and required additional treatment, compared with 45% of the type A male subjects. After 3 years, 9% of the type B males had died, in comparison with only 3% of the type A men; similar but less pronounced differences were found for the alcoholic women. The type B men and women were also found to have greater polydrug use at 1 and 3 years. Babor and colleagues[20] recognized that the type A and type B could represent two generational cohorts: Type A were 10 years older (44.9 versus 34.7 years) and could represent the traditional alcoholics who reached adulthood in the early 1960s. These people used fewer drugs and had less antisocial behavior partially by virtue of the prevailing social climate when they were introduced to alcohol as adolescents. Additional analysis of the data was performed by sorting patients into younger and older cohorts within each subtype, and the same pattern of differences in defining characteristics, personality variables, and posttreatment adjustment was observed for the within-age cohorts.

In the past year, an interesting debate has centered on the hypothesis of type I and type II alcoholism described by Cloninger and associates.[21] Vaillant[12] calls for reexamination of this dichotomy on several issues. One of Vaillant's strongest arguments is that Cloninger's model, which suggests the genetic transmission of alcoholism, has a strong potential bias in that the environmental effects of parental alcoholism are not distinguished from the genetic effects of parental alcoholism: "Is it the heavy genetic loading or the dysfunctional household that leads to early onset and antisocial features of the probands of alcoholism?" Vaillant then reports data from his longitudinal studies that suggest that the age of onset of alcoholism and the degree of antisocial symptoms were correlated with disturbed family environment but quite independent of the presence or absence of a hereditary link to alcoholism.

Our view is that there are two emerging typologies, as described by Babor and colleagues,[22] who acknowledge Vaillant's arguments as well as the lack of conceptual and operational specificity in Cloninger's concepts. However, they maintain that in the work of both Vaillant and Cloninger as well as the work of Jellinek, Schuckit, Goodwin, and others, there is a consistent pattern of alcoholism. According to Babor and associates, "many alcoholics conform to a pattern characterized by familial alcoholism, childhood attentional and conduct problems, early onset of alcohol abuse, a more rapid and severe course of alcoholic symptomatology, and a less sanguine prognosis. Many alcoholics also conform to a different pattern characterized by less familial and personal vulnerability factors than by environmental conditions that support heavy drinking. When these people develop alcohol dependence the course is less severe and the outcome much better presumably because they benefit from a stronger base of internal and external resources."

Although not exactly a "typology," the DSM-III-R and DSM-IV distinction between alcohol abuse and alcohol dependence disorders raises a question about the longitudinal course of patients classified by this method. Hasin and colleagues[23] report on 180 men classified as having alcohol abuse or dependence. Four years later, of 71 men initially diagnosed with alcohol abuse, 70% reported indicators of alcohol abuse only; 30% reported alcohol dependence with or without abuse. Of the 109 men initially diagnosed with alcohol dependence, 46% remained dependent 4 years later and 54% indicated abuse only. Although longer followup would be more revealing, this study suggests that alcohol abuse does not necessarily lead to alcohol dependence.[23]

Recovery

One of the most vital issues in the course of alcoholism is the recovery process. To the extent that we can find elements common to recovery, it may be possible through treatment, AA, or expanded use of community models to facilitate the recovery of alcoholics and prevent the beginning or progression of the disease process. How we define and operationalize recovery strongly influences findings and conclusions. For example, Vaillant and Milofsky[24] showed that recovered alcoholics with the most stable abstinence (mean of 10 years) did not differ significantly from never-abusing men in psychosocial adjustment, but men with less than 3 years of abstinence did not seem different from active alcoholics. One of the most common findings in the recovery literature is the high percentage of men who recover without treatment. In their study of 55 abstinent men, Gerard and Saenger[25] reported that only 16 began their abstinence during clinic treatment. Vaillant reports that 70% of the yearlong abstinence experiences among his Core City men were independent of clinical interventions. From a Canadian survey of alcohol abusers who recovered for a year or more, Sobell and Sobell[26] reported that 82% recovered without treatment but only 18% reported using

alcohol-related treatment including AA. In examining those treatments associated with abstinence, Vaillant reported that people who were "ever abstinent" as well as those who were "securely abstinent" were more likely to have rated AA or an alcoholic clinic to be important in their abstinence process, and only small numbers reported psychotherapy to be effective. Interestingly, among Vaillant's Harvard sample of alcohol abusers, an extremely high rate of psychotherapy was used (collectively, the 26 men received approximately 5000 hours of psychotherapy), but for only two of these men was psychotherapy associated with abstinence or a return to asymptomatic drinking. This tendency of middle-class and college-educated alcoholics to seek psychotherapy as opposed to other treatments that might be more likely to result in abstinence is reminiscent of the work of Hollingshead and Redlich.[27]

Vaillant reports on those nontreatment factors associated with abstinence. The most common nontreatment factor that men reported as contributing to abstinence was the development of a substitute dependence. These varied from the use of candy to benzodiazepines (only 10%), to prayer, meditation, hobbies, gambling, and chain smoking. The next most common nontreatment factor that men endorsed in the Vaillant study was the use of either religion or AA. This factor was followed closely by the development of a new love relationship. Vaillant also notes that having something to lose if they continued to abuse alcohol was a major factor in recovering. This, in part, explains the relatively more favorable prognosis for physicians in terms of both spontaneous recovery and response to treatment; the threat of loss of a medical license is a strong motivator for treatment. In Vaillant's study, nearly half of the men described medical consequences as a major factor resulting in abstinence, a finding consistent with clinical experience.

Concluding that these factors are interrelated and are embodied in many of the self-help recovery programs organized along an AA model, Vaillant further explored what type of individual in the ever-abstinent group was most likely associated with the use of AA. High attendance as contrasted with low attendance was associated with Irish ethnicity, blackouts, morning drinking, binge drinking, and a warm childhood environment. By contrast, less frequent users of AA were those who reported a higher degree of maternal neglect and had a verbal IQ score of less than 80. In differentiating nontreatment factors associated with abstinence versus a return to social drinking, Vaillant reported that abstinence was more closely associated with severe medical consequences, AA attendance, and new love relationships. By contrast, a return to social drinking was associated with compulsory supervision.

Summarizing some of his work with AA attendance, Vaillant[2] states: "Put differently, the alcoholics who were socially stable premorbidly tended to become abstinent without AA; but if the socially unstable alcoholics were to recover, frequent AA attendance appeared to be an important intervening variable."

Addressing the issue of whether a specific defining life event was the trigger for the resolution of alcoholic problems without treatment versus a cognitive appraisal process in which the pros and cons of continued drinking were evaluated, Sobell and colleagues[28] interviewed 182 subjects who had at least short-term recovery from alcoholism without formal treatment. The majority (57%) of recoveries were characterized as involving a cognitive evaluation in which the benefits of abstinence were perceived as outweighing continued drinking and the adverse consequences were not worth the benefit of drinking. Spousal support was reported as the main factor contributing to the maintenance of abstinence.[28] This is consistent with the literature showing positive family milieus and social support as significant factors associated with positive outcomes in both treatment and natural recovery studies.[29, 30]

Women and Gender

The preponderance of the early literature focused on alcoholism in men. Vaillant's study included only men, and although Jellinek's study included a small sample of women, only the data regarding men were reported. In recent years there has been an interest in alcoholism in women, with a broad range of foci including the course of the disorder. The renewed interest in and study of alcoholism among women come from at least three different sources. Vannicelli and Nash[31] reported a clear sex bias in their review of the alcoholic treatment outcome literature. They reported that only 95 (37%) of the 259 studies reviewed had described female or mixed-sex samples that were monitored for at least 6 months. Only 30 of these studies had distinguished between the sexes in the presentation of data. From the beginning of the Epidemiological Catchment Area project, it was apparent that

alcoholic women accounted for nearly 20% of the alcoholic group, higher than previously estimated.[32] Finally, both clinical and community experiences highlighted the concept of the "hidden alcoholic" among the female population and noted that gender role and societal barriers made it less likely that women would seek treatment, particularly early in their course of illness.[33]

Several issues are particular to the clinical course of alcoholism in women. As stated earlier, the boundaries between drinking, heavy drinking, problematic drinking, alcohol abuse, and alcohol dependence can be more diffuse than rigid. This issue may have particular relevance in studies of women's drinking. Long observed is a direct relationship between exposure to alcohol and alcoholism,[34] as well as between the percentage of a population that drinks regularly and problematic drinking. In this regard, during the past 40 years there has been a rise in drinking among women, particularly among college-educated women, and reports are beginning to show a gender parity in alcohol dependence among certain occupational groups.[35, 36] This raises the issue of a cohort effect in studies of gender differences and alcoholism. If the number of women drinkers has increased during the past 30 years, we might anticipate increases in problematic drinking or alcoholism among women. Although the Epidemiological Catchment Area project validated the more common prevalence of alcoholism and drug abuse among men as compared with women, that project was begun nearly 15 years ago and may not have detected these changes.

More relevant to this review is the issue of whether alcoholism in women has a different course than it does in men. Currently, little is known about the life course of alcoholism in women. Studies such as those by Vaillant, which tracked alcoholic men for extended periods, have not been carried out with alcoholic women. Consequently, this section focuses on studies of alcoholic women and men that are either cross-sectional in design or longitudinal but covering a relatively brief time period and including smaller samples. This section offers descriptions of alcoholic women and men before the onset of alcoholism, during the early stages of the disorder, and finally during the later stages and the recovery from alcohol abuse. As is true of all reports of gender differences, one must bear in mind that these patterns do not represent all alcoholic women and men.

GENDER-SPECIFIC PATHWAYS TO ABUSIVE DRINKING

A number of factors differentiate the history of alcoholism in men versus women. In a prospective longitudinal study that assessed subjects before the onset of problem drinking, Jones[37, 38] found that low self-esteem and impaired coping in the junior-high and high-school periods predicted later problem drinking in women but not men. In retrospective studies, alcoholic women more often than alcoholic men reported a family history of alcoholism,[39] histories of depression and eating disorders,[40, 41] and a history of receiving psychiatric treatment for conditions other than alcoholism.[42] In contrast to this picture of internalizing disorders primary to alcohol abuse in women, men may have higher rates of externalizing disorders (e.g., conduct disorder, antisocial personality disorder) before the onset of alcohol abuse. Finally, research suggests that alcoholic women report histories of childhood sexual abuse more often than do normal control women.[43] A recent follow-up study of substantiated cases of child abuse or neglect found that victimization was predictive of alcohol abuse among women but not among men. The relationship between childhood victimization and subsequent alcohol abuse in women was found even when controlling for parental substance abuse, childhood poverty, and race.[44]

It is important to note that gender differences in depression, eating disorders, and antisocial behavior are not unique to alcoholics. Few studies have made efforts to control for gender differences in the general population when comparing alcoholic men and women.[45] Nevertheless, recognition of gender-specific psychiatric conditions predating and co-occuring with alcoholism is relevant for designing effective treatment interventions.

GENDER-SPECIFIC PATTERNS OF ABUSIVE DRINKING

Many differences have been noted in the drinking patterns of alcoholic men and women. The onset of regular drinking and the onset of heavy drinking are later for alcoholic women than alcoholic men.[46, 47] Using retrospective reports, Schuckit and colleagues[48] explored the time course of the development of alcohol-related problems in alcohol-dependent men and women. Although the order of appearance of alcohol-related problems was generally similar for men and women, some interesting differences were noted. For example, aggressive acts (e.g., throwing things when intoxicated or striking a family member) and binge drinking, when reported, occurred later for women than men, and feelings of guilt and the formation of rigid drinking patterns, when reported, happened earlier for women than men. In addition to differences in timing of drinking and drinking problems, alcoholic men and women differ in the quantity and quality of their drinking. Men drink more alcohol than women and are more likely to drink continuously (fewer periods of abstinence), daily, and in binges.[46, 49, 50]

The social context of abusive drinking also differs by gender. Alcoholic women more than alcoholic men report drinking alone at home or with a significant other.[46, 51] In contrast, alcoholic men have more gregarious drinking styles. They are more likely than women to report drinking primarily with friends and acquaintances.[49] The more solitary drinking by women is likely a result of two factors: the greater stigma associated with alcoholism in women[47] and the greater risk of victimization from drinking in settings such as bars.[52]

Related to gender differences in the social context of drinking, alcoholic men and women report differences in the function of their drinking. In one of the few studies that included a nonalcoholic comparison group, Olenick and Chalmers[49] found that men more often than women reported using alcohol to help them feel relaxed in social situations and to ease and improve communication with others. This pattern was consistent for the alcoholic group and the control group. An interaction was found for the tendency to use alcohol to improve mood. Although alcoholic women more than alcoholic men reported drinking to enhance or alter their mood, the gender difference was reversed for the control group. Reliance on the mood-enhancing properties of alcohol was a feature that distinguished alcoholic women from nonalcoholic women and from alcoholic men.

Alcoholic women may use drinking to regulate mood variations resulting from exogenous or endogenous factors. Alcoholic women are more likely to see their drinking as a response to life problems, whereas alcoholic men are more likely to view their drinking as a source of problems.[53] Additionally, women alcoholics may use drinking to regulate changes in mood associated with the menstrual cycle. Alcoholic women, more than controls, have reported increased drinking before the onset of their monthly menstruation.[54] In all, these findings suggest that alcoholic women, more than alcoholic men, use alcohol to regulate or enhance their feelings.

Interesting differences are evident in reports of the social consequences of alcoholism for men and women. For men, public life is more likely to be affected. More than alcoholic women, men experience legal and career consequences such as arrests and job loss.[55, 56] For alcoholic women, family life is more often disrupted. More alcoholic women than men are separated or divorced.[55] Husbands of alcoholic women were more likely to end a marriage than were wives of alcoholic men.[57]

Although not thoroughly investigated, it is likely that these findings regarding the consequences of drinking are cohort and class specific. As employment outside the home and public drinking increase among women, women may increasingly face legal and career consequences. As summarized by Gomberg,[58] younger problem-drinking women were more likely to drink publicly and to face legal consequences for their drinking than were middle-aged problem-drinking women. Similarly, the finding that husbands of alcoholic women were more likely to leave the marriage than were wives of alcoholic men may well be specific to socioeconomic status. Women are not as likely to have the economic resources to leave unsatisfying relationships as are men.

GENDER-SPECIFIC FEATURES OF TREATMENT AND RECOVERY

Even though women have a later onset of problem drinking, they enter alcohol treatment at about the same age and with the same severity of symptoms as men.[59] The route to alcohol treatment tends to be more direct for men than for women. Women, more often than men, are likely to reach alcohol abuse treatment via a general physician[60] in response to health problems.[61] Women experience serious medical complications associated with heavy drinking (e.g., cirrhosis of the liver) after drinking less (controlling for body weight) and for fewer years than men.[62]

Data have suggested that women are underrepresented in alcohol treatment services,[63] but this pattern may be changing. A study of abstinence-based alcohol and drug treatment in the United States revealed that women make up 31% of inpatients and 27% of outpatients.[64] Similarly, the 1992 triennial survey of AA members revealed that 35% of members were female.[65] Thus, the percentage of people using recovery services who are women (27% to 35%) is similar to the percentage of alcohol-abusing individuals who are women (20% to 33%).[32, 66] It may be, however, that these relatively older estimates of the prevalence of women in the U.S. alcoholic population[32, 66] are no longer valid. Thus, the apparent increased representation of women in alcohol treatment services may simply reflect increases in the percentage of alcoholics who are women.

Response to treatment may differ by gender. In a meta-analysis of alcoholism treatment follow-up studies, women had better treatment outcomes for the first 12 months but men showed more improvement in longer-term outcomes.[66]

An interesting gender difference has been noted in the relationship between marital status and treatment outcome. In a short-term follow-up of alcoholics after inpatient treatment, Schneider and colleagues[56] found that marriage was *predictive* of relapse for women but *protective* of relapse for men. This pattern is consistent with a finding by Wilsnack and colleagues that separation or divorce predicted a *decrease* in problem drinking among women.[68] The negative relationship between marriage and recovery in alcoholic women may be due to the fact that, among heterosexual couples, alcoholic women are more likely than alcoholic men to be married to an alcoholic with whom they drink.[69, 70] Thus, the husbands of alcoholic women may be less supportive of their spouse's abstinence than are the wives of alcoholic men.[53]

Conclusion and Future Directions

Perhaps one of the strongest endorsements for AA and addiction treatment programs is that it has become increasingly difficult to examine a natural history from a treatment course of addictive disorders because of the widespread presence of these programs. Despite substantive critique, it is also clear that many individuals achieve sobriety through the standard treatment programs offered. It is also clear that women differ from men in their drinking careers as well as pathways and responses to treatment and recovery. Future research should further our developing knowledge of the course of alcoholism with the newer methods in mental health services research. Using large databases, we may shed light on what type of patient responds to what type of treatment(s), at what point in the couse of illness, with what outcome, and at what costs and benefits.

The answers to these questions may provide new insight into the design of current programs and the outreach and follow-up efforts needed to help people achieve stable recovery. Through this process, mental health services research can inform clinical practice to maximize efficacy and contain costs.

REFERENCES

1. Schuckit MA, Smith TL, Anthenelli R, Irwin M: Clinical course of alcoholism in 636 male inpatients. Am J Psychiatry 150(5):786–792, 1993.
2. Vaillant G: The course of alcoholism and lessons for treatment. In Grinspoon L (ed): Psychiatry Update: The American Psychiatric Association Annual Review, Vol III. Washington, DC, American Psychiatric Press, 1984, pp 311–319.
3. McCord W, McCord J: Origins of Alcoholism. Stanford, CA, Stanford University Press, 1960.
4. Kammeier ML, Hoffmann H, Loper RG: Personality characteristics of alcoholics as college freshmen and at time of treatment. Q J Stud Alcohol 34:390–399, 1973.
5. Pettinatti HM, Superman H, Maurer HS: Four-year MMPI changes in abstinent and drinking alcoholics. Alcoholism: Clin Exp Res 6:487–494, 1982.
6. Jellinek EM: The Disease Concept Of Alcoholism. New Brunswick, NJ, Hillhouse Press, 1960.
7. Lemere F: What happens to alcoholics? Am J Psychiatry 109:674–676, 1953.
8. Kendall RE, Staton MC: The fate of untreated alcoholics. Q J Stud Alcohol 27:30–41, 1966.
9. Drew LRH: Alcoholism as a self-limiting disease. Q J Stud Alcohol 29:956–967, 1968.
10. Vaillant GE: The Natural Course of Alcoholism. Cambridge, MA, Harvard University Press, 1983.
11. Vaillant G: Is there a natural history of addiction? Addictive States. New York, Raven Press, 1992, pp 41–57.
12. Vaillant G: Evidence that the Type 1/Type 2 dichotomy in alcoholism must be reexamined. Addiction 9:1049–1057, 1994.
13. Sundby P: Alcoholism and Mortality. Oslo, Universitets Forlaget, 1967.
14. Goodwin DW, Crane JB, Guze SB: Felons who drink: An eight year follow-up. Q J Stud Alcohol 32:136–147, 1971.
15. Bratfos O: The Course of Alcoholism: Drinking, Social Adjustment and Health. Oslo, Universitet Forlaget, 1974.
16. Morey LC, Skinner HA: Empirically derived classifications of alcohol-related problems. Recent Dev Alcohol 5:145–168, 1986.
17. Zucker RA: The four alcoholisms: A developmental account of the etiologic process. In Rivers PC (ed): Alcohol and Addictive Behavior. Lincoln, NE, University of Nebraska Press, 1987, pp 27–83.
18. Cloninger CR: Neurologenetic adaptive mechanisms in alcoholism. Science 236:410–416, 1987.
19. Babor T, Dolinsky Z, Meyer R, et al: Types of alcoholics: Concurrent and predictive validity of some common classification schemes. Br J Addict 87:1415–1431, 1992.
20. Babor T, Hofmann M, Delboca F, Hesselbrock M: Types of alcoholics, I: Evidence for an empirically derived typology based on indicators of vulnerability and severity. Arch Gen Psychiatry 49:599–608, 1992.
21. Cloninger CR, Bohman M, Sigvardsson S: Inheritance of alcohol abuse: Cross-fostering analysis of adopted men. Arch Gen Psychiatry 38:861–868, 1981.
22. Babor T, Longabaugh R, Zweben A, et al: Issues in the definition and measurement of drinking outcomes in alcoholism treatment research. J Stud Alcohol 12:101–111, 1994.
23. Hasin D, Grant B, Endicott J: The natural history of alcohol abuse: Implications for definitions of alcohol use disorders. Am J Psychiatry 147:1537–1541, 1990.
24. Vaillant GE, Milofsky ES: Natural history of male alcoholism. IV. Paths to recovery. Arch Gen Psychiatry 39:127–133, 1982.
25. Gerard DL, Saenger G: Outpatient Treatment of Alcoholism: A Study of Outcome and Its Determinants. Toronto, University of Toronto Press, 1966.
26. Sobell LC, Sobell MB: Cognitive mediators of natural recoveries from alcohol problems: Implications for treatment. Symposium on Therapies of Substance Abuse: A View Towards the Future. Annual Meeting of Association for Advancement of Behavior Therapy, New York, 1991. Cited in Sobell LC, Sobell MB, Toneatto L, Leo GI: What triggers the resolution of alcohol problems without treatment? Alcohol Clin Exp Res 17:217–224, 1993.
27. Hollingshead AB, Redlich FC: Social Class and Mental Illness. New York, John Wiley & Sons, 1958.
28. Sobell LC, Sobell MB, Toneatto T, Leo GI: What triggers the resolution of alcohol problems without treatment? Alcohol Clin Exp Res 17:217–224, 1993.
29. Moos RH, Finney JW, Chan D: The process of recovery from alcoholism. V. Comparing spouses of alcoholic patients and matched community controls. J Stud Alcohol 43:888–909, 1982.
30. Tuchfeld BS: Spontaneous remission in alcoholics: Empirical observation and theoretical implications. Stud Alcohol 42:626–641, 1981.
31. Vannicelli M, Nash L: Effect of sex bias on women's studies on alcoholism. Alcohol Clin Exp Res 8:334–336, 1984.
32. Anthony JC: The epidemiology of drug addiction. In Miller NS (ed): Comprehensive Handbook of Drug and Alcohol Addiction. New York, Marcel Dekker, 1991, pp 55–86.
33. Sandmaier M: The Invisible Alcoholics: Women and Alcohol Abuse in America. New York, McGraw-Hill, 1980.
34. Mulford HA: Drinking and deviant drinking, U.S.A., 1963. Q J Stud Alcohol 25:634–650, 1964.
35. Flaherty JA, Richman JA: Substance use and addiction among medical students, residents and physicians. Psychiatr Clin North Am 16:189–197, 1993.
36. Mercer PW, Khavari KA: Are women drinking more like men? An empirical examination of the convergence hypothesis. Alcohol Clin Exp Res 14:461–466, 1990.
37. Jones MC: Personality correlates and antecedents of drinking patterns in adult males. J Consult Clinical Psychol 32:2–12, 1968.
38. Jones MC: Personality antecedents and correlates of drinking patterns in women. J Consult Clin Psychol 36:61–69, 1971.
39. Midanik L: Familial alcoholism and problem drinking in a national drinking practices survey. Addict Behav 8:133–141, 1983.
40. Helzer JF, Pryzbeck TR: The co-occurrence of alcoholism with other psychatric disorders in the general population and its impact on treatment. J Stud Alcohol 40:219–224, 1988.
41. Higuchi S, Suzuki K, Yamada K, et al: Alcoholics with eating disorders: Prevalence and clinical course. A study from Japan. Br J Psychiatry 162:403–406, 1993.

42. Dahlgren L, Myrhed M: Alcoholic females I: Ways of admission of the alcoholic patient. Acta Psychiatr Scand 56:39–49, 1977.
43. Miller BA, Downs WR, Gondoli DM, Keil A: The role of childhood sexual abuse in the development of alcoholism in women. Violence Vict 2:157–172, 1987.
44. Widom CS, Ireland T, Glynn PJ: Alcohol abuse in abused and neglected children followed-up: Are they at increased risk? J Stud Alcohol 56:207–217, 1995.
45. Mello N: Some behavioral and biological aspects of alcohol problems in women. In Kalant OJ (ed): Alcohol and Drug Problems in Women: Research Advances in Alcohol and Drug Problems, vol 5. New York, Plenum, 1980, pp 263–298.
46. Blankfield A: Female alcoholics. II. The expression of alcoholism in relation to gender and age. Acta Psychiatr Scand 81:448–452, 1990.
47. Beckman LJ, Amaro H: Personal and social difficulties faced by women and men entering alcoholism treatment. J Stud Alcohol 47:135–145, 1986.
48. Schuckit MA, Anthenelli RM, Bucholz K, et al: The time course of development of alcohol-related problems in men and women. J Stud Alcohol 56:218–225, 1995.
49. Olenick N, Chalmers D: Gender-specific drinking styles in alcoholics and nonalcoholics. J Stud Alcohol 52:325–330, 1991.
50. Orford J, Keddie A: Gender differences in the functions and effects of moderate and excessive drinking. Br J Clin Psychol 24:265–279, 1985.
51. Horn JL, Wanberg KW: Symptom patterns related to excessive use of alcohol. Q J Stud Alcohol 30:35–58, 1969.
52. Fillmore K: Women's drinking across the adult life course as compared to men's. Br J Addict 82:801–811, 1987.
53. Thom B: Sex differences in help-seeking for alcohol problems: 2. Entry into treatment. Br J Addict 82:989–997, 1987.
54. Beckman LJ: Reported effects of alcohol on the sexual feelings and behavior of women alcoholics and nonalcoholics. J Stud Alcohol 40:272–282, 1979.
55. Robbins C: Sex differences in psychosocial consequences of alcohol and drug abuse. J Health Soc Behav 30:117–130, 1989.
56. Schneider KM, Kviz FJ, Isola ML, Filstead WJ: Evaluating multiple outcomes and gender differences in alcoholism treatment. Addict Behav 20:1–21, 1995.
57. Beckman LJ: Women alcoholics: A review of social and psychological studies. J Stud Alcohol 36:797–824, 1975.
58. Gomberg ESL: Gender issues. Recent Dev Alcohol 11:95–107, 1993.
59. Smart RG: Female and male alcoholics in treatment: Characteristics at intake and recovery rates. Br J Addict 74:275–281, 1979.
60. Weisner C, Schmidt L: Gender disparities in treatment for alcohol problems. JAMA 268:1872–1876, 1992.
61. Gomberg ESL: Alcoholic women in treatment: New research. Substance Abuse 12:6–12, 1991.
62. Blume SB: Women and addictive disorders. In Miller NS (ed): Principles of Addiction Medicine. (Section XVI: Women, Children, and Addiction). Washington, DC, American Society of Addiction Medicine, 1994, pp 1–16.
63. Blume SB: Chemical dependency in women: Important issues. Am J Drug Alcohol Abuse 16:297–307, 1990.
64. Miller NS, Hoffmann NG: Addiction treatment outcome. In Miller NS (ed): Treatment of the Addictions: Applications of Outcome Research for Clinical Management, vol 12. New York, Haworth Press, 1995, pp 41–55.
65. Alcoholics Anonymous: Comments on AA; Triennial Survey, 1992. New York, AA World Services, Inc, 1992.
66. Williams GD, Stinson FS, Parker DA, et al: Demographic trends, alcohol abuse and alcoholism 1985–1995. Alcohol, Health, and Research World 11:80–91, 1987.
67. Jarvis T: Implications of gender for alcohol treatment research: A quantitative and qualitative review. Br J Addict 87:1249–1261, 1992.
68. Wilsnack SC, Klassen AD, Schur BE, Wilsnack RW: Predicting onset and chronicity of women's problem drinking: A five-year longitudinal analysis. Am J Public Health 81:305–318, 1991.
69. Dahlgren L, Myrhed M: Alcoholic females II: Causes of death with references to sex differences. Acta Psychiatr Scand 56:81–91.
70. Williams CN, Klerman LV: Female alcohol abuse: Its effects on the family. In Wilsnack SC, Beckman LJ (eds): Alcohol Problems in Women: Antecedents Consequences, and Intervention. New York, Guilford Press, 1984, pp 280–312.

Consultation/Liaison: An Intervention in Drug and Alcohol Addiction

Ondrej Chudoba, MD

Sooner or later, addicted patients come into contact with a healthcare provider. This contact might be directly related to the addiction for which they are seeking treatment or might be initiated because of medical, surgical, or psychiatric consequences of the addiction or because of an illness different from the addiction or its consequences. Addicted patients can be seen in an outpatient clinic, an emergency room, or an inpatient ward. A patient's addiction might be identified in any of these settings, thus generating a consultation with the addiction psychiatry consult/liaison service.

When asked to consult under these circumstances, one has to keep an open mind about all the aspects of this complex situation:

1. The healthcare provider who is requesting the consultation and his or her reasons and goals
2. The patient, his or her addiction, and his or her goals (e.g., is the patient seeking help or is the patient in denial?)
3. The surrounding environment and circumstances in which the interaction between the healthcare provider and patient is occurring at the time of the consultation
4. The consultant

The consultation can be carried out in five different settings: (1) internal medicine service, (2) surgical service, (3) obstetrical/gynecological service, (4) psychiatric service, and (5) child and adolescent service.

Following is a separate analysis of each setting with a discussion of the different roles and aspects of the protagonists and the elements involved. In each setting, one has to consider (1) the healthcare provider originating the consultation, (2) the patient, object of the consultation, (3) the environment, and (4) the consultant who is being asked to help in the treatment of the patient.

Medical Setting

In a medical setting, a patient is being treated for an objective medical problem identified as the principal diagnosis—for example, a bleeding ulcer, pneumonia, uncontrolled diabetes, or heart attack. During the course of the treatment, the patient's healthcare provider has either started to suspect or made the diagnosis of addiction and has requested a consultation.

HEALTHCARE PROVIDER

First, before meeting a patient, it is advantageous to discuss the case with the patient's healthcare provider to get an understanding of what he or she wants and is expecting from the consultant. One has to remain alert for underlying issues that are not initially clear but that might be the main reason for the consultation. An example might be a resident in a university setting who has admitted a patient with chest pains secondary to cocaine dependence and who feels strongly that he wants to transfer this patient from his service to avoid having to take care of him because of his countertransference.

One does need to keep in mind at all times that the goal is to treat the patient and that at any given moment there might be that opportunity to do so. Sometimes part of the treatment is educating healthcare providers about addiction and what addiction means for patients. It also implies educating patients or their families about addiction. Understanding what the healthcare provider really is asking from the consultant helps to improve treatment and facilitates the act of liaison. The consequence is that the patient's treatment is improved.

PATIENT

Once we have discussed the case with the healthcare provider and we are armed with a better understanding of the reason why we have been asked for a consultation, when approaching a patient we should bear in mind that the patient needs to feel respected, needs to feel validated, and needs to perceive empathy on part of the consultant. Sometimes—and it is not a rare occurrence—the patient does not know about the consultation with addiction psychiatry and is surprised when we first introduce ourselves. For this reason, it is very important on the initial interview with patients that we make them feel that we are there to help; we must establish a relationship of mutual respect and clearly offer help.

Before going into the room to interview the patient, it is useful if possible to review the chart of the present episode. Additional information, if there is time, can be obtained from the old charts or from other sources of information. For example, in most hospitals nowadays, much information is stored in computers with easy access at any terminal. For example, one can access a listing of the medication that a patient has been receiving from the pharmacy. It can sometimes be surprising how many times a patient might have been prescribed Tylenol with codeine or antianxiety agents by different physicians or clinics for a long time and without question. After talking with the healthcare provider and obtaining all possible accessory information from present and previous charts or other sources of information, one enters the room to see the patient. It is necessary to introduce oneself, explain clearly the reason for being there, and then listen and be able to speak the patient's language. One needs to try to understand the way the patient is dealing with this interview and with the whole experience of the illness for which he or she is being treated.

The most important aspects of the initial interview are that patients feel that the physician listens to them, has respect for them, and is willing to treat them with dignity. Once rapport is established between the patient and the consultant, the first step is obtaining a thorough history. Patients who are honest and admit to the problem of addiction are easier to treat than are those in denial. In both cases, however, if patients feel that they are receiving help and are respected, they will slowly open up and be able to talk about their addiction. After a clear history is obtained from the patient, a physical examination is performed to search for objective signs of addiction that help establish the diagnosis and the severity of the addiction and its consequences.

For purposes of discussion, we can temporarily divide this scenario into acute and chronic situations. In an acute situation, we are being asked to see a patient who might be addicted to opiates and might be in heroin withdrawal. In that case, the first steps of treatment are to address the signs and symptoms of withdrawal and help the patient stabilize. On the other hand, in a chronic situation, there is no acute urgent medical necessity and we are asked to interview the patient when a diagnosis of addiction has been established and when the patient has expressed his or her desire to follow a particular addiction treatment program after treatment for the medical condition.

In both acute and chronic cases, it is of great importance to establish the drugs of addiction, the amount used by the patient, and the frequency of use. Patients frequently are unreliable in their responses to these questions and minimize their drug use. One helpful idea is to request the patients' help in searching their belongings or to ask them to bring all the medications that they are taking. It is often surprising to search a patient's belongings on admission to an internal medicine ward and to find prescription bottles of benzodiazepines, Tylenol with codeine, and other legal medications that have been used by the patient in an addictive way.

TREATMENT PLAN

Once the history is obtained and a diagnosis is established, a treatment plan has to be offered. It is essential that not only the healthcare provider but also the addicted patients themselves know what the treatment plan is, agree with it, have a clear understanding of who plays what role, and agree, even in writing sometimes, on all these points.

In many cases, when patients are in pain because of their illness, the single most important aspect of the initial treatment of their addiction is to establish a clear schedule for narcotic analgesics or nonnarcotic analgesics or, as the case may be, for methadone detoxification at the same time.

As mentioned earlier, patients and their physicians must be aware of the schedule and agree with it. An important and useful aspect of it is to try to avoid prescribing medication to be taken as needed. As-needed dosing opens the doorway to patients' manipulating their dosage, persuading nurses and residents on call at night who do not know them well to obtain a medication for reasons other than its main therapeutic indication. One way of dealing with this is by writing down the medication schedule and having the patient agree with it, then reviewing it initially perhaps every 12 hours and then once a day when the patient is stable.

Objective signs of withdrawal from opiates are as follows:

1. Tachycardia
2. Hypertension
3. Dilated pupils
4. Lacrimation, rhinorrhea, goose flesh, and diaphoresis

If a patient has two or more of these signs, consider withdrawal as a possible cause. Give methadone, 10 mg orally initially. Evaluate the patient 4 hours later and repeat the dose if indicated. Do this during the first 24-hour period. Most patients need between 20 and 40 mg/24 hours to stabilize. On day 2, repeat the total dose of day 1 and then decrease methadone by 5 mg every 3 days. It is helpful to establish one physician as the only one who changes this schedule. Patients can have two possible responses to this type of treatment: (1) They agree with it and treatment advances or (2) they become upset and manipulative, in which case treatment becomes difficult and complicated not only by the issue of the narcotic analgesics or methadone detoxification but also in terms of other aspects of their medical treatment. This is common in patients who have a diagnosis of personality disorder or its traits.

When interacting with patients, it is essential to establish a relationship based on mutual trust and to ensure that patients perceive the consultant and their physicians as honest and straightforward. Nothing sabotages the treatment of addicted patients more than trying to fool them, telling them that one thing will be done and then doing another.

ENVIRONMENT

The next factor to keep in mind is the circumstances surrounding patients: first, being treated by their healthcare providers, and second, being seen in consultation by the addiction psychiatrist. The question to be answered is, if this environment is not conducive to success in treatment or because of environmental factors, is there a high risk of failure? On an inpatient ward, for example, the best plans can fail if, during the night shift, the physician on call or the nursing staff are not sympathetic but at the same time are honest and firm and try to do things in a way different from that planned and agreed on with a patient and his or her physician.

Another example can be given for an outpatient setting. If we have the opportunity to see patients for 30 to 60 minutes once a week but then for the rest of the week they return to their family and their neighborhood, where they are surrounded by other addicted people and drug dealers, it is rare that they will be able to successfully complete treatment on an outpatient basis.

CONSULTANT

A final factor to consider is oneself, the consultant. It is impossible to be neutral in interactions with patients and their healthcare providers. One has to be capable in a professional way of keeping an objective distance from the conflicts into which one might step and to try objectively and honestly to offer help without promising that which cannot be guaranteed, but extending the hope of treatment. It is important to explain to patients for what reasons a decision is made—for example, to give or not to give methadone, to increase or not to increase the dose. No matter how complicated, stressful, or intense the situation, the goal is to help patients to obtain treatment. This is the center of focus and the first and most important reason why you are being sought for consultation.

Surgical Setting

In a surgical setting, a consultant has to keep certain ideas in mind when asked by a surgeon to evaluate a patient for addiction. If the patient is hospitalized, acute trauma frequently is the reason—for example, a motor vehicle accident, falling down the stairs while under the influence, or a mugging. In such cases, the most frequent problem that surgeons encounter is the acute onset of withdrawal. This is one of the main reasons why surgeons ask for a consultation.

HEALTHCARE PROVIDERS

The healthcare provider, in this case the surgeon, is most likely requesting a consultation to obtain help in stabilizing a patient and controlling his or her withdrawal symptoms. As discussed in other chapters, alcohol, opiates, and benzodiazepines cause the most serious of these withdrawal symptoms. It is important in this case to provide treatment of the intensity and frequency necessary to make patients feel comfortable to a certain degree and to have objective evidence that patients are showing no signs or symptoms of withdrawal.

This goal poses a problem in that patients might take advantage and demand higher doses than needed for stabilization. This is a very difficult situation to clarify because patients with chronic addiction to opiates do have pain even though they might be on a very high dose of methadone. Many physicians and other healthcare providers reason that if a patient is already receiving methadone, he or she does not need to receive any other narcotic analgesic. This is not true, however. In this case, methadone is being given to patients to return them to a stable baseline, but not enough of a dose is given to prevent pain as a result of trauma or surgery.

For this reason, it is important to educate both the healthcare providers and patients about the aspects of pain management in chronically opiate-addicted patients. Patients addicted to other substances suffer as much pain as any other human being. It is necessary once again to establish a very clear schedule of analgesics, to consider the dose and the frequency, and to have clear communication between the healthcare provider, the patient, and oneself. All three parties must agree that the goals of treatment are to (1) stabilize patients from withdrawal and (2) manage their pain.

CONSULTANT

In this kind of a surgical setting, the future treatment of patients' addiction has a secondary role until patients are surgically stable and their physicians believe that they do not have to continue under their care. Until that moment, the role of the consultant is that of a supportive member of the treatment team trying to help establish an environment that is conducive to the conclusion of surgical treatment. Again, specific to the surgical setting, withdrawal and pain management are the two main issues in the initial treatment of addicted patients.

INPATIENT ENVIRONMENT

The environment that surrounds surgical patients is highly technical—tubes, machines, and so forth. The surgeons are usually very busy and have little time to sit at the bedside of patients and explain in detail all the aspects of what is going on. As mentioned earlier, it is also common for patients to have been admitted to the hospital for acute trauma but never to have considered, until that moment, the idea of seeking treatment for their addiction.

PATIENT

For this reason, a very important role of the consultant is to take the time to be supportive of what the patient is undergoing, to be able to listen and speak the patient's language, and to give help in this time of crisis. For this reason, one of the variables that has importance is the time spent with patients. If one can find enough time to sit down and listen to patients' stories and to validate their suffering from both the trauma and the addiction, these circumstances may present themselves as a golden opportunity or a catharsis for patients, when they can be motivated to seek treatment for their addiction.

This is facilitated by explaining to patients what is happening in both the surgical aspects of their trauma and their withdrawal, what can be done for both, and what is being done. Many times patients are scared and fearful of the unknown. They do not comprehend the surgical treatment or the goals of treatment and withdrawal stabilization. Under these circumstances, patients substitute the lack of information for their own fantasies and goals. They do not know what chances they have once they are discharged from the surgical ward.

If one explains these opportunities and takes time to establish good rapport during the days and weeks that patients might be on a surgical ward, it is not uncommon for these patients to find themselves motivated and desiring treatment for their addiction.

Again, it is very common to find a tendency among the healthcare providers to blame patients for their problems, to see them as guilty, and to view all their suffering as secondary to what they have done to themselves. With this kind of approach, it is hard for healthcare providers to give empathic treatment. In such instances, a consultant can help to establish, through education, a better understanding of these patients' tragedy and as a result improve the treatment that they do receive.

OUTPATIENT ENVIRONMENT

Our discussion of the surgical setting has until now focused on acute trauma. In another aspect of the surgical setting are patients who are being seen in an outpatient surgical clinic or in a surgeon's office in anticipation of elective surgery. While taking a complete history, a surgeon might have begun to suspect the possibility of addiction. The surgeon then requests a consultation to establish or confirm the diagnosis and obtain help with the treatment.

This setting is similar to the medical setting. Here, one has to consider whether the addiction is a danger to the patient if he or she undergoes surgery and, in view of this being an elective procedure, whether it should be postponed until the patient has been withdrawn from the drug of addiction or has received treatment for the addiction and is clean or sober.

Once again, it is essential that close communication between the surgeon, the patient, and the consultant be established and that whatever plan is agreed on, all three parties feel comfortable with it and feel that they have contributed actively, that their opinions have been voiced and heard and accepted.

SUMMARY

Before finishing this segment on addicted patients in a surgical setting, I want to emphasize once again the problem of pain. In summary, pain is a very frequent cause of requests for consultation and of very difficult treatment of addicted patients. One has to keep in mind and focus on the fact that patients, no matter how high their maintenance methadone dose,

do suffer from pain. They might need analgesics to control their pain, whether nonsteroidal anti-inflammatory drugs or narcotic analgesics.

It is important to make scheduled treatment frequency and dosage known to all treating personnel. I recommend not using as-needed doses because they open a door to manipulation and difficulties in the relationship between patients and the staff taking care of them. After the cause of pain has been treated, the pain medication must be carefully tapered off. Then, in a second step, detoxification from methadone or establishment of a methadone maintenance dosage is undertaken if appropriate.

In difficult situations such as in elderly patients who have a long-standing history of cancer and who are being treated for multiple metastases, after careful consideration of all options and their consequences, even though one worries about addiction, one might consider allowing such patients to continue narcotic pain medication. A consultation with the anesthesiology pain control service, if available, is always a possibility and should be taken advantage of for improved pain management.

Obstetrical/Gynecological Setting

Approximately 85% of the women who suffer addiction are of childbearing age. The proportion of female addicts has steadily increased, particularly among young women. Certain data report that in 1981, 10% of addicts were female, and that figure rose to 19% in 1989. Therefore, one has to keep in mind that the number of pregnant addicts will most likely increase in the future. Addiction and certainly opiate dependence are serious problems because they affect not only a woman who is addicted but also her fetus and, later, her child.

PATIENT

Women who have addiction usually do not receive antenatal care. In one study, the first antenatal visit was on average at 28 weeks. These women also do not continue in antenatal care; the rate of dropouts is high.

In this setting, one can be consulted at any moment in the antenatal period, during labor, or even postnatally. Addicted patients in this setting have in common with addicted patients in a surgical setting that they do not have access to the healthcare system because of lack of motivation to stop drug use. The diagnosis of addiction is instead considered because of a positive result on a urine toxicology screen or because of signs or symptoms of withdrawal. For this reason, most of the time, one sees such patients in acute circumstances. The most definite method of diagnosing heroin or poly-drug addiction is by urine toxicology screens or the observation of early signs and symptoms of abstinence.

Once the diagnosis is made, one has to keep in mind that pregnant women addicted to her-oin are almost impossible to detoxify and, sec-ond, that abstinence may produce fetal distress that may be more harmful than passive depen-dence. For this reason, it is recommended that methadone maintenance treatment be initiated and that this, with adequate prenatal care, has the best outcome for both a mother and her fetus.

A complete medical history, keeping in mind the possibility of polydrug use, is essential in establishing a successful treatment program. Pregnant women addicted to cocaine also pre-sent problems. The number of women of childbearing age who use cocaine is increasing, and cocaine does cause prenatal compications. Also noted is an increase in addicted women who use both opiates and cocaine. In general, all pregnant addicted women, regardless of the drug that they are using, are to be considered at a higher risk of abnormal pregnancy, labor, and delivery.

MEDICAL AND OBSTETRICAL CONSEQUENCES

The use of drugs during pregnancy has both obstetrical and medical complications. Drug use in pregnancy, added to the lack of prenatal care, is difficult to treat. Among the complica-tions, infections, mostly sexually transmitted diseases, account for a high percentage of the medical complications and affect not only a pregnant addict but her fetus. Among these infections, one of the most dangerous is ac-quired immunodeficiency syndrome (AIDS). Certain studies show that about 80% of the infants and children diagnosed with AIDS have been born to women who have risk fac-tors for human immunodeficiency virus (HIV). Currently, the issue of mandatory HIV testing of all pregnant females has become a subject of heated debate. Among other medical prob-lems are other types of bacterial infections, hepatitis, and cardiac problems. Among obstet-rical complications are abortion, intrauterine death, abruptio placentae, placental insuffi-ciency, premature labor, preeclampsia, and postpartum hemorrhage.

THE ADDICTED NEWBORN

Fetal problems as a result of addiction are also common. For example, low-weight infants have all the problems related to prematurity, and of course, addicted neonates must fare withdrawal. In addition to their obstetrical problems, these patients have multiple social problems and special needs such as adequate nutrition for them and their babies, all factors that have to be considered. Once these patients are identified, it is best to collaborate with all healthcare providers involved in their treat-ment and plan an approach that addresses all of these problems and implements a solution. Patients must participate actively in this pro-cess and agree with the solutions. If they do not, the resulting high rate of noncompliance sabotages the best treatment plans.

After delivery, addicted neonates present with a wide array of withdrawal symptoms. Between 60% and 80% of babies born to drug-addicted women present with withdrawal. These infants should be admitted to a special care nursery for observation. Some of them present with withdrawal as soon as 1 hour after delivery; in others, withdrawal symptoms become manifested as much as 1 week later. Among the main withdrawal symptoms are jitteriness, irritability, abnormal crying, poor feeding, convulsions, and respiratory distress.

METHADONE MAINTENANCE PROGRAM

There is still some debate about the efficacy of detoxifying pregnant women from metha-done. Nowadays, it seems clear that a metha-done maintenance program for pregnant women is the treatment of choice. It stabilizes patients, diminishes the amount of illegal drugs used, and improves compliance with an-tenatal care. The medical and obstetrical com-plications of drug addiction thus can be better treated for both the mother and her child.

Many doctors question the use of methadone because they think that it will adversely affect a fetus, but research has shown that metha-done is less harmful for a fetus than illegal opiates because its levels do not fluctuate as do those of illegal opiates. Because of this, the amount of intrauterine withdrawal is de-creased. It has also been noted that the birth weight and the prematurity weight, as well as withdrawal symptoms, are more favorable in newborns that have been maintained on methadone. One might say that the safety of methadone has been established for addicted pregnant women and that methadone also helps their neonates, but approximately 60% of the infants who have received methadone in utero will develop withdrawal symptoms and will need treatment. Treatment of these babies is discussed later under the setting of the child and adolescent.

Drug-dependent women who are receiving methadone maintenance and who were receiving methadone before becoming pregnant can be continued on the same dosage. Those who have had no previous methadone maintenance and are treated for the first time when already pregnant should be admitted to an inpatient ward, where the correct amount of methadone should be established. Most patients are controlled on a daily dose of 20 to 40 mg of methadone. This dose sometimes has to be somewhat higher during pregnancy, and the increase depends on factors such as polysubstance dependence or continued use of heroin although receiving methadone. Pregnancy interferes with normal pharmacokinetics, and for this reason, the dose has to be titrated until patients are stabilized.

COCAINE AND ALCOHOL ADDICTION

Addiction to cocaine or alcohol during pregnancy is difficult to diagnose unless one has a high degree of suspicion. It is essential to identify the problem so that treatment can be initiated. Pregnant women who use cocaine during pregnancy have an increased rate of intrauterine growth retardation, preterm delivery, and low-birth-weight neonates. The teratogenic effects of alcohol are well known. Fetal alcohol syndrome and fetal alcohol effects are among the leading causes of mental retardation in the Western world.

SUMMARY

Addicted pregnant women are very difficult patients, and their treatment is complex because they present with a high risk of medical and obstetrical problems, as do their fetuses. Also complicating their care are the psychosocial problems that affect a woman of childbearing age who is addicted and pregnant.

Another problem that at times generates a consultation is overdose. In this situation, extreme care must be taken, and if the decision to give naloxone is considered, one has to be very conservative to avoid precipitating a severe acute withdrawal, which in a pregnant woman can be dangerous for her fetus. Clinical judgment has to be used for titration of the correct naloxone dose.

Psychiatric Setting

Co-occurrence of a major mental illness and addiction is increasingly common in a psychiatric setting. Studies have confirmed the comorbidity of psychiatric disorders and substance disorders. Drug use should always be suspected when a patient's symptoms change or become more intense or sudden treatment resistance is noted in a previously well-controlled patient. When asked in consultation by a psychiatrist to evaluate a patient for addiction, one has to consider the possibility that a patient's signs and symptoms are a consequence of the addiction only or the possibility of two different diagnoses, in another words, a dual diagnosis. The establishment of a clear diagnosis is of utmost importance because the treatment and the success or failure of it depend on a well-established diagnosis.

ESTABLISHING THE DIAGNOSIS

The treatment of addicted patients is very difficult, and one has to approach these patients with a great deal of empathy and understanding. From the history and from old medical records, one can sometimes obtain clear objective evidence of a long-standing psychiatric diagnosis years before the patient became addicted. In such cases the addiction interferes with the treatment of the mental illness and worsens this illness. It is helpful to explain to patients that it might be almost impossible to treat their illness with any degree of success until their addiction is addressed. These extremely difficult patients are very resistant to treatment and have a high rate of failures. On the other hand, addiction might be the first illness, and as a result of it the patient might have become mentally ill—for example, psychosis secondary to marijuana use that does not abate after marijuana use is discontinued. It is essential to take time to sit down and listen to patients.

THEORY OF SELF-MEDICATION

One issue that causes a great deal of conflict is the theory of self-medication. Patients perceive that their drug is the only thing that helps them to control the symptoms. It is not uncommon for schizophrenic patients to report that their cocaine euphoria helps them control the voices of the auditory hallucinations that otherwise have never been controlled. One has to understand such patients are very resistant to treatment for this same reason. It is one's duty to confront such a belief by informing patients that the findings of studies on this subject do not confirm this but on the contrary show a significant deterioration under these conditions. Again, one has to be honest and to educate patients about their addiction and mental illness and how they interact to complicate their treatment.

INITIATING A TREATMENT PLAN

One has to be able to negotiate treatment with patients and try to accommodate their current status without causing that same treatment to suffer from this negotiation. One has to accept that many patients will not engage in treatment for their addiction in this setting or, if they do so, will have multiple relapses and treatment failures. Essential to the outcome of treatment is the establishment of rapport between the consultant and the patient, as well as with the primary mental healthcare provider. Without establishing this rapport, the treatment cannot advance. The method for establishing this rapport has no clear guidelines or rules except to take time and to try to understand the patient. This understanding can be facilitated by thoroughly reviewing the present illness and obtaining a past history of medical and psychiatric illnesses, a social history, and a family history. Additional information can be obtained from family meetings if a patient is willing to accept these meetings and authorize them.

THE CONSULTANT

Again, the central point is listening to the patient and trying to determine what the illness—the mental illness a part from addiction—means for the patient. What does addiction mean for the patient, what resources and coping mechanisms does the patient have, and how does addiction fit into them? One must try to understand what would be helpful for this patient and how help and hope can be offered in an acceptable form. Because patients sometimes do not voice their needs or desires, one must try to reach a conclusion about these from information obtainable through different ways mentioned earlier. Once obtained, all this information has to be looked at in the context of the patient's environment and circumstances, because if the patient's environment and circumstances at the time of the consultation are not taken into account, treatment will again be at a high risk of failure.

More than in any other setting, in this one the consultant has to be ready to try to understand the patient's idiosyncratic way of dealing with this problem and the world at large. It is necessary to approach patients so that rapport can be established at the same time with empathy and respect, never in a controlling way and never taking care of the "situation," no matter how well intentioned and how right the healthcare providers can be in their diagnosis and treatment plan. All treatment interventions must be based on the patient's agreement, understanding, and willingness to participate. At other times, one is requested in consultation to treat either the acute intoxication or withdrawal from alcohol or drugs. In these circumstances, one has to remember that these two can present as psychiatric illnesses and that their signs and symptoms can be confused with those of a psychiatric disorder. Studies have shown that the medical and psychiatric population has a high prevalence of alcohol and drug dependence but that in the alcoholic and drug-addicted population, the prevalence of psychiatric disorders is less common.

DEPRESSION

An important consideration is the high prevalence of depression in alcoholic or addicted patients. Some studies have reported that as many as 98% of alcoholics at some point in their life history have depressive symptoms, and about 33% meet criteria for persistent depression for a period of 2 weeks or longer. When asked in consultation to see such a patient, one cannot make the diagnosis of a major depression or of depression as a result of the addiction at that one given moment in time. The only way to establish the diagnosis is by considering the possibility and observing a patient for a long period, preferably while that patient is receiving treatment for addiction. When the depression is of such intensity that it interferes with this treatment for addiction, the recommendation would be to initiate antidepressant medication even though the diagnosis might not be clear.

GERIATRIC PATIENTS

One interesting patient population that can often be encountered in this setting as well as in a medical and surgical setting is the geriatric population. Alcohol and drug dependence among the elderly is common, and it is very much underdiagnosed.

Addiction in this case is frequently to prescribed medications of the sedative type as well as hypnotics, benzodiazepines, and other over-the-counter medications. These cause severe side effects in this population, manifested in the clinical setting as dementia, depression, and anxiety. One has to have a high level of suspicion and to consider that these symptoms might result from either alcohol or drug use. The diagnosis can be established with urine toxicology screens, as well as a complete history focusing on what medications the patient is receiving, because again, the addiction commonly is to prescription medication.

If the diagnosis is established as a result, not only does the treatment have a significant impact on the lifestyle of the patient, but unnecessary diagnostic procedures and treatments related to an erroneous diagnosis are avoided.

While treatment for addiction is in progress, one has to remain alert for coexisting psychiatric illnesses, because these are common in the geriatric population. For example, affective and anxiety disorders, dementia, and delirium are common.

Child and Adolescent Service

THE NEWBORN

In child and adolescent services, because of the nature or the age of the patient, treatment has its own difficulties. In neonates, who might present with withdrawal symptoms because of addiction of their mother, one has to consider two different aspects. One is the syndrome of abstinence, and the other is the behavioral characteristics. The neonatal abstinence syndrome due to opiates is a generalized disorder with characteristic signs and symptoms of central nervous system disorders, hyperirritability, gastrointestinal dysfunction, and respiratory distress among others.

The behavior is also characterized by frantic sucking of fists or thumbs, difficulty with feeding, tremors that may be mild to severe, and high-pitched crying. The majority of these symptoms appear within 72 hours. The behavioral characteristics appear to be a lack of affect on part of the baby, and these babies seem to be less responsive to visual stimulation.

As a result, the ability to interact with the environment appears to be decreased, and these babies are socially less responsive during the first few days of life.

The importance of this situation must be explained to the mother to help her understand what her child is experiencing. She must receive empathic supportive treatment because studies have demonstrated that these mothers have a decreased affect for their neonates and are detached from them by behaviors that do not promote bonding. During this difficult period in the life of a mother and her baby, it is of great help to advise, support, explain, and educate to improve the interaction between mother and child.

CHILDREN

Children with fetal alcohol syndrome or fetal alcohol effects show characteristic findings: mental retardation, craniofacial abnormalities, growth retardation, and malformation of organs. Behaviorally, these children show attention deficits and are easily distracted.

Children exposed to cocaine in utero show low birth weight and growth retardation. These children also show impairment of orientation, motor coordination, and control of behaviors.

Another serious aspect of addiction in childhood is sexual or physical abuse. One has to remain alert for this possibility, because the diagnosis is frequently overlooked.

TREATMENT PLAN

In all the foregoing situations, when asked to consult, one has to organize a comprehensive treatment plan. Such a plan has to address the following aspects of the situation:

1. The addicted woman, the mother of the newborn child, not only needs treatment but also needs help with her social problems (housing, food, baby-care skills, and so forth).

2. Addicted children also benefit from this two-pronged approach. They need treatment for their withdrawal and for the medical consequences of being exposed to a drug in utero, as well as assessment and treatment of all the behavioral abnormalities that they manifest as a result of the passive addiction in utero. For this, it is advisable to recruit the help of a child psychiatrist, because these problems do not resolve in a short time and need long and intensive treatment.

3. The environment surrounding these patients frequently is chaotic and without any established structure or support. Public or private agencies can offer the resources these patients lack. The work of the consultant can be summarized in identifying the multiple aspects that need to be addressed and organizing a multidisciplinary team that can initiate and continue a comprehensive treatment plan focused on helping the child grow in as healthy a manner as possible.

THE ADOLESCENT

Older children who themselves have become addicted or adolescents with a history of addiction present extreme difficulties for a consultant who is asked either to establish the diagnosis or to initiate treatment. These patients are surrounded by an environment and circumstances that hinder positive rapport and block the advancement of treatment. These patients often have family background of addiction, suffer from poor social skills and structure in their daily lives, do not have support by other family members, and lack motivation to engage in treatment.

In adolescents or older children, the acute aspect of treatment—the withdrawal or detoxification after overdose—is essentially similar to that of adults, keeping in mind the body weight and the dosage. The problems in this aspect of treatment are similar to those in a medical setting, but where this setting takes on characteristics of its own, as mentioned earlier, is in the psychological and social aspects.

In summary, adolescent patients are difficult because of the environment and circumstances that surround them, and these have to be addressed as one of the main factors in treatment. The best way to do so is with a treatment team approach, as explained earlier. The team needs to be multidisciplinary and should address all issues—the patient, the patient's family, the patient's neighborhood, and the school—because all these influence a patient's behavior and motivation for treatment.

One must also consider the legal aspects of treating patients who are not adults and must keep in mind the confidentiality that these patients expect. This issue complicates treatment, unhappily, even more. No specific treatment guidelines have been established.

BIBLIOGRAPHY

American Psychiatric Association: Diagnostic and Statistical Manual of Mental Disorders, 4th ed. Washington, DC; American Psychiatric Association, 1994.

Anthenelli RM: The initial evaluation of the dual diagnosis patient. Psychiatr Ann 24(8): 407–411, 1994.

Burton RW, Lyons JS, Deveus M, et al: Psychiatric consultations for psychoactive substance disorders in the general hospital. Gen Hosp Psychiatry 13:83–87, 1991.

Chang G, Carroll KM, Behr HM, et al: Improving treatment outcome in pregnant opiate-dependent women. J Subst Abuse Treat 9:327–330, 1992.

Drake RE, McLaughlin P, Pepper B, et al: New Directions for Mental Health Services, no 50. San Francisco, Jossey-Bass, 1991, pp 3–12.

Finnegan LP: Treatment issues for opioid-dependent women during the perinatal period. J Psychoactive Drugs 23(2):191–201, 1991.

Galanter M, Egelko S, DeLeon G, et al: Crack/cocaine abusers in the general hospital: Assessment and initiation of care. Am J Psychiatry 149:810–815, 1992.

Guze SB, Cloninger R, Martin R, et al: Alcoholism as a medical disorder. In Rose R, ed. Alcoholism: Origins and Outcome. New York, Raven Press, 1988, pp 83–94.

Hyman SE: Manual of Psychiatric Emergencies, 2nd ed. Boston, Little, Brown & Co, 1989.

Lam SK, To WK, Duthie SJ, et al: Narcotic addiction in pregnancy with adverse maternal and perinatal outcome. Aust N Z J Obstet Gynecol 32(3): 216–221, 1992.

Levin FR, Weddington WW, Haertzen CA, et al: A substance abuse consultation service: Characteristics of patients and pedagogical potential. NIDA Res Monogr 105:291–292, 1991.

Little BB, Snell LM, Klein VR, et al: Maternal and fetal effects of heroin addiction during pregnancy. J Reprod Med 35(2): 159–162, 1990.

Miller NS: Epidemiologies of psychiatric and addictive comorbidity. Psychiatr Clin North Am 16(1):3–16, 1993.

Miller NS, Belkin BM, Gold MS: Alcohol and drug dependence among the elderly: Epidemiology, diagnosis and treatment. Compr Psychiatry 32(2): 153–165, 1991.

Miller NS, Mahler JC, Belkin BM, et al: Psychiatric diagnosis in alcohol and drug dependence. Ann Clin Psychiatry 3(1): 79–89, 1991.

Raundal E, Vaglum P: Different intake procedures: The influence on treatment start and treatment response—a quasi-experimental study. J Subst Abuse Treat 9:53–58, 1992.

Regier DA, Farmer ME, Rae DS, et al: Comorbidity of mental disorders with alcohol and other drug abuse: Results from the Epidemiologic Catchment Area (ECA) study. JAMA 264:2511–2518, 1990.

Schuckit MA: Evaluating the dual diagnosis patient. Drug Abuse and Alcoholism Newsletter. 17(10): 1–4, 1988.

Spelman J: Interventions for hospitalized addicted patients through psychiatric consultation. Psychiatr Ann 24(8): 424–426, 1994.

Thom B, Brown C, Drummond C, et al: Engaging patients with alcohol problems in treatment: The first consultation. Br J Addict 87:601–611, 1992.

Benzodiazepines, Other Sedative, Hypnotic, and Anxiolytic Drugs, and Addiction

Steven M. Juergens, MD

Sedative, hypnotic, and anxiolytic drugs are central nervous system (CNS) depressants traditionally used to reduce anxiety or to induce sleep. The focus of this chapter is the benzodiazepines (BZPs) (Table 18–1), the most commonly used drugs of this class in medical and psychiatric practice. They are also the most commonly used *addictive* drugs in medical and psychiatric practice. They are valuable agents whose addictive properties should not damn but rather limit their use. The appropriate use—as well as the recognition, management, and treatment of physiological dependence and addiction to these substances—is important, and the clinical judgments required can be difficult and subtle.

Other Sedative, Hypnotic, and Anxiolytic Agents

The barbiturates and barbiturate-like substances (Table 18–2) have been largely supplanted by the BZPs in clinical practice. Secobarbital, pentobarbital, and amobarbital are under the same federal controls as morphine but are available on the street from drug dealers. Methaqualone is no longer manufactured in the United States.

Except for the anticonvulsant actions of phenobarbital and its congeners, the barbiturate and other barbiturate-like drugs have a low therapeutic index and low degree of selectivity. Therefore, the therapeutic effect of sedation or anxiolysis is accompanied by CNS depression. Other disadvantages compared with BZPs are that barbiturates induce hepatic enzymes, causing more drug interactions; they produce more tolerance, are more reinforcing, have greater severity of withdrawal, and are more lethal in overdose. Unfortunately, there is evidence of some increase in their use where BZPs have become more regulated (e.g., the use of triplicate prescription forms).[1]

Buspirone is an azapirone approved for the treatment of anxiety disorders and is unrelated to the BZPs or barbiturate and barbiturate-like drugs. It acts as an agonist or partial agonist on serotonin type 1A receptors, but its mechanism of action is incompletely understood. It appears not to have withdrawal symptoms, does not reinforce drug-taking behavior, and causes little psychomotor impairment; therefore, it seems to have the lowest addiction potential compared with the BZPs, barbiturates, and barbiturate-like drugs.[2]

Zolpidem is a rapid-onset, short-duration imidazopyridine hypnotic that acts at the

Table 18–1. PHARMACOKINETIC PROPERTIES OF BENZODIAZEPINES

Generic Name (Trade Name)	Dosage Equivalent (mg)	Onset of Action	Relative Lipophilicity	Active Substances	Elimination Half-Life (Hours)*
Clonazepam (Klonopin)	0.25	Intermediate	+½	Clonazepam	18–50
Alprazolam (Xanax)	0.5	Intermediate	+++	Alprazolam	6–20
Triazolam (Halcion)	0.5	Fast	+++	Triazolam	1.7–3.0
Lorazepam (Ativan)	1.0	Intermediate	++½	Lorazepam	10–20
Estazolam (ProSom)	2.0	Intermediate	++	Estazolam	8–24
Diazepam (Valium and others)	5.0	Fast	++++	Diazepam Desmethyldiazepam	30–100
Clorazepate (Tranxene)	7.5	Fast	++++	Desmethyldiazepam†	30–100
Chlordiazepoxide (Librium and others)	10.0	Intermediate		Chlordiazepoxide Desmethylchlordiazepoxide Demoxepam Desmethyldiazepam	5–100
Oxazepam (Serax)	15.0	Slow	++	Oxazepam	5–12
Flurazepam (Dalmane)	30.0	Fast		Flurazepam Hydroxyethylflurazepam Desalkylflurazepam	50–100
Temazepam (Restoril)	30.0	Slow	+++	None	10–12
Quazepam (Doral)	30.0	Fast	++++++	Quazepam Oxyquazepam Desalkylflurazepam‡	20–120

*Elimination half-life represents the total for all active metabolites.

†Clorazepate is a product that is converted in the stomach to desmethyldiazepam, the active substance in the blood.

‡Desalkylflurazepam is identical to N-desalkyl-2-oxoquozepam.

Adapted from Cowley DS, Roy-Byrne PP, Greenblatt DJ: Benzodiazepines: Pharmacokinetics and pharmacodynamics (1985). In PP Roy-Byrne, DS Cowley (eds): Benzodiazepines in Clinical Practice: Risks and Benefits. Washington, DC, American Psychiatric Association, 1991; with additional information from Greenblatt DJ: Benzodiazepine hypnotics: Sorting out the pharmacokinetic facts. J Clin Psychiatry 52(Suppl):4–10, 1991.

gamma-aminobutyric acid (GABA) complex as the BZPs do but is not a BZP. It has little effect on the stages of sleep and few, if any, anxiolytic, anticonvulsant, and muscle relaxant effects. Dose-related side effects include dizziness, headache, nausea, and diarrhea, which limit escalation of dose.[3] However, zolpidem is positively reinforcing and does decrease psychomotor performance and impair memory similarly to triazolam.[4] Although withdrawal is claimed to be minimal, there is evidence of rebound effects on discontinuation, as with BZPs.[3]

Table 18–2. BARBITURATE AND BARBITURATE-LIKE MEDICATIONS AND DOSE EQUIVALENCIES (PHENOBARBITAL 30 MG = DIAZEPAM 10 MG)

	Generic Name	Trade Name	Dose Equivalent (mg)
Barbiturates	Amobarbital	Amytal	100
	Butabarbital	Butisol	100
	Butalbital	In Fiorinal and Esgic	100
	Pentobarbital	Nembutal	100
	Secobarbital	Seconal	100
	Phenobarbital	Luminal	30
Others	Meprobamate	Miltown, Equanil, Equagesic	400
	Glutethimide	Doriden	250
	Chloral hydrate	Noctec, Somnos	500–1000
	Ethchlorvynol	Placidyl	750
	Methaqualone	Quaalude	300

Data Regarding Benzodiazepine Addiction

The clinical and descriptive data regarding BZP addiction are surprisingly inadequate. The data most often have little clinical context and are often quite nonspecific.[5] There are case reports of BZP addiction[6] and reports documenting groups of BZP-addicted patients, largely from addiction treatment centers.[7] About 1% to 3% of the population of the Western world have received continuous BZP therapy for more than 1 year, with substantially higher rates of use among women than men and among older than younger populations.[8] The National Household Survey of 1992[9] estimated that in the United States, 1,806,000 people (0.9%) used a sedative and 3,046,000 people (1.5%) used a tranquilizer "nonmedically" in the past year, with men and those age 35 years and older having the highest percentage of misuse. It is difficult to translate data such as these into estimates of addiction, but significant chronic use clearly occurs, and empirical evidence demonstrates abuse and addiction.

Two patterns of BZP addiction are most prominent: (1) use of only BZPs for long periods and (2) use of BZPs in the context of multiple drug or alcohol addiction. In the latter example, BZPs may or may not be the primary addicting drug. The multiple drug/alcohol users are younger, take higher doses, and are more likely to escalate their use of the BZP, but the patients who use BZPs only may have more difficulty with withdrawal symptoms. Addiction to BZPs as part of a polydrug or alcohol addiction is most common, and primary BZP addiction is said to be rare,[7] but this has been challenged by chemical dependence professionals, and the information supporting that conclusion is inadequate.[5]

Pharmacokinetics and Pharmacodynamics

The pharmacokinetic properties of the sedative-hypnotics are important considerations in evaluating their addiction potential. The kinetic properties of BZPs (which apply to the barbiturate and barbiturate-like drugs as well) that may contribute to the abuse liability and persistent self-administration of these drugs are summarized in Table 18–3. Drugs that are potent positive reinforcers or that cause the development of physical dependence and withdrawal symptoms have the most potential for abuse and addiction.

Because all BZPs rapidly enter the brain tissue once they are in the circulation, the onset of action of BZPs relates to their absorption from the gastrointestinal tract. The most rapidly absorbed BZPs (i.e., diazepam) may produce more euphoria and be more reinforcing than others.[2]

The more highly lipophilic BZPs (see Table 18–1) are also rapidly distributed to peripheral tissue and have high volumes of distribution (i.e., diazepam). Therefore, after single doses, the duration of action is shorter, and this factor may be reinforcing as well.[10]

The rate of elimination after multiple doses is related to the elimination half-life of the parent drug and its metabolites (see Table 18–1). BZPs with a shorter elimination half-life and little accumulation (i.e., lorazepam and alprazolam) present more chance of developing

Table 18–3. KINETICS AND ABUSE POTENTIAL

Properties that increase potency as a reinforcer:
  High intrinsic pharmacological activity of drug
  Rapid absorption
  Rapid entry into specific brain regions
  High oral bioavailability
  Low protein binding
  Short half-life
  Small volume of distribution
  High clearance
Factors that promote physical dependence:
  High intrinsic pharmacological activity of drug
  Cumulative drug load (dose, frequency, duration of treatment)
  Small volume of distribution
  Long half-life
  Low clearance
Factors that promote appearance of the withdrawal syndrome:
  High intrinsic pharmacological activity of drug
  Short half-life
  High clearance
  Rapid exit from specific brain regions
  Small volume of distribution

From Coppell HD, Sellars EM, Busto U: Benzodiazepines as drugs of abuse and dependence. In Cappell HD, Glaser FH, Israel Y, et al (eds): Recent Advances in Alcohol and Drug Problems, vol 9. New York, Plenum, 1986, p 63.

withdrawal or rebound symptoms if doses are missed, spaced too far apart, or abruptly discontinued. Continued use may therefore be related to this negatively reinforcing quality.[10]

Pharmacodynamic factors may also be important. The differences in potency correlate with receptor-binding affinity (i.e., alprazolam binds with greater affinity and is more potent than diazepam). Higher-potency agents are associated with more seizures on withdrawal and may induce more severe physical dependence.[11]

ADDICTION PROPERTIES

BZPs and other sedative, hypnotic, and anxiolytic drugs are addicting. Substances that are addicting cause (1) reinforcement, because there appears to be a good concordance between drug self-ingestion and reinforcing effects; (2) physiological dependence, evidenced by tolerance and the negative reinforcement of withdrawal; and (3) adverse effects on the person's life.[2] The *Diagnostic and Statistical Manual of Mental Disorders,* 4th edition (DSM-IV),[12] diagnostic criteria for substance dependence operationalize the expression of these qualities and fit the traditional definition of addiction, emphasizing the compulsive use of the substance resulting in physical, psychological, or social harm to the user or others affected by the user's behavior and continued use despite that harm.[13] Addiction is characterized by preoccupation with acquisition of the substance, often with a pattern of relapse after abstinence or an inability to reduce use. Physiological dependence (evidence of tolerance or withdrawal) is specified if present in DSM-IV but is not insisted on or sufficient for the diagnosis.

REINFORCING EFFECTS

The addiction liability of sedatives, hypnotics, and anxiolytics can be assessed by examining the reinforcing effects of these drugs, with the assumption that the reinforcing effects are correlated with drug self-ingestion.[2]

Although in studies that use "normal" and mildly anxious subjects, BZPs are not preferred over placebo,[14] they are reinforcing for large populations. In anxious subjects who seek treatment, a significant proportion find diazepam to be a positive reinforcer.[15] Normal volunteers who drink lightly (less than 5 drinks per week) and moderately (an average of 11 drinks per week),[16] abstinent alcoholics and sons of alcoholics,[14] and occasional recreational users of illicit sedatives without physical dependence, as well as sedative abusers,[5] have reinforcing responses to BZPs.

Barbiturates, meprobamate, and methaqualone appear to have more euphoric or reinforcing properties than do BZPs.[14]

Various BZPs appear to have different relative addiction liability in substance abusers. Diazepam, lorazepam, triazolam, and alprazolam have relatively high addiction liability, whereas oxazepam, halazepam, clorazepate, and possibly chlordiazepoxide do not. The speed of onset of pleasurable effects is an important factor in addiction potential.[14]

PHYSIOLOGICAL DEPENDENCE

Tolerance. Tolerance to the sedative effects of BZPs develops over several days to weeks. Tolerance to anxiolysis does not usually occur, yet some patients do develop a need for higher doses of BZPs over time for anxiolysis. Tolerance to amnestic and psychomotor effects occurs but may be incomplete and variable among patients.[17]

Withdrawal. DSM-IV lists a single set of diagnostic criteria for withdrawal from any sedative, hypnotic, or anxiolytic (Table 18–4). Clinicians can specify "with perceptual disturbances." Sudden withdrawal can be life threatening. With barbiturate and barbiturate-

Table 18–4. DIAGNOSTIC CRITERIA FOR 292.0 SEDATIVE, HYPNOTIC, OR ANXIOLYTIC WITHDRAWAL

A. Cessation of (or reduction in) sedative, hypnotic, or anxiolytic use that has been heavy and prolonged.
B. Two (or more) of the following, developing within several hours to a few days after criterion A:
  (1) Autonomic hyperactivity (e.g., sweating or pulse rate greater than 100)
  (2) Increased hand tremor
  (3) Insomnia
  (4) Nausea or vomiting
  (5) Transient visual, tactile, or auditory hallucinations or illusions
  (6) Psychomotor agitation
  (7) Anxiety
  (8) Grand mal seizures
C. The symptoms in criterion B cause clinically significant distress or impairment in social, occupational, or other important areas of functioning.
D. The symptoms are not due to a general medical condition and are not better accounted for by another mental disorder.

Specify if: **With Perceptual Disturbances**

From the American Psychiatric Association: Diagnosis and Statistical Manual of Mental Disorders, 4th ed. Washington, DC, American Psychiatric Association, 1994, p 266.

like drugs, persons using the equivalent of 400 mg/day pentobarbital may have mild symptoms (i.e., anxiety, involuntary twitching of muscles, coarse intention tremors, weakness, sweating, and insomnia); persons who have been using the substance in the range of 800 mg/day (or more) for more than 40 days usually experience psychosis, convulsions, or delirium that resembles alcoholic delirium tremens. Symptoms appear within a day of abstinence. Seizures are usually grand mal, appear on the second or third day, and are often multiple, unlike alcohol withdrawal. The psychosis develops on the third to eighth day and may last as long as 2 weeks. The time course of the onset and duration of the symptoms is earlier and shorter with short-half-life drugs than with the longer-half-life drugs. Agitation and hyperthermia can cause exhaustion, cardiovascular collapse, and death. Users of dosages exceeding 800 mg/day may experience anorexia, delusions, hallucinations, and repeated seizures and could have cardiovascular collapse and death. Most symptoms appear in the first 3 days of abstinence, with seizures occurring before the onset of delirium on the second or third day.[18]

Patients withdrawing from BZPs may report other symptoms (Table 18–5). Seizures, persistent tinnitus, delirium, confusion, and psychotic symptoms have been reported but are uncommon.[11] Mania and obsessive-compulsive

Table 18–5. COMMONLY OBSERVED WITHDRAWAL SYMPTOMS

Anxiety
Irritability
Insomnia
Fatigue
Headache
Muscle twitching or aching
Tremor, shakiness
Sweating
Dizziness
Concentration difficulties
*Nausea, loss of appetite
*Observable depression
*Depersonalization, derealization
*Increased sensory perception (smell, sight, taste, touch)
*Abnormal perception or sensation of movement

---

*Symptoms more likely to represent true withdrawal rather than an exacerbation or return of original anxiety.
From Roy-Byrne PP, Nutt DJ: Benzodiazepines in Clinical Practice: Risks and Benefits. Washington, DC, American Psychiatric Association, 1991, p 138.

---

disorder have been reported to have been triggered with withdrawal as well.[19]

In evaluating the physiological dependence on BZPs, distinguishing withdrawal from relapse and rebound is difficult. Withdrawal is defined as "new" time-limited symptoms that are not part of the original anxiety state and that begin and end depending on the pharmacokinetics of the BZPs, relapse as reemergence of the original anxiety state, and rebound as an increase in anxiety that exceeds original baseline levels and may be a combination of relapse and withdrawal.[19] With abrupt discontinuation, symptoms begin the day afterward with short- and intermediate-half-life drugs, within 3 to 8 days with long-acting BZPs, and are most severe between 2 and 18 days after withdrawal, again depending on half-life.[20] With gradual taper of BZPs, the withdrawal syndrome is the most severe in the last quarter of the taper with short-half-life BZPs, but it is the most severe in the first week off BZPs in those taking long-half-life BZPs. The withdrawal syndrome for the most part remits by 3 to 5 weeks after the taper. However, persistence of isolated symptoms such as tinnitus may last months.[21, 22]

The vast majority (>90%) of long-term (greater than 8 to 12 months) users of BZPs experience withdrawal whether withdrawn slowly or rapidly.[21–23] Gradual taper of alprazolam after long-term treatment of panic disorder results in significant rebound of panic and anxiety, with symptoms exceeding pretreatment levels in more than 50% to 90%, depending on how rebound is measured.[22] Withdrawal does not appear to worsen if a BZP is used longer than 1 year, suggesting a threshold duration of treatment beyond which further BZP exposure has little pharmacological influence on the withdrawal experience.[21, 23] The incidence of withdrawal appears to be less in short-term users (< 6 to 8 months), although withdrawal can develop within weeks, especially if higher doses of high-potency agents are used.[11] One study of patients with panic reported a 50% incidence of withdrawal or rebound after only 8 weeks of treatment with alprazolam that was tapered over 4 weeks.[24]

The inability of patients on long-term BZPs to discontinue them because of withdrawal is of concern. Even with a slow withdrawal procedure over 1 month, more than one third of subjects are unable to discontinue BZPs.[21, 22]

Withdrawal reactions with BZPs are reported to be more likely or more severe if the drug is (1) rapidly eliminated, (2) highly potent, (3) discontinued abruptly rather than gradually tapered, (4) used in relatively high doses, and (5) used chronically on an as-needed basis rather than a fixed-dose schedule[19] or if the patient (1) has traits of dependence and neuroticism, (2) had mild to moderate alcohol use, (3) is less educated, (4) has more panic, anxiety, and depression at baseline,[22, 23] (5) has a prior history of alcohol or drug abuse, and (6) feels that he or she is addicted, weak, and "hooked" on these drugs.[19] The effect of half-life and dose on withdrawal is mitigated when the BZP is gradually tapered.[11, 21] Regarding various BZPs, withdrawal reactions appear to be most severe with quickly eliminated high-potency BZPs (e.g., alprazolam, lorazepam, triazolam), intermediate with quickly eliminated low-potency BZPs (oxazepam) and slowly eliminated high-potency BZPs (clonazepam), and mildest with slowly eliminated low-potency BZPs (e.g., diazepam, clorazepate, chlordiazepoxide).[25]

The management of sedative, hypnotic, and anxiolytic withdrawal is discussed in Chapter 42.

ADVERSE EFFECTS

Impairment of Memory. BZPs can induce memory problems. Most studies show that the ability to learn new information is impaired (anterograde amnesia) after BZP administration. This impairment apparently occurs by disrupting the process of taking information from temporary, short-term memory and transferring it to some kind of longer-term memory storage (the consolidation phase).[11]

Anterograde amnesia is increased with increased dose, faster absorption, intravenous administration, and higher potency of the BZPs. Tolerance to the anterograde amnesia occurs but is not complete. In chronic users, transient amnesic effects can occur related to postdose, peak BZP levels.[17] The elderly are more sensitive to the effects of BZPs on memory.[11]

Some evidence indicates that patients have a significant improvement in measures of memory and cognitive functioning after discontinuation of BZPs. Family and staff note that elderly patients who discontinue use of BZPs are brighter, more energetic, less dysphoric, and substantially more intellectually alert than while taking the drug.[26]

The increased sensitivity of the elderly may be partly attributed to a lower baseline performance in the elderly; thus, an equal decrement in a younger and an older patient would be more noticeable and have more serious consequences in the elderly patient.[11] In the elderly, BZPs are the drugs that most commonly exacerbate underlying dementia and may cause excess morbidity. The cognitive impairment often appears to develop insidiously as a late complication of a drug initially prescribed at a younger age. Some elderly patients may be given other drugs to treat side effects of the BZPs, such as neuroleptics given to patients who develop confusion while taking BZPs.[27]

BZP-induced memory problems may be unrecognized by patients, family, or clinicians, and the true incidence is unknown. People suffering from such memory problems may conclude that nothing worth remembering had happened if they are unable to recall events. In the elderly, memory problems may be blamed on aging rather than BZP use.

Cognitive and Psychomotor Effects. BZPs also impair cognitive and motor functioning with acute and chronic dosing, although the effects of chronic administration are not consistent in experimental subjects.[11] Sedation, drowsiness, ataxia, incoordination, vertigo, and dizziness are common side effects related to dose and individual susceptibility. Tolerance to these effects develops, although it may not be complete.[11] Impaired visual spatial ability and sustained attention deficits have been found in long-term BZP users, and patients are often unaware of their reduced ability.[28] Being elderly, using alcohol, using high doses of BZP, and taking other drugs (e.g., anticholinergics) are associated with increased sensitivity of cognitive and psychomotor effects.[11]

Risk of Deleterious Events. BZPs may impair specific driving skills, but such effects are not consistent from person to person and may depend on dose and time of administration. One study[29] compared two groups of patients with generalized anxiety disorder treated with diazepam, 5 mg three times daily, or buspirone, 20 mg/day for 4 weeks, by administering a weekly driving test. Diazepam significantly impaired control of lateral position for 3 weeks and speed control for 1 week, whereas buspirone showed no such effects. Elderly patients taking BZPs have a significantly increased risk of injurious motor vehicle accidents and a substantially increased relative risk with higher doses.[30]

The elderly have a significantly increased risk of falling and hip fracture in current users of long-half-life BZPs, and this risk does not dissipate after the first 30 days of therapy, indicating no development of tolerance to the impairment.[31] Short-half-life BZPs also pose considerable hazards to older patients because significantly incapacitating psychomotor effects occur in the first few hours after drug administration, putting patients at risk for falling should they need to void or to get out of bed for any reason.[32]

Other Psychiatric Problems. Behavioral disinhibition reactions with various BZPs may occur, usually associated with higher doses and pretreatment level of hostility. Cases of delirium have been reported with triazolam, usually at high doses in the elderly.[33]

Studies show that significant anxiety and depressive psychopathology remain in many long-term BZP users while they are using BZPs. However, patients who are able to withdraw successfully from long-term BZP treatment have significantly improved anxiety and depression scores compared with pretaper baseline,[21] implying that BZPs may worsen depression and anxiety long term. Depression and interdose anxiety have been noted to emerge with BZP therapy.[11] Gains with agoraphobia using alprazolam and exposure therapy are lost after treatment but maintained in patients treated with exposure therapy alone. Therefore, the use of BZPs may impair therapeutic progress long term.[34] Deterioration in mood and social behavior in subjects taking BZPs has been noted by raters but not by the subjects themselves; thus, negative effects may be difficult to elicit by self-report.[35]

BZPs can be a complicating factor in those patients with prior or current chemical dependence. Although existing studies have methodological difficulties, BZP abuse and dependence appear greater among alcoholics and addicts.[11] The development of alcohol or other drug addiction after primary BZP dependence, although reported less often than the reverse, has been observed,[36, 37] implying causation. Suicide attempts are linked with BZPs in many studies, and adverse effects on mood in use and withdrawal lead some to consider that BZPs foster suicidal thinking and action.[38] Substantial social and occupational impairment has been associated with BZP addiction as well.[6]

The high rate of withdrawal symptoms with BZP use and many patients' inability to discontinue BZPs, as described earlier, must also be considered an adverse consequence of BZP use that causes significant discomfort and may cause life disruption.

The high-potency short-half-life BZPs may have more adverse effects.[11] Wysowski and Barash[39] report that adverse behavioral reactions in patients receiving triazolam, reported to the Spontaneous Reporting System of the Food and Drug Administration, considering the extent of use, were 22 to 99 times those of temazepam for confusion, amnesia, bizarre behavior, agitation, and hallucinations. Higher doses and elderly age were associated with more reactions, but the higher incidence occurred even when high-dose cases were removed from analysis.

Overview of Therapeutic Uses, Concerns, and Addiction Issues

BZPs are used for a wide variety of indications. Their use in alcohol withdrawal is addressed elsewhere in this text. They are also used as anticonvulsants and muscle relaxants, but these uses are not reviewed here.

Panic disorder is treated with BZPs, with alprazolam being the most well studied, although it appears that many BZPs, if given in equivalent doses, may be effective acutely.[40] The usual dose range used is the equivalent of 2 to 10 mg of alprazolam daily.[40] However, there is concern about the efficacy of long-term use of BZPs for panic disorder. One study demonstrated that at 1-year follow-up, patients with panic disorder originally treated with imipramine or placebo fare as well as patients treated with alprazolam without the problems of physical dependence, difficulty with discontinuation, and concerns of developing addiction that alprazolam or other BZP therapy entails.[22]

BZPs have been used for the treatment of acute and chronic generalized anxiety/dysphoria. This is often an indistinct syndrome that may coexist with other anxiety, affective disorders, and medical disorders; may be a subsyndromal form of other anxiety, affective disorders, and medical disorders; or may represent an underlying personality disorder.[40] Acutely, BZPs may be used for severe anxiety when immediate symptom relief is necessary. The equivalent of diazepam, 10 to 30 mg/day, is the usual dose. They are best used intermittently during periods when the symptoms are most severe, at the lowest effective dose for the shortest periods possible. Long-term use is generally contraindicated. Some of these patients may fare better with antidepressant medications, other antianxiety medications such as buspirone, or other forms of psychosocial interventions. Because chronically dysphoric or personality-disordered patients may have more difficulty with BZP addiction and discontinuation of BZPs, caution is necessary.[11, 19, 21, 22]

BZPs are often combined with antidepressants in patients with depression and anxiety for initial short-term symptomatic relief. Alprazolam has been shown effective in milder outpatient depressions but is not considered a primary pharmacological treatment, and in general, BZPs have not proved to be effective antidepressants.[40]

BZPs are used as an adjunct to neuroleptics in treating patients with schizophrenia with active psychotic symptoms if they have an unsatisfactory response to neuroleptics alone, for patients with akathesia due to neuroleptics, and in treatment of tardive dyskinesia. They are an adjunct to lithium in treating patients with bipolar disorder.[41] The long-term use of BZPs in these populations has not been adequately studied.

BZP hypnotics are used for transient insomnia using the lowest effective doses available (i.e., flurazepam, 15 mg; triazolam, 0.125 mg) in a time-limited fashion, usually for 2 to 3 weeks.[42] Tolerance to the sedative effects develops within that time, especially with short-half-life agents.[11] Rebound insomnia (intense worsening of sleep above baseline levels after withdrawal of BZP) may develop after short-term use. This may lead patients to request to continue the BZP for sleep, which should be avoided. Tapering the hypnotic may attenuate the symptoms of rebound insomnia.[42] Parasomnias including rapid-eye-movement behavior disorder, periodic limb movements during sleep, sleepwalking, and night terrors may be treated with BZPs, but a careful diagnostic workup is needed because treatment is often long term and relapse of the parasomnias with discontinuation may be high.[42]

When patients are maintained on BZPs, physiological dependence and other adverse effects, including addiction, can develop. Lack of clear diagnosis without defined measures of benefit and projected time course of treatment may lead to indiscriminate use. Once continual use is begun, a cycle of dependence, withdrawal, continued treatment, and further dependence may develop, and many patients are unable to withdraw completely from the BZP.[2, 22]

Long-term use beyond detoxification is almost always a contraindication to the use of BZPs in those patients with prior or active chemical dependence. Patients with chemical dependence often have symptoms of anxiety or dysphoria and have often been placed on BZPs.[11] BZP dependence and addiction appear greater among alcoholics[14] as well as those patients with previous high-dose sedative-hypnotic drug use.[11] Opioid addicts commonly use BZPs, often to augment the euphoriant effects of the opiates.[11] Persons addicted to cocaine and other stimulants may use and become addicted to BZPs to ease the "crash" of the rapid decline in euphoria.[11] Physicians may take an inadequate substance use history, or they may lack understanding of cross-addiction and the chronic and negative effects of addiction. These factors may account for why these patients are placed on BZPs.[38]

In prescribing BZPs, one needs to weigh carefully the potential therapeutic benefit against the near certain risk of developing physical dependence, acute and chronic toxicity, and addiction. In a vast majority of cases, use should be short term (< 2 to 4 months) on as low a dose as is effective. Longer-term use should regularly be reevaluated to ensure that continued BZP use is appropriate and without problems. DuPont[43] elucidated a checklist to determine appropriate continuation of BZP use:

1. The diagnosis, distress, and disability warrant use.
2. The BZP is effecting a positive therapeutic response with appropriate doses, and the patient has no other drug or alcohol addiction.
3. The patient has no evidence of any BZP-induced problem.
4. A family member or significant other can confirm the effectiveness of BZP use and the lack of impairment and addiction.

If diagnosis, effectiveness, and lack of problems are confirmed, continued use may be indicated, but if problems are identified or the patient wants to stop, BZP discontinuation is indicated.[43] These criteria draw a line between problematic and nonproblematic use, but in practice this determination may not be so clear. Clinicians vary on their judgment about diagnostic implications for the use of BZPs. There is no clear consensus on length of treatment for many disorders. Use of increased amounts or other substances is often difficult to detect secondary to denial or inadequate history taking. The adequacy of response may be unclear because symptoms may fluctuate or comorbidity may complicate evaluation of the effectiveness of the BZP.[11] Toxic behavior may be subtle, unobtrusive, or attributed to other causes, and thus the physician or the patient is unaware of problems caused by BZPs. Physicians vary in their ability to recognize the diagnosis of addiction. Patients may not have a monitor or may disagree with the monitor, or the monitor may be in denial or unaware of problems. Additionally, problems may develop only after years of use[6]; thus, long-term vigilance is necessary.

The determination of addiction is easier in patients who use BZPs in the context of addiction to multiple drugs or alcohol or if patients show clear escalation of the dose of BZP. Adverse consequences of addiction are often obvious in their lives: illicit use, escalation of doses, use of BZPs to induce intoxication, use in combination with alcohol and other substances, and failure to inform the physician of the circumstances and purpose for which the drugs are used.

More difficulty is encountered when diagnosing addiction in those patients who have developed problems in the context of long-term sedative, hypnotic, and anxiolytic treatment (which is with BZPs in the vast majority of cases), usually for a preexisting psychiatric condition.[5, 6] Physical dependence occurs in those who are taking stable doses of BZPs within the therapeutic range without abuse of alcohol or other drugs and without any BZP-caused problems. This physical dependence is demarcated from addiction.

DSM-IV[12] criteria for substance dependence are adequate to make a diagnosis of BZP dependence. One failing, however, is that the criteria do not emphasize areas that are potentially problematic in BZP-dependent patients, such as worsening of affective or anxious symptoms, memory loss, psychomotor difficulties, or behavioral disinhibition, although these issues can cause problems in major life areas. The toxic behaviors may be subtle, unobtrusive, or attributed to other causes, and thus the physician, family, friends, or patient is not aware that the problems are caused by BZPs, making diagnosis difficult.

BZPs may be continued by physicians who have diagnostic uncertainty about their causing problems. Additionally, patients may not want to discontinue BZPs and, if withdrawn, may worsen clinically because of withdrawal symptoms, at least transiently. Other psychopathology, not BZP dependence/addiction, may be thought of as a cause of problems, and thus the BZPs may be continued and trials of other medications or therapies attempted instead of insisting on BZP abstinence and consideration of chemical dependence treatment.

When patients on BZPs continue to be symptomatic with psychiatric symptoms or to develop problems that could be secondary to BZPs, the BZP is potentially causative or is exacerbating the difficulties. To evaluate this uncertainty, often the only means available is to taper the patient off BZPs.

If adverse effects are recognized or the patient or the physician would like the BZP tapered but because of withdrawal the patient has significant difficulty and thus continues the use, then DSM-IV[12] criteria are met for the group using BZPs only, for a diagnosis of BZP dependence. It is recognized that this group may be different from multiple-drug-addicted patients but still seen as having substance dependence or addiction. This group of patients who begin taking BZPs as prescribed for chronic dysphoria and over time develop problems or abuse appear to represent the most common presentation of BZP dependence.[5]

When prescribing BZPs, a physician should initiate a process of informed consent, including a discussion with the patient, on initiation of treatment, about the effects of these drugs on memory, psychomotor effects including concerns about driving (especially in the first few weeks of initiating or increasing treatment), and the development of physical dependence and addiction.

Treatment Considerations

Beyond detoxification, little has been written about treatment for BZP and other sedative, hypnotic, and anxiolytic dependence. Treatment decisions depend on diagnosis. If a DSM-IV[12] diagnosis of substance dependence is established, either with sedatives, hypnotics, and anxiolytics alone or in the context of alcohol or multiple-drug dependence, then chemical dependence treatment is recommended and other psychiatric treatments are added if a patient has comorbid conditions. If a patient has physical dependence without other adverse effects, then a decision may be made between the clinician and the patient to continue treatment or to detoxify from these drugs and try alternative treatments if necessary for comorbid conditions. Treatment with BZPs should be for the briefest period warranted by the patient's condition.[11]

If a patient is not faring well and whether BZPs are a factor is uncertain, then withdrawal is favored, with observation off BZPs for at least 6 weeks to allow the effects of withdrawal/rebound to be differentiated from relapse. Some have argued that there is a protracted withdrawal syndrome that lasts several months, and thus observation off BZPs needs to be prolonged to make that distinction.[44]

Combining an abstinence-based, educational, and self-help model of chemical dependence treatment with appropriate adjunctive psychotherapeutic and psychopharmacological help in patients with comorbid chemical dependence and anxiety disorders can be effective clinically. If a patient continues to feel anxiety while off BZPs, addressing nutritional and lifestyle issues (i.e., abstinence from caffeine and nicotine, good sleep hygiene, regular appropriate exercise), cognitive/behavioral treatment, relaxation training, biofeedback, assertiveness training, support, and education about anxiety may help.

Conservative use of medication in chemically dependent patients is indicated because medication increases one's reliance on an external, rather than internal, locus of control. However, it is recognized that the symptoms of panic and anxiety can be debilitating and medication is often needed. Alternatives to the BZPs include buspirone and tricyclic antidepressants for generalized anxiety disorder; specific serotonin reuptake inhibitors, tricyclic antidepressants, and monoamine oxidate inhibitors are alternatives for panic disorder and agoraphobia.

Rarely should BZPs be used if a patient has a history of chemical dependence. In certain circumstances, other treatments are ineffective or not tolerated and the consequences of not treating are profound for a patient. If one considers using BZPs in such a case, a second opinion by a psychiatrist with expertise in addictions is warranted. If BZPs are used, clear documentation of rationale, close monitoring by a physician to observe for signs of deterioration or relapse, and short-term intermittent use are advised.

BZPs are unique in that they are the only addicting drugs used routinely in medical practice. They can be effective medication, but close monitoring by a physician is necessary and the possible complications of physical dependence, adverse effects, and addiction need to be weighed and respected.

REFERENCES

1. Weintraub M, Singh S, Byrne L, et al: Consequences of the New York state triplicate benzodiazepine prescription regulation. JAMA 266:2392–2397, 1991.
2. Roache JD: Addiction potential of benzodiazepines and non-benzodiazepine anxiolytics. In Stimmel B (ed), Erickson CK, Javors MA, Morgan WW (Guest eds): Addiction Potential of Abused Drugs and Drug Classes. Binghamton, NY, Haworth Press, 1990, pp 103–128.
3. Zolpidem for insomnia. Med Lett Drugs Ther 35:35–36, 1993.
4. Evans S, Funderburk F, Griffiths R: Zolpidem and triazolam in humans: behavioral and subjective effects and abuse liability. J Pharmacol Exp Ther 256:1246–1255, 1990.
5. Cole JO, Chiarello RJ: The benzodiazepines as drugs of abuse. J Psychiatr Res 24:135–144, 1990.
6. Juergens SM, Morse R: Alprazolam dependence in seven patients. Am J Psychiatry 145:625–627, 1988.
7. Busto U, Sellars EM, Naranjo CA, et al: Patterns of benzodiazepine abuse and dependence. Br J Addict 81:87–94, 1986.
8. Balter MB, Manheimer DI, Mellinger GD, Uhlenhuth EH: A cross-national comparison of antianxiety/sedative use. Curr Med Res Opin 8:5–20, 1984.
9. National Household Survey on Drug Abuse: Population Estimate 1992 CDHHS Health Service. Rockville, MD, Substance Abuse and Mental Health Service Administration, Office of Applied Studies, 1993.
10. Cowley DS, Roy Bryne PP, Greenblatt DJ: Benzodiazepines: Pharmacokinetics and pharmakodynamics. In Roy-Byrne PP, Colwey DW (eds): Benzodiazepines in Clinical Practice: Risks and Benefits. Washington, DC, American Psychiatric Association, 1991, pp 21–32.
11. American Psychiatric Association Task Force Report: Benzodiazepine Dependence, Toxicity and Abuse: A Task Force Report of the American Psychiatric Association. Washington, DC, American Psychiatric Association, 1990.
12. American Psychiatric Association: Diagnostic and Statistical Manual of Mental Disorders, 4th ed. Washington, DC, American Psychiatric Association, 1994.
13. Rinaldi RC, Steindler EM, Wilford BB, et al: Clarification and standardization of substance abuse terminology. JAMA 259:555–557, 1988.
14. Ciraulo DA, Sarid-Segal O: Benzodiazepine: Abuse liability. In Roy-Byrne PP, Cowley DS (eds): Benzodiazepines in Clinical Practice: Risks and Benefits. Washington, DC, American Psychiatric Association, 1991, pp 157–174.
15. deWit H, McCracken SM, Uhlenhuth EH, Johansen CE: Diazepam preference in subjects seeking treatment for anxiety. NIDA Res Monogr 76:248–254, 1987.
16. deWit H, Pierri J, Johansen CE: Reinforcing and subjective effects of diazepam in nondrug-abusing volunteers. Pharmacol Biochem Behav 33:205–213, 1991.
17. King DJ: Benzodiazepines, amnesia and sedation: theoretical and clinical issues and controversies. Hum Psychopharmacol 7:79–87, 1992.
18. Kisnad H: Sedative-hypnotics (not including benzodiazepines). In Miller NS (ed): Comprehensive Handbook of Drug and Alcohol Addiction. New York, Marcel Dekker, 1991, pp 477–502.
19. Roy-Byrne PP: Benzodiazepines in Clinical Practice: Risks and Benefits. Washington, DC, American Psychiatric Association, 1991, pp 133–153.
20. Busto U, Sellars EM, Naranjo CA, et al: Withdrawal reactions after long-term therapeutic use of benzodiazepines. N Engl J Med 315:854–859, 1986.
21. Schweizer E, Rickels K, Case G, Greenblatt DJ: Long-term therapeutic use of benzodiazepines: II. Effects of gradual taper. Arch Gen Psychiatry 47:908–915, 1990.
22. Rickels K, Schweizer E, Weiss S, Zavodnick S: Maintenance drug treatment for panic disorder. II. Short- and long-term outcome after drug taper. Arch Gen Psychiatry 50:61–68, 1993.
23. Rickels K, Schweizer E, Case G, Greenblatt DJ: Long-term therapeutic use of benzodiazepines: I. Effects of abrupt discontinuation. Arch Gen Psychiatry 47:899–907, 1990.
24. Pecknold JC, Swinson RP, Kuch K, Lewis CP: Alprazolam in panic disorder and agoraphobia: Results from a multicenter trial: III. Discontinuation effects. Arch Gen Psychiatry 45:429–436, 1988.
25. Wolf B, Griffiths RR: Physical dependence on benzodiazepines: Differences within the class. Drug Alcohol Depend 29:153–156, 1991.
26. Salzman C, Fisher J, Nobel K, et al: Cognitive improvement following benzodiazepine discontinuation in elderly nursing home residents. Int J Ger Psychiatry 7:89–93, 1992.
27. Larson EB, Kukull WA, Buchner D, Reifler BV: Adverse drug reactions associated with global cognitive impairment in elderly persons. Ann Intern Med 107:169–173, 1987.
28. Golombeck S, Moodley P, Lader M: Cognitive impairment in long-term benzodiazepine users. Psychol Med 18:365–374, 1988.
29. van Laar W, Volderts E, van Willigenburg A: Therapeutic effects and effects on actual driving performance in chronically administered buspirone and diazepam in anxious outpatients. J Clin Psychopharmacol 12:86–95, 1992.
30. Ray WA, Fought RL, Decker MD: Psychoactive drugs and the risk of injurious motor vehicle crashes in elderly drivers. Am J Epidemiol 136:873–883, 1992.
31. Ray WA, Griffin MR, Downey W: Benzodiazepines of long and short elimination half-life and the risk of hip fracture. JAMA 262:3303–3307, 1989.
32. Fisch HU, Bakir G, Karlaganis G, et al: Excessive motor impairment two hours after triazolam in the elderly. Eur J Clin Pharmacol 38:229–232, 1990.
33. Rothschild AJ: Disinhibition, amnestic reactions, and other adverse reactions secondary to triazolam: A review of the literature. J Clin Psychiatry 53:69–79. 1992.
34. Marks I, Swinson R, Basoglu M, et al: Alprazolam and exposure alone and combined in panic disorder with agoraphobia. A controlled study in London and Toronto. Br J Psychiatry 162:776–787, 1993.
35. Griffiths RR, Bigelow GE, Liebson I: Differential effects of diazepam and pentobarbital on mood and behavior. Arch Gen Psychiatry 40:865–873, 1983.
36. Allgulander C, Borg S, Vikander B: A 4–6 year follow-up of 50 patients with primary dependence of sedative and hypnotic drugs. Am J Psychiatry 141:1580–1582, 1984.
37. Wolf B, Grohmann R, Biber PM, et al: Benzodiazepine

abuse and dependence in psychiatric inpatients. Pharmacopsychiatry 22:54–60, 1989.

38. Miller NS, Gold MS: Introduction—benzodiazepines: A major problem. J Subst Abuse Treat 8:3–7, 1991.

39. Wysowski DR, Barash D: Adverse behavioral reactions attributed to triazolam in the Food and Drug Administration's spontaneous reporting system. Arch Intern Med 151:2003–2008, 1991.

40. Cowley DS, Dunner DL: Benzodiazepines in anxiety and depression. In Roy-Byrne PP, Cowley DR (eds): Benzodiazepines in Clinical Practice: Risks and Benefits. Washington, DC, American Psychiatric Association, 1991, pp 137–156.

41. Cohen S: Benzodiazepines in psychotic and related conditions. In Roy-Byrne PP, Cowley DS (eds): Benzodiazepines in Clinical Practice: Risks and Benefits. Washington, DC, American Psychiatric Association, 1991, pp 59–71.

42. Pascually R: Benzodiazepines and sleep. In Roy-Byrne PP, Cowley DS (eds): Benzodiazepines in Clinical Practice: Risks and Benefits. Washington, DC, American Psychiatric Association, 1991, pp 37–56.

43. DuPont RL: A practical approach to benzodiazepine discontinuation. J Psychiatr Res 24:81–90, 1990.

44. Ashton H: Protracted withdrawal syndromes from benzodiazepines. J Subst Abuse Treat 8:19–28, 1991.

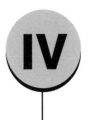

TREATMENT APPROACH

Integration of Addiction and Psychiatric Treatment

Kenneth Minkoff, MD

Previous chapters described the significant prevalence of psychiatric symptoms in the addiction population and substance disorders in people with psychiatric disorders. As it has become increasingly clear that dual diagnosis is an expectation more than an exception, the demand has increased for integrated treatment interventions to address substance disorders and psychopathology simultaneously in any treatment setting.

Despite this growing demand, numerous systemic, philosophical, and clinical barriers have inhibited the emergence of integrated treatment programs.

Systemic Barriers

Addiction and psychiatric services and funding are separated at federal, state, and local levels. Clinicians have commonly been trained in addiction *or* mental health, not both. Comorbid disorders in either setting are often underdiagnosed and undertreated; difficult patients, therefore, may frequently be bounced back and forth between service systems in what Ridgely and colleagues[1] termed "ping-pong therapy." Integrated programming models have been lacking owing to lack of programmatic and fiscal collaboration between agencies at the state and local levels.

Philosophical/Ideological Barriers

Long-standing separation of service systems has resulted in systems that have quite distinct ideologies, clinical philosophies, and treatment methods. These distinct ideologies often appear to be irreconcilable.[2] During the past three decades, for example, the public mental health system has espoused the deinstitutionalization ideology[3, 4] in which programmatic success has often been measured by reductions in hospital census and shifts in levels of care. Case managers attempt to control patients' behavior or to cushion consequences of that behavior, in order to avoid hospitalization. Substance addiction has been regarded as a problem behavior that may precipitate relapse rather than as a distinct disorder requiring specific and intensive treatment. By contrast, the addiction system, during the same time period, has evolved a recovery ideology, emphasizing the need for addicted individuals to ask for as much help as possible in order to attain sobriety and initiate the recovery process. The cornerstone of treatment has been to *encourage* addicted individuals to enter and remain in long-term inpatient treatment programs to promote the initiation of this process (Minnesota model). Simply put, deinstitutionalization ideology encourages patients to use scarce resources only to the extent necessary to remain out of the hospital; recovery ideology encourages patients to be given as much help as they *ask for* in order to promote recovery.

Additional philosophical barriers are associated with intersystem differences in the way treatment is provided and conceptualized. The mental health system has traditionally been organized according to a medical model, in which treatment is based on the results of scientific research, provided by a hierarchically organized team of professionals under the direction of a physician and geared to addressing and ameliorating objective symptoms of biological (or biopsychosocial) illness, often with primary reliance on the use of medication. In contrast, the addiction treatment system, as typified by 12-step programs, has been organized according to a peer-supported "spiritual" recovery model. In this model, treatment is based on the results of collective experience rather than science and is directed by peers rather than professionals. It emphasizes spiritual growth rather than objective, measurable symptom reduction and regards the use of mind-altering medication as antithetic to recovery. Because of these significant differences in philosophy, efforts to develop integrated programs are often diverted by heated battles between addiction and psychiatric staff. Psychiatrists and other mental health professionals may find it difficult to communicate as equals with recovering paraprofessional counselors who direct addiction treatment in many settings. Twelve-step programs have in fact been likened to cults in the psychiatric literature,[5] whereas many addiction settings oppose or do not permit the use of appropriately prescribed psychotropic medication.

Clinical Barriers

As has been noted in prior chapters, individuals with comorbid substance disorders and psychopathology often present a confusing clinical picture that can defy the diagnostic acumen of even the most skilled clinician. Patients with a dual diagnosis can be grouped into at least three major categories:

1. Complicated chemical dependence. Substance-dependent individuals with observable psychopathology that is largely or completely substance induced (e.g., alcoholics who become suicidal while intoxicated and remain depressed and hopeless in early sobriety while facing the reality of what they have lost because of their alcoholism).

2. Substance-abusing mentally ill. Individuals with significant axis I psychiatric disorders who meet DSM-III-R criteria for substance abuse because their use of substances exacerbates symptoms, interferes with medication, or inhibits recovery but does not meet criteria for substance dependence.

3. Substance-dependent mentally ill. Individuals with significant axis I disorders who also have DSM-IV diagnosable substance dependence.

Clinicians who are trained in only one type of disorder often have difficulty distinguishing complicated chemical dependence from the other two categories. Clinicians often struggle to distinguish which type of disorder is primary or secondary, in order to make an appropriate disposition or to determine which disorder is more important to treat. Addiction and mental health clinicians may battle over whether a patient is "really a psych patient" or "really an alcoholic." Programs are rarely available to treat both disorders simultaneously with equal intensity and to accept patients without knowing in advance which type of diagnosis is primary.

In addition to these diagnostic and disposition difficulties, the separate service systems have evolved differences in clinical approach that are difficult to reconcile in integrated programs. These difficulties are often subtle but may result in significant interference with the accessibility and effectiveness of dual-diagnosis services.

CASE MANAGEMENT VERSUS DETACHMENT

The nature of the clinical relationship in the mental health system is the provision of case management and care. Psychiatrically ill patients receive individual service plans that identify a list of problems or deficits that need attention, and treating clinicians and case managers are responsible for providing what the patients need in order to remain stable and not return to the hospital.

By contrast, the nature of the clinical relationship in the addiction system has been defined as empathic detachment. The role of the counselor is to engage empathically with the addicted individual but to detach from assuming responsibility for his or her sobriety. Patients are expected to recognize that they have a problem and then ask for help; the counselor must try to provide what is asked for.

In the mental health system, if a patient does not fare well, the case manager is responsible for changing the treatment plan to make the patient better (i.e., take the patient to Alcoholics Anonymous [AA], find the patient a job); in the addiction system, if a patient does not fare well, the patient is responsible for recognizing the need to ask for additional help (e.g., getting a sponsor, going to more meetings, choosing to enter a halfway house).

In this regard, addiction clinicians may regard mental health clinicians as enablers, doing more of the work of recovery than patients; mental health clinicians, on the other hand, may regard the addiction system as uncaring, because patients may be asked to assume responsibilities they cannot handle and may consequently be allowed to decompensate or become homeless.

SUPPORT VERSUS CONFRONTATION

Relief Versus Pain

Similarly, the mental health system is oriented to providing support to patients to make their lives easier and to provide treatment (often medication) for relief of painful symptoms. In the addiction system, clinicians frequently attempt to find ways to confront patients who are in denial of their addiction and to view suffering as necessary for both the onset and progress of recovery. Addiction is viewed as a disease in which individuals compulsively avoid painful feelings and in which efforts to relieve the painful consequences of the illness without addressing the underlying disease process only serve to continue the progression of the disease.

This dilemma takes many forms. For psychiatrists, one of the more significant conflicts involves the prescription of medication. Patients who report that anxiety or depression is causing them to continue to use alcohol may be given medication by a psychiatrist oriented to providing relief; an addiction clinician might confront patients that no relief is possible until sobriety is attained, recommend admission to a treatment program, and emphasize nonpharmacological means of dealing with painful feelings even after sobriety is attained.

Even when clinicians attempt to integrate these approaches, the intervention may not be performed properly. For example, a psychiatric day program that has struggled for many months to support patients who repeatedly come to the program intoxicated may suddenly confront such patients by discharging them outright from the program; alcoholic schizophrenic patients may be confronted by refusing to give them intravenous fluphenazine unless they stop drinking. Confrontations of this type are often provoked by frustration and lead only to deterioration of patients' clinical status and their relationship with treaters. Conversely, addiction clinicians attempting to support patients with psychiatric disabilities may fail to create appropriate treatment limits or expectations and then feel burned out by their efforts to work with those individuals.

Trends Toward Integration

Although in many locations the extensiveness of the barriers discussed earlier appears to be insurmountable, a number of trends in the past decade are fostering the possibility of service integration.

Systemic. Increased recognition of the prevalence of dual disorders has led to collaborative interagency efforts to promote services integration. In the mid-1980s, the Alcohol, Drug Abuse, and Mental Health Administration (ADAMHA) commissioned a series of reports to identify needs for treatment, training, and research for young adults with serious mental illness and substance disorders.[2, 6] This led to the funding, in 1987, of 13 demonstration programs for integrating treatment systems and methods to enhance services for patients with a dual diagnosis.[7] Since 1987, ADAMHA (incorporating the National Institute of Mental Health, National Institute on Alcoholism and Alcohol Abuse, and National Institute on Drug Abuse), and, since 1993, the Substance Abuse and Mental Health Services Administration (SAMHSA) have continued to prioritize funding of research demonstrations to promote service integration.

Ideological. Since the mid-1980s, there has been a growing recognition in the mental health system of the need for a new ideology[4] and a gradual shift from an emphasis on deinstitutionalization to an emphasis on recovery and consumer empowerment. *Recovery* is defined as a process of inner growth that is associated with increased acceptance of illness, increased ability to make healthy choices about treatment, and increased motivation and hope.[8–10] The concept of recovery from mental illness proceeds in distinct stages, as defined by longitudinal research[8] and by self-report literature.[9] Long-term outcome studies have demonstrated the possibility of more significant symptomatic improvement than was previously supposed.[11] The mental health consumer movement has grown in power in almost every state, demanding a more recovery-focused rehabilitation-oriented, client-centered service system emphasizing consumer choice and responsiveness to consumer requests rather than a more paternalistic case management approach to correcting deficits.[10] At the same time that the mental health system has begun to incorporate recovery concepts, the addiction system has begun to explore the possible need for case management in the treatment of recidivist or homeless substance addicts.

Clinical and Diagnostic. With the advent of DSM-III in 1980, the psychiatric community more clearly recognized the independent status of substance disorders. The DSM-III-R (1987) diagnosis of substance dependence deemphasized withdrawal and tolerance and substituted the concept of addiction based on compulsive behavior as demonstrated by lack of ability to control substance abuse in the presence of clear harmful consequences. This disease concept is more consonant with the disease concept described in the 12-step recovery programs. The latter half of the 1980s has seen an explosion of research on the underlying neurochemistry of the disease of addiction and the emergence of addiction psychiatry as a distinct subspecialty. Both of these trends have supported the idea that substance disorders can be viewed as independent, primary disorders even when they coexist with other psychiatric illnesses.

At the same time, there is growing recognition in the addiction recovery community that individuals with addiction may suffer from other independent psychiatric disorders and may require psychotropic medication. AA literature on the use of medication has supported this view.[12]

Developing a Model for Integrating Psychiatry and Addiction Treatment

As a result of the trends described in the previous section, it has been possible to develop an integrated philosophical approach to the simultaneous treatment of addictive and psychiatric disorders and to use this integrated philosophy as a cornerstone for the design and implementation of integrated treatment interventions, programs, and systems.

Minkoff[13] described an integrated psychiatric and addiction unit in which staff were trained in the application of the disease and recovery model to both addiction and major mental illness. Both substance dependence and major mental illness are viewed as examples of chronic biological mental illnesses, which share common characteristics: chronicity, incurabil-

ity, propensity to relapse, potential for deterioration without treatment, potential for stabilization with regular treatment, and deficit symptoms that must be addressed via long-term rehabilitation. Individuals who suffer from these diseases also share common reactions and resistances that interfere with treatment compliance and therefore become a focus of treatment effort: denial, anger, despair, shame, guilt, failure, and stigma, affecting not only the individual but his or her entire family.

For both types of disorders, according to this model, a process of recovery can be defined, with characteristic phases for each disorder: acute stabilization, engagement, prolonged stabilization/maintenance, rehabilitation/recovery. Individuals with dual disorders must negotiate these phases for each disorder but usually do not do so simultaneously; one illness (usually the mental illness) is commonly stabilized before the process of engagement for the substance disorder begins.

Consequently, the process of engagement itself has received significant attention in the psychiatric literature. Osher and Kofoed[14] divided the engagement phase into engagement, persuasion, and active treatment.

Using concepts derived from the Prochaska model of precontemplation-contemplation, Drake and colleagues[15] expanded the conceptualization of the engagement process. Although these researchers described engagement sequences for substance disorders, these stages of engagement are often applicable to the process of engagement for individuals with serious psychiatric disorders as well.

The value of an integrated treatment philosophy is that it creates a context in which barriers to integration can be addressed to make integrated treatment possible. In this model, both substance disorders and psychiatric disorders are primary when they coexist, and each disorder requires specific and appropriately intensive assessment, diagnosis, and treatment. Assessment of substance disorders in individuals with psychiatric illness requires application of DSM-IV diagnostic criteria just as for individuals without psychiatric illness. Assessment of psychiatric diagnosis in individuals with substance disorders requires similar application of DSM-IV criteria when the substance use is stabilized (usually for a period of 1 to 2 weeks). Secondary comorbid disorders are defined as those disorders whose symptoms resolve when the primary disorder is at baseline (e.g., a patient with bipolar disorder who uses alcohol only when manic or an alcoholic who is suicidal only when drunk).

Because the two disorders are primary, treatment mainly involves simultaneous application of treatment interventions for each disorder, with appropriate modification for the nature of the treatment setting and accompanying disability. Thus, 12-step interventions for addiction and psychopharmacological interventions for mental illness are regarded as collaborative, not competitive or inconsistent. In addition, addiction treatment for individuals with psychiatric disability usually needs to be *more* intensive not less intensive, because it is more difficult for psychiatrically impaired individuals to acquire and use sobriety skills. However, although the content may be the same, the format must be modified to accommodate for disability.

Similarly, this model permits an integrated treatment relationship. Because both mental illnesses and addiction have associated disabilities, case management and care for individuals with either disorder are needed; because both illnesses require active participation by the patient in a program of recovery, patients (consumers) must be empowered to make choices about their participation in treatment, even when those choices may not be good ones. Every individual must be approached with an appropriately individualized mixture of case management and empathic detachment about each disease. Given that recovery for both illnesses is a shared goal, philosophical battles about the best approach can be redefined as clinical discussions about the best approach for a particular individual, based on an individualized assessment of diagnosis, phase of recovery, and levels of acuity, severity, disability, and motivation for treatment associated with each disease.[16]

DEVELOPMENT OF AN INTEGRATED CARE SYSTEM

Because patients with a dual diagnosis are presenting with increasing frequency throughout both the addiction system and the mental health system, attempts to achieve services integration by developing individual dual-diagnosis programs are unlikely to adequately address the magnitude of the problem. Rather, principles of integration must be applied throughout both service systems so that a truly integrated system of care can evolve. Minkoff[16] applied the integrated disease and recovery model described in the previous section to the development of a conceptual framework for describing such an integrated care system. This framework is built on two key concepts: individualized treatment matching and programmatic specificity.

The need for individualized treatment matching derives from the fact that patients with a dual diagnosis are variable in their clinical presentations and treatment needs, both cross-sectionally and longitudinally. Going beyond the three major categories described earlier in this chapter (complicated chemical dependence, substance-addicted mentally ill, substance-dependent mentally ill), patients with a dual diagnosis can be further categorized for treatment-planning purposes—using the integrated disease and recovery model—based on diagnosis, phase of recovery, and level of acuity, severity, disability, and motivation for treatment associated with each disease.

To develop a comprehensive integrated care system, therefore, it is necessary to ensure that integrated treatment resources are available to serve dual-diagnosis patients of any type. Rather than developing a completely new set of programs, however, a more economical approach would be to enhance the capacity of existing programs to serve specific dual-diagnosis populations and then develop a smaller number of sophisticated integrated programs to serve the patients who are most difficult or complex.

Thus, in this model, the development of a comprehensive dual-diagnosis care system involves assigning a program-specific role in the total care system to each existing program and then identifying unique integrated program models at each phase of treatment or recovery to address the needs of patients who would otherwise fall through the cracks. The array of programs in this care system is illustrated in Table 19–1. The following discussion provides an overview of the elements of this care system, followed by a description of individual integrated program models that have already been developed.

ADDICTION SYSTEM

In the addiction system model, existing addiction treatment programs, whether providing acute stabilization (detoxification), rehabilitation, or ongoing recovery support, can be enhanced through staff training and education and through the provision of psychiatric consultation to make generic addiction treatment services available to individuals with most nonpsychotic mood and anxiety disorders, posttraumatic stress disorders, and personality disorders, as well as more severe mental illnesses that are well stabilized on nonaddictive

Table 19–1. MENTALLY ILL SUBSTANCE ABUSERS AND ADDICTION SYSTEM OF CARE

Phases of Recovery	Integrated Case Management Teams			
	Addiction System	Integrated Programs	Mental Health System	
Acute stabilization	**Detoxification** Addiction and personality disorder Addiction with anxiety, depression, or stable mental illness Mental health evaluation included	**Specialized Detoxification** Detoxification for patients on complex medications who are stabilized Detoxification for patients who are suicidal or threatening when intoxicated	**Acute Psychiatric Unit** Acute mental illness and detoxification if needed Substance evaluation and education included	
Engagement and active treatment	**Short-Term Inpatient Rehabilitation** Addiction Addiction and personality disorder Addiction and PTSD Addiction and depression, anxiety Addiction and stable mental illness Mental health education included	**Short-Term** Inpatient and/or integrated day treatment Dual-diagnosis program Psychiatric illness ⟷ addiction Diagnostic dilemmas Addiction and unstable mental illness Addiction and PTSD	**Long-Term Day Therapy** Chronic mental illness Severe personality disorder Severe PTSD Severe dissociative disorder Substance abuse education and support for all patients **Outpatient/Day Treatment Engagement and Treatment** Groups for addictions/ substance abuse	**Long-Term State Hospital** Severe chronic mental illness Substance education Support education Support for all patients Addiction rehabilitation program for chronic patients too sick for standard rehabilitation
Ongoing support and relapse prevention *Residential*	**Addiction Halfway Houses and Sober Houses** Addiction and personality disorder Severe addiction Addiction and depression, anxiety Addiction with stable mental illness; capable of independent living Mandated sobriety	**Residential** Dual-diagnosis residence Support for both mental illness and addiction Expectation of sobriety, with some flexibility	**Psychiatric Residences (wet, damp, or dry)** Chronic mental illness and can't live independently Substance abuse sobriety policies and education included, may or may not be required Engagement—focused	
Ambulatory	**For Addiction Support** 12-step programs and addiction clinics All addicted except unstable psychiatric illness	**Outpatient** Double-trouble 12-step programs	**Dual-Diagnosis Treatment Groups** Outpatient dual-diagnosis relapse prevention groups in mental health clinics and day programs	

PTSD = posttraumatic stress disorder.

medication without severe associated disability. Also necessary is for each program to develop the capacity to assess patients to identify which patients can be treated in those settings and which must be referred to more psychiatrically sophisticated settings.

MENTAL HEALTH SYSTEM

Similarly, existing programs in the mental health system can be enhanced through appropriate training and consultation to provide initial substance disorder assessment, stabilization, engagement programming, and referral services to patients who are presenting for psychiatric treatment and who may have coexisting substance problems. In addition, substance use education and assessment interventions can be incorporated into generic programming for all patients.

Programs that provide long-term care or rehabilitation services to individuals with severe psychiatric disabilities (whether in public hospitals, day programs, or residential settings) may need to develop active addiction treatment modules specific for their patients, because patients with severe disabilities usually cannot be accommodated in addiction settings. These modules may take the form of a time-limited (6 to 12 weeks) day program with a full schedule of didactics and discussion groups and skill training sessions focusing on attaining and maintaining sobriety, followed by an extended aftercare relapse-prevention group component. Patients suffering relapse could repeat the modular program at intervals.

INTEGRATED PROGRAM MODELS

Programs that provide particular capacity to offer integrated services are available for each phase of recovery in the comprehensive service system and are beginning to be described and studied in the treatment literature.

INTEGRATED CASE MANAGEMENT AND OUTREACH

The longitudinal course of many patients with a dual diagnosis is characterized *not* by continuous involvement with a single integrated dual-diagnosis program but by multiple treatment episodes in multiple settings, often with little continuity or connection. Patients with a dual diagnosis are more likely to be persistently or intermittently homeless or to have other types of housing instability[17, 18] and are more likely to be treatment noncompliant,[19] criminally involved,[20] and behaviorally disruptive.[21] Thus, although patients may at times receive *integrated* dual-diagnosis treatment, they are often more likely to receive *parallel* treatment (treating both disorders simultaneously in different settings) or *sequential* treatment (treating each disorder serially in different settings). In order to enhance both the engagement of clients and the continuity of care through multiple treatment episodes in both care systems, integrated case management/outreach programs have been developed. One such model is the continuous treat-

ment team program developed in New Hampshire,[22] in which cross-trained multidisciplinary staff, including at least one addiction specialist and a psychiatrist, provide outreach, case coordination, and direct treatment to the most difficult-to-engage patients with a dual diagnosis. Related program models have received federal grant funding for demonstration projects, specifically with homeless populations, and involve direct provision of outreach and treatment services on the streets, in shelters, and in transitional housing.[23–25] Although most residential programs have attempted to limit substance use, efforts have been made to engage homeless patients with a dual diagnosis by providing integrated case management and outreach in "wet" residences, where active substance use is permitted (though not encouraged).[26] In general, data from these demonstration projects indicate that continuity of integrated case management is associated with improved outcome over time.

INTEGRATED ACUTE STABILIZATION

Willens and colleagues[27, 28] described a dual-diagnosis detoxification program funded jointly by addiction and mental health treatment funds to provide enhanced psychiatric support to treat patients who require detoxification and do *not* require hospitalization but whose level of acute or chronic psychopathology prohibits treatment in a standard detoxification program.

INTEGRATED ENGAGEMENT

In addition to the outreach engagement programs described earlier, models have been proposed for engagement and active treatment of substance addicts in traditional psychiatric settings.[29, 30] Sciacca[31] described a group process for mobilizing clients in any psychiatric setting from complete denial through incremental stages of treatment readiness until the clients make a commitment to abstinence and can determine whether specific addiction treatment interventions are necessary to attain sobriety.

INTEGRATED ADDICTION AND PSYCHIATRIC TREATMENT

Minkoff[13] described an integrated psychiatric and addiction unit, which now also incorporates integrated day hospital and crisis residential program components. In this model, the unit provides a full addiction program *and* a full psychiatric program, and the unit treats exclusively addiction and exclusively psychiatric patients as well as patients with a dual diagnosis; all staff are therefore cross-trained. Patients with dual diagnoses receive stabilization and assessment for both disorders simultaneously by a cross-trained clinical team. Patients are then placed in a combined or mixed program for addiction or psychiatric engagement or treatment, depending on individual needs. Patients may be moved from one program to the other as their clinical status and willingness to participate change, but they keep the same clinical team throughout.

DUAL-RECOVERY ANONYMOUS

The growth in acceptance of both the reality of dual diagnosis and the need for prescribed medication in many individuals participating in 12-step recovery programs has resulted in the emergence of various dual-recovery or "double-trouble" meetings and programs.[32] The *Dual Recovery Book*[33] is essentially the equivalent of a "Big Book" for individuals with dual disorders, providing not only an assortment of case studies but also a framework for how dual recovery works and how to organize dual-recovery 12-step meetings. Incorporation of dual-recovery meetings (or equivalent) into a program of generic 12-step meetings can provide individuals with a dual diagnosis with a comfortable forum to discuss psychiatric medication, symptoms, disability, and stigma in a recovery context.

Conclusion

In conclusion, although the barriers to integration described at the beginning of this chapter are still present in many if not most settings, substantial progress in the integration of psychiatric and addiction treatment is being made. Advances have been made in both the conceptualization of integrated philosophies and systems and in the development of innovative integrated program models. As these program models are further studied and refined, our capacity to provide a comprehensive integrated addiction and mental healthcare system will continue to expand and develop.

REFERENCES

1. Ridgely MS, Goldman HH, Willenbring M: Barriers to the care of persons with dual diagnosis: Organizational and financing issues. Schizophr Bull 16:123–132, 1990.
2. Ridgely MS, Goldman HH, Talbott JA: Chronic Mentally Ill Young Adults with Substance Abuse Problems: Treatment and Training Issues. Rockville, MD, Alcohol, Drug Abuse, and Mental Health Administration, 1986.
3. Bachrach LL: The context of care for the chronic mental patient with substance abuse. Psychiatr Q 58:3–14, 1987.
4. Minkoff K: Beyond deinstitutionalization: A new ideology for the postinstitutional era. Hosp Community Psychiatry 38:945–950, 1987.
5. Galanter M: Cults and zealous self-help movements: A psychiatric perspective. Am J Psychiatry 147:543–551, 1990.
6. Ridgely MS, Osher FC, Talbott JA: Chronic Mentally Ill Young Adults with Substance Abuse Problems: Treatment and Training Issues. Baltimore, University of Maryland School of Medicine, 1987.
7. Teague GB, Schwab B, Drake RE: Evaluation of Services for Young Adults with Severe Mental Illness and Substance Use Disorders. Arlington, VA, National Association of State Mental Health Program Directors, 1990.
8. Strauss JS, Harding CM, Hafez H, et al: The role of the patient in recovery from psychosis. In Strauss JS, Boker W, Brenner HD (eds): Psychosocial Treatment of Schizophrenia. Toronto, Canada, Huber, 1987.
9. Deegan P: Recovery, the lived experience of rehabilitation. Psychosoc Rehab J 11:11–19, 1988.
10. Anthony W: Recovery from mental illness: The new vision of services researchers. Innovations and Research 1:1, 13–14, 1991.
11. Harding CM, Brooks GW, Ashikaga T, et al: The Vermont longitudinal study of persons with severe mental illness, II: Long-term outcome of subjects who retrospectively met DSM-III criteria for schizophrenia. Am J Psychiatry 144:727–735, 1987.
12. Alcoholics Anonymous: Living Sober. New York, Alcoholics Anonymous World Services, 1961.
13. Minkoff K: An integrated treatment model for dual diagnosis of psychosis and addiction. Hosp Community Psychiatry 40:1031–1036, 1989.
14. Osher FC, Kofoed L: Treatment of patients with psychiatric and psychoactive substance abuse disorders. Hosp Community Psychiatry 40:1025–1030, 1989.
15. McHugo GJ, Drake RE, Burton HL, Ackerson TH: A scale for assessing the stage of substance abuse treatment in persons with severe mental illness. J Nerv Ment Dis 183:723–728, 1995.
16. Minkoff K: Program components of a comprehensive integrated care system for seriously mentally ill patients with substance disorders. In Minkoff K, Drake RE (eds): Dual Diagnosis of Major Mental Illness and Substance Disorder. San Francisco, Jossey-Bass, 1991.
18. Drake RE, McLaughlin P, Pepper B, et al: Dual diagnosis of major mental illness and substance disorder. An overview. In Minkoff K, Drake RE (eds): Dual Diagnosis of Major Mental Illness and Substance Disorder. Minkoff K, San Francisco, Jossey-Bass, 1991.
19. Drake RE, Wallach MA: Substance abuse among the chronically mentally ill. Hosp Community Psychiatry 40:1041–1046, 1989.
20. Schutt RK, Garrett GR: Social background, residential experience, and health problems of the homeless. Psychosocial Rehabilitation Journal 12:67–70, 1988.
21. McCarrick AK: Manderscheid RW, Bertolucci DE: Correlates of acting-out behaviors among young adult chronic patients. Hosp Community Psychiatry 44:259–261, 1985.
22. Drake RE, Antosca LM, Noordsy DL, et al: New Hampshire's specialized services for the dually diagnosed. In Minkoff K, Drake RE (eds): Dual Diagnosis

of Major Mental Illness and Substance Disorder. San Francisco, Jossey-Bass, 1991.

23. Dexter RA: Treating homeless and mentally ill substance abusers in Alaska. Alcohol Treat Q 7:25–30, 1990.

24. Kline J, Harris M, Bebout RR, et al: Contrasting integrated and linkage models of treatment for homeless, dually diagnosed. In Minkoff K, Drake RE (eds): An Overview in Dual Diagnosis of Major Mental Illness and Substance Disorder. San Francisco, Jossey-Bass, 1990.

25. Hannigan T, White A: Housing hard-to-place mentally ill women—350 Lafayette Transitional Living Community. Status report of Programs of Columbia University Services. New York, Columbia University, 1990.

26. Blankertz L, White KK: Implementation of rehabilitation program for dually diagnosed homeless. Alcohol Treat Q 7:149–164, 1990.

27. Wilens TE, O'Keefe J, O'Connell JJ, et al: A dual diagnosis detoxification unit, I: Organization and structure. Am J Addict 2:91–98, 1993.

28. Wilens TE, O'Keefe J, O'Connell JJ, et al: A public dual diagnosis detoxification unit: II: Observation of 70 dually diagnosed patients. Am J Addict 2:181–192, 1993.

29. Kofoed L, Kania J, Walsh T, et al: Outpatient treatment of patients with substance abuse and coexisting psychiatric disorders. Am J Psychiatry 143:867–872, 1986.

30. Carey K: Substance use reduction in the context of outpatient psychiatric treatment. Community Mental Health J, in press.

31. Sciacca K: An integrated treatment approach for severely mentally ill individuals with substance disorders. In Minkoff J, Drake RE (eds). Dual Diagnosis of Major Mental Illness and Substance Disorder. San Francisco, Jossey-Bass, 1991.

32. Bricker M: The Evolution of Mutual Help Groups for Dual Recovery. TIE Lines [The Information Exchange], New York, 1994.

33. The Dual Disorders Recovery Book. Center City, MN, Hazelden Educational Materials, 1993.

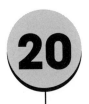

20

Implementing a Dual-Diagnosis Program and Treatment Outcome

Zack Zdenek Cernovsky, PhD, CPsych •
Maureen Pennington, MD, FRCP

Substance use in persons with psychiatric disorders exacerbates psychopathology and complicates the medical treatment of the associated mental illness.[1-5] Complications associated with substance use range from poor cooperation or compliance with pharmacotherapy or other therapies to, in some cases, an increased risk of tardive dyskinesia. For example, Dixon and colleagues,[6] in a study of a sample of 75 hospitalized schizophrenics, found that substance users had significantly higher tardive dyskinesia scores than nonusers.

Several investigators estimate the proportions of substance use within the psychiatric population to be as high as 40% to 80%.[1-4] Many factors may influence these rates, such as the availability and price of various addictive substances, the location of various halfway houses, and outpatient or day treatment clinics for the deinstitutionalized patient population. Patients with a severe psychiatric illness are frequently placed into semisupervised or unsupervised halfway housing or are required to attend day treatment or outpatient activities in mental health centers located within the inner city, at sites where illegal drugs or alcohol are readily available and where these patients are exposed to unfavorable peer pressure and maladaptive behavioral models.

Contemporary problems involved in treatments for patients with a dual diagnosis were discussed by Ries.[7] Ries described the majority of existing treatment facilities as adopting either a serial or a parallel treatment model. In the serial model, patients with a dual diagnosis are first treated only for one of two psychiatric disorders at a time. For example, a schizophrenic patient is stabilized mentally on a psychiatric ward and then referred to an addiction program. The parallel model involves concurrent but separate treatments—for example, the patient is housed on a psychiatric unit but attends a day program at an addiction unit either within the same institution or at a different but nearby institution.

Although these alternatives may be well suited for some subgroups of patients, they present serious disadvantages. Personal values and beliefs held by staff of addiction treatment units and staff of other psychiatric wards may be dramatically dissonant, with potentially negative repercussions on treatment outcomes. For example, a general psychiatric staff might counsel an alcoholic schizophrenic patient to continue taking antipsychotic medication and to drink only in moderation. Their approach might be based on the assumption that long-term effects of alcohol use on schizophrenics are the same as on the moderate social drinkers without mental illness. An addiction treatment unit staff is often likely to insist on complete abstinence from any psychoactive substances and, perhaps, rigidly insist on regular attendance at meetings of Alcoholics Anonymous (AA). Any drug, including prescribed antidepressant or antipsychotic medications, might be considered by some AA members as a hindrance to recovery from substance dependence rather than a help. Psychiatric symptoms per se might be incorrectly interpreted as signs of secretive ongoing alcohol or drug intake.

Many patients never stabilize sufficiently from either a chemical dependence or a major psychiatric disorder to participate fully in a serial or parallel treatment model. Ries[7] proposed a vision of integrated models that would concurrently apply the expertise from both treatment specialties and simultaneously address both disorders.

In our experience, the treatment of addicts with a concurrent major psychiatric illness cannot be successful unless carried out by staff with expertise in both addictions and general psychiatry. This becomes obvious within each of the four consecutive stages of treatment, as outlined in the following paragraphs.

Diagnostic Reevaluation

DIAGNOSIS

A thorough diagnostic reexamination is needed within the first days of a patient's stay on the ward. Detailed individual interviews and outside reports help to establish whether psychotic symptoms preceded substance use or have ever been present during years (or months) of complete abstinence from addictive chemicals. Occasionally, on the basis of new data, those diagnosed as suffering from schizophrenia are more appropriately reclassified as suffering from a substance-induced psychosis. Alternatively, patients who were diagnosed as chemically dependent and referred for addiction treatment only, with a note that they have been "treatment resistant," despondent, reclusive, socially isolated, or lacking in basic social skills, might be found, in a detailed psychodiagnostic examination, to suffer from a concurrent psychiatric disorder such as depression, panic disorder, adjustment reaction, or, occasionally, untreated schizophrenia.

Individual interviews for the purpose of differential diagnosis and reevaluation, social history interviews by addiction unit staff, and

personality assessments by clinical psychologists all help gradually to develop a trusting personal relationship between patients and the treatment team. A therapeutic ward atmosphere is fostered, and it in turn can rekindle a chronic patient's hope of gaining long-term control over both addictive behaviors and other problematic psychiatric symptoms.

MEDICATION

Medication as prescribed to patients elsewhere frequently needs reassessment. A previous prescription might have been given on the basis of an acute symptomatic presentation involving intensive substance intake. Symptoms may change considerably once a patient is fully detoxified.

The goal is to support patients pharmacologically to attain optimal functioning during their stay in an addiction treatment program and during the subsequent postdischarge period. Medications must be periodically reviewed and, if appropriate, dosages readjusted. Ongoing monitoring of patients' behavior by experienced psychiatric staff is essential.

TREATMENT GOALS AS SEEN BY THE PATIENTS

Diagnostic reevaluation involves eliciting patients' account of their specific expectations on the treatment process, goals, and outcomes. Therapeutic trust and alliance cannot develop unless patients feel that their viewpoints and opinions are heard and respected. Patients' cooperation is more adequate and extensive if they see the process as being oriented toward their own goals. Although an individual patient's initial goals may be considered inappropriate or maladaptive by staff, peer pressure from fellow patients and structured therapeutic group activities provide numerous opportunities for reconsideration of the recovery plan.

Schizophrenics with predominantly negative symptoms as well as some other dually diagnosed patients may display extremely passive attitudes and may be reluctant to formulate their own treatment goals or expectations unless amply provided with exhortations, repeated directions, and structured support from staff. Much encouragement, patience, and prompting may be needed. Some feel confused, uncomfortable, or embarrassed when asked about private personal goals. While providing encouragement and emotional support, it is also important to avoid pressuring patients. A deadlock can often be resolved by suggesting to patients that their particular goal, at this time, may be "to clarify personal goals" in life in a preliminary manner only and that the treatment program is designed to help with this problem.

LABORATORY TESTS

In general, the staff's contacts with patients in the first days on the ward should focus on assessment rather than treatment and should be primarily of a supportive and nurturant nature, emphasizing positive feedback to patients. Although this may be arduous, it is almost always helpful to identify and emphasize positive aspects of a patient's situation. This is particularly true of the feedback given about the results of laboratory (urine and serology samples) and psychological tests. Human immunodeficiency virus (HIV) seropositivity, hepatitis, and diabetes are not uncommonly diagnosed in the chemically dependent psychiatric population. For some, this information is dramatically upsetting and emotionally difficult to cope with. It reassures patients to be praised repeatedly for constructively participating in addiction treatment, for facing serious physical illness sober and free of addictive drugs, and for enhancing physical health and long-term outcome by actively participating in a personal recovery process.

PSYCHOLOGICAL TESTING

Interpretations of profiles on standard psychological tests, as described in various handbooks of clinical test instruments, have traditionally focused on the pathological, negative, and socially undesirable aspects of a patient's personality. The findings were rarely or only reluctantly and with misgivings communicated to patients. A few authors of these interpretational handbooks have noted that such feedback, given directly to patients, is often morally condemning, emotionally devastating, and perhaps detrimental to recovery efforts.

A laudable exception to this trend is the interpretative guide for the Minnesota Multiphasic Personality Inventory (MMPI) provided by Kunce and Anderson.[8] These authors have developed balanced hypotheses about potentially positive aspects of elevated MMPI scales. Within their system, particular personality traits can be interpreted as having both negative and positive potential (as stumbling stones that can be transformed into stepping stones), depending on life choices. Statistical support for some of their hypotheses comes from Cernovsky's[9] MMPI study of long-term outcomes in treated addicts.

It is at least as important to emphasize patients' areas of strength as to warn them about potential weaknesses and problems. Most of our dually diagnosed patients have previously been tested in various institutions by clinical psychologists; however, only a very few of them have ever received professional, helpful feedback about their test profiles (i.e., about their personality structure).

Although primarily developed for the MMPI, some of the approaches proposed by Kunce and Anderson may be equally applicable to other standard tests currently used in addiction settings, such as the Millon Clinical Multiaxial Inventory. Research in this area should be given a great priority, especially with a patient population that tends to view their illnesses as hopeless. Extensive, constructive, and positive feedback promotes trust in staff expertise and benevolence and strengthens patients' faith that their own constructive attitudes may lead to some measure of personal satisfaction and success in life.

SOCIAL HISTORY

Even the most reclusive patients usually appreciate the opportunity to review their life story in the presence of a warm, supportive, nurturant, and encouraging staff member. It may be the case that emphasis should be placed less on securing an accurate personal history than on determining which areas are currently emotionally important to a patient and which areas are too painful to approach directly. To a trained observer, this is often more obvious from subtle changes in nonverbal behavior than from words.

Dually diagnosed patients may occasionally provide us with fantasies in lieu of factual information. For example, an extensively educated but addicted artist suffering from a concurrent major mental illness discussed in length a satanic ritual sexual abuse experience he supposedly underwent as a child. He produced numerous drawings to document his experiences. We were unable to corroborate or disprove the history because he could not provide names of persons who could confirm his alleged ritual victimization experiences.

Two other patients repeatedly referred to their military experience with the U.S. Armed Forces during the wars in Vietnam and Korea, yet both seemed unfamiliar with the most basic military terminology. An ill-timed, premature, and excessively confrontative approach by staff is of limited value, in many of these cases, because it too often is interpreted by patients as an indirect rejection or personal degradation by staff. Allowing patients, in the initial stages of treatment, to verbalize their stories or fantasies comfortably may provide indirect but valuable psychological information about their personal values, ideal self-image, personal obsessions, and perhaps sexual orientation or unresolved sexual issues.

Far from aiming only at producing a written and coherent history, social history-taking sessions serve to demonstrate to the patients the staff's warm and supportive interest in their own review of past events and their personal emotional impact. A safe and relatively nonpunitive opportunity is offered for patients to revise their life goals and tentatively formulate new directions.

Treatment

More than two decades ago, Goldstein[10] called attention to the discrepancy between the prognosis of YAVIS and non-YAVIS patients. The acronym *YAVIS* was suggested by Schofield[11] and refers to the young, attractive, verbal, intelligent, and successful patient who is usually welcome by therapists. These patients tend to be well educated, introspective, cooperative, and verbally skilled and are likely to form a mutually satisfactory therapeutic relationship with staff. In contrast, non-YAVIS patients might be physically ordinary or clearly disadvantaged, reticent, elderly or middle aged, intellectually dull or sluggish, poorly educated, and of low socioeconomic status.

Many therapists are not pleased to accept non-YAVIS clients, and several factors are at the root of their misgivings. The traditional insight-based psychotherapies were not designed for non-YAVIS patients. The success rates of these therapies on similar groups tend to be low. Given their history of failures with traditional treatment approaches, non-YAVIS patients, especially those with concurrent diagnoses of chemical dependence and major psychiatric illness, are frequently labeled as treatment resistant or unsuitable for traditional psychological therapies. They may be deemed unsuitable for traditional addiction treatment programs and lost among the numerous other deinstitutionalized mentally ill but untreated persons.

Although some may be young, verbal, attractive, and intelligent, various other behavioral characteristics of dually diagnosed patients adversely affect their ability to participate in traditional treatments and to develop a harmonious and trusting relationship with staff. These frustrating behavioral characteristics include those discussed next.

LIMITED COOPERATION

A patient's illness as well as personal values and beliefs might obstruct or prevent collaborative work. For example, schizophrenic patients with extensive negative symptoms might declare that they are "too sick to have a therapy session," or a paranoid patient might vigilantly sit and listen in group therapy sessions without ever uttering a single comment or might limit participation to common social platitudes and cliches. Some dually diagnosed male patients who grew up in urban ghettos may consider cooperation in a therapeutic setting as a threat to their personal independence and role as a male. Some comply in a most superficial and perfunctory manner that is detrimental to treatment success.

LIMITED INSIGHT

Poor insight is one of the most common symptoms of major mental illness. Therefore, insight-oriented therapies or insight-based psychoeducational interventions tend to have a very limited value for those suffering from chronic psychotic illnesses. Unlike in other chemically dependent populations, changes within a patient's system of values, beliefs, or cognitive schemata of his or her social environment do not predictably result in personal recovery from addictive behaviors.

SOCIAL WITHDRAWAL

The reclusiveness of some schizophrenic patients, their direct or indirect avoidance of emotional intimacy, and their tendency to evade social confrontation or interaction may be deeply frustrating to therapists who strive to engage them emotionally with warm and nurturant support. By its very nature, social withdrawal also obstructs group therapies that focus on self-disclosure and depend on the spontaneous emotional support and active participation of group members.

ACUTE PSYCHOPATHOLOGY IN TRANSIENT DECOMPENSATIONS

It is possible for some dually diagnosed patients to decompensate temporarily when exposed to the stresses of individual or group therapy sessions during addiction treatment. In such cases, it is recommended that treatment be interrupted to allow the patient to restabilize, either with medication or, if necessary, also by transfer to a ward specialized in handling acutely ill psychotic patients.

NEW TREATMENT APPROACHES

Traditional insight-oriented or confrontational approaches to addiction treatment (e.g., those based on a combination of transactional analysis, educational videos, and relaxation training) are not suited to be the exclusive treatment modus for those dually diagnosed patients who suffer from a major and chronic psychiatric illness. Neither are insight-based treatments that target problems other than chemical dependence appropriate for this population. As already mentioned, this issue led Goldstein[10] to call for developing and implementing new therapies specifically designed to be effective with non-YAVIS patients. Some of these new approaches are suitable for the dually diagnosed clientele. Liberman and colleagues[12] eloquently and in much detail described an approach tailored specifically for chronic psychiatric populations. Although their approach was not originally designed for addiction treatment of dually diagnosed patients, its components are sufficiently flexible to allow relevant modifications.

Liberman and associates' approach is suitable for small groups of patients. It emphasizes repeated rehearsal of a wide variety of constructive behavioral patterns. Techniques include role playing, positive feedback, and gradual approximations toward more ideal behavior. Training sessions coach patients to select appropriate partners for social interactions, to pay close attention to various verbal and nonverbal cues in the behavior of their conversation partners, to use appropriately nonverbal behaviors, to provide positive feedback to others, and to articulate simple requests in socially harmonious ways.

The therapist might include successful patients from past weeks in a group with novice patients to provide constructive peer pressure, to generate positive expectations of treatment outcome, to address indirectly the patients' resistance to treatment, and to provide constructive behavioral models for target behaviors. The therapist has to provide ongoing positive feedback and encouragement in all sessions to compensate for the behavioral monotony and relative inexpressiveness of some chronic patients. The format of the sessions may follow the concise summary provided in Table 20–1. Therapists must have training in and practical experience with psychological theory of behavior modification.

In our particular application of Liberman's model to chemically dependent patients with major psychiatric disorders, behavioral rehearsals focus on acquisition and extensive use of addictive substance refusal skills, on selection of alternative social supports and leisure activities, and on skills involved in building healthy self-esteem. The drug and alcohol refusal skills training, based on behaviorial rehearsals, has elsewhere been shown to be successful with immature population groups such as schoolchildren.[13] Through repeated rehearsals, patients acquire semiautomatic behavioral patterns effective in refusing alcohol or other drugs, deflecting peer pressure, and selecting alternative partners free of alcohol and addictive drugs for social activities.

Patients may be taught, via behavioral modeling and rehearsals, a personalized repertoire of new behaviors to use when under emotional stress, in lieu of alcohol or addictive drugs. These behaviors may include searching for emotional support from appropriate friends or acquaintances, planning leisure activities, practicing self-esteem–building inner speech, and seeking professional help. Various aspects of self-esteem building and of self-reinforcement generally are sketched, in the form of small behaviorial steps, in a self-report inventory developed by Heiby.[14] These steps can serve as a useful basis for behavioral rehearsals in group therapy settings with selected groups of dually diagnosed patients. Thus, patients may be trained to praise and reward themselves for specific personal assets or for socially constructive behaviors such as giving positive feedback to others or staying sober and free of addictive drugs.

Some of the techniques of behavioral rehearsal developed by Liberman's team were specifically designed for resistant patients, including those who are relatively incoherent, distractible, and thought disordered (see details in Liberman and coworkers' book).[12] Particularly supportive, tactful, and nonconfrontative staff with abundant personal patience are needed with some of these procedures.

Discharge Planning

An important component of predischarge activities is evaluation of patients' satisfaction

Table 20-1. STEPS INVOLVED IN TYPICAL TREATMENT SESSIONS IN PATIENTS WITH DUAL DIAGNOSIS

What to Do	How to Do It
Give an introduction to social skills training.	Welcome patients, introduce yourself, and give a brief description of the purpose and methods used in training.
Introduce new patients.	Put new patients at ease by asking whether they would prefer being called by their first or last names.
Solicit orientation from experienced patients, who can explain the skills training to new patients.	Fill in any gaps, if necessary, and select patients who are clear, coherent, and upbeat to give the orientation.
Reward patients for their contribution to the orientation.	Use praise liberally while looking and smiling at patients.
Check homework assignments (if any).	Get the details of the actual performance, determine obstacles and impediments to generalization, and record the results on progress notes.
Help each patient pinpoint a particularly difficult situation or a related interpersonal problem, goal, and scene for this session.	Help patients operationalize their problems by asking "what," "with whom," "where," and "when." Watch for problems such as inappropriate nonverbal cues: face, hands, eyes, posture.
Target the scene and the interpersonal situation for dry-run role playing.	Help the patient select and plan the situation; get details from the patient.
Set up the scene.	Enlist others to act as role players, rearrange furniture, and get props.
Give instructions for the scene.	Coach the patient and role players; clarify short-term and long-term goals of this rehearsal.
Act out the scene as a dry run.	Watch the patient carefully, looking for deficits and assets in verbal and nonverbal performance. Keep the scene brief.
Give positive feedback.	Find something to praise immediately, solicit positive and corrective feedback from other patients, and use a blackboard or an easel to record information.
Assess receiving, processing, and sending skills.	Ask the patient what the other person said and felt, what the patient's short-term and long-term goals were in the situation, what alternatives were available to reach the goal, and which one would help to reach the goal.
Use a model.	Select a model for similarity to the real person. Ask the patient to annotate the skills demonstrated by the model.
Ensure that the patient has assimilated the demonstrated skills.	Ask the patient to report on the model's performance.
Use another model.	Use this option if the real person in the patient's life is unpredictable or would respond with more resistance than the first model.
Give instructions to the patient for the next rehearsal or rerun.	Concentrate on one or two behaviors that need improvement. Ask the patient to pinpoint the behaviors that are to be improved.
Rerun the scene.	Use coaching, with hand signals and whispered prompts, and give immediate praise.
Give summary positive feedback.	Give immediate positive feedback. Also enlist others in praising the patient. Be specific in praising the improved behavior patterns. Use an easel or a blackboard to point out improvement over the earlier performance.
Give real-life assignments.	Make out assignment cards, with clear, very simple instructions. Discuss anticipated obstacles.
Choose another patient for the training and repeat the steps.	Ask for a volunteer first. Select someone if no one volunteers.

Adapted from Liberman RP, Derisi WJ, Mueser KT: Social Skills Training for Psychiatric Patients. New York, Pergamon Press, 1989, pp 82–83.

with various aspects of the treatment program. Many dually diagnosed patients have difficulties articulating their impressions or organizing their ideas on these issues. The existing treatment satisfaction questionnaires (see, for example, Larsen and colleagues' article[15]) help to overcome these obstacles and to quantify patients' responses. The use of these tools also promotes the development of a trust-

ing bond with patients as needed for long-term follow-up, relapse prevention, and successful maintenance of dually diagnosed patients in community settings.

Dually diagnosed patients need to be carefully connected to various community resources. It is important to link these patients to as many viable sources of social support in their community as possible. In cases of particularly vulnerable and ill-equipped patients, readmission for a short stay on a treatment unit may be planned for and scheduled to take place several months after discharge. This valuable preventive measure makes patients feel less abandoned on discharge, gives them confidence in future support, and provides them with an extensive time interval to test newly acquired skills. Patients benefit from an opportunity, during the short term readmission, to reconsider those behaviors that proved ineffective in the community setting and to further enlarge a personal repertoire of strategies for a life free of addiction.

Follow-up and Outcome Evaluation

The least expensive form of deinstitutionalization consists of abandonment of chronic mental patients in the community, usually in the slums of inner cities. Although financially attractive, the approach leads to an unacceptable quality of life, exposure to undesirable peer pressures, and an increased risk of untimely death. Regular postdischarge contact between patients and the treatment facility staff is necessary to support dually diagnosed patients' involvement in socially desirable emotional support systems such as traditional self-help groups, leisure activities, community clubs, adult education classes, and community groups. Although more costly, this ongoing relationship greatly enhances favorable treatment outcomes over years.

The individual long-term outcome of treatment depends on numerous factors, including particular treatment approaches, the personal skills of the therapists involved, the addiction severity, the severity of mental illness, and the quality and availability of social support systems such as AA in the community. One-year follow-up data from an integrated treatment program using a mixed approach (including both insight-oriented and behavior rehearsal techniques) indicated that patients with dual diagnoses had lower rates of complete posttreatment abstinence than addicts free of other psychiatric disorders (9.1% vs. 26.9%). However, the former had higher proportions of partial improvement—that is, of continued but distinctly less frequent substance use (72.7% vs. 59.3%) than did the latter.

When all types of outcomes were combined to obtain average outcome values, dually diagnosed patients did not significantly differ from other substance users; the overall success rate of treatment was comparable.[16] It is possible that dually diagnosed patients exposed to integrated treatment programs find it more difficult than do other chemically dependent persons to avoid alcohol and other addictive drugs completely, perhaps because of psychotic symptoms, unstable moods, or associated intrapsychic problems. However, their overall treatment outcome may be as favorable, on the average, as the outcomes of chemically dependent persons without mental illness.

REFERENCES

1. Galanter M, Castaneda R, Ferman J: Substance abuse among general psychiatric population. Am J Drug Alcohol Abuse 14:211–235, 1988.
2. Kay SR, Kalanthara M, Meinzer AE: Diagnostic and behavioral characteristics of psychiatric patients who abuse substances. Hosp Community Psychiatry 40:1062–1064, 1989.
3. Lehman AF, Myers CP, Corty E: Assessment and classification of patients with psychiatric and substance abuse syndrome. Hosp Community Psychiatry 40:1019–1025, 1989.
4. Miller NS, Ries RK: Drug and alcohol dependence and psychiatric populations: The need for diagnosis, intervention, and training. Compr Psychiatry 32:268–276, 1991.
5. Schuckit M: Clinical implications of primary diagnostic groups among alcoholics. Arch Gen Psychiatry 42:1043–1049, 1985.
6. Dixon L, Weiden PJ, Haas G, Sweeney J: Increased tardive dyskinesia in alcohol abusing schizophrenic patients. Compr Psychiatry 33:121–122, 1992.
7. Ries R: Clinical treatment matching models for dually diagnosed patients. Psychiatr Clin North Am 16(1):167–175, 1993.
8. Kunce JT, Anderson WP: Normalizing the MMPI. J Clin Psychol 32:776–780, 1976.
9. Cernovsky ZZ: Es scale level and correlates of MMPI elevations. J Clin Psychol 40:1502–1509, 1984.
10. Goldstein AP: Psychotherapeutic Attraction. New York, Pergamon Press, 1971.
11. Schofield W: Psychotherapy, The Purchase of Friendship. Englewood Cliffs, NJ, Prentice Hall, 1964.
12. Liberman RP, Derisi WJ, Mueser KT: Social Skills Training for Psychiatric Patients. New York, Pergamon Press, 1989.
13. Jones RT, McDonald DW, Fiore MF, et al: A primary preventive approach to children's drug refusal behavior: The impact of rehearsal-plus. J Pediatr Psychol 15:211–223, 1990.
14. Heiby EM: A self-reinforcement questionnaire. Behav Res Ther 20:397–401, 1982.
15. Larsen DL, Atkinson CC, Hargreaves WA, Nguyen TD: Assessment of client/patient satisfaction. Evaluation and Program Planning 2:197–207, 1979.
16. Cernovsky ZZ, Smith DW, Pennington M: Correlates of long term treatment outcomes in treated addicts with and without dual diagnosis. Data from an unpublished program evaluation report, prepared in 1993 (in press).

Intervention for Drug/ Alcohol Addiction in Acute Psychiatric Presentations

Norman S. Miller, MD

The importance of intervention for acute psychiatric presentations for addictions treatment referrals cannot be overstated. An acute psychiatric illness or symptoms often are a part of the presentation of an addicted patient's first contact with psychiatric professionals. Patients are highly unlikely to become abstinent alone and need continuing treatment. In fact, studies indicate that successful treatment outcome is strongly correlated with the duration of continuing care. The longer that an addict with or without another psychiatric comorbidity participates in a treatment program, the greater the probability of maintaining abstinence and other improved measures of treatment outcome.[1] Addictions treatment programs and case manager programs find improved outcome with continued participation with the treatment services. Continuous abstinence is obtained for 88% of those who attend 12 months of continuing care after inpatient addictions treatment and 93% of those who used an outpatient program. Treatment outcome studies also find significantly reduced medical utilization, enhanced employment performance, and fewer legal complications after discharge from the treatment program.[1]

Emergency room physicians need to keep in mind the possible long-term benefits of treatment for patients with addiction problems and to refer appropriately.

Presentations of Addicted Patients in Acute States

Patients with addiction disorders present to the emergency room with medical, surgical, and psychiatric complications.[2, 3] Addiction-related emergency room visits or hospitalizations may result from infectious causes such as endocarditis, hepatitis, cellulitis, cutaneous abscesses, aspiration pneumonia, and human immunodeficiency virus (HIV) infection. Other presentations include trauma due to motor impairment or violent behavior. Psychiatric drug-induced states include psychosis, depression, withdrawal, or suicidal and homicidal thoughts. This chapter specifically addresses the psychiatric manifestations and assessment, as well as indications for detoxification and treatment of different substances.[4]

Drug-related hospital emergency room cases are sampled longitudinally in the United States in the Drug Abuse Warning Network (DAWN).[5] DAWN is a large-scale drug data collection system that is sponsored by the National Institute on Drug Abuse (NIDA). Morbidity data are obtained from hospital emergency rooms, and mortality data are collected from medical examiners' offices. For all drugs, the highest rates were observed for persons between 18 and 44 years of age. The lowest rates were in the oldest age group, 45 years of age and older.

Although females between the ages of 6 and 29 had higher rates of all drug-related emergencies than their male counterparts, males were more likely than females to experience drug-related emergencies that involved cocaine, heroin/morphine, or marijuana/hashish. Many of the female drug-related emergencies involve drugs such as tranquilizers and sedatives. Cocaine was implicated in the most emergencies per 100,000 population for both sexes and in all four age groupings. Males in the two middle age groupings, 18 to 29 and 30 to 44 years of age, had approximately 90 cocaine-related emergencies per 100,000 men. Women 18 to 29 years of age were more likely than 30- to 44-year-old women to have been affected by cocaine. For 18- to 29-year-old women, there were 59 cocaine-related emergencies per 100,000 women.[5]

For all drug-related emergencies, San Francisco had the greatest proportion of emergencies per 100,000 population (812) in 1990. New Orleans ranked second, with 520, and had the most cocaine-related emergencies, followed by Newark, Philadelphia, and New York. Emergencies that implicated heroin/morphine occurred most frequently in San Francisco, followed by Philadelphia.[5]

The rates for those psychiatric patients with an addiction comorbidity who use psychiatric emergency services exceed 50% to 80% of the total seen.[6, 7] A study of 247 chronically mentally ill patients committed for emergency involuntary hospitalization in a public intensive treatment unit revealed that almost 40% had positive urine toxicology for drugs including alcohol, barbiturates, cannabis, cocaine, methadone, opiates, phencyclidine, and stimulants.[8] Patients with positive results of screens were more likely to live alone or to be homeless, to be committed for making threats, and to have a diagnosis of organic mental disorder or substance use disorder. Patients with negative results of a screen were more likely to live in a supervised setting, to be committed for actions such as assaults and suicidal behavior, and to have a diagnosis of schizophrenia or other psychotic disorder.[8]

The periodicity of presentations of those patients with drug use and addiction was studied in 630 consecutive cases of drug overdose from October 1987 to March 1990.[9] A significant curve was obtained for a 24-hour period, with a peak time of presentation at 6:32 PM. Significant periodic rhythms were noted for cocaine, opiates, alcohol, analgesics, marijuana, and benzodiazepines. Also, a 4.8-hour periodic rhythm was noted for cocaine, marijuana, and alcohol. The most common drug reported was alcohol (n = 232), followed by cocaine (n = 181), opiates (n = 100), analgesic agents (n = 59), phencyclidine (n = 45), marijuana (n = 44), and benzodizepines (n = 41).[9]

Psychiatric Manifestations of Drugs and Alcohol

COCAINE

Cocaine remains a common drug that precipitates use of emergency services and complicates other psychiatric disorders. Cocaine is a central nervous system stimulant that produces identifiable states of intoxication and withdrawal. Although acute intoxication is characterized by hyperactivity, euphoria, and impaired judgment, most patients who arrive for emergency treatment are chronic users. The picture of chronic intoxication is one of pervasive and paniclike anxiety, paranoia (often auditory and visual hallucinations), and intense depression. Chronic cocaine users frequently feel out of control and express desperation, often accompanied by suicidal or homicidal thoughts/intents. As a consequence, violence is a relatively high risk among cocaine addicts.[3, 10, 11]

HALLUCINOGENS

Hallucinogens remain commonly used drugs—particularly among adolescents and young adults. Cannabis is still the second most used drug in the United States and is responsible for various adverse consequences due to its addictive use. These include mood disturbances of anxiety (paniclike), depression, memory loss, and impaired motor coordination and mental judgment. Lysergic acid diethylamide (LSD) continues to be used, and "bad trips" are not uncommon precipitants of emergency services. Adverse consequences of LSD include emotional lability, visual hallucinations, and depersonalization. Other hallucinogens include psilocin, psilocybin, and dimethyltryptamine, the use of which has a clinical presentation similar to LSD effects.[3, 10, 11]

Organic solvents are found throughout the United States and are used fairly frequently by the young. Sources of these drugs are organic solvents found in gasoline, glues, polishes, and aerosols, among others. These drugs can produce psychiatric symptoms that are similar to those described earlier for the other hallucinogens.[3, 10, 11]

Use of these drugs can be dangerous and can induce frightening and paranoid states in users—particularly chronic addicts. The potential for violence, directed at both oneself and others, is high. Emergency services are common sites for those who are under their intoxicating influence. In addition, psychiatric disorders are complicated by their use, and psychiatric disorders must be differentiated from the psychiatric manifestations of these drugs. The combination of psychotic disorders and drug-induced states is also quite common, because schizophrenics use hallucinogens with regularity.[3, 10, 11]

OPIATE NARCOTICS

Narcotics in the form of heroin, meperidine, methadone, oxycodone, and codeine also remain drugs commonly used by those who present to emergency services. Intravenous heroin use remains stable throughout the United States. Patients present with a myriad of psychiatric complications that include panic, anxiety due to withdrawal, and depression due to the sedating effects of narcotics. A common source is physicians who prescribe many of these medications and whom narcotic addicts pursue to obtain these drugs. Intoxication from these drugs is recognized by the altered mental state with cloudy sensorium, memory defects, and passivity.[3, 10, 11]

SEDATIVE-HYPNOTICS

Identification of adverse consequences of these drugs remains underrecognized. Benzodiazepines, particularly, because of chronic use, lead to serious but sometimes subtle complications. These are in actuality sedating drugs, and they induce depressed mood and impaired sensorium (memory loss). Because they produce pharmacological dependence in virtually all who use them for more than a few weeks, they induce rebound anxiety from their chronic use. Paniclike anxiety and apprehension accompany withdrawal states from benzodiazepines, along with various other symptoms. Because benzodiazepines are used as therapeutics, their toxicity is either tolerated or rationalized by the user and physician. However, studies clearly show that chronic use leads to a loss of efficacy and increased toxicity. Physicians in emergency departments are urged to consider benzodiazepines as a source of the presenting psychiatric symptoms.[12, 13]

ALCOHOL

Alcohol remains the drug most commonly used by those who use emergency services. Alcohol addiction presents with many adverse consequences that precipitate crises and use of emergency services. The adverse consequences are from effects of intoxication and withdrawal from alcohol. Acute intoxication interferes with judgment, coordination, mood, memory, and other aspects of mental states.

Emergency room physicians need to be cognizant of inebriated patients' potential for violence. Violence is typically associated with acute intoxication in the form of suicidal or homicidal thoughts or actions and accidents. Studies show that the leading risk factor for completed suicide is alcoholism and that 25% of alcoholics commit suicide.[14] Moreover, alcohol use is implicated in a large percentage of suicides. Other studies show that alcohol use is associated with the majority of homicides and that more than 50% (conservative estimates) of those convicted of homicide are alcoholics.[14]

Alcohol complicates many psychiatric conditions by worsening the clinical presentation. As many as 50% of those with schizophrenia are also alcohol dependent, and 80% of those with antisocial personality disorder are alcohol dependent. Studies conclude that the prognosis and course of these psychiatric disorders are affected by alcohol dependence. Many find that compliance with psychiatric treatments is reduced, recidivism with increased numbers of hospitalizations is greater, and psychopathology with increased depression and psychotic symptoms is more severe.[15]

Chronic alcohol use itself leads to other psychiatric states such as alcoholic hallucinosis, Wernicke's syndrome, and alcoholic dementia. These conditions are sometimes confused with other psychiatric disorders and must be differentiated for purposes of prognosis and treatment.[2, 3]

Assessment and Interventions for Detoxification

ASSESSMENT OF WITHDRAWAL POTENTIAL AND DETOXIFICATION

An assessment of all psychiatric patients in crisis should include urine or blood toxicology testing for drugs and alcohol and a Breathalyzer test for alcohol. The elements of denial, minimization, and rationalization arising in the addictive illness make literal self-report unreliable. Also, asking collateral sources, such as parents, friends, and spouses, about a patient's alcohol and drug use is often useful in determining the nature and extent of alcohol and drug use.[3, 10, 11]

COCAINE

Withdrawal from cocaine is not ordinarily of medical consequence but can be of significant psychiatric consequence because of the anxious and depressive states that are induced by chronic cocaine use. Although vital signs are often normal during withdrawal from pure cocaine use, they still may be elevated because cocaine addicts frequently use alcohol concurrently with cocaine or have used cocaine recently (sympathomimetic hypertension). The clinical examination may reveal pupillary dilatation, fine positional tremor of the upper extremities, agitation, and suspiciousness. Auditory and visual hallucinations may also occur.[3, 10, 11]

Withdrawal from cocaine does not generally require medications, except for symptomatic relief of anxiety and depression. A short course of benzodiazepines may be indicated, because these symptoms are usually short lived. Antidepressants are not indicated for cocaine-induced depression. Supportive psychotherapy may also be indicated.[3, 10, 11]

HALLUCINOGENS

Withdrawal from these drugs does not produce significant alterations in vital signs. Withdrawal is more an expression of the psychiatric effects, which include agitation, terrifying feelings and thoughts, anxiety, depression, agony, desperation, and hopelessness.[3, 10, 11]

Supportive therapy such as reassurance and a protective, low-stimuli environment may be necessary. Pharmacological agents can be used for agitation, such as benzodiazepines (diazepam) or neuroleptics (haloperidol).[3, 10, 11]

OPIATE NARCOTICS

Withdrawal itself can be identified by mild elevations in blood pressure and pulse, yawning, rhinorrhea, lacrimation, piloerection (goose bumps), abdominal cramps and diarrhea, muscle cramps, and joint and bone pain. Unlike withdrawal from alcohol and other sedative-hypnotics, withdrawal from narcotics is medically benign. However, it should be treated because of the relative inability for a narcotic addict to tolerate abrupt withdrawal.[3, 10, 11]

Generally, clonidine can be used for treatment during the period of withdrawal from opiates. However, methadone may be used in certain cases such as in patients who have severe, concurrent medical or psychiatric problems or are being withdrawn from methadone.[3, 10, 11]

SEDATIVE-HYPNOTICS

Withdrawal from benzodiazepines is also significant and must be evaluated in all users. The withdrawal course can be estimated according to the half-life of the drug—that is, peak period of withdrawal is 2 to 3 days for alprazolam and 5 to 6 days for diazepam.[3, 10, 11]

The withdrawal syndrome is characterized by anxiety, depression, tremors, mild tachycardia and hypertension, agitation, seizures, visual hallucinations, and delirium. Typically, not all these manifestations are present in all users, although anxiety and depression are very common.[3, 10, 11]

Longer-acting preparations of benzodiazepines are preferred over short-acting preparations to enhance the smoothness of withdrawal and to level out the peaks and troughs. Diazepam or chlordiazepoxide can be used. Also, phenobarbital may be used as a substitute in those who have a history of withdrawal seizures. Generally, anyone receiving benzodiazepines for longer than a few weeks should be tapered with substitution. A predominance of studies shows that in virtually all users, pharmacological dependence develops within weeks.

ALCOHOL

Assessment and treatment of alcohol withdrawal are essential. A careful history is indicated in anyone who is intoxicated or is in alcohol withdrawal, because the best predictor of future withdrawal is past withdrawal. Vital signs and clinical status are reliable indicators of severity of withdrawal at the time of assessment and for 3 to 4 days during the withdrawal period. Blood pressure and pulse are typically elevated above normal for the individual and sometimes are in the abnormal range. The clinical examination may reveal agitation hypervigilance and coarse tremor of the upper extremities in many cases of significant withdrawal.

Most patients in alcohol withdrawal do not

require medications for withdrawal complications. Clinicians can select those patients who require medications and hospitalization on the basis of history of previous withdrawal, vital signs, and clinical status. If a patient has no previous history of seizures, delirium tremens, or associated medical/psychiatric problems, withdrawal can proceed with only supportive measures. Otherwise, vital signs and clinical state can be observed for 3 to 4 days until resolved.

Suggested medications for alcohol withdrawal include diazepam, lorazepam, chlordiazepoxide, phenobarbital, and clonidine. The medications are chosen on the basis of target symptoms such as withdrawal seizures, elevations in vital signs, and level of agitation.

Interventions

The approach to addicted patients requires skill and knowledge of the nature and prognosis of addictive illnesses. Of primary importance is that addiction be regarded as an independent illness. The causes of addictive illness are not known, but the best available evidence reveals a biological basis for addictive use of drugs and alcohol. A caveat is that alcoholics or drug addicts are more likely to accept recommendations and suggestions if they are told they have an illness rather than a moral problem.[16, 17]

An important perspective to use is that underlying conditions do not cause addictive use of drugs/alcohol and probably do not cause significant use of drugs/alcohol. What generally happens is that addicts rationalize their drug/alcohol use by complaining that they drink because of depression, anxiety, or other reasons. However, studies show that these are frequently consequences of alcohol/drug use and not causes.[15–17]

The cardinal manifestations of drug and alcohol addiction are defense mechanisms—denial, minimization, rationalization, and projection. Addicts mysteriously and, partly unconsciously, deny drug use despite direct evidence such as a positive drug screen or Breathalyzer or a collateral source that confirms alcohol use. Addicts frequently project responsibility for their problems onto someone or something else, such as "a series of misunderstandings and bad breaks."[15–17]

These defense mechanisms are best confronted with evidence of the consequences of the addictive use of drugs and alcohol. The denial can be penetrated with concrete examples. It is best to avoid judgmental attitudes and accusations, which tend only to increase the denial and defensiveness. In addition, addicts are more likely to accept the confrontation if it is coupled with an explanation and offering of treatment for the addiction. In fact, confrontation without the hope of treatment should be avoided. Effective addiction treatment is available and should be offered to addicted patients.[15–17]

Those addicts who also have another psychiatric disorder such as chronic mental illness or affective and anxiety disorders require a careful and thoughtful evaluation. It works best when addictive and other psychiatric disorders are considered as independent of each other but with important interactions affecting each other. A full discussion is beyond the scope of this chapter. However, the following are general principles to be used as guidelines in evaluation of comorbidity.[18, 19] Alcohol and other sedating drugs can cause depression during intoxication, and the same substance may cause anxiety, hallucinations, and delusions during withdrawal. Stimulants and other hallucinogens can cause anxiety, hallucinations, and delusions during intoxication and depression during withdrawal.

Referrals for Drug/Alcohol-Addicted Patients

Patients who present in an addictive crisis are generally referred to one of three treatment settings. Dependent on the patient's presentation and needs, they should be referred for detoxification, for addictions treatment, or to a setting that can address comorbid issues.

DETOXIFICATION

Detoxification can generally be conducted on an outpatient basis. Compliance with treatments and abstinence from drugs and alcohol ultimately determine the level of care needed. If associated medical or psychiatric problems exist, inpatient detoxification may be indicated. Detoxification may be accomplished on a specialized unit devoted to detoxification or on a medical unit.[3, 10, 11]

ADDICTIONS TREATMENT

Clearly, a large number of patients present with psychiatric symptoms due to only drug or alcohol intake. If addictive disorders are considered as independent in producing psychiatric symptoms, unnecessary referrals to psychiatric care are avoided. Importantly, the treatment is specific for addictive disorders. Further evaluations may be conducted for other, concomitant psychiatric disorders. Most programs in the United States approach addictions with a 12-step method of abstinence-based treatment that uses cognitive/behavior techniques during the treatment experience. The 12-step method encourages participation in 12-step recovery groups such as Alcoholics Anonymous (AA) and Narcotic Anonymous (NA) while in treatment and after discharge.[1, 20]

Treatment outcome studies have found that at 1 year after discharge from abstinence-based treatment programs, 50% of the patients have continuous abstinence from alcohol and drugs. The studies have found that it is important for patients to attend continuing care in the treatment program and 12-step programs. One-year abstinence rates of 80% to 90% are achieved when weekly participation in continuing care and AA meetings follows the treatment program after discharge.[1, 20]

TREATING PSYCHIATRIC COMORBIDITY IN ADDICTIVE DISORDERS

Various models have been proposed and are being implemented to treat psychiatric comorbidity. These are termed *dual-focus, serial, parallel,* and *integrated* models. The dual-focus model provides additional tracts for dually focused patients in a specialized psychiatry setting within the addiction milieu. The serial model is the traditional practice of treating the psychiatric comorbidity in a psychiatry setting and then transferring to an addiction setting for treatment of the addictive disorders. A major disadvantage is that chronically mentally ill patients do not fare well in the confrontative and active group participation used in the addiction treatment settings. The parallel model is a newer practice in which patients primarily reside in a psychiatric setting and are sent to an addiction setting for addiction treatment. In the serial and parallel models, the staff and sites are separate and patients must contend with both. The integrated model is an attempt to provide addiction and psychiatric treatments in the same milieu by the same staff. Patients receive a core approach to the treatment of both categories of disorders because the staff are trained in psychiatric and addictive treatments.[21]

The integrated approach is gaining significant popularity in treating those chronically mentally ill patients with an addictive disorder. In this model, patients are assigned a case manager who integrates the total care. Patients are closely monitored longitudinally for compliance and outcome. Psychiatric and addiction services are integrated by the case manager.[22] Referring physicians need to consider the pros and cons of the different comorbid treatment settings when making referrals.

REFERENCES

1. Hoffmann NG, Miller NS: Treatment outcomes for abstinence-based programs. Psychiatr Ann 22(8):402–408, 1992.
2. Hoffman RS: The impact of drug abuse and addiction on society. Emerg Med Clin North Am 8(3):467–481, 1990.
3. Slaby AE, Martin SD: Drug and alcohol emergencies. In Miller NS (ed): Comprehensive Handbook of Drug and Alcohol Addiction. New York, Marcel-Dekker, 1991, pp 1003–1030.
4. Miller NS: Principles of Addiction Medicine. Washington, DC, American Society of Addition Medicine, 1994.
5. Kopstein A: Drug abuse related emergency room episodes in the United States. Br J Addict 87:1071–1075, 1992.
6. Raskin VD, Miller NS: The epidemiology of the comorbidity of psychiatric and addictive disorders: A critical review. J Addict Dis 12(3):45–57, 1993.
7. Elangovan N, Berman S, Meinzer D, et al: Substance abuse in psychiatric patients admitted to the emergency room. Proc West Pharmacol Soc 34:29–30, 1991.
8. Sanguineti VR, Brooks MO: Factors related to emergency commitment of chronic mentally ill patients who are substance abusers. Hosp Community Psychiatry 43(3):237–241, 1992.
9. Raymond RC, Warren M, Morris RW, Leikin JB: Periodicity of presentations of drugs of abuse and overdose in an emergency department. Clin Toxicol 30(2):467–478, 1992.
10. Swart GL, Hargarten SW: Emergency department management of intoxication with drugs of abuse. In Miller NS, Gold MS (eds): Pharmacological Therapies of Drug and Alcohol Addiction. New York, Marcel-Dekker, 1994.
11. Chang G, Kosten TR: Emergency management of acute drug intoxication. In Levinson JH, Ruiz P, Millman RB (eds): Substance Abuse: A Comprehensive Textbook. Baltimore, Williams and Wilkins, 1992, pp 437–444.
12. Rickels K, Schweizer B, Case WG, Greenblatt DT: Long-term therapeutics use of benzodiazeprines. I. Effects of abrupt discontinuation. Arch Gen Psychiatry 47:899–907, 1990.
13. Schweizer B, Rickels K, Case WG, Greenblatt DT: Long-term therapeutic use of benzodiazeprines. II. Effects of gradual discontinuation. Arch Gen Psychiatry 47:908–915, 1990.
14. Miller NS, Mahler JC, Gold MS: Suicide risk associated with drug and alcohol dependence. J Addict Dis 10(3):49–61, 1992.
15. Miller NS, Mahler JC, Gold MS: Psychiatric diagnosis in alcohol and drug dependence. Ann Clin Psychiatry 3(1):79–89, 1991.
16. Miller NS, Gold MS: The psychiatrist's role in integrating pharmacological and nonpharmacological treatment of addictive disorders. Psychiatr Ann 22(8):436–440, 1992.

17. Miller NS, Gold MS: Dependence syndrome of critical analysis of essential features. Psychiatr Ann 2:282–290, 1991.
18. Schuckit MA: The history of psychotic symptoms in alcoholics. J Clin Psychiatry 43:53–57, 1982.
19. Schuckit MA. Alcoholism and other psychiatric disorders. Hosp Community Psychiatry 34:1022–1027, 1983.
20. Miller NS, Millman RB, Keskinen BA: Treatment outcome at six and twelve months for cocaine. Adv Alcohol Subst Abuse 9(3/4):101–120, 1990.
21. Minkoff K: An integrated treatment model for dual diagnosis of psychoaddiction. Hosp Community Psychiatry 40:1041–1045, 1989.
22. Drake RE, Noodsy DL: Case management for people with coexisting severe mental disorder and substance use disorder. Psychiatr Ann 24(8):427–431, 1994.

Engagement and Persuasion

Lial Kofoed, MD, MS

Treatment efforts for patients with substance use disorders have often suffered more from the difficulty of getting patients into treatment than from lack of efficacy of the treatments themselves. A patient's interest in treatment or ability to engage in it is sometimes erroneously viewed by clinicians as a trait, rather than a state, characteristic. This viewpoint leads to a sort of nihilism among clinicians, reflected in such statements as the common consultation result, "The patient is not motivated for treatment at this time" or "The patient was offered, but would not accept, treatment." Although at one level these statements are undoubtedly true, they serve primarily to relieve the treating or consulting clinician of any further sense of responsibility for the patient's treatment rather than to provide useful information about a clinical course of action.

Fortunately, there has been increasing awareness of the need for and the efficacy of therapeutic strategies intended specifically to help patients accept their need for treatment. This chapter first presents an overview of some of the factors that make it difficult for patients to accept needed treatment, including specific focus on the complications produced by the comorbidity of substance use and other psychiatric disorders. Next follows a review of approaches to engagement and persuasion that show promise in helping patients overcome discouragement, denial, and fear and accept appropriate treatment.

Barriers to Treatment Acceptance

DEMORALIZATION

Demoralization is the first significant barrier to acceptance of treatment. Frank, in his superb work *Persuasion and Healing*, suggested that demoralization was a universal experience of all individuals seeking care. Demoralization was seen as a loss of the individual's sense of efficacy and sense of hope and future, and Frank pointed out that all types of healing encounters incorporated methods to combat demoralization.

It is not difficult to imagine how protracted substance addiction could produce demoralization. The profound social and economic losses and personal failures associated with substance use disorders are overwhelming and often are incomprehensible to patients. Their denial complicates demoralization by producing a blind spot to the true cause of difficulty, making it impossible for patients to come to grips with the nature of their problem and their treatment needs.

Demoralization and Psychiatric Comorbidity

Demoralization in patients with a dual diagnosis may be particularly worsened by the psy-

214

chiatric condition. The hopelessness, discouragement, and apathy of major depressive disorders; the disorganization and false attribution of causation of the psychotic paranoid disorders; or the seemingly uncontrollable intrusive affects and memories of posttraumatic stress disorder, when combined with the denial and the social and economic losses produced by both substance addiction and psychiatric disorders, inevitably produce profound demoralization.

DENIAL

The phenomenon of denial is universal in patients with substance use disorders. The development and elaboration of denial are relatively easy to understand. Schuckit[2, 3] provided evidence that a principal mechanism that predisposes individuals to a higher risk of alcoholism is enhanced ability to tolerate alcohol. He found that at a given blood level, adult male children of alcoholics are less impaired psychologically and have less body sway than children of nonalcoholics. Other work suggests that patients with alcoholism experience a more euphoric response from the benzodiazepine alprazolam than patients without alcoholism.[4] Essentially, then, individuals who ultimately develop substance use disorders are likely to be those whose initial experiences of alcohol or drug use are subjectively especially positive.[5]

Furthermore, given the slowly developing nature of these disorders (with, perhaps, the exception of volatile forms of cocaine such as crack), most individuals continue to use their intoxicant(s) of choice for months to years before encountering any significant consequences. (Of particular note is the challenge of nicotine dependence, in which personally experienced and compelling consequences, which are usually medical, may not occur for decades.)

The universal manifestation of denial, then, is a fairly straightforward consequence of the inability of the human organism to easily accept that a negative consequence is really a result of a pleasurable activity in which it has been engaging for months to years with no apparent problems. Expecting the connection between substance use and eventual consequence to be made easily is a lot like expecting to teach a rat to run a maze by rewarding it with food the next day rather than immediately on completing the maze correctly.

The clinical response of patients who are charged with driving while intoxicated exemplifies this phenomenon. Several studies suggest that the chance of arrest on a given drunk driving occasion is less than 0.5%.[6, 7] Most individuals will have driven drunk dozens to hundreds of times before their first arrest. Thus, the common response "That policeman must have had it in for me—I've been in a lot worse shape before and never been arrested" is, in fact, a true statement of the patient's experience and exemplifies the first stage in the evolution of denial.

State-specific learning contributes to the further development of denial. Memory does not generalize easily from the intoxicated to the sober state nor conversely. Thus, a consequence experienced while sober is relatively quickly forgotten as intoxication proceeds. A fight that occurs while intoxicated is not clearly remembered when sober and does not easily influence a patient's sober perception of the life problems that his or her intoxication has caused. The amnestic properties of some intoxicants, notably alcohol and benzodiazepines, may also produce blackouts that leave no recall of events during an intoxicated episode, again interfering with connection of cause and consequence.

Although relatively early in the course of these disorders denial stems from fairly straightforward cognitive and learning principles, matters become more complex and difficult as substance use disorders progress. As consequences and losses continue to accumulate, the connection between use and consequences becomes more compelling, and failed efforts at control occur again and again.[5] With this growing awareness and repeated failures to gain control comes a sense of shame and guilt that is often overwhelming. As losses accumulate, the need to avoid the shame and guilt becomes a primary psychological motivator, and denial undergoes a metamorphosis from a straightforward cognitive/behavioral phenomenon (the inability to connect remote causes and recent consequences) to a true primary defense mechanism in the dynamic sense: Denial becomes a mechanism to avoid intolerable feelings of shame and guilt. As denial assumes the dimension of a primary defense mechanism, other primitive defenses may also surface in the service of the same goal. Projection, with resultant paranoid and suspicious behavior, and somatization are commonly encountered.

Denial and Psychiatric Comorbidity

When this psychological picture is complicated by additional psychiatric pathology, clinical intervention becomes even more challenging. For example, if a patient with a substance use disorder also suffers paranoid schizophrenia, then the use of projection in the service of maintaining denial becomes exaggerated. A patient with depression, suffering both shame and guilt from consequences of substance addiction and shame and guilt as symptoms of depression, experiences even greater difficulty in overcoming denial and accepting needed substance addiction treatment. This illustrates one of the compelling reasons why early diagnosis and treatment of comorbid psychiatric illness are essential to promote successful treatment of substance use disorders in patients with a dual diagnosis.[8]

Treatment Approaches

ENGAGEMENT

Engagement has been defined as "the process of convincing patients that the . . . agency or provider has something desirable to offer them."[9] Engagement is often considered as the second phase in the treatment of patients with a dual diagnosis, after stabilization.[10] Engagement is perhaps best conceptualized as therapeutic efforts specifically aimed at combatting the extreme demoralization and resultant nihilism so frequently encountered in patients with a dual diagnosis. Much of what is judged as treatment refusal or unreadiness for treatment stems from this demoralization, and it is unrealistic to expect this multiply learned and reinforced demoralization to disappear spontaneously.

Engagement may be served by many approaches. To effectively engage dual-diagnosis patients using the tools of psychotherapy, clinicians must combat demoralization by conveying their belief that things can get better. This may be convincingly communicated through attitudes, through appropriate sharing of other professional experiences in which similar patients have improved, and through practical education and advice. Perhaps the core requirement for effectively engaging patients is the clarity of the clinician's own belief that treatment can be effective. Patients are only too quick to identify nihilism in the therapist, whether it is expressed in terms of treatment refusal or premature limit setting or in more subtle or countertransferential ways in the course of treatment. For instance, a patient readmitted for treatment failure may be approached nihilistically or may be hopefully reminded that lasting recovery seldom occurs after a single treatment but may well occur after two or three.

Case management and social assistance approaches, such as help in obtaining necessities such as food or shelter, may be substantially remoralizing. Appropriate assistance in accessing entitlement programs may similarly help. Occasions for socialization and recreation or vocational opportunities may be helpful.[11]

Confrontation is a much-discussed and little-understood therapeutic technique pertinent to both the engagement and persuasion phases of treatment. The goal of confrontation is to help patients understand hard truths that they have been avoiding. Rather than perceiving confrontation to be punitive or angry, I consider confrontation to be direct but nonjudgmental and find it is often appropriate to share the affect of concern as part of a confrontative interchange. I think of what I would say to a trusted colleague about a patient and then just say this to the patient. This way I can directly, accurately, and concisely share my concerns but avoid either overdisplay or underdisplay of affect and do not provoke any sense of power struggle with the patient.

Engagement and Psychiatric Comorbidity

Effective pharmacological or behavioral treatment of acutely distressing symptoms, often accomplished during hospitalization for detoxification and stabilization, may be substantially remoralizing. The need to provide symptom relief in the interests of combatting demoralization and therapeutic nihilism is a major reason why I argue against the common practice of delaying psychiatric diagnosis as long as possible in assessing patients with complex problems that include substance addiction. Although the diagnostic process is more complex and less reliable in patients with a dual diagnosis than in the absence of the complication of substance addiction, convincing evidence shows that criteria-based diagnoses are reasonably reliable and valid in the first weeks after detoxification.[12, 13] Guided by these tentative diagnoses, prompt initiation of appropriate pharmacological or behavioral treatments helps improve the cognitive capacity of patients early in the engagement effort, communicates a very real attempt to offer help in a meaningful way, and may produce significant enough improvement to help substantially in the engagement process.

Limit setting must be approached cautiously during the engagement phase. Any limits must take into account a patient's current understanding and capabilities and must be clearly communicated. Contingencies for failure to observe limits must be nonpunitive and must not lead to termination of treatment during the engagement phase. The entire intention of engagement is to engage patients sufficiently for therapeutic efforts, including limit setting, to subsequently and successfully proceed.

Engagement, Persuasion, and Coercion

Coercive approaches may help engagement efforts. In some cases, avoiding a legal, employment, or family consequence may be the only benefit of treatment that a patient is able to understand. Deferred sentencing, in which a legal consequence is held in abeyance as long as treatment participation is acceptable, can be a useful way to enhance treatment acceptance and involvement. Outpatient commitment, usually with inpatient involuntary commitment held in abeyance, can also be helpful.

It also seems clear that denial affects an individual's ability to accept needed treatment, because accepting treatment is an admission of need for treatment and hence of the reality of the underlying disorder. This is why many clinicians experienced with substance use disorders do not believe that self-motivated or voluntary treatment is particularly essential and why many such clinicians are comfortable working with patients mandated to treatment or even in some circumstances helping to ensure that a mandate to treatment occurs. When denial is a true primary defense mechanism, truly voluntary treatment is clearly an impossibility. Although some clinicians have believed that voluntary patients are likely to have better treatment outcomes, little evidence supports this belief in either primary or dually diagnosed patient populations. Rather, available evidence suggests that patients with legal or employee assistance mandates have as good or better treatment outcomes than putatively voluntary patients. This is probably because in a supportive treatment environment, where the issue is recovery rather than blame, it becomes more possible for patients to move away from denial, regardless of how they got into the treatment environment. If one reviews the first five steps of Alcoholics Anonymous (AA) in view of this understanding of denial, it is easily seen that these steps serve a similar purpose in allowing individuals to accept responsibility for their recovery without immediately being overwhelmed by guilt and shame, and subsequently provide a structure for relieving these feelings by acknowledging wrongs and correcting them to the extent possible.

PERSUASION

Once patients have been engaged in treatment, the process of modifying denial begins. This translates practically into the process of convincing these patients to accept a long-term abstinence-oriented treatment component.[9, 14, 15]

The process of persuasion requires that patients be engaged and be somewhat stabilized, so that they are not in acute crisis, they are not unapproachably demoralized or nihilistic, and their severe cognitive and affective symptoms have been somewhat ameliorated. Persuasion can occur in diverse settings, using various techniques, and is defined by its goal rather than its method.

In individual therapy, persuasion requires that the clinician be able to present the diagnosis and the need for abstinence-oriented treatment nonjudgmentally, with clarity and certainty. The way physicians typically present a diagnosis and treatment plan is to summarize the findings, provide the diagnosis, and talk about the therapeutic implications of the diagnosis and the prognosis with and without treatment. A diagnosis of heart disease, depression, or breast cancer usually is presented in a caring, nonjudgmental fashion. Perhaps because of our societal ambivalence about substance addiction, it seems difficult to provide findings and a prognosis and to avoid seeming judgmental in our discussions of these diagnoses. It is important to remember that we can make these diagnoses reliably, that we do know the therapeutic implications, that we know the prognosis for these disorders with and without treatment, and that those afflicted with these illnesses suffer as intensely as any patients and both require treatment and often benefit from it.

The job of persuasion is to bring home to individual patients the ways in which they have demonstrated a need for treatment, not to teach them DSM-IV diagnostic criteria. Thus, in the process of persuasion, it is important to explore with individuals their experience with alcohol or drugs, reviewing times when they may have used them when they didn't really wish to, or when they used more than they intended, or when others pointed out to them problems from use that they might not have recognized.

Involvement in peer groups, including both groups devised specifically for persuasion and existing naturalistic fellowships such an AA or

Narcotics Anonymous, may increase the efficacy of persuasive efforts.[15] Despite our best efforts, many patients remain suspicious that professionals are likely to overdiagnose and to recommend treatment because of economic incentives; that is, after all, how we make our living. Occasional well-publicized scandals, including past national publicity about inappropriate admissions of adolescents to substance addiction treatment programs, has been cited by patients in support of this belief (which, of course, also supports their denial). The stories and opinions of unpaid peers are considerably more credible, and it is much more difficult for patients to support denial by questioning the motivations of these peers. The modeling of personal acceptance of a substance use disorder in one's life, the caring and lack of judgmentalism that are modeled in the best fellowship meetings, and the personal disclosures of experiences and knowledge gained in a process of overcoming denial can be deeply moving for many patients in early recovery.

During this phase of treatment, it is often appropriate to begin some limit setting around substance use. The intent of limit setting here is not necessarily to attain stable abstinence (although if this occurs it is certainly desirable), nor is it to use relapse in a punitive or rejecting fashion. Rather, a patient's struggles to honor these limits can be an extremely important and valuable part of the persuasion process. Discussion of relapses and failures and what they mean about the role of intoxicants in a patient's life can be very important in overcoming denial. As part of this discussion, I find it helpful to use as a core definition of substance addiction the concept that the lesion really is one of control of substance use [5, 14, 16] rather than models of compulsion or constant use. The lesion of control of use is often partial but can almost always be demonstrated from a patient's own experience. Once this definition is accepted, I frequently use an illustrative metaphor for this partial lesion of control, comparing any continued intoxicant use to throwing matches on a pile of rags in the attic. The first match may not catch, but every match is a risk, and if the rags do catch fire then the house inevitably burns down.

Persuasion and Psychiatric Comorbidity

Although in some circles there is still controversy about the need for abstinence in treatment of some categories of primary substance use disorders, there seems to be little controversy about the need for abstinence from the addicting substances in patients with a dual diagnosis (the single exception to this may be use of methadone maintenance in dual-disordered patients with severe opiate dependence). Relapse of either the psychiatric or the substance addiction disorder frequently produces destabilizing reverberations (medication noncompliance, missed appointments, failure to pay bills or maintain housing[17]), leading to relapse of the other disorder as well. Thus, the risks of relapse are even higher in patients with a dual diagnosis than in primary substance-addicted patients. Recent evidence suggests that the presence of severe axis I illness may in fact impair the ability to control alcohol use even in the absence of other risk factors. Drake and Wallach,[18] in a 4-year follow-up of a group of patients with schizophrenia who at initial evaluation used alcohol with no evidence of problems, found a high rate of development of alcohol-related problems in the intervening 4 years, with most of their subjects having either decided to stop drinking because of their problems with alcohol or still clearly drinking in a problematic pattern at the follow-up. Thus, available data support the choice of abstinence-oriented treatment for patients with a dual diagnosis, and persuasive efforts should maintain this focus.

Some patients and some psychiatrically uninformed counselors may have difficulty distinguishing between drugs of addiction and drugs necessary for treatment of psychiatric illness, most of which have little or no addiction liability. Early and explicit discussion and education about this issue minimizes confusion and noncompliance.

As in patients with primary substance use disorders, persuasive efforts in patients with psychiatric comorbidity are markedly enhanced by appropriate group approaches. One extremely valuable site for persuasion groups is the inpatient general psychiatry unit. On most psychiatry units, between 40% and 60% of patients have a dual diagnosis, but unit staff are often unclear about appropriate unit roles and programming in treatment of such patients. They often become frustrated by attempting too much, with subsequent disappointment and disillusion when patients do not (because they cannot yet) respond.[19] In fact, the general psychiatry unit is an excellent site for stabilization, engagement, and persuasion efforts. On the inpatient unit, acute symptoms are controlled as promptly as possible, continued use of intoxicants is (ideally) ceased or at least diminished, and inpatients are faced with the fact that things have gone badly enough that they required admission, producing a greater acceptance of the patient role and a greater amenability to influence.[15] Additionally, on the unit at the same time are many other patients whose substance use has also contributed to their need for hospitalization and who are at different places in their understanding and acceptance of their substance use disorders. The combination of symptom stability, sobriety, influenceability, and the presence of an ideally constructed peer group illustrates the importance of establishing persuasion groups in every inpatient general psychiatry unit.

I have found it helpful to establish criteria for inclusion in a persuasion group, in order both to acknowledge the possibility of arbitrary error and in the process to help minimize defensiveness. Patients are told, (1) "You have said that you have problems with alcohol or drug use," or (2) "Staff think alcohol or drug use may have contributed to your need for hospitalization," or (3) "For other reasons, staff think you might have problems with alcohol or drug use," or (4) You used to have problems with alcohol or drug use." I note that objective support of the first criterion can often be obtained by alcohol and drug screening on admission. Despite substantial data that alcohol or drug use contributes to a plurality of acute psychiatric admissions,[17] toxicological screening remains underused while we illogically but consistently screen for much less frequent complications such as thyroid disease. The fourth criterion was developed because the periods preceding and following psychiatric hospitalization are usually times of high relapse risk even for patients in stable recovery, and reviewing experience in the peer group can be a helpful support to continued sobriety. The group also offers patients with experience with the recovery process an opportunity to share this and provides both support for their identity as a recovering person and a helpful demystification of the process of recovery for other patients.

Such groups can be conducted in various ways. Some have been run in a primarily psychoeducational mode, whereas others have attempted to mix more individualized discussion and sharing with basic facts about diagnoses and their treatment implications. Outpatient persuasion groups can also be extremely useful, although the problem of continued substance addiction can be challenging to address. Generally, once at the persuasion phase, it seems reasonable to expect patients to be free of acute intoxication when attending groups, even if complete abstinence has not been obtained.

AA and other recovery fellowships can also be helpful parts of the persuasion process, if the right match of group and patient can be found. The sharing of individual experience, the nonjudgmentalism about alcoholism demonstrated, and the fact that AA is a fellowship and members clearly have no incentive to encourage unnecessary treatment may help some patients come to accept treatment even when they have been suspicious of the motives of the professionals they've encountered. Conversely, some patients may not tolerate the social pressures of AA attendance. Some AA groups do seem judgmental about psychiatric diagnoses, and some are discouraging of pharmacotherapy even though these are clearly not official positions of the AA organization. Thus, when referring to AA or other 12-step fellowships, it is advisable to be familiar with particular groups and to refer to them to avoid inadvertently encouraging a kind of inverse denial in which denial focuses on the psychiatric component of the dual diagnosis. It is often helpful to discuss in advance the possible conflicts and different information a patient is likely to hear in AA, to minimize experiences of cognitive dissonance and possible rejection of psychiatric treatment.

Training

Clinicians working with patients with a dual diagnosis are well advised to seek out formal or experiential training with one of the growing number of clinicians who have been able to work successfully with this population of patients and to be familiar with the clinical research literature that suggests that guarded optimism about treatment outcome is in order.[20–22] Exposure of psychiatric residents to effective dual-diagnosis treatment programming helps prevent the development of inappropriately nihilistic attitudes and should be considered an essential part of general psychiatry residency training.

Summary

Demoralization and denial are barriers between substance-addicted patients and the treatments they need. Patients' demoralization and nihilism are therapeutically approached using various techniques that promote engagement, "the process of convincing patients that the . . . agency or provider has something desirable to offer them."

Once patients become engaged in a therapeutic effort, individual and group persuasion techniques are used to modify denial and convince patients to accept a long-term abstinence-oriented component of their treatment plan. Available evidence suggests efficacy of engagement and persuasion efforts and supports the benefits of subsequent specialized dual-diagnosis treatment.

REFERENCES

1. Frank JD: Persuasion and Healing. A Comparative Study of Psychotherapy, 2nd ed. Baltimore, Johns Hopkins Press, 1973.
2. Schuckit MA: Subjective responses to alcohol in sons of alcoholics and control subjects. Arch Gen Psychiatry 41:879–884, 1984.
3. Schuckit MA: Genetics and the risk of alcoholism. JAMA 54:2614–2617, 1985.
4. Cirualo DA, Barnhill JG, Grenblatt DJ, et al: Abuse liability and clinical pharmacokinetics of alprazolam in alcoholic men. J Clin Psychiatry 49:333–337, 1988.
5. Goldsmith RK: An integrated psychology for the addictions: Beyond the self-medication hypothesis. J Addict Dis 12:139–154, 1993.
6. Beitel GA, Sharp MC, Glauz WD: Probability of arrest while driving under the influence of alcohol. J Stud Alcohol 36:109–116, 1975.
7. Selzer ML, Vinokur A, Wilson TD: A psychosocial comparison of drunken drivers and alcoholics. J Stud Alcohol 38:1294–1312, 1977.
8. Kofoed L: Assessment of comorbid psychiatric illness and substance disorders. New Dir Ment Health Serv 50:43–55, 1991.
9. Osher FC, Kofoed LL: Treatment of patients with psychiatric and psychoactive substance abuse disorders. Hosp Community Psychiatry 40:1025–1030, 1989.
10. Kofoed L: Outpatient vs. inpatient treatment for the chronically mentally ill with substance use disorders. J Addict Dis 12:123–137, 1993.
11. Drake RE, Noordsy DL: Case management for people with coexisting severe mental disorder and substance use disorder. Psychiatr Ann 24:427–431, 1994.
12. Corty E, Lehman AF, Meyers CP: Influence of psychoactive substance use on the reliability of psychiatric diagnosis. J Consult Clin Psychol 61:16170, 1993.
13. Penick EC, Powell BJ, Liskow BI, et al: The stability of coexisting psychiatric syndromes in alcoholic men after one year. J Stud Alcohol 49:395–404, 1988.
14. Atkinson RM: Persuading alcoholic patients to seek treatment. Compr Ther 11:16–24, 1985.
15. Kofoed LL, Keys A: Using group psychotherapy to persuade dual-diagnosis patients to seek treatment. Hosp Community Psychiatry 39:1209–1211, 1988.
16. Clark WD: Alcoholism: Blocks to diagnosis and treatment. Am J Med 71:275–286, 1981.
17. Safer DJ: Substance abuse by young adult chronic patients. Hosp Community Psychiatry 38:511–514, 1987.
18. Drake RE, Wallach MA: Moderate drinking among people with severe mental illness. Hosp Community Psychiatry 44:780–782, 1993.
19. Pinsker H. Addicted patients in hospital psychiatric units. Psychiatr Ann 13:619–623, 1983.
20. Drake RE, McHugo GJ, Noordsy DL: Treatment of alcoholism among schizophrenic outpatients: 4-year outcomes. Am J Psychiatry 150:328–329, 1993.
21. Hanson M, Kramer TH, Gross W: Outpatient treatment of adults with coexisting substance use and mental disorders. J Subst Abuse Treat 7:109–116, 1990.
22. Kofoed L, Kania J, Walsh T, et al: Outpatient treatment of patients with substance abuse and coexisting psychiatric disorders. Am J Psychiatry 143:867–872, 1986.

Treatment of Comorbid Disorders with a Case Manager Approach

Robert E. Drake, MD, PhD •
Douglas L. Noordsy, MD

Substance use disorder frequently complicates the course of severe mental disorder (SMD). Compared with those who have SMD alone, those with dual disorders (SMD and substance addiction) are prone to various adjustment difficulties and negative outcomes. These include medication noncompliance, inability to participate in rehabilitation, suicide, homelessness, violent behavior, rehospitalization, incarceration, human immunodeficiency virus (HIV) infection, and early mortality.[1-5] On the other hand, those who attain stable remission of a substance disorder appear to have similar risk status as those who are abstinent.[6] Therefore, there has been great interest in early intervention and assertive treatment of substance use disorder for patients with SMD.

Since the initial reviews of the problem of dual disorders in the mid-1980s,[7] the difficulties of providing mental health and substance addiction services in parallel treatment systems

have been evident. Clinicians, program administrators, researchers, and policy makers have advocated integrated approaches to treatment in which mental health and substance addiction interventions are combined within the same program and tailored specifically to meet the needs of this population. Evidence continues to accumulate that integrated approaches are effective.[8, 9] For example, we reported that more than 60% of a group of 18 patients with schizophrenia and alcoholism achieved stable remission after 4 years of integrated treatment through an intensive case management team.[9]

Case Management for People with Dual Disorders

The optimal methods for integrating substance addiction and mental health treatments for this population are not yet clear. Most experts have recommended case management because people with dual disorders are often not engaged in services and have diverse service needs.[10, 11] For example, nearly all of the 13 National Institute of Mental Health demonstration programs for young adults with co-occurring serious mental illness and substance

The work for this chapter was supported by grants from the Robert Wood Johnson Foundation (13539), the National Institute of Mental Health (R18-MH46072 and K02-MH00839), and the National Institutes on Alcohol Abuse and Alcoholism (R01-AA08341 and U01-AA08840). An earlier version of this chapter appeared in *Psychiatric Annals*, volume 24, 1994, and is reprinted with permission of the publisher.

addiction, funded between 1987 and 1990, included some form of case management.[12] These demonstrations consistently showed that case management could be used to integrate treatments and that dually disordered clients could be successfully engaged in community-based services.[13] Several large research projects currently in the field are investigating the effectiveness of these case management interventions. These include studies headed by Sara Corse in Philadelphia, Susan Essock in Connecticut, Maxine Harris in Washington, DC, Jeanette Jerrell in California, Marlene Pelser in Maine, Al Santos in South Carolina, and our group in New Hampshire. Results from these studies should help during the next few years to clarify the optimal delivery of case management for people with dual disorders of SMD and substance addiction.

The aim of this chapter is to summarize current clinical experiences with the delivery of substance addiction treatments to persons with SMD through case management. Several themes are consistent across programs. First, these teams tend to be multidisciplinary and include clinicians with backgrounds in psychiatry, nursing, case management, substance addiction, and rehabilitation. Second, the teams use assertive outreach and culturally relevant programming to engage dually disordered clients in community-based services that include substance addiction treatment. Third, because many of the clients are initially in a premotivational state with regard to their substance disorder and are not receptive to an abstinence-oriented intervention, the teams use motivational approaches to prepare clients for active substance addiction treatments. Fourth, substance addiction treatment involves a longitudinal process, and most clients respond to a consistent, long-term approach rather than to a short-term intervention. Fifth, substance addiction treatment is offered in the context of comprehensive services, such as those described in the community support system model.[14] There is less agreement about many other issues such as the optimal caseload size for these teams, mechanisms of training in dual disorders, the use of involuntary interventions, and the use of inpatient and residential services.

In the remainder of this chapter, we elaborate on the style of case management and some of the specific case management interventions for substance addiction that we have found to be helpful to dually disordered clients. We recommend multidisciplinary teams, as described earlier. The teams have varying caseload sizes, from 10 clients per clinician for the most disengaged clients with the greatest needs, such as those who are homeless, to as many as 35 clients per clinician for more stable clients. The teams generally meet each day and use a shared-caseload model in which several clinicians relate to each client. The shared-caseload model allows clients to express preferences and to relate to more than one provider. It also enables clinicians to cover for each other, to increase the intensity of services during crises, to provide support among team members, and to share education across disciplines.

The teams provide substance addiction interventions that are specific to a client's stage of treatment, as described by Osher and Kofoed.[15] That is, interventions vary in relation to whether a client is in the engagement, persuasion, active treatment, or relapse prevention stage. Indeed, the primary purpose of conceptualizing the treatment in terms of stages is that it helps clinicians to plan potentially appropriate interventions. Within each stage, multiple interventions are offered to recognize and respect clients' individual coping styles and preferences for treatment, to maximize clients' participation in treatment, and to follow our belief in using the shared decision-making model.

STAGE 1: ENGAGEMENT

Engagement begins when a dually disordered client is referred for treatment. The goal of engagement is to form a trusting relationship, or working alliance, which enables the case manager or team to support a client through substance addiction treatment. A number of interventions may facilitate the engagement process: practical assistance, empathic interviewing, crisis intervention, forming an alliance with the family or other social network members, and ensuring that legal constraints are sensible. Most of these grow out of recognizing the validity of a client's world view. In other words, the relationship is initially built on helping the client to achieve ends that he or she identifies as important.

Throughout engagement, team members relate to a client using the techniques of motivational interviewing.[16] This involves acceptance, expressing empathy, listening carefully, reflecting a client's views back, and understanding a client's conceptualization of his or her situation in life.

Working with the family and other stakeholders from the beginning is also helpful because dually diagnosed clients are often entangled in multiple systems (e.g., family, welfare, housing, legal, and vocational) in ways that unintentionally produce adverse consequences. For example, the family may want to help but is inadvertently reinforcing substance addiction; the court may remand a client to an inpatient substance addiction program that is inappropriate for the client's mental condition and stage of treatment; and the housing or vocational system may exclude a nonabstinent client from potentially helpful services.

JASON: AN EXAMPLE OF ENGAGEMENT

Jason was a 24-year-old single man with diagnoses of bipolar disorder and marijuana dependence. At the time of referral, he was completely noncompliant with his prescribed mood stabilizer and relied instead on marijuana and a benzodiazapine to control his manic symptoms. He used marijuana throughout the day and took the benzodiazepine erratically, sometimes trading it with his drug dealer for marijuana. He had had multiple hospitalizations for dangerous and threatening behavior. He lived with a girlfriend, and their baby was due in 2 months. He was angry with his previous treatment team for hospitalizing him and insisting that he abstain from marijuana and take medications.

His new case management team made it clear that it was Jason's role to decide whether his pattern of marijuana use was problematic or not. Various team members played basketball and went hiking and mountain biking with Jason, activities he had previously enjoyed. The goals were to build shared positive experiences that capitalized on Jason's strengths and to rekindle his interest in activities less compatible with substance use. The team psychiatrist contained the benzodiazepine use by prescribing small quantities, while reinforcing Jason's ability to recognize his symptoms. The psychiatrist made frequent home visits that included pill counts to communicate a firm limit on medication use.

Jason quickly shifted into discussing his guilt about marijuana use, citing his family's disapproval, his pending fatherhood, and a younger sister who had quit marijuana use when she became a mother. A team member who had recently become a father engaged Jason in anticipating the pleasures of fatherhood and helped him develop goals around

being a parent. Meanwhile, another team member made contact with his parents and his girlfriend and began educating them about Jason's illnesses and supporting their efforts to set clear limits around his behaviors in their home. Jason expressed paranoia when his girlfriend whispered concerns to team members during home visits, but this was minimized by discussing all issues openly with him.

STAGE 2: PERSUASION

When a working alliance has formed, the clinician or team begins to help a client to develop motivation for an abstinence-oriented intervention. The goal of persuasion is to prepare a client for active change strategies. Once again, we recommend paying careful attention to clients' preferences. Some clients prefer individual interventions, some peer-group experiences, and others multiple family groups. The core experiences in this phase of the treatment are (1) enabling a client to rekindle hopes and goals for making a better adjustment and (2) allowing a client to explore, at his or her own pace, the barriers to achieving those goals. The great majority of clients are ambivalent about their use of drugs. With support and hopefulness, clients inevitably recognize that their use of alcohol and drugs constitutes an important barrier to attaining their goals and become motivated for active substance addiction treatment.

During persuasion, several interventions are possible. The core individual counseling approach is motivational interviewing, which aims to establish a sense of discrepancy, or cognitive dissonance, between clients' current situation and goals.[16] Discussions avoid confrontation and argumentation while supporting clients' developing sense of self-efficacy. Peer group discussions similarly aim to help clients explore the influence of alcohol and drugs in their lives in a safe, supportive environment.[17] Family psychoeducation and multiple family groups help families understand the interplay between mental illness and substance addiction and to achieve consistency in reinforcing movements toward abstinence. Other social network interventions may also enable clients to find a network that supports abstinence rather than substance addiction. Skill-building activities, such as social skills training and vocational activity, help clients to gain hope, confidence, competence, new supports, and new activities.

One critical adjunctive intervention during

persuasion is helping clients to achieve control of the co-occurring psychiatric disorder. Many, if not most, dually disordered clients fail to take their medications regularly and have poor symptom control. Parenteral or closely monitored antipsychotic medications are often helpful. Other medications need to be used more judiciously with actively substance-addicted clients, but all medication regimens require a careful plan and close monitoring for these clients. Symptom control usually improves further with abstinence, but medication compliance often helps to reduce symptoms and to increase participation in substance addiction treatment.

From the beginning of treatment, we recognize that sustained abstinence requires that clients change many aspects of their life—cognitions, beliefs, habits, behaviors, friends, and often living situations. Interventions in many of these areas can begin even before clients are consciously working on abstinence. Progress in these related areas helps to create a hopeful attitude and motivation for achieving stable abstinence.

DEBRA: AN EXAMPLE OF PERSUASION

Debra was a 21-year-old woman who was diagnosed with schizoaffective disorder and polysubstance dependence. At the time of referral, she had dropped out of school, lost several jobs, and was sharing an apartment with several drug-using friends. She spent nearly all her time using drugs or sleeping. Her father had obtained guardianship for her finances because of her drug use. He was frustrated by attempts to direct Debra's money toward basic needs rather than drug use.

The case manager found Debra an apartment of her own, helped her move her belongings, and provided assistance in obtaining basic furnishings and utensils. The team's vocational specialist helped her obtain supported employment. She performed well on the job but was fired after several months when she was found getting high during a coffee break.

Debra soon developed a relationship with a man but reported difficulty being with her boyfriend for long periods of time because of paranoia. The case manager helped Debra develop the discrepancy between her goal of maintaining this relationship and the use of hallucinogens, which she reported worsened the paranoia.

Debra found that she could control paranoia by taking her antipsychotic regularly and avoiding drug use. She became abstinent from drugs but started drinking heavily with her boyfriend instead. Rather than criticizing her alcohol use, the team supported her decision to abstain from drug use and discussed her drinking episodes openly with her. She was also helped to develop new relationships with peers who were not using drugs.

Debra soon began reporting depressive and obsessional symptoms. Her hypersomnia became more prominent. She ruminated about every interaction with her boyfriend and feared he would leave her. The team psychiatrist prescribed a serotonin reuptake inhibitor, which was marginally helpful. She obtained another job but left it within a month because of obsessional fears at work. The individual counseling now focused on developing a discrepancy between her desire to appear functional to her boyfriend and her desire to share alcohol use with him.

As Debra was developing motivation for changing her alcohol use, she stated that she only drank heavily because her boyfriend did. She began cutting down gradually. However, when her boyfriend broke off the relationship, her alcohol consumption increased markedly. She angrily reported that her depressive, obsessional, and psychotic symptoms were out of control. The team helped her make the connection between substance use and symptoms and provided intensive support. When 2 days of abstinence led to a dramatic reduction in symptoms, Debra developed a clearer understanding of this relationship and began considering active treatment strategies.

STAGE 3: ACTIVE TREATMENT

After several months of exposure to persuasion-stage interventions, most clients adopt the goal of abstinence and are ready for active, abstinence-oriented strategies. At this point, individual targets identified during the longitudinal process of assessment and based on the biopsychosocial model of addiction are attacked by specific intervention strategies.[18] For example, some specific targets might be social anxiety, hopelessness, boredom, cognitive expectations that alcohol alleviates insomnia, lack of structured activities, spending time with drug users, and living in a high-risk situation. Again, these interventions can be conducted in individual, group, or family settings, depending on a client's preferences. Interventions are considered empirical trials, with regular reviews of progress. Failures lead to a reconsideration of the problem and the intervention plan rather than to blaming a client or discouragement.

We recommend cognitive-behavioral and social network approaches in all of these settings. Clients with SMD find these interventions attractive and respond to them. For example, with appropriate supports, they are able to identify high-risk situations, to learn and practice skills, and to try them in the real world. Because substance addiction is an environmentally sensitive disorder, actively repairing social networks and building new supports during this phase are also helpful. Our colleagues at Community Connections in Washington, DC, have developed manuals that describe in detail, with many clinical examples, the cognitive-behavioral and social network interventions that case managers can use effectively during this stage.

A number of other interventions may be helpful during active treatment. Some clients fit into the existing self-help system in the community. This is particularly true for those with affective disorders rather than schizophrenic disorders.[19] We encourage clients to go to work during this stage, using a model of supported employment that involves rapid placement and individualized supports.[20] We also involve families in behavioral treatments at this stage, and these interventions sometimes involve a community reinforcement approach, in which families participate as active reinforcers of abstinence. Many clients also elect to use disulfiram during this stage to avoid the impulsive use of alcohol. Monitored use can be accompanied by specific reinforcers.

Laboratory monitoring is essential in building a credible dual-disorder program, particularly so during the active treatment stage. Clients appreciate the concrete markers of progress and assistance with the compulsion to use substances secretly. We recommend using random urine screens and saliva tabs for alcohol.

BUD: AN EXAMPLE OF ACTIVE TREATMENT

Bud was a 52-year-old man with diagnoses of chronic schizophrenia and alcohol dependence. He reported heavy drinking since his teenage years and did not become interested in abstinence until he developed pancreatitis, alcoholic hepatitis, gastritis, and general malaise. He was referred to the dual-diagnosis team during an inpatient detoxification, so team members met him in the hospital to develop a treatment plan. Because he had failed several previous inpatient alcoholism treatments, the inpatient team had referred him to an outpatient evening alcoholism treatment program. Members of the dual-diagnosis team agreed to help with transportation. Disulfiram was suggested, but Bud declined, insisting that he could manage craving.

After a few days in the evening program, Bud dropped out and returned to drinking a quart of vodka daily. He had attended a few Alcoholics Anonymous (AA) meetings in the hospital but declined the team's offers to attend community meetings, stating that the members were all lying and that the meetings increased his craving for alcohol. He lost his supported employment for missing work. Team members stayed involved, seeing him even when he was intoxicated. He expressed hopelessness about ever stopping his drinking and told team members that they were wasting their time trying to help. He began forgetting his evening antipsychotic dose, and hallucinations returned. He agreed to a plan to take all of his antipsychotic in the morning, improving compliance and symptom control.

He soon stated his desire to become abstinent again. Options were reviewed, and he now accepted a trial of disulfiram. After initial abstinence, he failed an appointment, so the team psychiatrist and a case manager made a home visit and found him drinking at his kitchen table. He reported that he had little reaction from disulfiram and expressed a desperate desire to continue taking it. During review of the risks of combining disulfiram and alcohol, Bud stated that death was not of concern to him, because he saw no other way out. After carefully considering the risks, the team decided to side with Bud's motivation and continue disulfiram on the condition that he become abstinent. Within 2 days, he returned to drinking, however, and agreed to discontinue disulfiram. Suicidal ideation was monitored closely.

Bud remained motivated for active treatment, stating that his drinking was unpleasant but that he could not overcome craving. Options were reviewed, and he chose a trial of naltrexone. He noted reduced craving and a reduction in alcohol consumption by 50% when taking 25 mg daily. His demoralization diminished. An increase to 50 mg was associated with no further improvement. A reanalysis of drinking behaviors revealed that morning "shakes" and a drinking partner staying in his apartment were strong cues to drink alcohol. Bud agreed to ask his acquaintance to leave. The case manager scheduled a general medical evaluation and provided transportation.

Bud again stated that abstinence was his goal. An outpatient detoxification was organized to get him through withdrawal. He was told he had the choice between alcohol and a benzodiazepine but could not combine the two. He was carefully educated about detoxification and signs of serious medical concern requiring immediate contact with the team. A long-acting benzodiazepine was prescribed to reduce risk of rebound withdrawal. Daily contacts were made for medication distribution, and vital signs were checked by the team nurse. After a day of abstinence, Bud drank the second day and the benzodiazepine was withheld. He returned to the detoxification plan the next day and successfully completed a 2-week taper.

Case management efforts initially focused on reducing cue reactivity by helping Bud to rearrange his apartment and get out more. He joined the case manager and other sober clients in shooting pool at the local community center and began accepting rides to AA meetings. His social network was expanded further by attending the dual-diagnosis group at the mental health center and reestablishing contact with his family. Social skills training that began in the group was extended in individual sessions, focusing on his social anxiety and loneliness. The vocational specialist helped him apply for several jobs.

STAGE 4: RELAPSE PREVENTION

Once clients have been abstinent for 6 months, treatment focuses on relapse prevention. The goals during this stage are to help clients remain aware of the dangers of alcohol and drug use, attend to specific risk factors, and reinforce behavioral changes. Clients again express individual preferences in this process. Some continue to reinforce abstinence by attending self-help groups. Others continue to attend dual-disorder groups in the mental health center, to discuss alcohol and drugs with their case managers, or to help in the dual-disorder program by serving as counselors or group leaders. Any of these strategies

can be successful. Laboratory monitoring should also continue.

Clients also use this stage to solidify their gains by adopting further health-promoting changes in their lifestyles. For example, many address addictions to caffeine and nicotine, take up regular exercise, and improve their diets during this stage. Some begin to pursue further education or better jobs. Many continue to work on repairing family relationships and establishing new social connections. Case managers provide support, advocacy, and skills training to facilitate these changes.

BRIAN: AN EXAMPLE OF RELAPSE PREVENTION

Brian was a 35-year-old man diagnosed with schizophrenia and alcohol and amphetamine dependence who lived with his parents. His abstinence began after a hospitalization for recurrent agitated behavior. The dual-diagnosis team helped Brian and his family to recognize the relationships between his substance use, agitation, and psychosis and to develop a coordinated plan to help Brian attain abstinence. He used a dual-diagnosis group, community self-help meetings, individual substance addiction counseling, and urine drug screens during active treatment.

Twice-monthly family meetings with Brian, his parents, and occasionally his siblings were central to his relapse prevention plan. These meetings addressed Brian's tendency to withdraw from treatment and to misinterpret symptoms. They allowed for early detection and intervention for high-risk behaviors. Brian and his family were educated about mental illness, substance addiction, and prodromal symptoms of relapse. They decided to maintain an alcohol-free household and to assist Brian with transportation to self-help meetings. Most important, the meetings helped his family members function as informed, contributing members of the treatment team.

Team members helped Brian and his family to identify risk factors for relapse into active substance use, agitation, and psychosis. Frequent insomnia was Brian's chief concern. Brian's mother expressed concern about his consumption of large volumes of coffee. Brian agreed that caffeine use frequently led to agitation and insomnia and decided to abstain. Several slips associated with insomnia led Brian's family to keep only decaffeinated coffee in the house for several months and help him identify caffeine-free soft drinks. Brian's sleep improved considerably.

Brian also identified chronic, intermittent neck, leg, and back pains that resulted in craving substance use. Evaluation by his family doctor was arranged, but no cause was found. Treatment with anti-inflammatory medication over the years had been minimally helpful. A trial of an antidepressant medication was initiated by the dual-diagnosis team psychiatrist and markedly reduced his somatic pain.

Conflict with family members also raised Brian's desire to use substances. Disagreements often centered around Brian's feeling that others resented his presence in the home. Boredom and lack of structured activities were also problems. Therefore, a plan was developed for Brian to take on responsibility for certain household chores. Brian felt proud of his contribution and the positive response he received from his parents.

After his family had been unable to get him to a few self-help meetings, Brian's attendance began to fall off. When this issue was raised in the family meeting, the case manager suggested that it might be time for Brian to assume greater responsibility for getting himself to meetings. Brian regularly reported craving substances in his dual-diagnosis group and on one such occasion considered calling his self-help sponsor. The group helped Brian to understand feelings of inadequacy and social inhibition that had prevented him from calling for help. He soon called the sponsor, who gave him a ride to a meeting that day, and they began attending meetings together regularly.

Urine drug screens were continued weekly throughout the relapse prevention period. When he was craving drug use, Brian found it helpful to know that he had a drug screen scheduled that could detect his use. He could get past the craving more easily knowing that he could not deceive his family and caregivers.

Summary

Case management for dually disordered clients integrates substance addiction treatment into the comprehensive community support program model. The approach to substance addiction intervention proceeds through stages of engagement, persuasion, active treatment, and relapse prevention, with various specific interventions in each stage. The interventions are flexible, individualized, and determined in part by clients' preferences. Based on a biopsychosocial model, individual, client-specific factors that sustain substance addiction are identified and targeted for interventions. Treatment includes empirical trials and reviews of progress at each step until stable abstinence is achieved. All stakeholders are involved in the process of identifying targets and implementing interventions.

REFERENCES

1. Alterman AI, Erdlin FR, McLellan AT, et al: Problem drinking in hospitalized schizophrenic patients. Addict Behav 5:273–276, 1980.
2. Bartels SJ, Teague GB, Drake RE, et al: Service utilization and costs associated with substance abuse among rural schizophrenic patients. J Nerv Ment Dis 181:227–232, 1993.
3. Cournos F, Empfield M, Horwath E, et al: HIV prevalence among patients admitted to two psychiatric hospitals. Am J Psychiatry 148:1225–1230, 1991.
4. Drake RE, Osher FC, Wallach MA: Alcohol use and abuse in schizophrenia: A prospective community study. J Nerv Ment Dis 177:408–414, 1989.
5. Yesavage JA, Zarcone V: History of drug abuse and dangerous behavior in inpatient schizophrenics. J Clin Psychiatry 44:259–261, 1983.
6. Zisook S, Heaton R, Moranville J, et al: Past substance abuse and the clinical course of schizophrenia. Am J Psychiatry 149:552–553, 1992.
7. Ridgely MS, Goldman HH, Talbott JA: Chronic Mentally Ill Young Adults with Substance Abuse Problems: A Review of the Literature and Creation of a Research Agenda. Baltimore, MD, University of Maryland Mental Health Policy Studies Center, 1986.
8. Kofoed LL, Kania J, Walsh T, et al: Outpatient treatment of patients with substance abuse and coexisting psychiatric disorders. Am J Psychiatry 143:867–872, 1986.
9. Drake RE, McHugo GJ, Noordsy DL: A pilot study of outpatient treatment of alcoholism in schizophrenia: Four-year outcomes. Am J Psychiatry 150:328–329, 1993.
10. Fariello D, Scheidt S: Clinical case management of the dually diagnosed patient. Hosp Community Psychiatry 40:1065–1067, 1989.
11. Drake RE, Teague GB, Warren RS: New Hampshire's dual diagnosis program for people with severe mental illness and substance abuse. Addiction Recovery 10:35–39, 1990.
12. Teague GB, Schwab B, Drake RE: Evaluating Programs for Young Adults with Severe Mental Illness and Substance Use Disorder. Arlington, VA, National Association for State Mental Health Program Directors, 1990.
13. Mercer-McFadden C, Drake RE: A Review of Demonstration Programs for Young Adults with Co-occurring Substance Use Disorder and Severe Mental Illness. Rockville, MD, Substance Abuse and Mental Health Services Administration, 1995.
14. Stroul BA: Community support systems for persons with long-term mental illness: A conceptual framework. Psychosocial Rehabilitation Journal 12:9–26, 1989.
15. Osher FC, Kofoed LL: Treatment of patients with psy-

chiatric and psychoactive substance abuse disorders. Hosp Community Psychiatry 40:1025–1030, 1989.

16. Miller WR, Rollnick S: Motivational Interviewing. New York: Guilford Press, 1991.

17. Noordsy DL, Fox L: Group intervention techniques for people with dual disorders. Psychosocial Rehabilitation Journal 15:67–78, 1991.

18. Drake RE, Mercer-McFadden C: Assessment of substance abuse among persons with severe mental disorder. In Lehman AF, Dixon L (eds): Double Jeopardy: Chronic Mental Illness and Substance Abuse. New York, Harwood Academic Publishers, 1995.

19. Noordsy DL, Schwab B, Fox L, Drake RE: The role of self-help programs in the rehabilitation of persons with mental illness and substance use disorder. Community Ment Health J (in press).

20. Becker DR, Drake RE: Individual placement and support: A community mental health center approach to vocational rehabilitation. Community Ment Health J 30:193–206, 1994.

Treatment of Addiction and Psychotic Disorders

Robert E. Murray, MD, PhD •
Richard K. Ries, MD

A substantial number of patients who suffer from addictive disorders have additional co-morbid psychiatric diagnoses. A number of these are relatively straightforward depressive, anxiety, and personality disorders. The needs of these patients can often be met by a focused psychiatric intervention delivered as an adjunct to standard addiction interventions.[1] However, a more severely affected group suffers from comorbid psychoses. This population may ultimately benefit from traditional addiction treatment but more likely requires amplified psychiatric interventions, modification of traditional addiction treatment modalities, and major psychiatric medications.[2, 3] Indeed, a great many psychotic patients may deteriorate in the presence of the social stress of a typical addiction treatment center or 12-step group meeting. They are often unable to respond to the empathic focus of interpersonal therapy and may misinterpret new information offered at a rapid pace, perhaps even incorporating it into disordered thought processes. It is the aim of this chapter to discuss the dual-diagnosis treatment of such seriously mentally ill chemically affected patients. An important aspect of this treatment is integration of psychiatric treatment with the traditional addiction treatment paradigm.

Why Do Psychotic Persons Use Alcohol/Drugs?

The use of mind-altering substances is a commonplace practice endorsed by all cultures. The use of these substances to enhance the pleasures we experience and our ability to function in various adverse circumstances has multiple historical roots. Such substances vary from the occasional social use of time-honored alcoholic beverages enhancing religious and social functions to more aggressive use celebrating marriage, rites of passage, and victorious encounters of many kinds. Such use becomes abuse when adverse consequences occur, increasing the frequency of accidents, fires, and wrongful deaths. Abuse becomes dependence when the use is driven by a compulsion or irrational need. Dependence, if untreated, usually produces a severe loss of function via self-destructive action, psychosis, dementia, or preoccupation with pursuit of the drug of choice to the exclusion of normal self-care and social responsibility. A range of substance use (from use to abuse to dependence) may occur in all diagnostic categories of DSM-IV. There is no unified theory that explains the complex interactions between psychoses and substance addiction; however, it should be recognized that the psychoactive effects of alcohol and other drugs are more likely to destabilize an already unstable (psychotic) mind than a more stable one.

National prevalence statistics such as those developed by the Epidemiological Catchment Area program show that persons with schizophrenia have an increased use of and dependence on alcohol and other drugs compared with persons without comorbid psychotic disorders.[4, 5] Other data indicate that those persons without a formal mental disorder who use alcohol, cocaine, or marijuana on a regular basis have an increased risk for psychotic experiences when screened for them. Studies of young adult chronically psychotic patients in urban mental health populations find substance abuse in more than 50% of cases. On the other hand, Rounsaville and colleagues found almost no cases of schizophrenia in their careful study of treatment-seeking cocaine or opiate abusers.[6] This may simply reflect that certain kinds of patients are found in certain kind of places. Screening criteria used by cocaine treatment facilities do not admit those patients with bizarre, psychotic, or clearly inappropriate behaviors. Thus, substance-using chronically psychotic patients are more likely to be found in urban case-managed populations such as those reported in the psychiatric "young adult chronic populations." Being familiar with the prevalence and nature of the presenting problems in a particular clinic or community is pragmatic for clinicians.

Traditional Treatment of Substance Use Disorders

Treatment of substance abuse and dependence uncomplicated by psychiatric comorbidity can be approached in various ways ranging from motivation enhancement to spiritually based recovery programs such as Alcoholics Anonymous (AA). The 12-step model provides recovering patients with a sober social support system and a means to restore spiritual equilibrium, because in the background of many addicts are circumstances that often begin the erosion of spiritual well-being and self-esteem. In general, addicts appear to be acting "in the past," reacting to current events within a belief system that was shaped in their younger years. The recovery process outlined by AA includes recognition of the past by encouraging making amends and a compiling self-inventory of character flaws, generating a paradigm for psychodynamic growth. This recovery process is well

described by an abundant literature but has had difficulty finding support in current biologically driven psychiatric literature. It has also been discussed though not broadly accepted within psychoanalytical literature (despite having a similar fundamental structure), perhaps a result of its popular origin. Recently, however, Cloninger reported data supporting a spiritual base to personality structure in mainstream psychiatric literature.[7]

This spiritual base has been interpreted by others as religion and deemed fundamentally objectionable either because it conflicted with their established religious beliefs or as a result of wholesale rejection of religion. Such individuals may find the support system they need within their religious faith or within alternative groups such as Rational Recovery. Rational Recovery endorses a rational emotive psychological approach and does not directly address spirituality.[8]

Three aspects of recovery—(1) commitment to abstinence, (2) psychodynamic restructuring, and (3) spiritual development—may emerge from a combination of 12-step participation and various therapies generally following a cognitive-behavioral or interpersonal model. Application of this treatment model in unmodified form requires intact cognitive/sensory functions; this requirement is often not met by patients with psychotic illness. Specific modifications necessary to cope with these deficits are addressed in this chapter.

Psychotic Disorders: Diagnosis and Classification

Psychotic symptoms may be (1) a result of substance use in a person otherwise not having a psychotic disorder, (2) a result of substance use by a person in whom psychotic symptoms may have existed before the substance abuse, or (3) not caused by substance use, although preexisting psychotic symptoms may be increased, altered, or temporarily decreased as a result of the use of substances.

Some researchers have attempted to characterize psychotic disorders as either primary or secondary to the use of substance. Certainly in the case of acute psychotic disorders, this classification facilitates an appropriate focus of treatment. However, in the case of chronic psychoses, many investigators have largely abandoned the primary/secondary differential. In the clinical forum, the historical information needed to establish diagnostic priority is frequently unavailable or unreliable or often does not lead to major differential assessment or treatment of patients who have long-term combined psychosis and substance use. Ries and coworkers developed a system of classifying psychiatric disorders as either low or high in severity, depending on severity and persistence of the mental illness.[9] Initial psychiatric severity is assessed in terms of patients' ability to perform basic functions and to communicate. For example, most psychoses are rated as high severity whereas most anxiety disorders are rated as low severity. Substance use is characterized on a separate axis that ranges from low (use/abuse) to high (dependence) in severity. Thus, patients may be represented on a 2 × 2 matrix into four categories: (1) low psychiatric/low substance (LL), (2) low psychiatric/high substance (LH), (3) high psychiatric/low substance (HL), and (4) high psychiatric/high substance (HH) (Fig. 24–1). This structural classification is instrumental in treatment matching.

Most severely mentally ill substance-affected patients fall into the HL to HH categories and are likely found in homeless populations and public mental health clinics. The LH categories (e.g., depression plus cocaine dependence) are often found in addiction treatment centers as characterized by Rounsaville and colleagues.[6]

DRUG-INDUCED PSYCHOTIC DISORDERS

Any drug of abuse, including alcohol, can induce psychotic symptoms if taken in sufficient quantity or for an extended period of time. In this section, the major drug categories are reviewed, with emphasis on common psychotic symptoms associated with their use or withdrawal.

Alcohol

DSM-IV[10] lists a number of psychiatric disorders induced by alcohol. They include alcohol intoxication, idiosyncratic intoxication, withdrawal delirium, hallucinosis, amnestic disorder, and dementia associated with alcoholism. However, because most patients with a dual diagnosis use various substances either at the same time or serially, attributing psychotic symptoms to specific drugs is often problematic. Alcohol hallucinosis is not commonly reported. Temporary drug-induced psychotic or paranoid symptoms 24 to 48 hours after using a combination of cocaine, marijuana, and alcohol are common. Attribution of specific symptoms of intoxicated patients to one drug among a set of abused drugs may not alter treatment decisions that are often directed at symptomatic relief and reestablishing autonomic homeostasis. Treatment of withdrawal syndromes in polydrug abuse often targets the most threatening of the presenting symptoms, with broad coverage of many possibilities and anticipation of an extended withdrawal with several phases reflecting the pharmacological profiles of all drugs ingested.

Alcohol is the psychoactive substance of abuse most available to any patient of any diagnosis and thus is usually the drug most commonly used by dually diagnosed populations. Its effects are noted in the context of suicide attempts, property destruction, and use of alcohol for transient relief of psychotic symptoms. Patients admitted in a state of intoxication may correctly evaluate themselves and conclude that they need help. Paradoxically, after detoxification, they often experience a flight into health and seek premature discharge.

Stimulants

Secondary to alcohol, marijuana and cocaine are the drugs most frequently used in the dually diagnosed population. Cocaine and other potent stimulants have well-documented roles in the induction of psychotic or severe paranoid symptoms. It is not uncommon to find patients with what appears to be an aggressive paranoid psychosis induced by cocaine. This is particularly true when freebase cocaine or crack is used. It should be pointed out, however, that the bulk of such patients have also

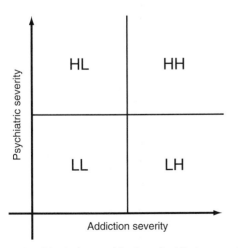

Figure 24–1. Matrix for psychiatric and addiction severity.

been using alcohol and often other drugs as well. Cocaine use is encountered in dually diagnosed patients in the following situations:

1. A brief but aggressive drug-induced paranoid psychosis in a chronic polydrug abuser who has been using cocaine and alcohol. These patients are typically admitted on involuntary status as a danger to others or themselves and usually respond within 24 hours to unit structure and brief use of antipsychotic, anticonvulsant, or benzodiazepine sedatives if needed.

2. A young chronic psychotic "street person" who has either schizophrenia or unstable bipolar disorder and who episodically abuses cocaine, alcohol, and marijuana. This type of use is usually not sustained, probably because of the difficulty in obtaining support for use of illicit drugs. If such patients have the "good luck" to obtain or be able to afford the use of crack for a few days, they often decompensate with an aggravation of their baseline psychotic or mood symptoms and are admitted on involuntary treatment status. Two things may occur simultaneously: (1) The patient may have stopped his or her baseline therapeutic psychiatric medications and (2) the use of crack and alcohol aggravates the baseline psychiatric disorder. These two processes obviously lead to the onset of active psychosis. It is somewhat paradoxical that psychotic patients should choose psychotomimetic drugs; nevertheless, some evidence shows that schizophrenic patients preferably abuse stimulants despite the apparent psychotomimetic effect.[11]

Shaner and colleagues studied 108 consecutive patients admitted with a diagnosis of schizophrenia. They found that approximately 30% of these otherwise unselected patients had used cocaine in the week before admission. Only two patients in this series were reported to be amphetamine abusers. Nevertheless, abuse of amphetamine-like stimulants may be an important factor in the genesis and maintenance of psychotic illness in selected chemical-abusing patient populations. The frequency of such use may depend to a great extent on local availability. The effect of amphetamines on schizophrenic patients is variable and in fact may be state dependent,[12] producing increased psychotic symptoms in some and decreased in others. Variables may include an unrecognized comorbid residual attention deficit disorder. Specific patient populations may be at increased risk for the psychotomimetic effects of amphetamines. In a controlled double-blind study, patients with borderline personality disorder were found to exhibit more psychotic symptoms after administration of an amphetamine challenge than did normal controls.[13]

Marijuana

Mathers and Ghodse documented psychotic symptoms attributed to marijuana in a controlled study.[14] Psychotic symptoms in patients presenting with positive urine cannabis screens were found to be of brief duration; no subgroup with chronic cannabis-induced psychosis could be identified. More enduring psychoses are more likely to be due to an underlying, independent psychotic disorder, most often schizophrenia. Thus, cannabis use may exacerbate psychotic symptoms in patients with major psychotic disorders such as schizophrenia, bipolar disorder, or other psychiatric conditions (discussed later). Psychotic syndromes lasting longer than 1 week after cessation of cannabis abuse should prompt strong consideration of a premorbid predisposition to an independent psychosis. The possible occurrence of psychotic symptoms due to ongoing marijuana chronic intoxication was not precluded but deemed less likely. It is well known that marijuana has a long half-life. Dual-diagnosis units encounter a small but regular number of chronic marijuana users who are admitted for depression and suicidal overdose. These patients have often used marijuana for 5 to 20 years and have become less and less functional in their relationships, jobs, and activities. Treatment of any psychotic component generally follows the model of treatment of brief reactive psychosis or appropriate treatment of an independent psychotic disorder.

Opiates

Although polydrug users abuse virtually any substance, the bulk of patients use alcohol, marijuana, and cocaine. Few psychotic patients use heroin on a regular basis. It appears that for patients with chronic unstable psychoses such as schizophrenia, the complex behavior to obtain money and drugs, inject the drugs, and repeat the cycle regularly is too difficult. More histories of heroin or other intravenous drug use are elicited from nonpsychotic patients. Little evidence shows that use of opiates leads to psychotic symptoms. Patients on methadone may manifest psychotic symptoms once their methadone dose decreases to a certain point. These patients are not usually found in dual-diagnosis programs, however.

Other Agents: Hallucinogens, Inhalants, Anesthetics, and Anticholinergics

As indicated by their very name, hallucinogens can induce psychotic symptoms. However, in recent years, relatively few patients with acute psychoses due to hallucinogens have been reported. More common are 23- or 24-year-old psychotic patients with an early history of heavy marijuana and hallucinogen use throughout their teenage years. Although these patients are admitted with a schizophrenia-like presentation, they often present with social skills not typical of schizophrenia. Their symptoms may appear more schizotypal—that is, less florid, more likely eccentric with odd or magical thinking and preserved alertness and attentiveness. These patients may respond to a trial of carbamazepine or benzodiazepines in an attempt to block kindled hallucinogenic experiences; paradoxically, neuroleptics may exacerbate symptoms.[15]

In certain populations, primarily adolescent, inhaled organic solvents are a drug of choice. Inhaled chemicals include aliphatic and aromatic hydrocarbons, alkyl nitrites, diethyl ether, and nitrous oxide obtained from a wide variety of sources accessible to adolescent experimentation. An intoxication resembling that with alcohol occurs, with disinhibition, psychosis (with high dose), and seizures. In adult treatment settings, inhalant use is important as a potential etiological agent in psychotic disorders and dementias resulting from the neurological degenerative processes occurring over time with these agents.[15]

Anticholinergic agents are common in many recreational drugs as well as many medical preparations. Anticholinergic abusers have used plants of the nightshade family as well as antiasthma inhalers, antiparkinson drugs, antihistamines, and amitriptyline. Psychotic patients prescribed antiparkinson agents for the treatment of neuroleptic-induced extrapyramidal symptoms are susceptible to abuse of these agents and occasionally develop drug-seeking behavior targeting these drugs. The desired effect is euphoria, then excitement, delirium, and psychosis. Acute treatment may include anticonvulsants or benzodiazepines; neuroleptics and any other agent that has intrinsic anticholinergic activity should be avoided.

A final category occasionally encountered is the dissociative anesthetics, most frequently phencyclidine. Patients using PCP present acutely with a bizarre aggressive psychosis rendering them oblivious to pain. Chronically psychotic patients tend not to use this class of drugs. These patients are typically found to be a member of an aggressive subculture such as a street gang. Repeated use of drugs of this class may result in dementia or chronic psychoses.[15] In patients presenting with apparent phencyclidine-induced psychosis, treatment with neuroleptic agents is indicated and may be necessary for a sustained period. It is important in the acute presentation to rule out anticholinergic delirium, a condition precluding the use of neuroleptics.

NON–DRUG-INDUCED PSYCHOSES

Non–drug-induced psychotic disorders are commonly associated with and exacerbated by chemical addictions. The common psychotic syndromes are briefly discussed next.

Schizophrenia

Schizophrenia is a syndrome characterized by (1) psychotic symptoms, (2) disturbance of functioning in work, social relationships, and so forth, (3) not being due to another disorder, and (4) continuous signs of the disturbance for at least 6 months. Symptoms are classified as positive or negative. Positive symptoms are generally easy to describe and quantitate. They are hallucinations and bizarre delusions that are generally mood noncongruent. The second set of symptoms, classified as negative, are hard to describe and quantify. They are often overlooked in clinical evaluations. Attempts to codify these characteristics have culminated in DSM-IV. This codification carefully separates schizophrenia from schizophreniform disorder on the basis of duration and from affective disorders and certain personality disorders (schizotypal, schizoid, and paranoid) on the basis of quantitative and qualitative differences. These attempts have met with substantial success and recognition from virtually all areas of psychiatry. Publication of DSM-III in 1980 led to a great increase in diagnostic uniformity. However, attempts to identify a unifying genotype have failed, and in fact, family studies of schizophrenic probands have shown an increased incidence of unipolar depression and schizoid and schizotypal personality disorders in first-degree relatives, suggesting the possibility of a continuous rather than discrete variation.[17] A unifying descriptive feature of the cluster A personality disorders plus the axis I diagnoses, schizophrenia, schizophreniform disorder, and schizoaffective disorder is a tendency to withdraw from close interpersonal relations. It is this characteristic that makes chemical addiction in this diagnostic group intensely resistant to traditional treatment; in fact, patients with any of these diagnoses may readily decompensate further when exposed to the group process of traditional treatment.

Schizophrenic patients are known to use alcohol, marijuana, cocaine, and nicotine frequently.[3, 18] Despite reports indicating that schizophrenic patients prefer stimulants to alcohol and others stating the opposite, no robust findings consistently support either hypothesis. It may be that schizophrenic patients tend to use the substances that are most readily available to them, and thus environment and opportunity tend to determine use patterns. Nonalcohol substance abuse among patients with a clear-cut diagnosis of schizophrenia tends to follow an intermittent pattern. It appears that regular and heavy use leads to decompensation, noncompliance with outpatient treatment, and hospitalization. These episodes are also key events precipitating progression of downward social drift, primarily through loss of housing.

Psychotic Affective Disorders

Bipolar affective disorder is also clearly characterized in DSM-IV. Two levels of symptoms are differentiated into bipolar I and II. The second, less severe form lacks frank psychotic features and is restricted to the development of hypomania rather than full mania, or bipolar I. Core features of mania are poor impulse control and overinvolvement in many kinds of problematic behaviors, including substance abuse, spending, sex, and criminal activity. Therefore, with mania more than other diagnoses, the question is asked, Is the substance abuse just a symptom of mania or is it really a separate problem? The answer to this question may guide clinicians to focus on different interventions. The concept of self-medication is frequently evoked for this diagnosis, implying use of alcohol to medicate hyperactive symptoms (discussed elsewhere in this text). The analogy with the medical treatment of mania with neuroleptics or benzodiazepines supports this concept. However, if medical treatment of mania in an addicted patient is considered adequate, a major risk occurs that an independent but interacting chemical addiction is consequently not treated. Additionally, manic patients frequently use alcohol or stimulants not to sedate a manic episode but to sustain their euphoric psychosis. This yields cycles of substance abuse, manic psychosis, and frequent hospitalization. Patients with this diagnosis may become extremely psychotic but may have long periods with essentially normal mental status. Thus, unlike schizophrenic patients, they may successfully participate in traditional chemical dependence treatment services. This population may avoid such treatment, however, by attributing their problems wholly to their mental illness. Corroboration of this belief by mental health professionals is an enabling factor. Other factors leading to avoidance of treatment include a relatively low level of substance abuse limited to alcohol and benzodiazepines. These low levels, however, may have a major and predictable role in precipitating and sustaining manic episodes.

Unipolar depression may also be accompanied by psychosis. Treatment is directed at acute stabilization, with appropriate use of antidepressants and neuroleptic agents or electroconvulsive therapy. These patients may also benefit from traditional addiction treatment services once stabilized with continued use of appropriate psychotropic agents.

Brief Reactive Psychoses

Brief reactive psychosis is induced by well-defined severe stress causing temporary psychotic behavior whose content usually reflects some aspect of the precipitating stress. Substance abuse may or may not be involved. Treatment involves acute stabilization with brief use of neuroleptics. Education about substance abuse is indicated, and in some cases more structured treatment is necessary if substance abuse has been sustained. Patients in this diagnostic group are susceptible to iatrogenic addiction to benzodiazepines.

Dissociative disorders and posttraumatic stress disorder have received increasing attention during the past 10 to 15 years. Many chemically addicted patients have histories of severe childhood sexual and physical abuse fostering the development of a dissociative defensive style.[19] Dissociative disorders may mimic active psychosis in certain patients. Patients who complain of voices or thoughts of control and who otherwise have nearly normal findings on mental status examinations and who were abused as children are likely candidates for dissociative disorders versus schizophrenia or other kinds of psychoses. This differential is important because these patients do not respond well to neuroleptics and frequently have significant axis II presentations as well. Behavioral disturbances frequently include self-mutilation. This group is particularly prone to abuse of prescription drugs, notably benzodiazepines, which seem to enhance the dissociative defense they successfully used as children, and thus are at risk of iatrogenic addiction. Although they may benefit from traditional addiction treatment, they initially are optimally treated within a specialized track limited to other patients with similar personality disorders before entry into the mainstream of addiction recovery.[9]

Organic Brain Damage

Organic brain damage may occur as a result of trauma, drug or alcohol ingestion, or other medical disorder. Patients with organic brain damage frequently have difficulties with cognition and impulse control, thus making rational decisions about substance use difficult. Psychotic symptoms in such patients often are disorganized and confused, resembling more of a delirium than a schizophrenic or manic picture. Thus, such patients may appear to have a case of extreme toxicity that is resistant to treatment. However, if a supportive environment is available, a highly structured, concrete approach may be successful. Pharmacological treatment of organically affected patients must be designed to enhance residual brain function. It is particularly important to recognize the potential cumulative anticholinergic effects on cognition and memory in these patients. The entire gamut of medications prescribed by physicians from many specialties may need to be assessed.[20] Subcortical dementia may present as aggressive dyscontrol and is best treated with low-dose neuroleptics and anticonvulsants, avoiding benzodiazepines and excessive use of medications with strong anticholinergic effects such as amitriptyline and diphenhydramine.

Specific Issues in the Treatment of Dually Diagnosed Patients

SOMATIC TREATMENT OF PSYCHIATRIC DIAGNOSES

Acute treatment of substance-abusing psychotic individuals may not be specific to their long-term psychiatric diagnosis. The use of benzodiazepines, barbiturates, beta blockers, and alpha-2 agonists is not substantially different in the treatment of withdrawal syndromes occurring in patients with and without a schizophrenic spectrum diagnosis. These medications can also be useful in the treatment of panic symptoms, mania, or the side effects of neuroleptic medications. However, both benzodiazepines and barbiturates are themselves potentially addicting and are relatively contraindicated in addicted patients.

The Role of Benzodiazepines

Benzodiazepines have increasingly been used in the management of psychoses and mania. They are both effective and free of extrapyramidal symptoms. Unfortunately, in chemically addicted patients, these drugs are often used inappropriately. It is not uncommon to find psychotic patients who have abused benzodiazepines by increasing doses or combining them with alcohol or other drugs. When these patients are treated in a traditional addiction treatment track, they are appropriately weaned from benzodiazepines. In addition, however, they are at risk of being told to discontinue appropriate treatment with effective nonaddicting psychotropic medications. The cycle of psychosis, iatrogenic addiction, and discontinuation of medication with return to psychosis may occur for many cycles unless addiction treatment and effective psychiatric evaluation and treatment occur simultaneously.

Neuroleptic Medications

The use of neuroleptic agents such as haloperidol or trifluphenazine in the treatment of enduring psychoses is well established, and such use does not lead to abuse or dependence. However, the need to minimize side effects through optimal dosing and selection of a neuroleptic agent is exceptionally important. The additional reduction in affective modulation (akinesia) or increase in agitated behavior (akathisia) may further increase a patient's difficulty in accessing community-based resources such as AA. Further, neuroleptic action may exaggerate the symptom of anhedonia, contributing to noncompliance.[21] Therapy with lithium or anti-convulsants as an adjunct to neuroleptic medication is an effective way of reducing neuroleptic dose and minimizing side effects and may be essential in some treatment-resistant patients.[22, 23]

Even with optimal neuroleptic selection and careful dosing, side effects may require medication. Benzodiazepines are often useful in treating such side effects and are sometimes indicated in dually diagnosed patients despite their potential for abuse and dependence. For those patients with akathisia, the beta antagonist propranolol is often effective without the accompanying risk of addiction. Other medications that may be useful for all the extrapyramidal side effects except tardive dyskinesia can be divided into those that are strongly anticholinergic (benzotropine, diphenhydramine, Artane) and those that have dopaminergic activity (amantadine and bromocriptine). The former may contribute to psychosis in those affected with an organic dementing process. Exacerbation of psychotic symptoms by dopaminergic agents has been reported in patients being treated with these agents for Parkinson's disease, as well as in patients with known psychotic disorders.[22, 23] Patients with a dual diagnosis are at risk for all of these problems and indeed may misuse these drugs in an attempt to obtain sedation or stimulation.[15] Objective monitoring of symptoms is therefore important to avoid undertreatment by the physician or abuse of medication by patient. In all cases, it is important to emphasize careful dosing and use of adjunctive valproic acid or carbamazepine to minimize the effective neuroleptic dose. In patients with tardive dyskinesia, this latter approach is the only treatment known to be effective.

Electroconvulsive therapy has also been documented as effective in the treatment of psychotic disorders.[24] Direct data referable to comorbid substance abuse are sparse, possibly because of exclusion of alcoholic patients from published studies. Comorbid alcoholism and schizophrenia have been reported by Zorumski to have favorable outcomes in the electroconvulsive treatment of depression.[25]

Somatic Treatment of Addiction

Pharmacological treatment of addiction may be classified as (1) substitution therapy (methadone), (2) antagonist therapy (naltrexone), (3) aversion therapy, and (4) selective neuroadaptive modulation.

Substitution Therapy. Methadone maintenance is an effective way to reduce harm to patients chronically dependent on opiates. Patients with chronic psychoses are minimally represented in this group. To some degree tobacco use may be another form of substitution therapy. Psychotic symptoms may emerge after the cessation of methadone or of tobacco. Use of tobacco is discussed more extensively in a later section.

Antagonist Therapy. The use of opiate antagonists has achieved some recognition in the treatment of opiate-dependent patients. As already noted, opiate dependence is uncommon among psychotic patients. Of pertinence to this chapter is the potential use of opiate antagonists in the treatment of nonopiate addictions, principally alcohol. This is currently at the stage of selected small population surveys.[26] Any positive effect presumably reflects a common final pathway of reinforcement between opiates and non–opiate-addicting substances. A major concern is motivating patients to take a medication that may induce dysphoria. Paradoxically, distinct beneficial effects of opiate blockade have been reported in schizophrenic patients with significant reduction in psychosis ratings,[27] possibly permitting reduction in neuroleptic dose. No studies of the treatment of alcohol abuse by opiate blockade in psychotic patients have been published. Several controlled, random studies of small groups of nonpsychotic alcohol-dependent patients have reported favorable outcomes.[27] However, in view of positive effects on psychotic symptoms in schizophrenic patients, future use of opiate blockade for the treatment of alcohol dependence in psychotic patients may be efficacious and practical. Both potential benefit for psychotic symptoms and reduction in alcohol craving and consumption may be associated with opiate receptor blockade.

Aversion Treatment. Aversion treatment has been reported to have some success in the treatment of substance abusers. The treatment of cocaine abuse alone and combined with alcohol abuse has been reported to have resulted in abstinence rates 18 months after treatment of 75% to 80%.[28] These recovery rates may to some degree reflect compliance with a program rather than any specific effect of the aversion treatment. No data concerning outcomes in patients with comorbid psychoses have been published. However, compensated psychotic patients have not been excluded from treatment in aversion treatment programs. Certain features of this approach are worth comment. Although multimodal treatment (therapy, 12-step support groups, and medication) is usually recommended, aversion does not fully depend on other modalities. Those patients who have chronic psychoses and who are unable to participate in traditional treatment may in fact benefit from the fairly concrete concepts relied on in aversion therapy. A significant limitation of the approach, however, is its relative specificity, requiring aversion to each drug and all of its variations—that is, bourbon, gin, beer, and wine all need to be treated if indicated. Perhaps an even greater obstacle to its widespread use is the general feeling among the traditional AA recovering community that it does not lead to lifestyle changes beyond abstinence that are deemed to be necessary for long-term recovery. This argument diminishes as the severity scale of mental illness increases (HL and HH), because the ability to make dramatic lifestyle changes of such persons may be more limited.

Disulfiram is an inhibitor of aldehyde dehydrogenase that yields enhanced sympathomimetic response to alcohol when taken before alcohol use. As such, it has aversive value. A similar intolerance to alcohol has been observed in individuals with certain genetic polymorphisms. These genetic polymorphisms may also reduce diathesis for alcohol dependence. This provides a supportive rationale in the use of disulfiram as a treatment for alcohol dependence. It is widely accepted that its role is within a structured, supervised program with the goal of obtaining sufficient abstinence to protect patients in the early recovery process from the destructive effects of intoxication. A Veterans Administration cooperative study has suggested that compliance with medication prescription was more important to the outcome than the actual medication received (placebo or disulfiram).[29] Disulfiram is also known to cause psychiatric symptoms. Larson and colleagues[30] reviewed the psychiatric effects of disulfiram and pertinent drug interactions in patients with comorbid psychiatric diagnosis. With prudent regard for potential medical and psychiatric risks, disulfiram (250 mg daily) is a useful adjunctive treatment for alcohol dependence in patients with comorbid psychotic disorders. Impaired cognition or active psychosis may produce deterioration of personal organization and judgment, precluding the use of disulfiram in more severely affected patients. Specific skills required include (1) the ability to understand the cause-and-effect relationship between the use of disulfiram, alcohol, and consequent symptoms; (2) an adequate ability to control impulsive actions to promote reflection before use of alcohol, and (3) an acceptable level of compliance when not drinking, as evidenced by attendance at program activities and medication compliance.

Treatment of Selective Neuroadaptation (Cocaine) in Psychotic Patients. As previously noted, cocaine use in chronically psychotic patients is frequent but intermittent. Even occasional use in vulnerable patients (i.e., bipolar disorder) is a major concern. Certainly, appropriate pharmacological management after recognized treatment strategy of established comorbid psychiatric diagnoses is indicated. Specific interventions altering the reinforcing value of cocaine use may also be of value. Several dopaminergic medications have been studied as putative agents of reversal of a postulated cocaine neuroadaptation.[31] These studies have been largely limited to open trials. Favorable results emanating from these trials may be a result of compliance more than any specific pharmacological action. Open trials of desipramine have also been cited as providing evidence of effective treatment of cocaine addiction. Several double-blind studies that have been completed have addressed the issue of pharmacological treatment of cocaine addiction with desipramine or amantadine.[31] These studies have reported mixed results; one study in fact suggested that the treatment of psychiatric symptoms with desipramine may have enabled the continuing use of cocaine.[31] The anticonvulsant carbamazepine has also been reported to reduce cocaine use in nonmotivated chronic cocaine abusers.[32] The role of carbamazepine in the treatment of motivated individuals is uncertain.

Treatment of Comorbid Medical Complaints

Comorbid conditions that have potential direct implications in the use of psychotropic medications include seizure disorders and cardiovascular and pulmonary disease. The opportunity to coordinate anticonvulsant therapy with anticonvulsant treatment of bipolar disorder is an example of killing two birds with one stone. The use of beta blockers may have positive effects (treatment of akathisia, panic symptoms) or negative effects (depression). Medications used in pulmonary disease (beta agonists, e.g., Alupent) may exacerbate mania and in fact may be sought out by patients with a predisposition to the use of stimulants. Pain control is an obvious topic that is addressed elsewhere in this text. The potentiation of anticholinergic psychotomimetic effect by nonpsychiatric medications such as cimetidine, digoxin, oxybutynin, and furosemide may be important in vulnerable patients, in particular elderly patients.[20] The perimenstrual time period is known to be a period of increased risk of relapse in premenopausal women. Pyridoxine may be useful in the treatment of premenstrual syndrome and in fact may have a broader role in maintaining serotonergic function.[33] These, of course, are only highlights from a complex list of interactive possibilities between substance abuse and medical treatment of comorbid conditions.

Tobacco Use

Tobacco use is clearly an issue of substance abuse and substance dependence; however, it is also an issue of self-medication. It is important that this latter aspect of tobacco use in patients with a dual diagnosis not be ignored. Social policy concerning tobacco use is rapidly changing in North America. Dually diagnosed patients have a high incidence of tobacco dependence, which is an expensive condition for many of these patients on limited incomes. Few controlled data exist concerning the influence of the powerful pharmacological agents included in tobacco on the symptoms of psychosis, on side effects of medications, or on the level of craving of alcohol or illicit drugs. Although adverse consequences are many (e.g., lung cancer) and well recognized, beneficial consequences also need to be identified. Among possible benefits, nicotine may reduce the risk of development of extrapyramidal symptoms.[34] Patients report its effectiveness in controlling symptoms of anxiety and feelings of boredom, and case reports of manic psychosis occurring after the cessation of cigarette use have been published.[35] Careful attention to the role of tobacco as an unplanned adjunctive medication is indicated. Tobacco addiction treatment has increasingly become part of standard alcohol/drug treatment. When and how this should develop in psychotic patients with dual disorders remains to be seen.

PSYCHOSOCIAL TREATMENT OF PSYCHOTIC PERSONS

Psychosocial as well as biological medication interventions are necessary in the treatment of psychotic dually disordered patients. Either as a consequence of or precedent to substance abusing, psychotic patients often have deficits in interpersonal skills and problems with housing/self-care and medication compliance. The magnitude of these problems usually requires a case manager in addition to a psychiatrist and whatever specific addictive interventions are designed. This multimodal team approach to long-term care has been described elsewhere.[18]

Psychotherapeutic Interventions

The AA program as a psychotherapeutic intervention with use of cognitive behavioral therapy was previously mentioned. As a specific variation of cognitive behavioral therapy, Miller[36] described motivational enhancement therapy. This modality has defined a nonconfronting style that enhances patients' own cognitive processing of their problem-solving options. It is applicable to both nonpsychotic and moderately compensated psychotic patients. The counting of small gains and acceptance of brief lapses as learning experiences is particularly applicable in the psychotic population. We use this approach both individually and in group activities in our large program with severely mentally ill dually diagnosed patients at Harborview Medical Center.[18]

Psychotherapy and rehabilitation of chronically psychotic and organically impaired patients should begin with task-oriented activities and should not require a great deal of abstract thinking, because this is by definition impaired. As a specific example, the use of structured work environments within treatment programs addresses the needs of restoring self-esteem and provides work "hardening" to potentially employable patients. At all times with any chosen modality, it is important to recognize and build on small gains. A general tendency of patients (and often the staff) is to become quickly discouraged after small gains are not quickly converted into total cures. Frequent supportive evaluation of demonstrable gains is a valuable tool that consolidates the gains and reinforces the need for a long horizon.

Nonpsychotic patients with a diagnosis of bipolar disorder, borderline personality disorder, posttraumatic stress disorder, dissociative psychosis, or panic disorder may benefit from more insight-oriented therapy, with careful attention to remaining within boundaries of reality. Linehan[37] described dialectic behavioral therapy for borderline persons as a structured means to accomplish these goals. We use much of this approach in our program. The role of empathic concern is a vital one. Equally important, however, is the recognition and interpretation of empathic failure. It is empathic failure occurring on a daily basis that affectively unstable patients cannot cope with.[38] When this failure occurs in a structured therapeutic setting, the opportunity to identify cognitive bias leading to such failure should not be missed. This requires that the therapist maintain a stable presence throughout the turbulence of the therapeutic interactions leading to empathic failure. Linehan emphasizes frequent contact (daily, by phone) to facilitate this stabilization.

Use of the classification system presented in Figure 24–1 is helpful in establishing a psychotherapeutic treatment plan. Patients with high psychiatric severity may benefit from more concrete approaches; those with high addiction severity may benefit from brief motivational enhancement to facilitate their early choices leading to recovery.

Family therapy has earned a well-respected place in the traditional treatment of addictions. Family therapy in patients with psychotic illnesses has been an area of controversy. In the 1970s, family therapy assumed a "blaming" posture, seeking to find a cause of the onset of severe mental illness within the family. Behavior patterns within the family were cited as the cause of deterioration leading to the now discredited schizophrenogenic family paradigm. It is now thought that genetic predispositions are overwhelming factors in the etiology of psychotic disorders, although schizophrenic patients seem to remain stable longer with the assistance of ongoing family therapy. The most useful model to follow is a psychoeducational model that supports the structure of the family in dealing with the illness that has drained the family's resources and initiated deterioration of intrafamilial strengths.[39] Information about the etiology, nature, and course of schizophrenia helps family members develop means to understand and anticipate the apparently uncontrollable process of psychotic illness. Family therapy has not been emphasized in the treatment of patients with a dual diagnosis. This is most likely because of far advanced familial deterioration by the time a patient fails in traditional psychiatric or traditional addictions treatment before entering an integrated dual-diagnosis treatment system. A carefully conducted nonjudgmental psychoeducational family program should be a major asset to those patients with a dual diagnosis with intact and available families.

Homelessness

The problem of homelessness is currently a major concern of public policy. This problem is endemic among the populations who are chronically psychotic and have substance abuse problems. Public policy has generated a patchwork of shelters in the central areas of most U.S. cities. Although these shelters are often of great value, certain seriously mentally ill patients may be victimized in these settings. Sedative psychotropic medications that may be effective in the treatment of psychotic symptoms may also impair the vigilance necessary to maintain health and safety in an environment containing a significant number of predatory individuals. Thus, what may be evaluated as "noncompliance with medications" may in fact be a strategy to prevent rape. Drake and Wallach[40] found that dually diagnosed patients compared with those with mental illness alone were younger, were more often male, and were less able to manage their lives in the community in terms of maintaining stable housing and regular meals. Probably for reasons similar to those leading to inadequate housing, psychotic patients are particularly prone to nutritional depletion owing to the complexities of meal preparation and obtaining adequate housing.

Administrative Issues

Administrative obstacles encountered in the treatment of dually diagnosed patients have been decreasing slowly. Only within the past year has the state of Washington made it possible for the same facility to be licensed for the treatment of both psychiatric and substance abuse disorders. The current national focus on cost effectiveness in medicine should logically result in additional administrative streamlining. Established administrative barriers were initially developed as a way to protect addicted patients from inappropriate diagnostic labeling in traditional psychiatric treatment centers and subsequent ineffective treatment. Comtois and colleagues[18] described a large outpatient program for severely mentally ill patients at Harborview Medical Center, Seattle, Washington. Included are details of administrative structure that follow the treatment guidelines suggested in this chapter and that attempt to integrate the contents of psychiatric and addictions treatment. Specifically described are progressive levels of care designed to meet the needs of a spectrum of patients. Flexibility is emphasized. The role of case managers in treatment decisions and internal monitoring of patient progress via structured rating forms is also emphasized. The psychiatrist's role is that of diagnostician, medication prescriber, team leader, and treatment plan reviewer. Traditional psychiatric training is required, as well as the development of more skills in administration and addiction disorders than is usually provided.[41] By incorporating psychiatric residents and fellows into dual-disorder treatment units, better training should occur.

REFERENCES

1. Ries RK, Miller NS: Dual diagnosis: Concept, diagnosis, and treatment. In Dunner DL (ed): Current Psychiatric Therapy. Philadelphia, WB Saunders, 1993, p 131.

2. Minkoff K: An integrated treatment model for dual diagnosis of psychosis and addiction. Hosp Community Psychiatry 40:1031–1036, 1989.
3. Aliesan K, Firth RC: A MICA program: Outpatient rehabilitation services for individuals with concurrent mental illness and chemical abuse disorders. J Appl Rehabil Counseling 21(3):25–26, 1990.
4. Reiger DA, Farmer ME, Rae DS, et al: Comorbidity of mental disorders with alcohol and other drug abuse. JAMA 264:2511–2518, 1990.
5. Lehman AF, Myers CP, Corty E, et al: Prevalence and patterns of dual diagnosis among psychiatric inpatients. Compr Psychiatry 35:106–112, 1994.
6. Rounsaville BJ, Anton SF, Carroll K, et al: Psychiatric diagnosis of treatment-seeking cocaine abusers. Arch Gen Psychiatry 48:43–51, 1991.
7. Cloninger CR, Svravic DM, Pryxbeck TR: A psychobiological model of temperament and character. Arch Psychiatry 50:975–990, 1993.
8. Galanter M, Egelko S, Edwards H: Rational recovery: Alternative to AA for addiction? Am J Drug Alcohol Abuse 19:499–570, 1993.
9. Ries R: Clinical treatment matching models for dually diagnosed patients. Psychiatr Clin North Am 16(1): 167–175, 1993.
10. American Psychiatric Association: Diagnostic and Statistical Manual of Mental Disorders, 4th ed. Washington, DC, American Psychiatric Association, 1994.
11. Shaner A, Khalsa M, Roberts L: Unrecognized cocaine use among schizophrenic patients. Am J Psychiatry 150(5):758–762, 1993.
12. van Kammen DP, Boronow JJ: Dextro-amphetamine diminishes negative symptoms in schizophrenia. Int Clin Psychopharmacol 3(2):111–121, 1988.
13. Schulz S: Amphetamine response in borderline patients. Psychiatry Res 15:97–108, 1985.
14. Mathers DC, Ghodse AH: Cannabis and psychotic illness. Br J Psychiatry 161:648–653, 1992.
15. Brust JC: Other agents: Phencyclidine, marijuana, hallucinogens, inhalants and anticholinergics. Neurol Clin 11:555–561, 1993.
16. Thombs DL: A review of PCP abuse: Trends and perspectives. Public Heath Rep 104:325, 1989.
17. Crow TJ: The demise of kraepelinian binary system as a prelude to genetic advance. In Cloninger CR, Gershon ES (eds): Genetic Approaches to Mental Disorders. Washington, DC, American Psychopathological Association Series, 1994, p 163.
18. Comtois KA, Ries RK, Armstrong HE: Case manager ratings of the clinical status of dually diagnosed outpatients. Hosp Community Psychiatry 45:568–573, 1994.
19. Brown GR, Anderson B: Psychiatric morbidity in adult inpatients with childhood histories of sexual and physical abuse. Am J Psychiatry 148(1):55–61, 1991.
20. Tune L, Carr S, Hoag E, Cooper T: Anticholinergic effects of drugs commonly prescribed for the elderly: Potential means for assessing risk of delirium. Am J Psychiatry 50:1756–1757, 1992.
21. Siris SG: Pharmacological treatment of substance-abusing schizophrenic patients. Schizophr Bull 16(1):111–122, 1990.

22. Wilcox JA, Tsuang J: Psychological effects of amantidine on psychotic subjects. Neuropsychobiology 23:144–146, 1990.
23. Wolkowitz-Owen M: Rational polypharmacy in schizophrenia. Ann Clin Psychiatry 5:79–80, 1993.
24. Avery D: Electroconvulsive therapy. In Dunner DL (ed): Current Psychiatric Therapy. Philadelphia, WB Saunders, 1993, p 524.
25. Zorumski CF, Rutherford JL, Burke WJ, et al: ECT in primary and secondary depression. J Clin Psychiatry 17:298–300, 1986.
26. Volpicelli JR, Alterman AI, Hayshida M, et al: Naltrexone in the treatment of alcohol dependence. Arch Gen Psychiatry 49:876–880, 1992.
27. Rapaport MH, Wolkowitz O, Kelsoe JR, et al: Beneficial effects of nalmefene augmentation in neuroleptic-stabilized schizophrenic patients. Neuropsychopharmacology 9:111–115, 1993.
27a. Froehlich JC, Li TK: Recent developments in alcoholism: Opioid peptides. Recent Dev Alcohol 11:187, 1993.
28. Frawley PJ, Smith J: One-year follow-up after multimodal inpatient treatment for cocaine and methamphetamine dependencies. J Subst Abuse Treat 9:271–286, 1992.
29. Fuller, RK, Branchey L, Brightwell DR, et al: Disulfiram treatment of alcoholism: A Veterans Administration cooperative study. JAMA 256:1449–1455, 1986.
30. Larson EW, Olincy A, Rummans TA, et al: Disulfiram treatment of patients with both alcohol dependence and other psychiatric disorders: A review. Alcohol Clin Exp Res 16:125–130, 1992.
31. Meyer RF: New pharmacotherapies for cocaine dependence revisited. Arch Gen Psychiatry 49:904, 1992.
32. Halikas J, Kemp K, Kuhn K, et al: Carbamazepine for cocaine addiction? Lancet 1(8638):623–624, 1989.
33. Bernstein AL: Vitamin B6 in clinical neurology. Ann N Y Acad Sci 585:250–260, 1990.
34. Newhouse PA, Hughes JR: The role of nicotine and nicotinic mechanisms in neuropsychiatric disease. Br J Addiction 86(5):521–526, 1991.
35. Benazzi F, Mazzoli M: Psychotic affective disorder after nicotine withdrawal. Am J Psychiatry 151(3):452, 1994.
36. Miller WR: Behavioral treatments for drug problems: Lessons from the alcohol treatment outcome literature. NIDA Res Monogr 137:167–179, 1993.
37. Linehan MM: Dialectical Behavior Therapy for treatment of borderline personality disorder: Implications for the treatment of substance abuse. NIDA Res Monogr 137:201–215, 1993.
38. Newman SJ: The housing and neighborhood conditions of persons with severe mental illness. Hosp Community Psychiatry 45:338–343, 1994.
39. Nichols MP, Schwartz RC: Family Therapy, 2nd ed. Boston, Allyn and Bacon, 1991.
40. Drake RE, Wallach MA: Substance abuse among the chronic mentally ill. Hosp Community Psychiatry 40(10):1041–1045, 1989.
41. Miller NS, Ries RK: Drug and alcohol dependence and psychiatric populations: The need for diagnosis, intervention and training. Compr Psychiatry 32(3):268–276, 1991.

Treatment of Addictive Disorders in Emergency Populations

Andrew Edmund Slaby, MD, PhD, MPH

The emergency room or crisis unit is for many individuals with addictive disorders their first encounter with the healthcare system. For some, it will remain their only contact. These emergency caregivers function as primary clinicians to manage acute drug crises, to serve as differential diagnosticians, to treat drug-related medical/psychiatric problems, and to refer elsewhere as needed.[1, 2]

Patients addicted to recreational and medicinal drugs present in medical crises such as overdose and withdrawal from opiate and central nervous system depressants (e.g., alcohol or barbiturates). In some instances, a medical emergency masquerades as a psychiatric problem. A person addicted to cocaine may present with overwhelming anxiety due to a stimulant-induced cardiac arrhythmia. An alcoholic may look demented but may be suffering a reversible cognitive deficit due to thiamine deficiency or a subdural hematoma. Many substance abusers are self-medicating affective or anxiety disorders.[3–9] Sustained abstinence is to be predicated on appropriate diagnosis specific management of the underlying disorder.[10] Although referral of patients with enduring histories of addiction to a 12-step program (Narcotics Anonymous, Cocaine Anonymous, Alcoholics Anonymous) is appropriate, only a fraction will comply.[11] Detoxification with an extended stay in a treatment center enhances compliance but does not guarantee it.

In the following sections, specific addiction-related emergencies are addressed and diagnosis-specific interventions provided where indicated.

Alcohol Amnestic Syndrome
(Korsakoff's Syndrome)

The alcohol amnestic syndrome develops after delirium tremens or insidiously.[1, 2] Although it most frequently occurs with alcoholic polyneuritis,[12] it also accompanies polyneuritis of pregnancy. Onset is seldom before age 35 years, and men, perhaps because of their greater prevalence of alcoholism, are more affected. Patients generally report years of use of alcohol and poor dietary intake, and convulsions are common. Peripheral neuropathy is minimal to quite severe. Short-term but not intermediate memory is disturbed (e.g., patients cannot remember the name of three objects after 10 minutes but do have a normal digit span), and confabulation is noted. The irreversible memory impairment is obviated if Wernicke's encephalopathy is aggressively treated in the early stages with thiamine. Prolonged heavy use of alcohol leads to a malabsorption syndrome even if dietary intake is sufficient. Prophylactic use of thiamine has significantly decreased the incidence of this condition.

Patients with this disorder are given 50 mg of thiamine three or four times a day, as well as a high-potency vitamin B complex, and withdrawn from alcohol. Massage of affected muscles is prescribed as tenderness subsides. Propranolol (Inderal) is used to manage violent outbursts if present.

Alcoholic Hallucinosis

Alcoholic hallucinosis is characterized by auditory hallucinations in a clear sensorium. In some instances, men are accused of homosexual indiscretions and women, of promiscuity. Fear may lead to panic and violence and even to litigious behavior. Onset is usually 1 to 2 weeks after cessation of alcohol use, and the disorder lasts weeks or years. It is believed by some[1] to occur in individuals with a predisposition to schizophrenia.[13]

Patients are generally in need of hospitalization to protect themselves from harm and are sedated with a benzodiazepine (e.g., 5 to 10 mg of lorazepam [Ativan]) or an antipsychotic (e.g., 5 to 10 mg of thiothixene [Navane]). Physical restraints may be required to protect patients and staff from harm. Patients should be medicated sufficiently to sleep through the night, and care taken to ensure adequate dietary and vitamin intake. Problems in care can be minimized by careful explanation of any procedures undertaken and assurance that a patient's room is well lit (including use of a night lamp).

Alcohol Idiosyncratic Intoxication

Some persons become severely intoxicated on small amounts of alcohol, as corroborated by serum ethanol levels. They act uninhibitedly and may impulsively harm themselves or others. Delirium, rage, hallucinations, and depression are also encountered. Onset is usually sudden, without recall for the behavioral change. The condition is more common in younger persons and is atypical of the behavior of the person when sober. Episodes last minutes to 24 hours or more. It is believed to be more common among people with an epileptic predisposition.

Untreated, these episodes tend to abate with sleep, without recall of the episode on awakening. Violent patients must be afforded protection from harm to themselves or others. In some instances, restraints or sedation with benzodiazepines is required (e.g., 5 to 10 mg of lorazepam).

Alcohol Intoxication

Acute management of patients intoxicated with alcohol entails both understanding of the management of acute toxic psychosis and awareness of the myriad of medical problems that may attend the condition.[14, 15] These include gastrointestinal bleeding, psychiatric disorders that are being self-medicated,[16-19] concurrent substance use disorders, diabetes, pancreatitis, acquired immunodeficiency syndrome (AIDS), tuberculosis, and subdural hematomas. Friends and relatives usually report that a patient drank to excess, and the report is corroborated by serum alcohol levels in excess of 100 mg/dl. Disinhibition is observed at lower levels; inhibition predominates at greater levels. Duration of behavior changes (e.g., self- and other-directed violence, distractibility, depression, irritability, rage, slurred speech, incoordination) is as long as 12 hours. Alcohol is metabolized at the rate of 1 ounce of 80-proof alcohol per hour; therefore, symptoms become more apparent as alcohol levels are rising than when falling.

Alcohol intoxication is a frequent concurrent condition with drowning, car accidents, airplane crashes, household accidents, frostbite, severe sunburn, and fractures. More than one fourth of suicides[5] and one half of murders occur after drinking. Victims of murders may themselves be intoxicated, leading them to take risks resulting in their deaths. Alcohol addiction is a risk factor for sexual and physical abuse of spouses and children, rape, and incest. Some individuals cannot cease drinking once they have commenced it. Others may for long periods abstain from drinking but are unable to terminate a pattern of periodic binges.

Medical conditions that may be contributing to the clinical presentation should be identified and provided diagnosis-specific treatment. Five to 10 mg of lorazepam or a similar-acting benzodiazepine is administered if sedation is required. Patients should be placed in well-lit rooms with minimal distractions and with physical restraints if needed. Those who are mildly intoxicated may respond to simple support and coffee. Risk of suicide[5] in diagnosed alcoholics is 60 to 120 times that in the rest of the population, with alcoholism contributing to about 25% of suicides.[5] Many individuals with primary anxiety disorders self-medicate with alcohol.[19] This latter group should receive nonaddicting anxiolytics to manage their condition,[20] such as buspirone (Buspar). In all instances, primary psychiatric conditions require diagnosis-specific treatment. Dually diagnosed patients can be recognized by onset of behavioral and psychological symptoms before alcohol use, lack of cessation of symptoms or intensification of symptoms after abstinence is obtained, and a family history of primary psychiatric disorders rather than substance addiction disorders.

Alcohol Withdrawal Delirium

Withdrawal delirium (so-called delirium tremens or DTs) occurs after sudden withdrawal of prolonged intake of sufficient amounts of a number of different central nervous system depressant drugs such as alcohol, barbiturates, and benzodiazepines.[21] Onset with alcohol alone is usually 2 to 10 days after cessation of use, with delirium lasting for hours to days. Death due to hyperthermia or circulatory collapse occurs in 4% to 20% of cases.[1, 2] Concurrent physical illness predisposes patients to the delirium and complicates the clinical picture. Emergency clinicians should evaluate patients for the presence of malnutrition, anemia, gastritis with hematemesis, cirrhosis, electrolyte imbalance, pneumonitis, profound dehydration, and subdural hematomas.

Vivid nightmares, panic attacks while falling asleep, illusions, hallucinations (particularly tactile), restlessness, disorientation, agitation, and psychosis may accompany the delirium. Patients tend to have a coarse, persistent tremor of the hands, dry lips, tachycardia, diaphoresis, elevated temperature and blood pressure, restlessness, and a coated tongue. Seizures occur, and patients may aspirate and die.

Patients must be well hydrated with intravenous fluid and provided thiamine and multivitamin preparations. Carbamazepine (Tegretol) is used to reduce the likelihood of seizures. Many substances are used for alcohol withdrawal delirium, including lorazepam, diazepam (Valium), chlordiazepoxide (Librium), paraldehyde, and chloral hydrate in doses sufficient to suppress symptoms without oversedation so that symptoms of an evolving epidural or subdural bleed are not missed. All

procedures should be explained to patients to minimize fear, and patients placed in well-lit rooms with minimal distractions to avoid the development of frightening distortions (illusions) of unfamiliar stimuli. Mechanical restraints may be required. Hematocrit, serum electrolytes, and blood urea nitrogen values are monitored to ensure that fluid replacement is adequate and physiological. Sedation is aimed at reducing agitation to allow peaceful sleep and comfortable rest and to prevent exhaustion. Intramuscular paraldehyde must be used with caution to prevent sterile abscesses and nerve damage. Need for further sedation should be reassessed with each dose to minimize oversedation. Sponge baths, cooling blankets, and aspirin have been used to reduce temperature. If blood loss is severe from esophageal varices or another source, replacement may be indicated. Infections require appropriate antibiosis. Blood pressure, temperature, and pulse are initially monitored every half hour until stable.

Benzodiazepine Withdrawal

Abrupt cessation of high doses of benzodiazepines used for a protracted period can lead to symptoms ranging from severe discomfort to delusions and seizures.[2, 21] Withdrawal signs and symptoms include anxiety, depersonalization, agitation, malaise, tachycardia, palpitations, perceptual distortions, and myalgia. When symptoms occur with rapid cessation, return to the initial dosage and withdraw more gradually. Symptoms tend to be most pronounced with short-acting benzodiazepines such as alprazolam (Xanax)[22] and lorazepam. In such instances, withdrawal may take weeks or even months.[23, 24] Buspirone is ineffective in the management of benzodiazepine withdrawal.[25]

Amphetamine and Other Sympathomimetic Intoxication, Delirium, and Delusional Disorders

Use of stimulant drugs, popularly referred to as "uppers," can lead to delusional disorders in a clear sensorium as well as a number of other signs and symptoms, not comporting to a specific psychiatric syndrome. Sudden cessation of amphetamine or cocaine[26–28] use leads to dysphoria and further drug seeking and in some cases suicidal depressions requiring immediate intervention.[29] Confusion, fragmented thinking, and dysattention can begin within 24 hours of use. Prolonged use may lead to paranoia. Amphetamine-like drugs may be taken alone or together with a sedating substance in the form of a speedball or "croak" intravenously. Chronic users of uppers and downers confuse clinicians in the emergency room by varying symptoms at times suggestive of schizophrenia. Paranoid schizophrenics may be addicted to stimulants, enhancing their symptoms and problems in management. Pupils are dilated but reactive, and blood pressure, heart rate, and temperature increased.

Uncomplicated intoxication with amphetamine-like substance abates rapidly with discontinuation of use. Most symptoms are gone within 6 hours. Chronic users may continue to be somewhat delusional for weeks or more unless treated with neuroleptics. Benzodiazepines are usually sufficient to ameliorate symptoms of anxiety. Desipramine and bromocriptine have been used to reduce cocaine craving after withdrawal.[30-34]

Stimulant addicts can be quite violent, even homicidal, and may require restraints.

Amphetamine Withdrawal

Sudden cessation of stimulant drugs such as cocaine and amphetamines may lead to profound depression and suicide.[29] Hypersomnia and fatigue, however, are more common.

If profoundly depressed after ceasing use, a patient is provided antidepressants for a few months or, if needed, electroconvulsive therapy.

Barbiturate and Similarly Acting Sedative-Hypnotic Withdrawal and Intoxication

Intoxication and withdrawal of sedative-hypnotics mimics a number of psychiatric symptoms including schizophrenia, depression, and anxiety disorder. Delirium tremens occurs if a chronic user of sufficient amounts stops use without sufficient medication to prevent withdrawal delirium and seizures.[35]

Patients generally have a long history of use of barbiturates and similarly acting drugs. Abuse of the shorter- and intermediate-acting ones is more common than addiction to drugs such as phenobarbital. It is difficult, as in most instances of recreational drug addiction, to elicit an accurate history of use. Patients may be withdrawn from alcohol, to which they readily admit use, only to suffer delirium tremens later from withdrawal of sedative-hypnotics, which they failed to reveal or were not asked about. Although different members of the sedative-hypnotic, barbiturate, and benzodiazepine classes of drugs vary in their metabolism, absorption rates, and distribution, they are quite similar in signs and symptoms of intoxication and withdrawal. Duration of withdrawal and severity of acute symptoms is dependent on duration of use, individual susceptibility, and type of drug used. Untreated, withdrawal from sedative-hypnotics, like that from alcohol, may be fatal.

Consumption of the equivalent of 400 mg or less a day of pentobarbital or secobarbital for less than a year is unlikely to present major problems on withdrawal. Cessation of 600 mg/day for as little as 3 to 4 weeks, however, may cause anxiety, tremor, nausea and vomiting, weakness, insomnia, and involuntary twitching. Discontinuation of 800 mg for the same period may result in delirium and grand mal seizures.[1, 35] Barbiturate withdrawal is similar to withdrawal from alcohol, with the exception that the coarse tremor seen with alcoholic withdrawal may be absent. Serum and urine screens are necessary to determine the putative agent. High doses of barbiturates cause death by respiratory depression. Severe opiate intoxication can be differentiated from barbiturate intoxication by use of naloxone or another opioid antagonist. Opioid antagonists have no effect on intoxication due to other drugs.

Signs and symptoms of barbiturate withdrawal include anxiety, insomnia, restlessness, irritability, dysattention, formication, paranoia, visual hallucinations, nausea, and vomiting. Psychomotor activity may either increase or decrease. Sexual and aggressive impulses are disinhibited. Intoxication is characterized by ataxia, slurred speech, incoordination, dysattention, and memory impairment.

The amount of barbiturate used daily is estimated by history and use of the barbiturate tolerance test. Patients are then withdrawn slowly using a dose of barbiturate that *just* produces toxic symptoms. Advocates of use of longer-acting barbiturates such as phenobarbital for withdrawal contend that the longer half-life reduces fluctuations in blood barbiturate levels and thereby decreases withdrawal symptoms. In addition, phenobarbital does not produce the high caused by shorter-acting barbiturates. Those who argue for the use of the shorter-acting barbiturates for withdrawal emphasize the flexibility afforded by substances that remain in the bloodstream for only 4 to 6 hours. Daily reduction in dose during uncomplicated withdrawal is 30 mg/day for phenobarbital and 100 mg/day for pentobarbital.

Inpatient hospitalization is recommended for both barbiturate and alcohol withdrawal because of the danger of medical complications.

Benzodiazepine Intoxication and Withdrawal

Withdrawal from long-term use of large doses of benzodiazepines produces signs and symptoms similar to withdrawal from alcohol and barbiturates unless carried out with caution over time.[21] Polysubstance users frequently combine use of benzodiazepines with alcohol, cocaine, or sedative-hypnotics. It is difficult to distinguish among these states without the aid of serum or urine screens. If withdrawal from benzodiazepines is responsible for the clinical picture of withdrawal, commence withdrawal with a dose sufficient to cause remission of symptoms and slowly decrease the daily dose. Weekly decrements of 0.125 mg or 0.25 mg may be needed to withdraw from alprazolam without discomfort.[23] If benzodiazepines are used with opiates, withdraw each independently to allow correct modulation of rate of withdrawal without symptoms.

Caffeine Intoxication

Individuals may present acutely with symptoms of a panic attack due to excess use of caffeine-containing substances such as coffee, tea, and chocolate. Individual tolerance varies.[36] For some, as little as one or two cups induce symptoms and any coffee in the afternoon disturbs sleep. In addition to anxiety, patients may have nausea, vomiting, diarrhea, tachycardia, palpitations, and cardiac arrhythmias. Symptoms abate within 24 to 48 hours of cessation of use. Benzodiazepines are helpful to mollify anxiety, restlessness, and irritability during the acute phase. Patients are well advised to avoid caffeine-containing products in the future if they are found particularly sensitive.

Cannabis Intoxication

Rarely, marijuana smoking leads to behavioral changes mandating emergency intervention. These behavioral changes can usually be attributed to one of four conditions: (1) An individual has smoked or ingested large amounts of a particularly potent variety such as refined hashish; (2) the marijuana used has been adulterated with another substance such as phencyclidine (PCP); (3) the patient's personality and expectations are such that mild symptoms or decreased inhibition leads to anxiety or panic; or (4) cannabis is used to self-medicate emerging schizophrenia, mania, or depression.[1, 2] The magnitude and character of response relate to set (expectation about what should occur), setting, personality, and dose. Most marijuana smokers do not seek medical intervention. Both marijuana and cocaine increase heart rate and blood pressure; when used together, the magnitude is greater than if either were used alone.[37]

Cannabis use can be a factor in persistent insomnia, underachievement in school, decreased drive and motivation, poor appetite, and problem behavior.[38, 39] Chronic use may require medical intervention for successful withdrawal and abstinence.[39] Withdrawal symptoms occur after as little as 21 days of use and include sweating, chills, tremulousness, wild dreams, and insomnia. Onset is usually within 10 hours of cessation of use, and withdrawal is complete in 96 hours. Symptoms of use mimic a number of psychiatric disorders and should be suspected when changes in a clinical state occur in any population at risk.[38] Suicide and homicide risk evaluation and management should be followed by diagnosis-specific treatment of any concurrent psychiatric or medical disorders. Anxiety and psychiatric symptoms directly related to cannabis use are treated with benzodiazepines and neuroleptics, respectively. Urine and serum drug screens are generally sufficient to identify polydrug use.[40]

Hallucinogen Use

Hallucinogens such as lysergic acid diethylamide (LSD), mescaline, and psilocybin may produce frightening distortions of perceptions, paranoia, and intense anxiety from use or after use owing to flashbacks.[2] The majority of hallucinogens are related structurally to serotonin (e.g., LSD) or catecholamines (e.g., mescaline). Cocaine or methedrine is sometimes mixed with a hallucinogen to provide extra stimulation. If strychnine is used as an adulterant, serious medical consequences including death may ensue. Hallucinogen hallucinosis typically occurs with a full alert state. Symptoms relate to the particular drug ingested, dose, duration of action, concomitant drugs used, medical state, premorbid personality, rate of onset of drug used, expectations of the drug used, and setting in which the drugs are taken. If symptoms persist, consideration should be given to the possibility that the drug was used by someone incipiently or already psychotic and to the possibility the drug precipitated psychosis in a genetically predisposed individual. Symptom onset is usually within 1 hour of use and resolves in 4 to 6 hours untreated. In some instances, it may last as long as 2 to 3 days.

Some symptoms are especially characteristic of hallucinogenic psychosis. Body images are often distorted, and kaleidoscopic and other visual hallucinations are dominant. Paranoia and other-directed violence are more characteristic of stimulants. Individuals using hallucinogens may perceive themselves as invulnerable or as possessing Promethean (or perhaps better said Icarian) strength and attempt to fly out of a window, plunging to their death. Synesthesias are characteristic. Colors may be tasted and sounds productive of color. Pseudohallucinations are seen. For instance, users see geometric forms that they know are not real. Hyperacusis, difficulty expressing thoughts, mood lability, increased vividness of both real and fantasized sensations, and feelings of having special insights or religious experiences are other perceptions.

Pupils tend to be reactive and dilated. Heart rate is increased, and a slight increase in blood pressure is noted. Incoordination and sweating may be observed.

Patients ideally are placed in well-lit rooms away from distracting noises and people. They should be repeatedly oriented to time, place, and date and assured that they are not going insane. This orientation process is sometimes referred to as "talking down." The presence of familiar people is comforting and facilitates recovery. Benzodiazepines are used for panic and anxiety. Neuroleptics with minimal anticholinergic properties, such as the high-potency, low-dose phenothiazines and thiothixine, should be used if psychotic symptoms are particularly disturbing. Chlorpromazine is helpful if it is documented that the patient has taken LSD. If a hallucinogen with more anticholinergic properties was used, however, the atropine-like effects of chlorpromazine may enhance both fear and visual hallucinations,

and its use with STP (2,5 dimethoxy-4-methyl-amphetamine) is not safe. If symptoms persist, a more severe underlying psychosis may be responsible.[41]

Flashbacks generally respond to oral anxiolytics such as alprazolam (1 to 2 mg) or small doses of an antipsychotic (e.g., 4 mg of perphenazine).

Opiate Intoxication

Opiate intoxication leads to psychiatric emergencies ranging from confused states to coma.[42] Although patients may protest that they have smoked, snorted, or taken intravenously only the purist opiate derivations, cost-conscious dealers in an economically tight environment may have cut the drug with a number of other substances to increase profit margin. In some instances, a substance use may prove lethal to the customer. The adulterants used complicate the clinical presentation, as do concurrent psychiatric and medical (e.g., AIDS, hepatitis, alcoholism) illness. Nausea is common after the first dose of opiates, but euphoria more often occurs subsequently. Drowsiness, apathy, constipation, and analgesia are common. Heart rate and body temperature are decreased, and speech slurred. Pupils are constricted unless overdose is severe, in which case dilation is seen. The face is flushed, and hypertension may be present. Meperidine (Demerol), like cocaine, causes muscle twitching and seizures in high doses. Narcotic antagonists such as nalorphine, naloxone, and levallorphan reverse the signs and symptoms of narcotic intoxication unless irreversible cerebral anoxia has occurred.

Opiate Withdrawal

Opiate users tend to seek drugs when in withdrawal and in so doing may feign medical illnesses such as a kidney stone in hope that a sympathetic physician may prescribe a narcotic such as morphine. Few narcotic addicts maintain sobriety. Methadone maintenance therapy may be all that can be hoped for. The drugs used and their dose, duration of use, and last use should be determined. Opiate withdrawal occurs with Talwin, Percocet, heroin, morphine, meperidine, Dilaudid, methadone, and Darvon.[43] If a patient is admitted to a treatment facility, a rectal and vaginal inspection should be included in the physical examination to search for hidden drugs. Inspection of needle marks provides clues to the last use. Withdrawal commences after abrupt cessation in 1 to 2 weeks after continuous use and commences pursuant to administration of an opiate agonist after therapeutic doses for 3 to 4 days. Symptoms generally become manifested within 6 to 8 hours after the previous dose, peak at 2 to 3 days, and have run their course by the seventh to tenth day. Death is uncommon for opiate withdrawal unless a patient has concurrent medical problems such as coronary artery disease. Urine and blood screens are used to distinguish opiate from other substance use withdrawal.

Common features of opiate withdrawal are anxiety, myalgia, nausea, hot and cold flashes, and craving for opiates. Patients yawn, perspire, and lacrimate. Pupils dilate and respond poorly if at all to light. Gooseflesh is seen, and heart rate and blood pressure are increased. Patients experience rhinorrhea and, if male, orgasm. They are restless and febrile, suffer diarrhea, often vomit, and are insomniac.

Methadone given in gradually decreasing doses based on the estimated use at cessation is provided because of its cross-tolerance with a number of opiates. Rate of withdrawal should never exceed 20% of the daily dose above 20 mg of methadone per day. Trimethobenzamide (Tigan) and hydroxyzine (Vistaril) are used if nausea and vomiting occur despite adequate opiate provision for other withdrawal symptoms. Individuals concurrently addicted to sedative-hypnotics or benzodiazepines experience symptoms of withdrawal unless a sedative-hypnotic or benzodiazepine is provided to prevent discomfort during withdrawal. Clonidine is often used to minimize withdrawal symptoms of opiates but is ineffective for withdrawal of benzodiazepines.[44]

Phencyclidine Intoxication

Angel dust (PCP) is a powerful hallucinogen with cholinergic, dopaminergic, and opioid properties.[45] In addition to its ability to induce violent behavior to the extent of homicide, it can cause death. Large doses result in status epilepticus and adrenergic crises, with respiratory failure as a late sequela. The drug may be taken orally or intravenously, snorted, or smoked. It can contaminate marijuana and other mind-altering drugs such as mescaline and LSD, causing a response to them far greater than the user anticipated.

Symptom onset is rapid and often confused with schizophrenia. Patients may be quite incapacitated, with considerable risk to themselves and others. The clinical picture of PCP intoxication is less dependent on a user's personality than the clinical presentations of other hallucinogens. Intoxicated individuals tend to be hostile, agitated, suspicious, and paranoid. Ataxia, paresthesias, and analgesia are characteristic, with pupils constricted or normal. Patients often experience a dissociation of somatic sensation. Temperature, heart rate, and deep tendon reflexes are increased, and the sensorium clouded. Position sense is impaired, and nystagmus occurs, initially horizontal and with time vertical. Rigidity, myoclonus, and muscle spasticity are also features.

PCP intoxication is a true medical emergency and may require care in a medical unit until a patient's physical condition is stabilized. Haloperidol and thiothixene are more effective than chlorpromazine, which may aggravate the clinical picture.[46] Diazepam is effective for symptomatic relief but may impede urinary removal of PCP. Cranberry juice and ascorbic acid are provided to acidify the urine and enhance excretion.[47, 48]

Vital signs are monitored, external stimuli reduced, and instrumentation avoided when possible. Serum half-life is 1 to 3 days in overdoses. Blood, urine, and gastric contents are obtained for analysis. Individuals are provided protection from harm by themselves or others. Cardiovascular or respiratory complications may require transfer to a medical venue.

Those who prefer diazepam for management argue that neuroleptics may induce dangerous hypotensive crises. Urine PCP levels do not predict hypotensive crises, drug interactions, or violent behavior.[49]

Volatile Nitrates

Volatile nitrates such as amyl nitrate (poppers, rush) are used to promote abandonment in art, sex, and dance and are especially popular in the gay subculture. Seldom does use of these substances result in symptoms that necessitate emergency psychiatric intervention.[1] Lightheadedness and alterations in consciousness generally pass quickly after cessation of use. Inverted T waves and a depressed ST segment may appear transiently on the electrocardiogram.

REFERENCES

1. Slaby AE: Handbook of Psychiatric Emergencies, 4th ed. Norwalk, CT, Appleton & Lange, 1994.

2. Giannini AJ, Slaby AE: Handbook of Overdose and Detoxification Emergencies. New York, Medical Examination Publishing Company, 1983.

3. Dulit RA, Fyer MR, Haas GL, et al: Substance use in borderline personality disorder. Am J Psychiatry 147:1002–1007, 1990.

4. Gukstien OG, Brent DA, Kamineo Y: Comorbidity of substance abuse and other psychiatric disorders in adolescents. Am J Psychiatry 146:1131–1141, 1989.

5. Murphy GE: Suicide and substance abuse. Arch Gen Psychiatry 45:593–596, 1988.

6. Roehrich H, Gold MS: Diagnosis of substance abuse in an adolescent psychiatric population. Int J Psychiatry 16:137–143, 986–987.

7. Slaby AE, Garfinkel LF: No One Saw My Pain. New York, Norton, 1994.

8. Steinberg DE: Dual diagnosis: Addiction and affective disorders. The Psychiatric Hospital 20:71–77, 1989.

9. Weiss RD, Mirin SM: The dual diagnosis alcoholic evaluation and treatment. Psychiatr Anna 19:261–265, 1989.

10. Mueser KT, Yarnold PR, Levinson DF, et al: Prevalence of substance abuse in schizophrenia: Demographic and clinical correlates. Schizophr Bull 16:31–58, 1990.

11. Zweben JE: Recovery oriented psychotherapy: Facilitating the use of 12-step programs. J Psychoactive Drugs 15:243–251, 1987.

12. Charness DS, Simon RP, Greenberg DA: Ethanol and the nervous system. N Engl J Med 321:442–454, 1989.

13. Drake RE, Osher FC, Noordsy DL, et al: Diagnosis of alcohol use disorders in schizophrenia. Schizophr Bull 16:57–67, 1990.

14. Cohen M, Kern JC, Hassett C: Identifying alcoholism in medical patients. Hosp Community Psychiatry 37:358–400, 1986.

15. Koranyi EK, Ravidrm A, Sequin J: Alcohol withdrawal concealing symptoms of subdural hematoma—a caveat. Psychiatric Journal of the University of Ottawa 15:15–17, 1990.

16. Bokstrom K, Baldin J, Langstrom G: Alcohol withdrawal and mood. Acta Psychiatric Scand 80:505–513, 1989.

17. Bulik CM: Drug and alcohol abuse by bulimic women and their families. Am J Psychiatry 144:1604–1606, 1987.

18. Dorus W, Kennedy J, Gibbons RD, Ravi SD: Symptoms and diagnosis of depression in alcoholics. Alcohol Clin Exp Res 11:152–156, 1987.

19. Kushner MG, Sher KJ, Beitman BD: The relation between alcohol problems and the anxiety disorders. Am J Psychiatry 147:685–695, 1990.

20. Meyer RE: Anxiolytics and the alcoholic patient. J Stud Alcohol 47:269–273, 1986.

21. Bustro U, Kaplan HL, Sellers EM: Benzodiazepine-associated emergencies in Toronto. Am J Psychiatry 137:224–227, 1980.

22. Juergens SM, Morse RM: Alprazolam dependence in seven patients. Am J Psychiatry 145:625–627, 1988.

23. Cantopher T, Oliveri S, Cleave N, et al: Chronic benzodiazepine dependence: A comparative study of abrupt withdrawal under propranolol cover versus gradual withdrawal. Br J Psychiatry 156:406–411, 1990.

24. Schweizer E, Case WG, Rickels K: Benzodiazepine dependence and withdrawal in elderly patients. Am J Psychiatry 146:529–531, 1989.

25. Schweizer E, Rickels K: Failure of buspirone to manage benzodiazepine withdrawal. Am J Psychiatry 143:1590–1592, 1986.

26. Estroff TW, Gold MS: Medical and psychiatric complications of cocaine abuse with possible points of pharmacological treatment. Controversies in Alcoholism and Substance Abuse 10:61–76, 1986.

27. Gawin FH, Ellinwood EH: Cocaine dependence. Annu Rev Med 40:149–161, 1989.

28. Gawin FH, Kleber HD: Abstinence symptomatology and psychiatric diagnoses in cocaine abusers. Arch Gen Psychiatry 43:107–113, 1986.

29. Raskin DE: Amphetamine use. J Clin Psychopharmacol 3:262, 1983.

30. Baxter LR: Desipramine in the treatment of hypersomulence following abrupt cessation of cocaine use. Am J Psychiatry 140:1525–1526, 1983.

31. Dackis CA, Gold MS, Sweeney DR, et al: Single-dose bromocriptine reverses cocaine craving. Psychiatry Res 20:261–264, 1987.

32. Gawin FH, Kleber HD: Cocaine abuse treatment: Open pilot trial with desipramine and lithium carbonate. Arch Gen Psychiatry 41:903–909, 1984.

33. Gawin FH, Kleber HD, Bydo R, et al: Desipramine facilitation of initial cocaine abstinence. Arch Gen Psychiatry 46:117–121, 1989.

34. Taylor WA, Gold MS: Pharmacologic approaches to the treatment of cocaine dependence. West J Med 152:573–577. 1990.

35. Epstein RS: Withdrawal symptoms from chronic use of low-dose barbiturates. Am J Psychiatry 137:107–108, 1980.

36. Gilliland K, Andress D: Ad lib caffeine consumption symptoms of caffeinism and academic performance. Am J Psychiatry 138:512–574, 1981.

37. Foltin RW, Fischman MW, Pedroso JJ, Pearlson GD: Marijuana and cocaine interactions in humans: Cardiovascular consequences. Pharmacol Biochem Behav 28:459–464, 1987.

38. Estroff TW, Gold MS: Psychiatric presentations of marijuana abuse. Psychiatr Ann 16:21–224, 1986.

39. Tenmont FS: The clinical syndrome of marijuana dependence. Psychiatr Ann 16:225–234, 1986.

40. Vereberg K, Gold MS, Mule SJ: Laboratory testing in the diagnosis of marijuana intoxication and withdrawal. Psychiatr Ann 16:234–241, 1986.

41. Bowers MB, Mazure CM, Nelson JC, et al: Psychotogenic drug use and neuroleptic response. Schizophr Bull 16:81–85, 1990.

42. Eisendrath SJ, Goldman B, Douglas J, et al: Meperidine-induced delirium. Am J Psychiatry 144:1062–1065, 1987.

43. Johnson DA, Bohan ME: Propoxyphene withdrawal with clonidine. Am J Psychiatry 140:1217–1218, 1983.

44. Charney DS, Heninger GR, Kleber HD: The combined use of clonidine and naltrexone as a rapid, safe, and effective treatment of abrupt withdrawal from methadone. Am J Psychiatry 143:831–837, 1986.

45. Giannini AJ, Giannini MC, Price WA: Antidotal strategies in phencyclidine intoxication. Int J Psychiatry Med 14:315–321, 1984.

46. Giannini AJ, Eishan MS, Loiselle RH, Giannini MC: Comparison of haloperidol and chlorpromazine in the treatment of phencyclidine psychosis. J Clin Pharmacol 29:202–204, 1989.

47. Allen RM, Young SJ: Phencyclidine-induced psychosis. Am J Psychiatry 135:1081–1084, 1978.

48. Castellani S, Giannini AJ, Adams PM: Physostigmine and haloperidol treatment of acute phencyclidine intoxication. Am J Psychiatry 139:508–510, 1982.

49. Khajawall AM, Erickson TB, Simpson GM: Chronic phencyclidine abuse and physical assault. Am J Psychiatry 139:1604–1606, 1982.

Anxiety Disorders and Addictions

Sajiv John, M.D. • Norman S. Miller, M.D.

Many alcohol- and drug-dependent persons display symptoms of anxiety at some stage in their illness. Studies have shown that 50% to 67% of alcohol-dependent men have high scores on state anxiety measures, with symptoms that can resemble generalized anxiety disorder, panic disorder, or phobic disorder. These figures are increased in the context of intoxication or withdrawal, with up to 80% admitting to repetitive panic attacks during these states.[1] Some workers have concluded that anxiety and addictive disorders are genetically linked, whereas others have postulated that persons with anxiety disorders are trying to self-medicate their symptoms with drugs or alcohol. Studies have also shown that it can be very difficult to distinguish between temporary syndromes related to intoxication or withdrawal and a coexisting independent anxiety disorder that may require long-term treatment.[2] Distinguishing between them is crucial, however, because treatment strategies are very different.

Epidemiology

The findings of the Epidemiological Catchment Area study provided support for the notion that psychiatric disorders are frequently associated with alcohol/drug disorders.[3] One third of the total population in that sample met lifetime criteria for one of the psychiatric diagnoses, and one third of those with one diagnosis also had a second psychiatric diagnosis. Alcohol dependence was the most common diagnosis made, affecting 13.7% of the population, and phobias were the next most common disorder, diagnosed in 12.8% of the population. These trends have been reproduced in the more recent National Comorbidity Survey,[4] which revealed total lifetime and 12-month prevalence rates for any anxiety disorder in the general population to be 24.9% and 17.2%, respectively. Both studies did establish comorbidity but did not address causality or attempt to make primary and secondary distinctions. This becomes an important issue, because alcohol and drug dependence can produce many of the psychiatric syndromes described in these studies. Conversely, alcohol and drug dependence may exist independently with these other disorders.

Some studies have shown high rates of anxiety in patients with drug or alcohol addiction. Stockwell and colleagues[5] reported that as many as 80% of their male inpatient alcoholic sample had agoraphobia or social phobia when last drinking. The more severely phobic men were found to be most dependent on alcohol, whereas those with no phobias were the least alcohol dependent. They also showed that dependence on alcohol and periods of heavy drinking were associated with an exacerbation of agoraphobia and social phobia. Subsequent periods of abstinence were associated with significant improvement in these anxiety states. Studies such as this one have usually focused on patients who are actively dependent or are in early withdrawal. It is currently believed that anxiety disorders coexist with addictive disorders at rates no different from that in the general population for anxiety disorders alone, irrespective of the degree of addiction. Similarly rigorous studies have shown no evidence that the rates of alcohol or drug addiction are greater in subjects with a lifelong anxiety disorder.[6]

Mechanisms

PHARMACOLOGICAL EFFECTS

Anxiety can occur during acute and chronic intoxication with stimulants such as cocaine or withdrawal from depressants such as alcohol. The mechanism underlying both these states is believed to be catecholamine discharge from the sympathetic nervous system. This catecholamine release produces symptoms that are indistinguishable from the classic features of anxiety.[7] Interestingly, lactate infusion produces panic attacks in alcoholics as well as in those with an innate vulnerability to panic attacks. Furthermore, alcoholics tend to have high lactate levels during intoxication, more evidence that chronic alcohol intake may have an etiological role in the development of anxiety.

THE SELF-MEDICATION HYPOTHESIS

Several workers have reported that when alcohol and anxiety disorders occur in the same person, as many as 40% to 60% of these individuals report anxiety as having preceded the alcohol problem.[8] These findings largely fueled the self-medication hypothesis, which essentially states that people with anxiety or depression self-medicate themselves with alcohol or drugs to obtain relief from their primary symptoms. Retrospective data analysis and subjective reports suffer major limitations in this area—addicts often rationalize their behavior, suffer from poor recall, and frequently use the defense of denial. More rigorous studies have shown that two thirds of the patients who said that their alcohol problem developed after the behavioral condition showed evidence of severe alcohol-related problems before other diagnosable anxiety syndromes were diagnosed.[9, 10] It is also well known that regular use of alcohol or drugs can worsen an underlying psychiatric disorder. Preoccupation with obtaining the drug, repeated withdrawal symptoms, poor compliance with prescribed medication or therapy, and the adverse psychosocial and medical consequences that an addict inevitably faces all can clearly worsen an underlying psychiatric condition such as an anxiety disorder. In the majority of cases, abstinence results in improvement in most anxiety symptoms. This normalization may sometimes be delayed several weeks, even a few months. Data generated before the onset of drug or alcohol dependence or after prolonged abstinence reveal little evidence of major anxiety syndromes.[11]

GENETICS

Alcoholism is a genetically influenced condition. The risk for alcohol abuse or dependence is three to four times higher in children of alcoholics than in comparison subjects. If persons at high risk are to develop alcohol disorders as a consequence of anxiety or if alcohol and anxiety are genetically linked, one would expect to find a higher than normal rate of anxiety disorders before the onset of alcohol dependence in the children of alcoholics. Studies that have assessed anxiety levels among children of alcoholics and adopted-away children of alcoholics have revealed a higher than normal rate of antisocial personality disorder, impulsiveness, and low self-esteem. Some studies have discovered higher levels of anxiety symptoms but not of anxiety disorders in these children. More long-term studies in this area are awaited. Further, when alcoholic twin pairs were observed over time, only the heavily drinking twin showed anxiety symptoms, suggesting that the anxiety was a pharmacological effect of chronic alcohol use and not an etiological factor. It is currently believed that there is no evidence that either of these groups, who are at high risk for developing alcoholism, are also at risk for developing anxiety disorders.[6, 12]

Other studies have assessed the prevalence of alcoholism in the biological relatives of persons with an anxiety disorder. They have focused on persons with panic disorder, phobic disorders, and generalized anxiety disorder. Although some have suggested a modest crossover in some pedigrees, in general they have not shown a consistent crossover between alcoholism and anxiety disorders. One study used structured personal interviews to evaluate the rate of major psychiatric disorders in 605 first-degree relatives of alcohol-dependent men and women. After controlling for several potential confounding variables, the rates of disorders among those interviewed included 3% for panic disorder, 1% each for agoraphobia and obsessive-compulsive disorder (OCD), and 2% for social phobia, with an overall rate for major anxiety disorder in first-degree relatives of 7%. These percentages are comparable to those expected in the general population.[6]

PSYCHOSOCIAL

Prolonged use of alcohol or drugs usually results in dysfunction and conflict in various areas such as family, work, and interpersonal relationships. Many alcohol- or drug-dependent men and women grow up in homes that lack a stable environment because of alcohol or drug use and antisocial personality disorder in their parents. Many alcohol or drug users may have cognitive deficits, including a fetal alcohol effect. Anxiety symptoms or a worsening of true anxiety disorder could occur as a consequence.[13]

Other factors complicate data interpretation. The criteria for alcohol and drug dependence have changed during the past few decades and are not applied in a consistent fashion. This clearly limits the conclusions that can be drawn from available data. Also, once assortative mating—in this context, the tendency of an alcohol or drug-dependent individual to select a spouse with alcohol, drug, antisocial, or other psychiatric problems—is considered, the rate of anxiety disorder in relatives of alcoholics decreases by about 10%. Therefore, finding anxiety disorders among alcohol-dependent individuals could be a result of a family history of anxiety disorder that is independent of alcohol problems.[6]

Clinical Features

Any of the anxiety disorders described in DSM-IV[14] can occur during intoxication or withdrawal. Phobias, panic disorder, and generalized anxiety disorder are described most commonly. DSM-IV refers to these states as substance-induced anxiety disorders, and they typically include prominent anxiety, panic attacks, or obsessions and compulsions occurring during or within 1 month of substance intoxication or withdrawal. These symptoms have to cause significant distress or impairment in social, occupational, or other important areas of functioning and should not occur exclu-

sively during the course of a delirium. Anxiety arising as a consequence of alcohol or drug use typically abates after a few days to weeks of abstinence. It may occasionally persist for a prolonged period (i.e., weeks to months) and therefore needs careful observation and follow-up.

Anxiety can also occur independently as a comorbid disorder. The clinical features of the anxiety syndrome induced by alcohol or drugs are identical to those in an anxiety syndrome arising de novo. It can therefore be very difficult to distinguish a true dual diagnosis from anxiety occurring as part of intoxication or withdrawal. DSM-IV criteria attempt to differentiate the two. Evidence that an anxiety disorder is not substance induced might include the following: The symptoms precede the onset of substance use; the symptoms persist for a substantial period after cessation of acute withdrawal or severe intoxication or are substantially in excess of what would be expected given the type or amount of the substance used or the duration of use; or there is other evidence of an independent non–substance-induced anxiety disorder (e.g., a history of recurrent non–substance-related episodes).

Treatment

Withdrawal symptoms always need to be treated. Close monitoring for serious complications such as seizures or delirium tremens during alcohol withdrawal is essential. Anxiety or depressive symptoms during withdrawal from alcohol are very common and usually transient. Benzodiazepines such as chlordiazepoxide (Librium) or lorazepam (Ativan) are often prescribed during this phase. Going "cold turkey" and suffering withdrawal symptoms or being made to suffer withdrawal for a condition that is perceived as a weakness of character has been shown not to contribute to motivation and has been shown to lead to a high treatment dropout rate. The major phase of withdrawal is typically 3 to 5 days for most drugs—for example, alcohol, heroin, and most short- and medium-acting sedative-hypnotics. Drugs with a longer half-life such as diazepam or methadone can manifest a withdrawal syndrome that begins later and lasts several days longer. High levels of anxiety generally continue to improve with continued abstinence, although such anxiety can occasionally persist as long as 3 months.

Despite the various approaches to the problem of addiction, the *12-step approach* remains a crucial part of treatment. The effectiveness of Alcoholics Anonymous (AA) may be accounted for by its thorough response to the addictive problem. AA provides cognitive strategies, compensatory psychological mechanisms, and intrapersonal and interpersonal resources to assist addicted persons in successfully negotiating the vicissitudes of human living.[15] Surveys of AA members show recovery rates of 44% at less than 1 year, 83% between 1 and 5 years, and 91% at greater than 5 years of weekly attendance at regular meetings. Cognitive-behavioral techniques in the 12-step treatment approach are effective for anxiety symptoms associated with addiction. Ultimately, the progression of the alcoholism or drug addiction will determine the prognosis of both disorders whether or not the anxiety is treated by other means.[16]

As mentioned earlier, the longer the anxiety persists during abstinence, the more likely it is that the patient has a true dual diagnosis. Treatment in this case is essentially the same as in an anxiety disorder occurring without coexisting alcohol or drug addiction, with some differences. Most of the discussion that follows focuses on the treatment of persons with generalized anxiety disorder, panic disorder with or without agoraphobia, and phobic disorder. A *cognitive-behavioral approach* is very effective for persons with both anxiety and addiction and is widely used for those with mild to moderate impairment. The major cognitive-behavioral techniques for panic and generalized anxiety disorders are breathing retraining, exposure to somatic cues, relaxation training, and cognitive restructuring to give the uncomfortable effects and physical sensations associated with panic a more benign interpretation. Techniques that have proved effective with phobic disorders include exposure (in vivo, individual or group), cognitive restructuring, and social skills training.[17] There are limited data available on management of OCD and addictive disorder. Clinical experience suggests that treatment of OCD with clomipramine or selective serotonin reuptake inhibitors (SSRIs) and specific behavioral techniques such as exposure procedures and response prevention in conjunction with a 12-step–based approach to the addiction is effective. A discussion of posttraumatic stress disorder (PTSD) and addiction can be found in another part of the book and is not addressed here in detail except to state that it is crucial to treat the addiction using the principles outlined earlier and not to assume that all symptoms are due to PTSD.

Medication remains an option for those who are significantly impaired by their anxiety after adequate time and involvement in a recovery program for addiction. A thorough evaluation to assess whether the individual is abstinent, using continuing treatment, or attending self-help meetings, and using other forms of addiction therapy is usually necessary before a diagnosis of psychiatric comorbidity can be definitely established. Medication can sedate and dull reactions to external stimuli; this may be countertherapeutic in a person recovering from an addiction. Some anxiety during abstinence is important for growth and recovery. An addict's ability to use the 12 steps of AA and to accept psychiatric advice depends on clear thinking and emotional balance. When medications are used, a specific target symptom should be the focus. Also, medication should always be tried in time-limited intervals such as weeks to months. A drug holiday should then be attempted to see if the medicine is still necessary. Benzodiazepines, if prescribed, are best used for short periods under close supervision to bring symptoms under control quickly and facilitate other treatment approaches.

Drugs such as diazepam (Valium), lorazepam, and alprazolam (Xanax) are very effective antianxiety agents but are best avoided because they are frequently used by addicts and also have a street value. Agents such as clonazepam (Klonopin, 0.25 to 0.50 mg two to three times a day) or lorazepam (10 to 25 mg two to three times a day) are effective and appear to have less abuse potential with lower street value. They are preferably avoided in the medium to long term because these patients are vulnerable to addiction. Drug seeking in the case of benzodiazepines is common and must be distinguished from true withdrawal. Drug seeking is generally characterized by attention and focus by the patient on the drug, a lack of objective withdrawal symptoms, and a reluctance to consider nondrug therapies for symptomatic relief.[16–18]

Most drug treatment today features antidepressants, both tricyclics and the SSRIs, and buspirone. Tricyclics and SSRIs have been shown to be effective in treating both anxiety and depression and can be used long term. Tricyclics, such as imipramine and nortriptyline, can produce sedation, hypotension, syncope, and other anticholinergic side effects. The SSRIs fluoxetine (Prozac), sertraline (Zoloft), and paroxetine (Paxil) can produce an initial increase in anxiety, sedation, insomnia, and gastrointestinal upset. Although both drugs are effective, SSRIs are gaining wider use because of their lower addiction potential, reduced anticholinergic effects, and lower risk of lethal effects in the event of an overdose. A withdrawal syndrome that is much milder than that produced by benzodiazepines has been described with most antidepressants including the SSRIs. Buspirone has been shown effective in treating mild to moderate anxiety and does not have addiction potential. In doses of 15 to 60 mg a day, it can significantly decrease anxiety symptoms in recovering addicts. It can also be given in combination with the SSRIs.[16–18]

Outcomes

Outcome studies have been very few. The ones that have appeared have been frequently criticized as suffering from poor methods. One focus of outcome studies has been the primary location of the patient (i.e., in an addiction setting or in a psychiatric setting). Studies have shown that in an *addiction setting*, the use of medication generally tends to be discouraged, although it is gaining more acceptance for legitimate independent psychiatric disorders. There is usually a waiting period for the pharmacological and addictive effects of the drugs to resolve or lessen before initiating pharmacotherapy. The exceptions are usually cases of documented schizophrenia or mania. Anxiety and depression are usually associated with addictive disorder and are believed to require no or sparing use of medication. Because of these expectations within therapy groups, patients with major mental illness such as schizophrenia, mania, and anxiety disorders such as OCD tend to be excluded unless they meet strict behavior control. These disorders also tend not to be diagnosed or treated unless they significantly interfere with function. Conversely, in a *psychiatric setting*, even though increasing reports of comorbid psychiatric and addictive disorders have appeared in recent years, studies show that addictive disorders continue to be underdiagnosed. The self-medication hypothesis continues to be a source of error in psychiatric diagnosis that leads to reduced rates and incomplete treatment for addictive disorders.[19]

A review summarizes treatment outcome data from 49 inpatient and 33 outpatient sites throughout the United States.[20] The data are from the Comprehensive Assessment and Treatment Outcome Research (CATOR), which is the largest independent evaluation service for addictions treatment in the United States. Most programs monitored are variations of the Minnesota model, but psychiatrically based and aversion therapy models are included as well. The sample consisted of 6508 American Society of Addiction Medicine (ASAM) level III patients (inpatients) and 1572 ASAM level II patients (outpatients). The results were as follows:

1. Both inpatients and outpatients were similar in their demographic characteristics, being largely composed of white men between the ages of 20 and 40, high-school educated, employed, and from middle-class to lower middle-class households.

2. The populations differed significantly in clinical characteristics, with more than twice as many of the inpatients being dependent on prescription drugs, stimulants, marijuana, or opiates in addition to alcohol.

3. A global clinical severity index was developed from the number of symptoms for alcohol and drug dependence, the patterns of use, and the most recent use. Forty percent of inpatients scored in the higher range, compared with only 20% of the outpatients. About a third of outpatients fell in the lowest range of this index, and only one in seven inpatients showed such low indications of severity.

4. Inpatients also had higher levels of medical problems and problems with vocational functioning before admission.

5. The 1-year abstinence rate when all cases, including noncontacted individuals, were included fell within the 45% to 60% range.

6. Both inpatients and outpatients who attended either AA or continuing-care programs were more likely to remain abstinent than nonattenders. Ninety percent of those who attended both AA on a weekly basis and aftercare for the entire year maintained their abstinence.

7. Analysis of those who suffered a relapse after the first 6 months revealed significantly higher stress levels than those who were able to maintain their abstinence during that period. Continuing care may be more appropriate to address some of this stress, whereas AA may be better at addressing issues of craving.

8. Both inpatients and outpatients showed significant decreases in posttreatment medical care use for expensive hospital services. Admissions for medical conditions were decreased by 50%.

Few studies have attempted to predict the role of a lifetime diagnosis of a major psychiat-

ric illness on the treatment outcome in an abstinence-based program. One such study[20] evaluated 6355 subjects from inpatient (78.4%) and
outpatient (21.6%) programs from 41 independent sites. The subjects received structured interviews to document treatment outcomes for
abstinence and the diagnosis of depressive disorder. A diagnosis of major depression did not
predict the abstinence rate at 1 year from alcohol and drugs (54.9% versus 54.4%). Attendance at continuing-care and AA meetings was
associated with significantly better abstinence
rates. Depressed patients were more likely to
be regular attenders.

REFERENCES

1. Brown SA, Irwin M, Schuckit MA: Changes in anxiety among abstinent male alcoholics. J Stud Alcohol 52:55–61, 1991.
2. Angst J, Vollrath M: The natural history of anxiety disorders. Acta Psychiatr Scand 84:446–452, 1991.
3. Robins LN, Locke BZ, Regier DA: An overview of psychiatric disorders in America. In Robins LN, Regier DA (eds): Psychiatric Disorders in America. New York, Free Press, 1991.
4. Kessler RC, McGonagle KA, Zhao S, et al: Lifetime and 12 month prevalence of psychiatric disorders in the United States. Results from the National Comorbidity Survey. Arch Gen Psychiatry 51(1):8–19, 1994.
5. Stockwell T, Smail P, Hodgson R, Canter S: Alcohol dependence and phobic states II. A retrospective study. Br J Psychiatry 144:58–63, 1984.
6. Schuckit MA, Hesselbrock V: Alcohol dependence and anxiety disorders: What is the relationship? Am J Psychiatry 151(12):1723–1734, 1994.
7. Miller NS: Psychiatric diagnosis in drugs and alcohol addiction. Alcohol Treat Q 12(2):75–92, 1995.
8. Weiss KJ, Rosenberg DJ: Prevalence of anxiety disorders among alcoholics. J Clin Psychiatry 46:3–5, 1985.
9. Morrissey ER, Schuckit MA: Stressful life events and alcoholism among women seen at a detoxification centre. J Stud Alcohol 39:1559–1576, 1978.
10. Vaillant G: The Natural History of Alcoholism. Cambridge, MA, Harvard University Press, 1983.
11. Schuckit MA, Montero MG: Alcoholism, anxiety, depression. Br J Addict 83:1373–1380, 1980.
12. Schuckit MA: Biological vulnerability to alcoholism. J Consult Clin Psychol 55:301–309, 1987.
13. Reich W, Earls F, Powell J: A comparison of the home and social environments of children of alcoholic and nonalcoholic parents. Br J Addict 83:831–839, 1988.
14. American Psychiatric Association: Diagnostic and Statistical Manual of Mental Disorders, 4th ed. Washington, DC, American Psychiatric Association, 1994.
15. Hopson RE, Beaird-Spiller B: Why AA works: A psychological analysis of the addictive experience and the efficacy of alcoholics anonymous. Alcohol Treat Q 12(3):1–17, 1995.
16. Miller NS: Pharmacotherapy in alcoholism. In Miller NS: Treatment of the Addictions: Applications of Outcome Research for Clinical Management. Binghamton, NY, Haworth Press, 1995, pp 129–152.
17. Hollander E, Simeon D, Gorman JM: Anxiety disorders. In Hales RE, Yudofsky SC, Talbott JA (eds): American Psychiatric Press Textbook of Psychiatry, 2nd ed. Washington, DC, American Psychiatric Press, 1994.
18. Miller NS: Pharmacological management of major comorbid psychiatric disorders in drug and alcohol addictions. Psychiatr Ann 25(10):621–627, 1995.
19. Miller NS, Gold MS: The psychologist's role in integrating pharmacological and nonpharmacological treatments for addictive disorders. Psychiatr Ann 22(8):436–440, 1992.
20. Miller N, Hoffman NG: Addictions treatment outcomes. In Miller NS: Treatment of the Addictions: Applications of Outcome Research for Clinical Management. Binghamton, NY, Haworth Press, 1995, pp 41–56.

Treatment of Addictive and Depressive Disorders

Christopher Sinnappan, MD •
Norman S. Miller, MD

Diagnosis of Addiction and Affective Disorders

Affective disorders are difficult to diagnose in the presence of addictive disorders. On the other hand, an addictive disorder in the presence of affective symptoms is not particularly difficult to diagnose. Addictive disorders frequently can emulate all the affective disorders. An intoxicated alcoholic can have all the signs and symptoms resembling a major depressive episode, and a detoxifying alcoholic can have the signs and symptoms resembling an anxiety disorder as found in DSM-IV. A crack cocaine addict who is intoxicated resembles a person with bipolar disorder having a manic episode. That same addict, when he or she crashes off the cocaine high, can become profoundly depressed and suicidal and can have feelings of helplessness and worthlessness. How does one make a diagnosis of an affective disorder in patients with addiction or a diagnosis of an addictive disorder in a setting of affective symptoms?

CLINICAL APPROACHES TO ALCOHOL-INDUCED SYMPTOMS

When considering alcoholism and depression, several reasons can be cited for the diffi- culty in diagnosing the two disorders. Alcohol can cause depressive symptoms.[1-4] Prolonged drinking can lead to signs of temporary serious depression.[5] The comorbidity of lifetime diagnoses of alcoholism and major depression is about 30% to 50%, as found in the Epidemiological Catchment Area Study.[6]

The first step in the diagnosis is to achieve abstinence of at least 2 to 4 weeks' duration before attempting to diagnose major depression.[7] Data on this natural course of alcoholism showed that 42% of inpatient male alcoholics had scores of 20 or greater on the Hamilton Depression Rating Scale on admission for alcohol treatment and that at 4 weeks only 6% continued to have such high Hamilton scores suggestive of major depression.[8] Another study, which looked at recently admitted alcoholics, showed that 32% on admission had major depressive disorder, but these patients had a 50% drop in their depressive symptoms in the first 3 weeks of abstinence.[9]

In one study, Brown and colleagues showed that depressive symptoms decreased rapidly among primary alcoholics versus those with a primary affective disorder. "A minimum of 3 weeks of abstinence from alcohol was needed to distinguish between groups with a primary alcohol dependence and a secondary affective disorder versus a group with a primary affective disorder and a secondary alcohol dependence." During that time, the former group had a 49% reduction in Hamilton depression scale scores, compared with a 14% reduction in Hamilton depression scale scores in the latter group.[10]

Addiction treatment must be the first step to help patients maintain sobriety and abstinence. It is only in the presence of several weeks of sobriety that a correct diagnosis of an affective disorder can be made. Depression in many alcoholics abates with abstinence and addiction treatment.[11]

SUICIDALITY

The caveat to this addiction-first treatment is a patient who is suicidal, homicidal, or medically unstable. The first two conditions require inpatient psychiatric admission for stabilization and for the protection of the patient and others. The last condition requires medical admission and treatment. An alcoholic's mood swings and depression must be taken seriously. Alcoholism carries a 10% to 15% risk of successful suicide completion, and addiction creates a higher risk for suicide attempt.[12] A patient's safety must be the primary consideration. Once a patient is psychiatrically and medically stabilized, addiction treatment must proceed at once.

DIAGNOSIS OF MAJOR DEPRESSION

After 2 to 4 weeks of abstinence, reevaluation of patients may reveal a concomitant diagnosis of major depression. It is important that this condition be treated. It is also important that patients, their families, physicians, and other staff not fall into the self-medication trap.[13] Physicians and patients frequently see addiction as caused by depression and not an independent disease process. Patients are more likely to seek treatment and maintain abstinence if they believe they have a disease.[13] If patients start to believe that they were depressed and that was why they began to drink, then the importance of treating the addiction wanes. Denial sets in rapidly. Denial is a primary process in which the addiction flourishes.[11] It is important that patients and physicians realize that they are dealing with two illnesses that are independent and require treatment.

In one study, a lifetime diagnosis of major depression was shown not to have a strong effect on addiction treatment outcome. In fact, the strongest correlation to addiction treatment outcome was found to be attendance in aftercare and self-support groups. No difference in legal outcomes, medical utilization, or psychosocial adjustment factors was found between depressed and nondepressed alcoholics.[14] Previous studies show that depressed alcoholics resemble nondepressed alcoholics more than they do depressed nonalcoholics.[15] Evidence seems to indicate that an addiction must be treated vigorously without regard to other affective disorders.

LABORATORY FINDINGS IN DIAGNOSIS OF ADDICTION

Although the diagnosis of addictive disorders and affective disorders is a clinical one, laboratory tests have an important secondary role in the clinical assessment. Laboratory tests can verify statements of use, relapse, and system damage due to chronic use.

An elevated gamma-glutamyl transferase (GGT) level can be found in two out of three alcoholics. GGT is a sensitive measure of drug and alcohol damage to the liver.[16] Elevated mean corpuscular volume (MCV) is noted in one fourth of alcoholics. A late sign of alcoholism, an elevated MCV shows the effect of alcohol on folate metabolism and its direct toxic effect on the bone marrow.[17]

One of ten alcoholics have increased uric acid levels. Alcohol metabolism leads to increased lactic acid production. Lactic acid competes with uric acid in the kidneys for excretion sites.[18] In 80% of individuals who drink heavily, one or more have an increased level of carbohydrate deficient transferrin (CDT). CDT is highly specific for heavy alcohol consumption and is not elevated in liver disease. It may be a useful marker in follow-up studies of alcoholics in treatment.[19]

A blood alcohol level (BAL) exceeding 150 mg/dl without any obvious signs of intoxication is diagnostic of alcoholism.[20] Such high BALs without symptoms indicate a high level of tolerance consistent with dependence. However, BALs indicate use during the past 2 to 12 hours only.

Urine toxicology tests for cocaine, heroin, methadone, phencyclidine, marijuana, benzodiazepines, and barbituates reflect a 1- to 3-day window of past use.[21] However, urine samples are difficult to obtain with honesty from addicts and are easily evaded. All urine toxicology tests should be supervised collections to ensure reliability of results. These urine tests are ways of determining compliance with treatment.

COLLATERAL SOURCES OF INFORMATION FOR DIAGNOSIS

It is important early in the course of treatment to involve the family and significant others of the patient. Information gained from them must be carefully transcribed. The family of a patient frequently have become enablers and codependents in the process of dealing with the patient's addiction. In this context, the family and the patient may continue to propose the self-medication hypothesis as an excuse for the addiction.

CASE EXAMPLE

Frank, a 34-year-old man with history of alcoholism in his family, presented to the inpatient psychiatric unit with depressed mood, suicidal ideation, and chronic alcoholism. In the emergency room, the psychiatrist had a conversation with his wife, who confirmed his heavy drinking history.

On admission to an inpatient psychiatric unit, Frank was convinced that the pressures of work and home had led to his depression, and he denied any alcohol problem. In a family meeting, with the treatment team, the patient, and his wife, the wife denied that her husband had a significant alcohol problem and supported her husband.

In this case example, the treatment team had to treat and educate not only the patient but also his wife. Involving the patient's support system helps with the diagnosis and treatment of the addictive and affective disorder. It is important that a patient's support system understand that the patient has two concurrent diagnoses and that both need treatment.

NEUROCHEMICAL BASIS OF CHEMICAL DEPENDENCE-INDUCED DEPRESSION

All drugs of addiction in some way increase the brain stimulation in the reward/drive/reinforcement areas of the brain or lower the brain's reinforcement thresholds. Species-specific survival drives (i.e., eating, drinking, sex, and shelter) are positively reinforced through the medial forebrain bundle and the mesolimbic system. The locus caeruleus extends neuroadrenergic fibers to the ventral tegmental area. The ventral tegmental area projects dopaminergic fibers into the nucleus accumbens. The GABAergic inhibitory fiber systems synapse onto the locus caeruleus and ventral tegmental area. Survival behaviors trigger this system and create satiety and positive reinforcement. Drugs of addiction are also positive reinforcers.[22]

Amphetamines and cocaine block the reuptake of dopamine into the presynaptic neuron from the ventral tegmental area to the nucleus accumbens.[23] The increase of dopamine in the cleft causes feedback inhibition of the dopamine cell firing. The increased dopamine in the cleft creates the equivalent of positive reinforcement of the system.[24]

However, the chronic use of stimulants, for example, cocaine, can lead to dopamine depletion.[25] Dopamine depletion leads to associated clinical symptoms such as low energy, depression, and intense cocaine craving.[26] It has been shown that dopamine agonists such as bromocriptine can relieve cravings.[27] In this way, cocaine and other stimulants create the neurochemical imbalance that leads to depression.

Alcohol's effect on the brain appears to be mediated by interaction with lipid membranes. Alcohol also appears to share sites of action with barbituates and benzodiazepines in the GABA receptors.[28] Alcohol induces the release of dopamine in the nucleus accumbens.[29]

Initial alcohol use has been shown to increase serotonin and its metabolite 5-hydroxyindoleacetic acid in the cerebrospinal fluid. This evidence explains the initial euphoria experienced with alcohol. Chronic alcohol use has been shown to decrease serotonin and its metabolite 5-hydroxyindoleacetic acid in the cerebrospinal fluid. This neurochemical change is the basis for the onset of depression in chronic alcoholics.[30]

Opiates bind to specific opiate receptors. Opiate receptors have been found on neurons in the ventral tegmental area. Opiates seem to provoke ventral tegmental area cells to increase dopamine activity, thus leading to positive reinforcement. However, chronic use leads to an endogenous opiate deficiency. This deficiency leads to feedback inhibition and downregulation of receptors. After detoxification, the endogeneous opioid systems may gradually return to normal or may not. This deficiency may lead to depression in recovering opiate addicts.[24] Opiates have direct inhibitory effects on neuroadrenergic systems in the brain. This action may increase the likelihood of depression in opiate addicts.[31]

Pharmacological Treatment of Depression in Alcoholics

TRICYCLIC ANTIDEPRESSANTS

This section describes the available data on the treatment of depression in alcoholics. In this age of new psychopharmacological medications, the knowledge of efficacy in the treatment of depression in addictions is limited. More research needs to be directed at the use of new medications in the addiction field. The best-studied class of antidepressants are the tricyclics, used in the treatment of alcoholism. In 1993, Nunes and colleagues, in an open trial of imipramine in 60 depressed alcoholics, found that 45% responded with improvement in mood and in drinking behavior. An additional 13% responded to increasing dose or to the addition of disulfiram. The average mean blood level was 368 ng/ml. This open trial showed that both depression and drinking behavior respond to imipramine. This was an open trial, however. Even the researchers suggest the possibility of a placebo effect. Double-blind placebo studies are needed.[32]

In 1991, Mason and Kocsis performed a randomized double-blind placebo-controlled trial of desipramine in depressed alcoholics. The depressed alcoholics showed significantly less depression on desipramine than on placebo. However, there were no group differences in the rate of nonsobriety. Patients receiving desipramine showed a trend toward longer periods of sobriety.[33] In this methodologically sound study, desipramine did not show a significant impact on increasing sobriety over placebo.

In 1975, Shaw and colleagues examined depressed alcoholics using placebo versus a chlordiazepoxide-imipramine study design in a randomized trial. No significant differences between pre-treatment and posttreatment measurements were found between groups. Both groups experienced decreases in depression rating scale.[34] However, this study failed to measure blood levels of antidepressants. Ciraulo and Jaffe, in their review, demonstrated that most studies failed methodologically by not measuring blood levels of antidepressants, by beginning medication in the postwithdrawal phase, when most abstinent alcoholics normally show the greatest decrease in depressive symptoms, and by failing to measure both depressive and drinking behaviors.[35] Methodologically sound studies are scarce. The need for more rigorous studies in the use of tricyclics is evident. Another problem with the use of tricyclic antidepressants with alcoholics is the high toxicity and lethality of mixing tricyclics with ethanol. This risk must be considered before the use of tricyclics in alcoholics.[36]

SEROTONIN REUPTAKE INHIBITORS

Another class of antidepressants that has been studied in alcoholics is the selective serotonin reuptake inhibitors (SSRIs) such as fluoxetine and citalopram. Naranjo and associates investigated citalopram, an SSRI, in 1991. In a double-blind placebo-controlled randomized trial, 40 mg/day of citalopram versus placebo was administered to nondepressed alcohol-dependent drinkers to investigate whether SSRIs had an inhibitory effect on the consumption of alcohol. A significant decrease (average decrease 17.5%) was observed in daily alcoholic drinks consumed by those on citalopram as compared with those on placebo. There was also a significant self-reported decrease in interest, desire, and craving for alcohol ($P < 0.05$). The percentage of days abstinent increased in the drug group (27.7%) compared with the placebo group (15.5%, with a $P < 0.01$). These findings show that SSRIs may act to decrease the urge to drink and to decrease the reinforcing effects of alcohol.[37]

In 1989, Naranjo and coworkers studied fluoxetine and its effect on alcohol intake. In this study, 29 men in the early stages of problem drinking were randomly assigned to receive fluoxetine, 40 mg/day or 60 mg/day or placebo for 4 weeks. The 60-mg/day group exhibited significant decreases in mean daily alcoholic drinks and decreased total drinks per 14 days but no significant increase in days of abstinence. Neither the 40-mg/day group nor the placebo group showed any difference on alcohol consumption.[38]

In 1990, Gorelick studied the effect of fluoxetine on the alcohol consumption of male alcoholics. In a double-blind placebo-controlled randomized trial, 10 subjects received fluoxetine (up to 80 mg/day) and 10 subjects received placebo for 28 days. The fluoxetine group had a 14% lower alcohol intake during the first week only. No significant effects were observed in the last 3 weeks. No differences were noted in results of Hamilton Depression and Anxiety Scales.[39] Gorelick and Naranjo and their groups failed to follow their studies beyond the 5-week period required for fluoxetine to achieve steady state.

All of the foregoing studies of SSRIs show decreases in the number of drinks consumed but fail to demonstrate an increase in the number of days of abstinence. In 1993, Cornelius and colleagues conducted an open trial with 12 patients with DSM-III-R diagnoses of both major depression and alcoholism. They received fluoxetine for 8 weeks with doses ranging from 20 to 40 mg/day. All 12 patients had reported prominent suicidal ideation on admission to the hospital. Statistically significant improvements were noted on measures of depression and postdischarge alcohol consumption. However, this was not a double-blind placebo-controlled study, and the sample population was limited to 12 patients.[40] These studies do point to the potential for SSRIs to treat both depressive symptoms and the alcohol consumption of depressed alcoholics.

What about other atypical antidepressants? In 1991, Tollefson and associates studied the effects of buspirone and its metabolite 1-pyrimidinylpiperazine (1-PP) in mixed anxious-depressive patients with alcoholism. In a randomized double-blind placebo-controlled trial of buspirone, 51 patients with a dual diagnosis received a maximum daily dose of 60 mg of placebo or 60 mg of buspirone by week 4. They were monitored for 24 weeks. Blood levels of buspirone and 1-PP were determined to confirm compliance. The results showed that at final study dose, 1-PP was significantly related to improvement in anxiety, global depressive symptoms, and number of days not using alcohol. Buspirone may be an effective treatment strategy in anxious or mixed anxious-depressive patients with comorbid alcohol dependence.[41] In another study of atypical antidepressants, Altamura and coworkers in 1990 studied the antidepressant and alcohol intake effect of viloxazine in 30 dysthymic patients in a placebo-controlled study. They received 400 mg of oral viloxazine daily for 12 weeks. The results showed significant alleviation of depression and reduced alcohol intake in the viloxazine group compared with the placebo group.[42] In 1991, Monti and Alterwain studied the effects of ritanserin in decreasing alcohol intake in chronic alcoholics. Five male patients were given 10 mg/day of ritanserin in a single-blind fashion for 28 days with placebo 7 days before and 15 days after ritanserin. The mean total score for depression and anxiety showed striking reductions during ritanserin use. They also reported decreased use of alcohol and craving for alcohol.[43] These studies of atypical antidepressants need to be replicated with larger numbers and in better-designed studies before the use of these drugs in depressed alcoholics can be advocated.

In 1987, Fawcett and colleagues reported on a double-blind placebo-controlled trial of lithium carbonate therapy for alcoholism. In this study, 104 subjects who met the criteria for alcohol dependence (DSM-III criteria) were treated with lithium and monitored for 12 months. The results revealed three groups: noncompliant subjects (0 to 7% abstinent), compliant subjects at subtherapeutic lithium levels (31% to 44% abstinent), and compliant subjects with therapeutic serum lithium levels (67% abstinent). There was no evidence that depressed alcoholics showed a better treatment response than nondepressed alcoholics or that lithium had any significant impact on the mood or social adjustment of alcoholics.[44] In 1989, Dorus and associates reported on a large (n = 457) double-blind placebo-controlled randomized trial of lithium carbonate (600 to 1200 mg/day) in alcoholics. They monitored the subjects for up to 1 year, dividing the alcoholic groups into those with a history of depression and those without a history of depression. The results reported showed no significant difference between alcoholics on lithium and those on placebo in the outcome measures such as number of alcoholics abstinent, number of days of drinking, number of alcohol-related hospitalizations, changes in the rating of severity of alcoholism, and change in severity of depression.[45] These studies show that the use of lithium carbonate to treat depressed alcoholics is not effective. The evidence for lithium's increasing abstinence is not supported.[46]

Treatment of Depression in Other Addictive Disorders

Several trials have investigated antidepressants in opioid addiction. Spensley gave doxepin to 27 methadone maintenance patients in an uncontrolled open trial. Of these, 93% (25/27) experienced symptom relief for depression, anxiety, and insomnia.[47] Woody and colleagues reported a double-blind study of doxepin in 35 patients receiving methadone maintenance. These patients had mild depressive symptoms on depression rating scales. The doxepin group showed improvement in the outcome measures of depression, anxiety, and heroin craving.[48] This study was seriously flawed, however, because of the initiation of methadone at the same time that the doxepin was started.[31] Titievsky showed success on the Hamilton Depression Rating Scale scores for depression and anxiety in a double-blind placebo-controlled study of doxepin in 46 patients receiving methadone maintenance.[50] Finally, Kleber and Weissman conducted an 8-week double-blind placebo-controlled study of 46 methadone maintenance patients who met the DSM-II criteria for depression. The patients were treated with a daily dose of imipramine between 150 and 225 mg. In this study, Kleber and Weissman found no difference between either group in depression because both groups showed substantial improvement in the depression rating scales.[51] The research on antidepressants in opioid addicts is limited to those on methadone maintenance because of the difficulty in retaining opioid-abstinent patients. Patients receiving methadone maintenance are likely to be more compliant. Methadone may mask depressive symptoms in these addicts.[51] Little research has been conducted on the use of SSRIs in depressed opioid addicts.

The treatment of cocaine addiction has not focused on dually diagnosed patients with major depression. Most research has looked at reversing the cocaine craving and anhedonia due to cocaine use. According to the dopamine hypothesis, chronic cocaine use results in dopamine and norepinephrine depletion, which leads to catecholamine postsynaptic receptor hypersensitivity.[52] It is believed that this receptor hypersensitivity leads to cocaine craving and anhedonia. Antidepressants were used to treat this craving and anhedonia. Giannini and coworkers found desipramine to be more effective than the active placebo diphenhydramine in reversing depressive symptoms in chronic cocaine users.[53] Gawin and colleagues, in a 6-week double-blind randomized trial of desipramine, lithium, and placebo, found that 59% of the group receiving desipramine achieved at least 3 consecutive weeks of abstinence, as compared with 25% for the lithium group and 17% for the placebo group. Gawin's group used desipramine at 2.5 mg/kg/day for 6 weeks.[54] Tennant and Rawson, who used lower doses (75 to 100 mg) for only 2 weeks, found no difference between groups receiving placebo versus desipramine.[55] Again, the data on SSRIs in cocaine addiction are not available. More research needs to address both opioid and cocaine addiction and affective disorders and their psychopharmacological treatment efficacy.

General Recommendations

First, it is important in the presence of a possible comorbid diagnosis of addictive and affective disorder to establish the proper diagnosis. A diagnosis of an affective disorder must be delayed until a patient can be evaluated after a 2- to 4-week period of abstinence. During this period, aggressive treatment of the addiction must be started. Confrontation of patients' denial of their addiction needs to be addressed. Acceptance of addiction as a separate and independent disease process by the patient and the physician is vital for the patient's recovery. Second, after the period of abstinence, if an affective disorder is diagnosed, then treatment of both disorders must continue. Treatment of addiction with an abstinence-based model with aftercare and self-support groups is the most efficacious method to achieve recovery. The use of psychopharmacological treatments in this comorbid population has been poorly researched. However, it is our recommendation that strong consideration be given to use of SSRIs in the treatment of depression in the presence of an addiction. The reduced side effect profile, the efficacy in treating depression in nonaddicted patients, and the relative safety of SSRI overdose in comparison with the tricyclics all are important reasons to use these medications first. Consideration must be given to the physiological differences in addicted as compared with nonaddicted patients. Alcohol causes increased hepatic microsomal enzyme activity, which leads to increased metabolism. This increased metabolism leads to decreased serum blood levels of antidepressants.[56] These mechanisms must be kept in mind when treating addicted patients for affective disorders, because nonresponse may be due to inadequate levels of antidepressant.

REFERENCES

1. Gibson S, Becker J: Changes in alcoholics' self-reported depression. Q J Stud Alcohol 34:829–836, 1973.
2. Mayfield DG: Psychopharmacology of alcohol: Affective change with intoxication, drinking behavior, and affective state. J Nerv Ment Dis 146:314–321, 1968.
3. Mayfield DG: Psychopharmacology of alcohol: Affective tolerance in alcohol intoxication. J Nerv Ment Dis 146:322–327, 1968.
4. Tamerin JS, Weiner S, Mendelson JH: Alcoholics' expectancies and recall of experiences during intoxication. Am J Psychiatry 126:1697–1704, 1970.
5. Schuckit MA: Genetic and clinical implications of alcoholism and affective disorder. Am J Psychiatry 143:140–147, 1986.
6. Regier DA, Farmer ME, Rae OS, et al: Comorbidity of mental disorders with alcohol and other drug abuse. Results from the Epidemiologic Catchment Area (ECA) Study. JAMA 264(19):2511–2518, 1990.
7. Petty F: The depressed alcoholic. Clinical features and medical management. Gen Hosp Psychiatry 14:258–264, 1992.
8. Brown SA, Schuckit MA: Changes in depression among abstinent alcoholics. J Stud Alcohol 49(5):412–417, 1988.
9. Dorus W, Kennedy J, Gibbons RD, et al: Symptoms and diagnosis of depression in alcoholics. Alcoholism 11(2):150–154, 1987.
10. Brown SA, Inaba RK, Gillin JC, Schuckit M, et al: Alcoholism and affective disorders: Clinical course of depressive symptoms. Am J Psychiatry 152(1):45–52, 1995.
11. Miller NS, Mahler JC: Alcoholics Anonymous and the "AA" model for treatment. Alcohol Treat Q 8(1):39–51, 1991.

12. Berglund M: Suicide in alcoholism. Arch Gen Psychiatry 41:888–894, 1984.
13. Miller NS, Chappel JN: History of disease concept. Psychiatr Ann 21(4):196–205, 1991.
14. Miller NS, Hoffman NG, Ninoneuvo F, Astrachan B: Lifetime diagnosis of major depression as a predictor of treatment outcome in inpatient abstinence based programs for alcohol/drug disorders. Arch Gen Psychiatry (in press).
15. Woodruff RA, Guze SB, Clayton PJ, Carr D: Alcoholism and depression. Arch Gen Psychiatry 28:97–100, 1973.
16. Gjerde H, Amundsen A, Skog OJ, Morland J, Aasland OG: Serum gamma-glutamyltransferase: An epidemiological indicator of alcohol consumption? Br J Addict 82:1027–1031, 1987.
17. Chick J, Kreitman N, Plant M: Mean cell volume and gamma-glutamyltransferase as markers in drinking in working men. Lancet 1:1249–1251, 1981.
18. Barnes HN, Aronson MD, Delbanco TL: Alcoholism—A Guide for the Primary Care Physician. New York, Springler-Verlag, 1987.
19. National Institute of Alcohol Abuse and Alcoholism: Screening for alcoholism. Alcohol Alert 8:1–4, 1990.
20. Criteria Committee, National Council on Alcoholism: Criteria for the diagnosis of alcoholism. Ann Intern Med 77:249–258, 1972.
21. Schwartz RH: Urine testing in the detection of drugs of abuse. Arch Intern Med 148:2407–2412, 1988.
22. Gold MS, Miller NS: Seeking drugs and alcohol and avoiding withdrawal: The neuroanatomy of drive states and withdrawal. Psychiatr Ann 22(8):430–435, 1992.
23. Miller NS, Gold MS: The relationship of addiction, tolerance, and dependence to alcohol and drugs: A neurochemical approach. J Subst Abuse Treat 4:197–207, 1987.
24. Wise RA: The neurobiology of craving: Implications for the understanding and treatment of addiction. J Abnorm Psychol 97:118–132, 1988.
25. Extein, Dackis. Brain mechanisms in cocaine dependency. In Washington, Gold (eds): New York, Guildford Press, 1987, pp 73–84.
26. Jaffe JH. Drug addiction and drug abuse. In Gilman AG, Rall TW, Nies AS, Taylor P (eds): The Pharmacological Basis of Therapeutics. New York, Pergamon Press, 1990.
27. Dackis GA, Gold MS: Bromocriptine as treatment of cocaine abuse. Lancet 1:1151–1152, 1985.
28. Carr L: The pharmacology of mood-altering drugs of abuse. Primary Care 3(20):19–31, 1993.
29. Miller NS, Gold MS: Drugs of Abuse: A Comprehensive Series for Clinicians, vol 2: Alcohol. New York, Plenum Press, 1991.
30. Ballenger JC, Goodwin FK, Major LF, et al: Alcohol and central serotonin metabolism in man. Arch Gen Psychiatry 36:224–227, 1979.
31. Gold MS, Redmund DE, Kleber HD: Noradrenergic hyperactivity in opiate withdrawal supported by clonidine reversal of opiate withdrawal. Am J Psychiatry 136:100–102, 1979.
32. Nunes EV, McGrath PJ, Quitkin FM, Stewart JP: Imipramine treatment of alcoholism with comorbid depression. Am J Psychiatry 150(6):963–965, 1993.
33. Mason BJ, Kocsis JH: Desipramine treatment of alcoholism. Psychopharmacol Bull 27(2):155–161, 1991.
34. Shaw JA, Donley P, Morgan DW, et al: Treatment of depression in alcoholics. Am J Psychiatry 132(6):641–644, 1975.
35. Ciraulo DA, Jaffe JH: Tricyclic antidepressants in the treatment of depression associated with alcoholism. J Clin Psychopharmacol 1:146–150, 1981.
36. Weller RA, Preskorn SH: Psychotropic drugs and alcohol: Pharmacokinetic and pharmacodynamic interactions. Psychosomatics 25:301–309, 1984.
37. Naranjo CA, Poulos CX, Bremren KE, Lanctot KL, et al: Citalopram decreases desirability, liking, and consumption of alcohol in alcohol-dependent drinkers. Clin Pharmacol Ther 51:729–739, 1992.
38. Naranjo CA, Kadlec KE, Sanhuenza P, et al: Fluoxetine differentially alters alcohol intake and other consummatory behaviors in problem drinkers. Clin Pharmacol Ther 47:490–498, 1990.
39. Gorelick DA, Paredes A: Effect of fluoxetine on alcohol consumption in male alcoholics. Alcohol Clin Exp Res 16(2):261–265, 1992.
40. Cornelius JR, Salloum IM, Cornelius MD, Perel JM, Thase ME, Ehler JG, Mann JJ: Fluoxetine trial in suicidal depressed alcoholics. Psychopharmacol Bull 29(2):195–199, 1993.
41. Tollefson GD, Lancaster SP, Montague J, Couse C: The association of buspirone and its metabolite 1-pyrimidinylpiperazine in the remission of comorbid anxiety with depressive features and alcohol dependency. Psychopharmacol Bull 27(2):163–170, 1991.
42. Altamura AC, Mauri MC, Girardi T, Paretta B: Alcoholism and depression: Placebo-controlled study with viloxazine. Int J Clin Pharmacol Res 10:293–298, 1990.
43. Monti JM, Alterwain P: Ritanserin decreases alcohol intake in chronic alcoholics. Lancet 1:337–360, 1991.
44. Fawcett J, Clark DC, Aagesen CA, et al: A double-blind, placebo-controlled trial of lithium carbonate therapy for alcoholism. Arch Gen Psychiatry 44:248–256, 1987.
45. Dorus W, Ostrow DG, Anton R, Cushman P, Collins JF, Schaefer M, Charles H: Lithium treatment of depressed and nondepressed alcoholics. JAMA 262:1646–1652, 1989.
46. Jefferson JW: Lithium: The present and the future. J Clin Psychiatry 51(Suppl 8):4–8, 1990.
47. Spensley J: The adjunctive use of tricyclics in a methadone program. Journal of Psychedelic Drugs 6:421–423, 1974.
48. Woody GE, O'Brien CP, Rickels K, et al: Depression and anxiety in heroin addicts: A placebo controlled study of doxepin in combination with methadone. Am J Psychiatry 132:447–450, 1975.
49. Weiss RD, Mirin SM: Tricyclic antidepressants in the treatment of alcoholism and drug abuse. J Clin Psychiatry 50(Suppl 7):4–9, 1989.
50. Titievsky J, Seco G, Barranco M, et al: Doxepin as adjunctive therapy for depressed methadone maintenance patients: A double-blind study. J Clin Psychiatry 43:454–456, 1982.
51. Kleber HD, Weissman MM, Rounsaville BJ, et al: Imipramine as treatment for depression in addicts. Arch Gen Psychiatry 40:649–653, 1983.
52. Gawin FH: Chronic neuropharmacology of cocaine: Progress in pharmacotherapy. J Clin Psychiatry 49 (Suppl 2):11–16, 1988.
53. Giannini AJ, Malone DA, Giannini MC, et al: Treatment of depression in chronic cocaine and phencyclidine abuse with desipramine. J Clin Pharmacol 26:211–224, 1986.
54. Gawin FH, Kleber HD, Byck R, et al: Desipramine facilitation of initial cocaine abstinence. Arch Gen Psychiatry 46:117–121, 1989.
55. Tennant FS, Rawson RA: Cocaine and amphetamine dependence treated with desipramine. In Harris LS (ed): Problems of Drug Dependence 1982. Rockville,

MD, National Institute on Drug Abuse, 1983, pp 351–355.

56. Ciraulo DA, Alderson LM, Chapron DJ, et al: Imipramine disposition in alcoholics. J Clin Psychopharmacol 2:2–7, 1982.

57. Extein IL, Gold MS: Hypothesized neurochemical models for psychiatric syndromes in alcohol and drug dependence. J Addict Dis 12(3):29–43, 1993.

58. Gold MS, Miller NS: The biology of addictive and psychiatric disorders. In Miller NS (ed): Center City MN: Treating Coexisting Psychiatric and Addictive Disorders. Hazelden Press, 1994, pp 35–49.

Psychopharmacotherapy for the Addicted Borderline or Antisocial Patient

John M. Davis, MD • Bradley M. Pechter, MD •
Philip G. Janicak, MD • Frank J. Ayd, Jr., MD

A great deal of comorbidity is associated with both borderline and antisocial personality disorders (BPDs and APDs). Addiction is perhaps one of the most striking comorbid features causing troubles for patients, clinicians, and society. Despite the difficulties in treating addicted patients, the psychopharmacotherapy of these comorbid disorders holds considerable hope and promise.

Gitlin suggested several practical approaches to the use of psychotropics with BPDs.[1] The identification of symptom clusters is particularly useful and suggests that the psychopathology of axis I and axis II disorders lies on a continuum. This approach fosters coherent application of established pharmacotherapeutic modalities to otherwise vexing problems. The same agents used to treat full diagnostic syndromes can be used when presentations show certain symptom clusters—for example,

- *Antipsychotics* for psychotic symptoms such as paranoia, hallucinations, or disorganized thought
- *Antidepressants* (e.g., selective serotonin reuptake inhibitors [SSRIs] and monoamine oxidase inhibitors [MAOIs]) for depressive symptoms, compulsivity, anxiety, or panic
- *Mood stabilizers* for presentations with mood instability

Several principles need to be followed when prescribing medications for addicts with BPD or APD:

- Patients must understand that prescribed medications are useful but not a panacea
- Always emphasize nonpharmacological, psychosocial treatments to be used concurrently
- Avoid polypharmacy (i.e., using more than one medication simultaneously for the same indication)
- If possible, avoid medications with adverse effects such as addiction potential, paradoxical disinhibition, lowering of the seizure threshold, or tardive dyskinesia
- Maintain proper *informed consent*[2, 3]

Addicted Patients

BORDERLINE PERSONALITY DISORDER

BPD is characterized in DSM-IV as "a pervasive pattern of instability of mood, interpersonal relationships, and self-image."[4] Those patients with BPD and addictions fare more poorly overall, as evidenced, for example, by less education and employment and more frequent prostitution and promiscuity.[5] Estimates vary, but perhaps 70% of patients with BPD are dependent on alcohol or drugs.[6–11] Women with BPD generally prefer alcohol and sedatives, whereas men prefer stimulants.[5] Impulsive behavior, which is a diagnostic criterion for BPD, often includes addiction or dependence. This overlap can cause diagnostic confusion and highlights the comorbidity of this disorder with addictions. Our clinical preference is to treat substance use disorders aggressively and to integrate this treatment with the treatment aimed primarily at the personality disorder. Some clinicians may prefer to focus on the BPD first and refer out for subsequent addiction treatment. We believe that this approach is not as strong and puts patients at risk for consequences of continued addictive behaviors.

We have found it useful to divide BPD into three symptom clusters:

- Impulsive, which includes self-injurious and aggressive actions
- Affective (including depressive and mood lability symptoms)
- Psychotic

Those patients showing the impulsive cluster symptoms may be most likely to have a concurrent addiction, but certainly those with affective or psychotic symptoms have their predicted share of comorbid substance dependence. Medications can be helpful, but no single agent is likely to be effective across all three symptom clusters.[12]

Research on BPD is compromised by diagnostic overlap with other disorders and the stably unstable nature of patients with BPD. Unfortunately but understandably, research on BPD often uses heterogeneous or small sample sizes. Even fewer studies focus on patients with BPD with comorbid addiction. Nevertheless, we endeavor to present research on medications that can be used in treating this dually diagnosed population. In keeping with our earlier discussion, we organize the information by treatment of symptom clusters.

Impulsive Cluster

As mentioned earlier, in our experience, the impulsive cluster is most often associated with an addiction. Behavioral dyscontrol is at the core of borderline, addictive behavior. Addiction can be thought of as both a self-injurious and interpersonally damaging set of behaviors. To counter this dyscontrol, many approaches have been tried. Links and colleagues, in a blind crossover study with a small sample, examined lithium, desipramine, and placebo

for patients with BPD.[13] They found lithium to be effective in BPD by decreasing suicidal symptoms and anger. Another mood stabilizer, carbamazepine, was found effective by other investigators.[14] Although some investigators have reported lithium to be effective in alcoholism,[15] this has not been replicated by others[16] and remains unproven. No investigators, to our knowledge, have suggested that lithium or any anticonvulsant/mood stabilizer is contraindicated in addicted patients. Synthesizing these observations leads us to conclude that mood-stabilizing agents may be a safe and effective treatment for addicted patients with BPD with impulsive features. An ancillary benefit of prescribing anticonvulsants in this population is that they may provide prophylaxis for alcoholic patients who have BPD and who are prone to seizures.

MAOIs also show some promise in the psychopharmacotherapy of BPD. In a multiple crossover study, Gardner and Cowdry compared alprazolam, carbamazepine, trifluoperazine, and tranylcypromine versus placebo.[14] Those patients on the MAOI tranylcypromine showed the most remarkable response compared with placebo. Interestingly, those patients on alprazolam were the most likely to show behavioral dyscontrol.[17] This finding, coupled with the ubiquitous clinical experience of addiction to alprazolam, argues strongly against the use of this agent (and arguably all benzodiazepines) in addicted patients with BPD.

The MAOI phenelzine was shown by Soloff and colleagues[18] to decrease hostility in BPD when compared with placebo and to relieve depression when compared with haloperidol. Although these findings are initially promising for the psychopharmacotherapy of BPD, the investigators ultimately found no significant benefit of phenelzine compared with placebo when given for an additional 4 months.

The SSRIs are a particularly promising group of medications. Studies have shown some benefit of the SSRIs with alcoholism[19] and in treating the impulsive symptom cluster of BPD. Most of the evidence for using SSRIs for BPD comes from open trials. Collectively, these studies show promise in treating the irritability and impulsive aggression of BPD.[20–25] Norden[26] specifically found improvement in addictive substance use (among other impulsive symptoms) in his study of fluoxetine in 12 patients with BPD without major depression. Salzman,[27] in a double-blind placebo-controlled study of fluoxetine for BPD, found a significant reduction in anxiety independent of the level of depression. We consider SSRIs a particularly promising class of agents with this group of dually diagnosed patients. Reward, mediated by serotonin and dopamine in the limbic system of the brain, may be the mechanism responsible for these effects.

SSRIs also have a significantly safer profile in overdose than tricyclic antidepressants (TCAs) or MAOIs. This advantage has obvious implications in treating patients with BPD and an addictive illness because they are at risk for overdose and suicide attempts.

Affective Cluster

The evidence for the use of TCAs in BPD is mixed. The strongest case is made for using TCAs in patients with a clear concurrent major depressive illness. Cole and colleagues[28] showed that five of six patients with *both* BPD and major depression responded to TCAs but patients with BPD without concurrent major depression did not respond. Some studies even suggest that treatment of BPD with TCAs can actually *increase* irritability and agitation.[29]

In a similar manner, imipramine and chlorpromazine were found by Klein and colleagues[30] to be useful in patients with emotionally unstable personalities. This syndrome is associated with ineffectiveness and excitability when patients are faced with minor stress and has many of the features noticed in addicts, including
- Pleasure seeking
- Impulsivity
- Social isolation
- Episodes of dysphoria

In this study, both agents were significantly more effective than placebo. Chlorpromazine effected improvement in 81% of cases and imipramine in 67%.

Lithium was found by Rifkin and colleagues[31] to stabilize affectively labile characters whose symptom cluster resembles BPD or cyclothymic disorders. These patients had long-standing problematical behaviors such as poor work histories and truancy, which also resembled BPD.

Psychotic Cluster

The practice of using antipsychotic agents for BPD has some proponents in the literature, but the use of these agents should be reserved for patients with BPD with clear psychosis. This can be manifested as paranoia, grandiosity, possibly catatonia, or loose, disorganized speech or thought processes. Some of these features can be precipitated or caused by psychoactive drugs and thus can muddle the diagnostic work. If psychosis can be explained *solely* on the basis of drug intoxication or withdrawal, antipsychotic medication should be a very limited palliative measure while the causative factor is addressed. Miller and colleagues note that depersonalization-derealization (a psychotic-type symptom) was commonly found in patients with BPD with no addiction (37%) or with concurrent alcohol-sedative addiction (28%) but rarely in patients with addictions to stimulants (5%).[5] With these general thoughts in mind, we next briefly review the literature on antipsychotic use in BPD and relate it specifically to addicted patients with BPD.

A few placebo-controlled studies support the use of antipsychotics in BPD. In one double-blind placebo-controlled study, thiothixene (mean dose = 8.7 mg/day) was found to be superior to placebo in controlling illusions, ideas of reference, and psychoticism.[32] This study population included patients with mixtures of BPD and schizotypal personality disorder. Overall, the BPD responded less than the schizotypal disorder to thiothixene. Cowdry and Gardner's multiple crossover design between trifluoperazine, tranylcypromine, carbamazepine, alprazolam, and placebo showed modest improvement for the five patients in the antipsychotic group who completed the trial.[33]

Haloperidol was found to be superior to both amitriptyline and placebo in treating the psychotic symptoms in a fairly large (n = 28 in each group) study of BPD.[34] Interestingly, depressive symptoms were improved by both haloperidol and amitriptyline. Thiothixene was found to be more effective than haloperidol in another study, but this population was less psychotic and included many patients with schizotypal personalities.[35] Finally, a 4-month continuation study using haloperidol, phenelzine, and placebo showed inferior results for haloperidol.[36] These patients showed a quicker decline and greater dropout rate while on haloperidol than on placebo and more depression than with phenelzine. Overall, no changes were noted on global assessment scales for the groups.

Open trials using antipsychotics in BPD, although less compelling individually, are much more numerous.[37, 38] Various antipsychotics are found to be effective (to various degrees) in BPD. Unfortunately, we are aware of no studies specifically aimed at addicted patients with BPD. Clozapine appears useful when significant psychosis is present in BPD.[39] Loxapine and chlorpromazine are reported by others to be efficacious.[40] Alprazolam has been reported to be ineffective and even detrimental (based on suicide or assaultive behaviors).[39] One study noted the use of antipsychotics to be associated with depressive symptoms,[41] and three patients who had BPD and who were receiving carbamazepine in a previously cited study[42] were removed after developing melancholia. It is unknown whether these trends would continue if the BPD were compounded by an addictive illness. Clinicians should be aware, however, of these potential problems and be prepared to alter pharmacotherapy and possibly start the patients on an antidepressant.

ANTISOCIAL PERSONALITY DISORDER

The clinical manifestations of addiction and APD overlap considerably. No distinct pharmacological approaches to treating APD have been formulated, but biological studies of aggression and violence may present a rational beginning. Evidence that type II alcoholics have low cerebrospinal fluid levels of 5-hydroxyindoleacetic acid (and thus low brain serotonin levels) suggests that these disorders may be benefitted by SSRIs. Evidence that SSRIs *reduce* impulsivity may quell some concern that these agents precipitate violence or suicidal ideation.[43] The use of lithium has met with mixed results in treating aggression and alcoholism but may warrant further investigation.[44, 45] At present, we recommend aggressive addiction treatment for those with concurrent APD. We are aware of no studies showing disulfiram or naltrexone to exacerbate aggression or impulsivity. These medications may be effective pharmacotherapy in this dually disordered population. Because most patients with APD are men, therapeutic approaches may need to be skewed appropriately.[46, 47]

REFERENCES

1. Gitlin MJ: Pharmacotherapy of personality disorders: Conceptual framework and clinical strategies. J Clin Psychopharmacol 13:343–353, 1993.
2. Ayd F: Psychopharmacologic treatment of personality disorders. Int Drug Ther Newsletter 25:1–2, 1990.
3. Janicak PG, Davis J, Preskorn SH, et al: Principles and Practice of Psychopharmacotherapy. Baltimore, Williams & Wilkins, 1993.
4. American Psychiatric Association: Diagnostic and Statistical Manual of Mental Disorders, 4th ed. Washington, DC, American Psychiatric Association, 1994.
5. Miller FT, Abrams T, Dulit R, Fyer M: Substance abuse in borderline personality disorder. J Drug Alcohol Abuse 19(4):491–497, 1993.
6. Baxter L, Edell W, Gerner R, et al: Dexamethasone suppression test and axis I diagnoses of inpatients with DSM-III borderline personality disorder. J Clin Psychiatry 45:150–153, 1984.
7. Akiskal HS, Chen SE, Davis GC, et al: Borderline: an adjective in search of a noun. J Clin Psychiatry 46:41–48, 1985.
8. Andrulonia PA, Glueck BC, Stroebel CF, et al: Borderline personality subcategories. J Nerv Ment Dis 1270:670–679, 1982.
9. Pope HG, Jonas JM, Hudson JL, et al: The validity of DSM-III borderline personality disorder: A phenomenological, family history, treatment response, and long-term follow-up study. Arch Gen Psychiatry 40:23–30, 1983.
10. Frances A, Clarkin JF, Gilmore M, et al: Reliability of criteria for borderline personality disorder: A comparison of DSM-III and the diagnostic interview for borderline patients. Am J Psychiatry 45:150–153, 1984.
11. Dulit RA, Fyer MR, Haas GL, et al: Substance abuse in borderline personality disorder. Am J Psychiatry 147:1002–1006, 1990.
12. New AS, Trestman RL, Seiver LJ: The pharmacotherapy of borderline personality disorders. CNS Drugs 2:347–354, 1994.
13. Volpicelli JR, Alterman AI, Hayashida M, et al: Naltrexone in the treatment of alcohol dependence. Arch Gen Psychiatry 49:876–880, 1992.
14. O'Malley SS, Jaffe AJ, Chang G, et al: Naltrexone and coping skills therapy for alcohol dependence. Arch Gen Psychiatry 49:881–887, 1992.
15. Dackis CA, Gold MS, Pottash ALC, Sweeney DR: Evaluating depression in alcoholics. Psychiatry Res 17:105–109, 1986.
15a. Fawcett J, Clark DC, Aagesen CA, et al: A double-blind, placebo-controlled trial of lithium carbonate therapy for alcoholism. Arch Gen Psychiatry 44:248–256, 1987.
15b. Kline NS, Wren JC, Cooper TB, et al: Evaluation of lithium therapy in chronic and periodic alcoholism. Am J Med Sci 268:15–22, 1974.
15c. Nagel K, Adler LE, Bell J, et al: Lithium carbonate and mood disorder in recently detoxified alcoholics: A double-blind, placebo-controlled pilot study. Alcoholism Clin Exp Res 15:982–990, 1991.
15d. Merry J, Reynolds CM, Bailey J, Coppen A: Prophylactic treatment of alcoholism by lithium carbonate: A controlled study. Lancet 4:481–482, 1976.
15e. Reynolds CM, Merry J, Coppen A: Prophylactic treatment of alcoholism by lithium carbonate: An initial report. Alcoholism Clin Exp Res 1:109–111, 1977.
16. Merikangas KR, Leckman JF, Prusoff BA, et al: Familial transmission of depression and alcoholism. Arch Gen Psychiatry 42:367–372, 1985.
16a. Dorus W, Ostrow DG, Anton R, et al: Lithium treatment of depressed and nondepressed alcoholics. JAMA 262:1646–1652, 1989.
16b. Pond SM, Becker CE, Vandervoort R, et al: An evaluation of the effects of lithium in the treatment of chronic alcoholism. I. Clinical results. Alcoholism Clin Exp Res 5:247–251, 1981.
17. Nunes EV, McGrath PJ, Quitkin FM, et al: Imipramine treatment of alcoholism with comorbid depression. Am J Psychiatry 150:963–965, 1993.
18. Nunes EV, Quitkin FM, Brady R, et al: Imipramine treatment of methadone maintenance patients with affective disorder and illicit drug use. Am J Psychiatry 148:667–669, 1991.

19. Gorelick DA: Serotonin uptake blockers and the treatment of alcoholism. Clin Pharmacol 267–282, 1991.

19a. Gorelick DA, Paredes A: Effect of fluoxetine on alcohol consumption in male alcoholics. Alcohol Clin Exp Res 16:261–265, 1992.

19b. Amit Z, Brown Z, Sutherland Z, et al: Reduction in alcohol intake in humans as a function of treatment with zimeldine: Implications for treatment. In Naranjo CA, Sellers EM (eds): Research advances in new psychopharmacological treatments for alcoholism. Amsterdam, Excerpta Medica, 1985, pp 189–198.

19c. Naranjo CA, Sellers EM, Jullivan JT, et al: The serotonin uptake inhibitor citalopram attenuates ethanol intake. Clin Pharmacol Ther 41:266–274, 1987.

19d. Naranjo CA, Sellers EM, Roach CA, et al: Zimeldine-induced variations in alcohol intake by non-depressed heavy drinkers. Clin Pharmacol Ther 35:374–381, 1984.

20. Coccaro EF, Astill JL, Herbert JA, et al: Fluoxetine treatment of impulsive aggression in DSM-III-R personality disorder patients. J Clin Psychopharmacol 10(5):373–375, 1990.

21. Cornelius JR, Soloff PH, Perel JM, et al: Fluoxetine trial in borderline personality disorder. Psychopharmacol Bull 26:151–154, 1990.

22. Cornelius JR, Soloff PH, Perel JM, et al: A preliminary trial of fluoxetine in refractory borderline patients. J Clin Psychopharmacol 11:116–120, 1991.

23. Markowitz PJ, Calabrese JR, Schulz SC, et al: Fluoxetine treatment of borderline and schizotypal personality disorder. Am J Psychiatry 148:1064–1067, 1991.

24. Norden MJ: Fluoxetine in borderline personality disorder. Prog Neuropsychopharmacol Biol Psychiatry 13:885–893, 1989.

25. Kavoussi RJ, Liv J, Coccaro EF: An open trial of sertraline in personality disorder patients with impulsive aggression. J Clin Psychiatry 55:137–141, 1994.

26. Norden MJ: Fluoxetine in borderline personality disorder. Prog Neuropsychopharmacol Biol Psychiatry 13:885–893, 1989.

27. Salzman C: Effect of fluoxetine on anger in borderline personality disorder (abstract). Neuropsychopharmacology 10(Suppl 1):826, 1994.

28. Cole JO, Salomon M, Gunderson J: Drug therapy in borderline patients. J Clin Psychiatry 25:249–254, 1984.

29. Schiff HB, Sabin TD, Geller A, et al: Lithium in aggressive behavior. Am J Psychiatry 139:1346–1348, 1982.

30. Klein DF: Importance of psychiatric diagnosis in the prediction of clinical drug effects. Arch Gen Psychiatry 16:118–126, 1967.

30a. Klein DR: Chlorpromazine-procyclidine combination imipramine and placebo in depressive disorders. Can Psychiatric Assoc J 11(Suppl 1):146–149, 1966.

31. Rifkin A, Quitkin F, Carrillo C, et al: Lithium carbonate in emotionally unstable character disorder. Arch Gen Psychiatry 27:519–523, 1972.

32. Goldberg SC, Schulz SC, Schulz PM, et al: Borderline and schizotypal personality disorders treated with low-dose thiothixene vs placebo. Arch Gen Psychiatry 43:680–686, 1986.

33. O'Malley SS, Jaffe AJ, Chang G, et al: Naltrexone and coping skills therapy for alcohol dependence. Arch Gen Psychiatry 49:881–887, 1992.

34. Soloff PH, George A, Nathan S, et al: Amitriptyline versus haloperidol in borderlines: Final outcomes and predictors of response. J Clin Psychopharmacol 9:238–246, 1989.

35. Serban G, Siegel S: Responses of borderline and schizotypal patients to small doses of thiothixene and haloperidol. Am J Psychiatry 141:1455–1458, 1984.

36. Cornelius JR, Soloff PH, George A, et al: Haloperidol versus phenelzine in continuation therapy of borderline disorder. Psychopharmacol Bull 29:333–337, 1993.

37. Teicher MH, Glod CA, Aaronson ST, et al: Open assessment of the safety and efficacy of thioridazine in the treatment of patients with borderline personality disorder. Psychopharmacol Bull 25:535–549, 1989.

38. Brinkley JR, Beitman BD, Friedel RO: Low-dose neuroleptic regimens in the treatment of borderline patients. Arch Gen Psychiatry 36:319–326, 1979.

39. Frankenberg FR, Zanarini MC: Clozapine treatment of borderline patients: A preliminary study. Compr Psychiatry 34:402–405, 1993.

40. Leone NF: Response of borderline patients to loxapine and chlorpromazine. J Clin Psychiatry 43:148–150, 1982.

41. Teicher MH, Glod CA, Aaronson ST, et al: Open assessment of the safety and efficacy of thioridazine in the treatment of patients with borderline personality disorder. Psychopharmacol Bull 25(4):535–549, 1989.

42. Gardner DL, Cowdry RW: Development of melancholia during carbamazepine treatment in borderline personality disorder. J Clin Psychopharmacol 6(4):236–239, 1986.

43. Mann J, Kapur S: The emergence of suicidal ideation and behavior during antidepressant pharmacotherapy. Arch Gen Psychiatry 48:1027–1033, 1991.

44. Sheard MH, Marini JL, Bridges CL, et al: The effect of lithium on impulsive aggressive behavior in man. Am J Psychiatry 133:1409–1413, 1976.

45. Schiff HB, Sabin TD, Geller A, et al: Lithium in aggressive behavior. Am J Psychiatry 139:1346–1348, 1982.

46. Zanarini MC, Gunderson JG, Frankenburg FR: Axis I phenomenology of borderline personality disorder. Compr Psychiatry 30(2):149–156, 1989.

47. Waldinger RJ, Frank AF: Clinicians' experiences in combining medication and psychotherapy in the treatment of borderline patients. Hosp Community Psychiatry 40(7):712, 1989.

Treatment of Addiction in Adolescent Populations

Catherine A. Nageotte, MD, MS Health
Services • Jacqueline M. Amato, MD

Psychoactive substance use among U.S. children and adolescents is a major public health problem. Child and adolescent psychoactive substance use and psychoactive substance use disorders rates in the United States were reported to be the highest in the industrialized world.[1] Alcohol-related motor vehicle accidents are the leading cause of death among U.S. adolescents aged 15 to 24 years, and elevated alcohol levels are often found in victims of suicide and homicide.[2] Adolescent psychoactive substance use renders enormous costs to American society including lost productivity and future earnings over the life span, motor vehicle accidents, highway safety program costs, crime and punishment costs, and healthcare costs. Every American is a stakeholder in the effort to better understand and prevent adolescent psychoactive substance use.

Psychoactive Substance Use Versus Addiction/Dependence—Nosological Perspectives

The continual development of definitions used to describe excessive use of alcohol and drugs reflects the current evolution of attitudes toward mental illness in general. Chemical de-

pendence, in particular, tends to provoke strong emotional responses.[3] The need for clarification of the terminology surrounding addiction becomes increasingly apparent as this disease becomes more prevalent within the adolescent population. Addiction is defined as follows: (1) a preoccupation with acquiring a substance that dominates the user's lifestyle, (2) compulsive use of drugs and alcohol despite adverse consequences, and (3) a pattern of relapse to use of drugs and alcohol after a period of abstinence or an inability to cut down use despite recurrent adverse consequences.[4]

The formal psychiatric classification system for adolescent addiction as well as for adult addiction is outlined in the *Diagnostic and Statistical Manual of Mental Disorders*, fourth edition (DSM-IV). The main category, substance-related disorders, is broken down further into two subgroups, the substance use disorders (substance dependence and substance abuse) and the substance-induced disorders (substance intoxication, substance withdrawal, substance-induced delirium, substance-induced persisting dementia, substance-induced persisting amnestic disorder, substance-induced psychotic disorder, substance-induced mood disorder, substance-induced anxiety disorder, substance-induced sexual dysfunction, and substance-induced sleep disorder).[5] Separate criteria sets define substance dependence, sub-

of adolescent addiction. Adolescence begins with the onset of puberty and presents a gamut of psychological and sociocultural challenges. According to Erikson, the primary task of adolescence is ego identity formation. Ego identity refers to one's sense of self and the capability to exhibit the capacity to function independently.[15]

Although this period of adolescent development is wrought with behavioral and emotional challenges, a minority of adolescents are actually disturbed. Evidence indicates that 80% of teenagers progress through adolescence without significant emotional turmoil and distress, but a significant minority (20%) do exhibit emotional and behavioral turmoil.[16] This evidence challenges the commonly held belief that adolescence is a period of chaos.

Distinguishing between normal and abnormal adolescent behavior can be challenging. Normal adolescents often exhibit extremes in behavior; however, if these are within the normal range, they do not interfere with an adolescent's functioning at school, work, or home. Experimentation with drugs and alcohol may be normative adolescent behavior. However, once this activity causes significant functional impairment at school, work, or home, the line between normative and serious use is crossed. Behaviors that indicate trouble include excessive hostility, major communication problems with parents or other authority figures, isolation, erratic habits, and abrupt changes in personality.[17]

Addicted adolescents may experience long-term biopsychosocial/developmental consequences. From a psychological perspective, these young people tend to perceive a low risk in experimenting with substances and are unconcerned about the long-term dangers of drugs. Addicted adolescents, like addicted adults, use denial to avoid coping with negative consequences of continued psychoactive substance use. Denial causes these individuals to acquire an unrealistic view of themselves and other people, places, and things.[17] Denial prevents internalization of personal responsibility, self-efficacy, and self-esteem. This, in turn, reinforces addictive behavior.

Epidemiology

Adolescent psychoactive substance use is quite prevalent. A survey conducted between 1975 and 1992 by the National Institute of Drug Abuse showed that 41% of high-school seniors reported illicit drug use (such as marijuana,

cocaine, LSD) at some time in their lives and 25% reported illicit drug use other than marijuana.[18] Eighty-eight percent of students reported use of alcohol by 12th grade; 51% had used it in the preceding month. By the eighth grade, 13% of the teenagers reported having drunk five or more servings of alcohol at one sitting; 21% of 10th graders and 28% of 12th graders reported similar use. Marijuana use was reported by 21% of 10th graders; this rose to 33% among seniors in high school. Cigarettes were the most commonly abused substance with 7% of 8th graders, 12% of 10th graders, and 17% of 12th graders smoking daily. Daily alcohol consumption was reported by 0.6%, 1.2%, and 3.4% of 8th, 10th, and 12th graders, respectively. By the 10th grade, 0.8% of the students reported using marijuana daily, and 0.3% of 8th graders reported daily use of inhalants.

The trends in adolescent drug abuse appear to vary with the drug. The number of adolescents smoking cigarettes in the preceding 30 days decreased from 38% in 1977 to 29% in 1981. Daily cigarette use dropped from 29% to 20% during the same time period. By 1984, only 19% of adolescents smoked daily; little had changed by 1992. The annual prevalence rate of alcohol use by high-school seniors rose from 85% in 1975 to 88% in 1979. During the same period, daily use of alcohol by the same group of adolescents went from 5.7% to 6.9%. These rates remained steady between 1985 and 1987, after which a slight decline in daily use (3.4%) was noted in 1992. Similarly, the annual and 30-day prevalence rates of marijuana use were steady between 1978 and 1979, and this was followed by a decline in 1980. By 1992, the annual marijuana use rate was 22%, compared with 51% in 1979. The annual rate of cocaine use increased from 6% in 1976 to 12% in 1979. This was followed by little or no change in prevalence rate between 1979 and 1985. However, the annual rate was 12.7% in 1986 and decreased to 3.1% in 1992.

The annual prevalence rate of LSD use showed a modest decline from 1975 to 1977. Between 1981 and 1985, the annual prevalence rate went from 6.5% to 4.4%. The rate increased to 5.6% by 1992; the trend appears to be rising.

Risk Factors

As outlined in Chatlos' biopsychosocial disease model, several risk factors serve to influence the development of adolescent addiction. In a study conducted by Dupre and colleagues,

55% of 64 adolescents were first given alcohol or drugs by a friend. The reported reasons for alcohol and drug use were "because it was cool, 30%; fun, 19%; everyone else did it, 19%; and peer pressure, 16%."[11] Other predictors of psychoactive substance initiation include previous participation in delinquent activities, low interest in conventional activities such as academics or religion, risk taking and impulsive behavior, poor relationship with parents, lack of access to healthy role models, parental psychoactive substance use, and lack of mentorship.[19]

The heritability of alcoholism gains credence from family, twin, and adoption studies. Fifty-four percent of identical twins and 38% of fraternal twins raised in the same family are concordant for alcoholism.[9] Studies have reported that sons of alcoholic fathers may be at a distinct disadvantage for developing alcoholism.[9] However, these studies fail to describe the degree to which risk for alcoholism can be attributed to genetic versus environmental factors. This question can only be answered by additional, hypothesis-driven research.

In addition to risk factors for adolescent psychoactive substance abuse, risk factors for future substance abuse have also been identified. Early age of psychoactive substance use initiation appears to be the single best predictor of subsequent abuse.[20] Other risk factors associated with future substance abuse include restrictive parental attitudes about drinking and alcohol use or, conversely, parental drug or alcohol-related problems.[21]

Assessment and Treatment of Adolescents with Psychoactive Substance Use Disorders

LEGAL ASPECTS

All states have specific regulations regarding the assessment and treatment of minors for mental health and psychoactive substance use problems. Consent for treatment must be provided by both the minor and parent or legal guardian unless the minor is committed. Emancipated minors (younger than 18 years and married, self-supporting, or a parent) can provide consent for treatment on their own behalf. Federal rules strictly regulate release of information that could identify a patient as a psychoactive substance user; both a minor's and parent's prior consent must be obtained

before such information may be released. If the minor is emancipated, he or she is able to provide necessary consent for release of information. Due process standards require that any patient treated for psychoactive substance use be informed of federal and state protective regulations at the time consent for treatment is obtained. Federal laws also strictly regulate admission of minors to methadone treatment.[22]

ASSESSMENT OF CHILD AND ADOLESCENT PSYCHOACTIVE SUBSTANCE USE DISORDERS

Clinical research continues to refine the systematic assessment of child and adolescent psychopathology, including psychoactive substance use disorders (PSUDs). The Diagnostic Interview Schedule for Children—Revised,[23] the Kiddie Schedule for Affective Disorders and Schizophrenia,[24] and the Diagnostic Interview for Children and Adolescents[25] all have demonstrated reliability and validity in generating DSM-III-R diagnoses and severity ratings for child and adolescent psychopathology. However, routine clinical use of these instruments is not feasible.

Several instruments devised for clinical use have acceptable psychometric properties and use a biopsychosocial assessment scheme. The Personal Experience Inventory (PEI) and the Chemical Dependence Assessment Scale (CDAS) are the two best-developed instruments for screening evaluation of adolescent psychoactive substance use; both are validated for use in clinical settings. The PEI is a standardized, self-report measure for 12- to 18-year-olds that identifies all forms of PSUDs, as well as related risk factors.[26] The CDAS is a self-report measure designed to describe and quantify adolescent drug use and psychological adjustment.[27] The Teen Addiction Severity Index (T-ASI) is a semistructured interview targeting six domains (substance use, school/employment status, family function, social relationships, legal status, psychiatric status) for development of a severity rating that may be sensitive to clinical change.[28] As such, the T-ASI can be used to assess treatment progress. The Drug Use Screening Inventory (DUSI) is a self-report instrument that profiles substance use involvement in conjunction with severity of disturbance in nine domains of functioning.[29] In addition to those domains assessed by the T-ASI, the DUSI addresses recreation, health status, and behavior patterns.

TREATMENT SETTING

Treatment of adolescents occurs in inpatient, residential (halfway house, group home), partial hospital/day treatment, and outpatient settings. The overwhelming majority (81.5%) of adolescents receive addiction treatment in an outpatient setting.[30] In the late 1980s and early 1990s, the American Society for Addiction Medicine (ASAM) and the National Association of Addiction Treatment Providers recruited adolescent and adult addiction treatment specialists to form consensus panels to develop addiction treatment placement criteria. Both panels defined three areas to be considered in addiction treatment planning and decision making: (1) level of care, (2) primary problem assessment dimensions, and (3) criteria for admission, continuing care, and discharge.[31]

The four levels of care differ from one another in three basic ways: (1) degree of direct medical management provided, (2) degree of environmental structure, control, and safety provided, and (3) degree of treatment intensity provided:

Level I—Outpatient treatment
Level II—Intensive outpatient/partial hospitalization treatment
Level III—Medically monitored intensive inpatient treatment
Level IV—Medically managed intensive inpatient treatment

The six primary problem dimensions to be assessed when making patient placement decisions and formulating individual treatment plans are (1) acute intoxication or withdrawal potential, (2) biomedical conditions and complications, (3) emotional and behavioral conditions or complications, (4) treatment acceptance/resistance, (5) relapse potential, and (6) recovery environment. A patient's progress with treatment should be evaluated according to the six problem dimensions to ensure ongoing comprehensive treatment planning. Once a patient's health status has improved within the current level of care, he or she is discharged to a less intensive level of care, according to the discharge criteria for each given level.

Medical management, the most intensive level of care, is necessary when an adolescent (1) poses severe withdrawal risk, (2) has a complicated or coexistent biomedical illness requiring 24-hour skilled nursing care, or (3) has a severe psychiatric illness requiring 24-hour psychiatric care, in addition to addiction treatment. Medically managed intensive inpatient treatment is typically provided in an inpatient hospital setting where full acute care services and intensive medical or psychiatric care services can be provided on site; 24-hour physician and nursing services and 16-hour/day professional counseling services must be available. Because most adolescents do not present with physical dependence or withdrawal symptoms nor the extent of physical deterioration seen in many adults, medically managed care for the management of withdrawal is rarely necessary.

Medically monitored intensive inpatient treatment is necessitated in the following situations: (1) if withdrawal symptoms are present or imminent but management does not require 24-hour nursing care, (2) biomedical complications of addiction require medical monitoring but not acute medical care (e.g., pregnancy), (3) the adolescent displays a mild to moderate risk of harm to self or others, requiring 24-hour monitoring, (4) addiction treatment resistance persists despite negative consequences of continued use, warranting 24-hour structure, or (5) either the environment poses threats to recovery that necessitate removal or the patient has been unable to maintain abstinence in a less restrictive addiction treatment setting. Medically monitored intensive inpatient treatment is typically provided in a free-standing licensed healthcare facility or specialty unit of a general or psychiatric hospital. A multidisciplinary team of addiction-credentialed clinicians provide a planned regimen of 24-hour evaluation and treatment services. Although full resources of an acute care or medically managed inpatient treatment service system should be available, it is not necessary to have them at the same site.

Intensive outpatient treatment is suitable in the following situations: (1) The adolescent does not exhibit overt symptoms of withdrawal risk, (2) the presence of a coexisting biomedical condition or complication is not severe enough to interfere with treatment, (3) the adolescent has a diagnosed but stable psychiatric disorder (i.e., attention-deficit hyperactivity disorder [ADHD], eating disorder) with minimal potential to interfere with addiction treatment, (4) treatment resistance is sufficient to require a structured treatment program but not sufficient to render outpatient treatment ineffective, (5) the adolescent is experiencing intensification of addiction symptoms and a high likelihood of relapse in a less structured program, or (6) the recovery environment is unsupportive but the adolescent has sufficient skills to cope if bolstered by program support.

Level II intensive outpatient treatment is typically provided in day treatment or partial hospitalization settings, outpatient psychiatric or addiction treatment clinics, or after-school programs. Weekly contact ranges between a minimum of 9 and a maximum of 20 hours.

Level I outpatient treatment is suitable when the following conditions are met: (1) No withdrawal risk is present, (2) if a biomedical condition or complication is present, it would not interfere with outpatient addiction treatment, (3) if psychiatric symptoms are present, the adolescent's mental status is stable enough to permit active participation in the treatment process, (4) the adolescent is willing to cooperate and attend all scheduled treatment activities but requires motivation and monitoring interventions, (5) the adolescent is able to maintain abstinence and recovery goals with minimal support, or (6) the adolescent has sufficient social skills to obtain necessary support for recovery and to become actively involved in community-based, self-help fellowship. Level I outpatient treatment is typically provided in outpatient addiction treatment clinics, outpatient psychiatric clinics, or school settings. Fewer than nine contact hours per week are provided.

TREATMENT ELEMENTS

The most frequently described adolescent addiction treatment elements include individual treatment planning, individual therapy, group therapy (self-help groups, relapse prevention, social skills training, addiction education), family therapy, pharmacotherapy, and intermittent drug toxicology testing. In practice, various models of addiction treatment form the conceptual basis for treatment programs; all were initially developed for adult addiction treatment and subsequently applied to adolescent addiction treatment.

The Individual Treatment Contract

Adolescents completing PSUD treatment indicated that devising a treatment contract was the single most therapeutic intervention that they had received.[32] In this study, the treatment contract was based on a problem list conjointly prepared by the adolescent and primary therapist during the initial treatment phase. The treatment contract specified long-term goals, based on the T-ASI domains, that were specific, sensible, achievable, and measurable. Individual treatment was provided by a team composed of a program coordinator who provided supervision to primary therapists responsible for direct contact with adolescent patients. Kaminer suggests that adolescent participation in devising a treatment contact enhances a patient's motivation and probability of engaging in behaviors that result in favorable treatment outcomes. Use of a treatment contract may mitigate attrition in that it offers adolescents an opportunity to exert some degree of control over the treatment process.

The Individual Treatment Plan

Development of an individual treatment plan prepares patients for the stages of treatment according to the stages of change model proposed by Prochaska and DiClemente: (1) precontemplation—no thought of change; (2) contemplation—thought but no action, start of intent to change; (3) action; and (4) maintenance.[33] The individual treatment plan should specify the goals and objectives of treatment and the specific treatment elements that will be used to accomplish these goals and objectives. The individual treatment plan should be reviewed with the patient at regular intervals to monitor treatment progress or lack thereof and to be updated when treatment goals and objectives are revised. The individual treatment contract, as described earlier, may be the most important part of the individual treatment plan in adolescent addiction treatment, the major difference being that adolescents are largely responsible for developing their treatment contract but the therapist is responsible for developing the individual treatment plan.

Individual Therapy

Individual therapy in addiction treatment may be most effective when it includes "all those interventions and roles a therapist must play in assuring that a substance abuser's physical and psychological needs are understood and managed."[34] The goal of individual therapy should be to support the initiation and maintenance of abstinence. Cognitive-behavior strategies may be particularly useful in helping adolescents identify substance addiction triggers and devise behavioral alternatives to mitigate these triggers. This process sets the stage for developing and negotiating the individual treatment contract with the therapist and family.

Family Therapy

Individual family therapy in which adolescents with PSUD and their families participate serves several functions. Early formation of a therapist-family relationship can mitigate adolescent treatment resistance by preparing both the family and adolescent patient for potential problems while actively engaging the family in the treatment process. An important family therapy goal is to identify and work out family conflicts before they become barriers to treatment. The family should actively negotiate components of the adolescent's treatment contract such as his or her adherence to parental limits and home responsibilities. Individual family therapy provides an opportunity for the therapist to identify other family members who may need treatment for PSUDs.

Multiple family group therapy is designed to work with groups of families who have an adolescent family member in addiction treatment. Goals for multiple family therapy include (1) educating the family about the role of the treatment program and the need to plan for relapse prevention and rehabilitation when needed, (2) examining the family relationships and determining what strengths and vulnerabilities might affect treatment and relapse prevention planning, (3) helping families help one another to cope with the shame and helplessness often related to having an adolescent with PSUD, (4) planning and cooperating with the families regarding treatment techniques for conflict resolution, and (5) providing families with information about PSUDs, community resources, and self-help groups for the adolescent and family members.[35]

Group Therapy

Group therapy is likely to be most effective when the aims, structure, roles of leaders and participants, inclusion and exclusion criteria for participants, and group process procedures are clearly defined. Although most adolescent PSUD treatment programs use some form of group therapy, it remains unclear exactly what types of group therapy are most effective and under what circumstances.

Both social skills training and relapse prevention groups are widely used in treatment of adolescent PSUDs. Both use a cognitive-behavioral approach to teach adolescents how to cope effectively with high-risk interpersonal situations that may lead to relapse. Specific skills taught include anger management, assertiveness training, effective oral communication, and thinking through a given behavior sequence to its likely outcome so that adolescents can determine how they should proceed and the related costs and benefits of doing

so. Several practitioners have developed skills manuals appropriate for adolescent use.

A1-Ateen is a self-help group specifically for adolescents with PSUDs or adolescents whose parents have PSUDs, or both. A1-Ateen incorporates the 12-step lifestyle change program and the 12 traditions of Alcoholics Anonymous, with some modifications. Although adolescents may benefit from participating in Alcoholics Anonymous, Kaminer recommends they be assisted in selecting appropriate sponsors so that they do not repeat morbid relationship patterns, especially those involving abuse.[36]

Pharmacotherapy

Given the fact that no reliable and valid studies exist on the use of pharmacotherapy in treatment of adolescent PSUDs, we must rely on clinical experience of those who regularly treat adolescents with PSUDs. Clinical experience suggests that there is no reason to assume that pharmacotherapy of adolescent PSUDs should be any different from that of adult PSUDs.[36] Clinicians need to be explicit and honest about lack of research evidence supporting use of pharmacological agents in the treatment of adolescent PSUDs when obtaining medication consent from adolescents and their parents/legal guardians. The main role for pharmacotherapy is detoxification of adolescents presenting with histories of tolerance or withdrawal from alcohol, barbiturates, and opioids. Protocols developed for detoxification of adults from these psychoactive substances should be used as treatment guides.

Methadone maintenance is the treatment of choice for pregnant adolescents addicted to heroin, as it is with pregnant women addicted to heroin. Methadone maintenance decreases the risk of human immunodeficiency virus infection associated with contaminated needle use as well as the risk for fetal distress associated with abrupt changes in serum levels, because methadone has a longer serum half-life than heroin. Nonpregnant adolescents younger than 18 years are required to have two documented failures with detoxification before methadone maintenance is offered; they must have an authorized adult sign an official consent form to be admitted to a methadone maintenance program.

Evidence supporting pharmacotherapy targeted to facilitate continued abstinence and recovery beyond the initial detoxification phase in adolescent PSUD treatment is also sorely lacking. Kaminer reported one case of facilitated cocaine abstinence by desipramine in an adolescent with 6-months follow-up that confirmed continued abstinence.[37] Even in studies examining pharmacological facilitation of abstinence and recovery in adults with PSUDs, it is not clear that continued abstinence and recovery can be attributed to pharmacotherapy versus other treatment elements. At this time, a prudent clinician should not pursue pharmacological facilitation of abstinence and recovery in treating adolescent PSUDs outside of a study protocol that has been reviewed and approved by an institutional review board.

Many adolescents with PSUDs are also diagnosed with depression at the time of initial assessment. If an adolescent with PSUD continues to meet diagnostic criteria for major depression after 2 weeks of psychoactive substance abstinence, a trial of antidepressant medication is warranted. Specific serotonin reuptake inhibitors (SSRIs) are preferable to tricyclic antidepressants because they are less cardiotoxic with overdoses and they lack sedative potentiation with alcohol; this is particularly important because the risk of suicide is high among adolescents with PSUDs.[37] SSRIs are also preferable for treatment of major depression in adolescents who are impulsive.

Lithium is the drug of choice for treatment of adolescents with bipolar disorders.[38] Lithium side effects in adolescents are similar to those reported by adults. Premedication workup and relative contraindications to lithium treatment of adolescents with comorbid bipolar disorder and PSUDs are no different from those of adolescents with bipolar disorder alone. As with adult women, female adolescents should have a negative result of a pregnancy test and should use some form of long-acting birth control (Norplant, Depo-Provera) before initiating lithium treatment (except in emergencies) because of lithium's association with increased risk of congenital cardiac anomalies for infants exposed during the first trimester. Adolescents with comorbid PSUDs and bipolar disorders need more frequent clinical and blood level monitoring than those with bipolar disorder alone because of their high risk for suicide and impulsive behavior.[36]

The use of medications with addicting properties, such as the benzodiazepines, to treat anxiety disorders in adolescents with PSUDs is not recommended. Evidence supporting pharmacological treatment of adolescents with panic disorder is nonexistent. Pharmacological treatment of obsessive-compulsive disorders (OCDs) in adolescents with clomipramine is well studied[39]; clomipramine has significant superiority over placebo in decreasing obsessive-compulsive symptoms in children and adolescents.[40] SSRIs such as fluoxetine may also be effective in reducing OCD symptoms in adolescents.[41] Although evidence supporting use of SSRIs over clomipramine is less definitive, SSRIs may be safer to use in adolescents with comorbid OCD and PSUDs because SSRIs lack sedative potentiation with alcohol and are less cardiotoxic with overdose.

No studies examining pharmacotherapy of eating disorders and comorbid-morbid PSUDs in adolescents have been reported. To date, no effective pharmacotherapy of anorexia has been reported. Antidepressants have short-term efficacy in decreasing the frequency of binging episodes in adults with bulimia nervosa.[41] Use of medication to treat adolescents with comorbid eating disorders and PSUDs should be considered only when nonpharmacological treatments have failed.

Neuroleptics continue to be the medications of choice for treating adolescents and adults with schizophrenia, whether or not they have comorbid PSUDs. Pharmacotherapy of adolescents with comorbid disruptive behavior disorders and PSUDs is discussed in Chapter 33.

Conclusions

Although evidence suggests that adolescent experimentation with psychoactive substances may be normative, we know that adolescent psychoactive substance use is a necessary, if not sufficient, causative factor in the biopsychosocial development of adolescent PSUDs. These disorders currently constitute a major threat to the health and well-being of U.S. adolescents. Without continued cooperation of concerned researchers, clinicians, parents, and advocates with policymakers and funding agencies, it is unlikely that randomized, controlled clinical trials of adolescent addiction treatment modalities will be funded and conducted. Without empirical evidence demonstrating adolescent addiction treatment efficacy and effectiveness, it remains unlikely that these services will achieve reimbursement parity with other forms of healthcare service used by adolescents. This would be particularly tragic given that a large proportion of adolescents with PSUDs also have comorbid psychiatric or chronic medical disorders.

Despite this lack of clear-cut empirical evidence, however, a body of adolescent addiction treatment knowledge continues to grow from contributions made by those clinicians who continue to care for these youth. Clinical experts were instrumental in devising a blueprint for clinician decision making in the form of the ASAM Patient Placement Criteria to ensure that addiction treatment services continue to be available, predictable, and reviewable. The development of alcohol and drug treatment standards by the Joint Commission, subsequent national accreditation, and development of patient placement criteria have succeeded in moving addiction treatment into the mainstream of healthcare services delivery.

REFERENCES

1. Johnston L, Bachman JG, O'Malley PM: National Trends in Drug Use and Related Factors Among American High School Students and Young Adults, 1975–1987. NIDA-DHHS Publication ADM-87-1587. Washington, DC, US Dept of Health and Human Services, 1987.
2. American Academy of Pediatrics Committee on Adolescence: Alcohol use and abuse: A pediatric concern. Pediatrics 79:450–453, 1987.
3. Miller NS, Gold MS: Dependence syndrome: A critical analysis of essential features. Psychiatr Ann 21(5):282–288, 1991.
4. Jaffe JA: Drug addiction and drug abuse. In Gilman AG, Rall TW, Nies AS, Taylor P (eds): The Pharmacological Basis of Therapeutics, 3rd ed. New York, Pergamon Press, 1990, pp 522–573.
5. American Psychiatric Association: Diagnostic and Statistical Manual of Mental Disorders, 4th ed. Washington, DC, American Psychiatric Association, 1994, pp 103–115.
6. MacDonald DI: Drugs, drinking and adolescence. Am J Dis Child 138(2):117–125, 1984.
7. Shedler J, Block J: Adolescent drug use and psychological health. Am Psychol 45:612–630, 1990.
8. Chatlos JC: Adolescent drug and alcohol addiction: Diagnosis and assessment. In Miller NS (ed): Comprehensive Handbook of Drug and Alcohol Addiction. New York, Marcel Dekker, 1991, pp 211–233.
9. Miller NS, Toft D: The Disease Concept of Alcoholism and Other Drug Addiction. Center City, MN, Hazelden Foundation, 1990, pp 1–35.
10. Bohn MH, Meyer RE: Typologies of addiction. In Galanter M, Kleber HD (eds): Textbook of Substance Abuse Treatment. Washington, DC, American Psychiatric Association, 1994, pp 11–24.
11. Dupre D, Miller NS, Gold MS, Rospenda K: Initiation and progression of alcohol, marijuana and cocaine use among adolescent users. Am J Addict 4(1):43–48, 1995.
12. Isralowitz R, Singer M (eds): Adolescent Substance Abuse: A Guide to Prevention. New York, Haworth Press, 1983.
13. Brent DA, Perper JA, Allman CJ: Alcohol, firearms, and suicide among youth. Temporal trends in Allegheny County, Pennsylvania, 1960–1983. JAMA 257(24):3369–3372, 1987.
14. Marttunen MJ, Aro HM, Henriksson MM, Lonnqvist JK: Psychosocial stressors more common in adolescent suicides with alcohol abuse compared with depressive adolescent suicides. J Am Acad Child Adolesc Psychiatry 33(4):490–497, 1994.
15. Brunstetter RW, Silver LB: Normal adolescent development. In Kaplan HI, Sadock BJ (eds): Comprehensive Textbook of Psychiatry, 4th ed. Baltimore, Williams & Wilkins, 1985, pp 1608–1613.
16. Offer D, Howard KI, Schonert KA, Ostrov E: To whom do adolescents turn for help? Differences between disturbed and nondisturbed adolescents. J Am Acad Child Adolesc Psychiatry 30(4):623–630, 1991.
17. Morrison MA, Smith TS: Psychiatric issues of adolescent chemical dependence. Pediatr Clin North Am 34(2):461–480, 1987.
18. Johnston LD, O'Malley PM, Bachman JG: Overview of Key Findings. National Survey Results of Drug Use from the Monitoring the Future Study, 1975–1993. NIH Publication 94-3809. Rockville, MD, US Dept of Health and Human Services, 1994, pp 5–26.
19. Kandel DB, Raveis VH: Cessation of illicit drug use in young adulthood. Arch Gen Psychiatry 46:109–116, 1989.
20. Blum RW: Adolescent substance abuse: Diagnostic and treatment issues. Pediatr Clin North Am 34(2):523–537, 1987.
21. Rogers PD, Harris J, Jarmuskewicz J: Alcohol and adolescence. Pediatr Clin North Am 34(2):289–303, 1987.
22. MacDonald DI: Patterns of alcohol and drug use among adolescents. Pediatr Clin North Am 34(2):275–288, 1987.
22. State Methadone Maintenance Treatment Guidelines. Washington, DC, Food and Drug Administration, 1992.
23. Costello E, Edelbrock C, Costello AJ: Validity of the NIMH Diagnostic Interview Schedule for Children: A comparison between pediatric and psychiatric referrals. J Abnorm Child Psychol 13:579–595, 1985.
24. Orvaschel H, Puig-Antich J, Chambers W, et al: Retrospective assessment of prepubertal major depression with the Kiddie-SADS-E. J Am Acad Child Psychiatry 21:392–397, 1982.
25. Wellner Z, Reich W, Herjanic B, et al: Reliability, validity, and parent-child agreement studies of the Diagnostic Interview for Children and Adolescents (DICA). J Am Acad Child Adolesc Psychiatry 26:649–653, 1987.
26. Winters K, Henly G: Personal Experience Inventory Test and Manual. Los Angeles, Western Psychological Services, 1988.
27. Oetting ER, Beauvais F: Epidemiology and correlates of alcohol use among Indian adolescents living on reservations. In Epidemiology of Alcohol Use and Abuse Among US Ethnic Minorities. NIAAA Publication ADM-89-1435. Washington, DC, US Dept of Health and Human Services, 1989, pp 323–373.
28. Kaminer Y, Bukstein OB, Tarter RE: The Teen Addiction Severity Index (T-ASI): Rationale and reliability. Int J Addict 26:219–226, 1991.
29. Tarter RE: Evaluation and treatment of adolescent substance abuse: A decision tree method. Am J Drug Alcohol Abuse 16:1–46, 1990.
30. Beschner GM: The problem of adolescent drug abuse: An introduction to intervention strategies. In Friedman AS, Beschner GM (eds): Treatment Services for Adolescent Substance Abusers. NIDA Publication ADM-85-1342. Washington, DC, US Dept of Health and Human Services, 1985, pp 1–12.
31. Hoffman NG, Halikas JA, Mee-Lee D, Weedman RD: Patient Placement Criteria for the Treatment of Psychoactive Substance Use Disorders. Washington, DC, American Society of Addiction Medicine, 1990, pp 61–107.
32. Kaminer Y, Tarter RE, Bukstein OB, Kabene M: Staff, treatment completers' and noncompleters' perception of the value of treatment variables. Am J Addict 1:115–120, 1992.
33. Prochaska JO, DiClemente C: Toward a comprehensive model of change. In Miller WR, Heather N (eds): Treat-

ing Addictive Behaviors: Processes of Change. New York, Plenum, 1986, pp 3–27.

34. Khantzian EJ: Psychotherapeutic interventions with substance abusers—the clinical context. J Subst Abuse Treat 2:83–88, 1985.

35. Bartlett D: The use of multiple family therapy groups with adolescent drug addicts. In Sugar M (ed): The Adolescent in Group and Family Therapy. Chicago, University of Chicago Press, 1986, pp 262–282.

36. Kaminer Y: Treatment selection and modalities. In Kaminer Y (ed): Adolescent Substance Abuse: A Comprehensive Guide to Theory and Practice. New York, Plenum, 1994, pp 197–256.

37. Kaminer Y: Psychoactive substance abuse and dependence as a risk factor in adolescent attempted and completed suicide. Am J Addict 1:21–29, 1992.

38. Carlson GA: Bipolar disorders in children and adolescents. In Garfinkel BD, Carlson GA, Weller EB (eds): Psychiatric Disorders in Children and Adolescents. Philadelphia, WB Saunders, 1990, pp 21–36.

39. Rapoport JL: Pediatric psychopharmacology: The last decade. In Meltzer HY (ed): Psychopharmacology: The Third Generation of Progress. New York, Raven Press, 1987, pp 1211–1214.

40. DeVeaugh-Geiss J, Moroz G, Biederman J, et al: Clomipramine hydrochloride in childhood and adolescent obsessive-compulsive disorder—a multicenter trial. J Am Acad Child Adolesc Psychiatry 31:45–49, 1992.

41. Ambrosini PJ, Bianchi MD, Rabinovich H, Elia J: Antidepressant treatments in children and adolescents. II. Anxiety, physical, and behavioral disorders. J Am Acad Child Adolesc Psychiatry 32:483–492, 1993.

Posttraumatic Stress Disorder and Addiction: What Are the Links?

Mary Langley, MD

This chapter is intended to provide an integrated approach to the treatment of posttraumatic stress disorder (PTSD) complicated by addiction. A fair amount of research data and clinical material for each disorder is available in isolation, but very few sound guidelines for an approach to the combined disorders is available in the literature to date. A practical guide to understanding each disorder in the context of the other is discussed, followed by clinical examples. A nomogram indicating recommended pharmacological decision-making methods is provided. Also included in this chapter is information about psychological theories of trauma and approaches that have been validated on the basis of sound psychosocial research. Finally, an integrated approach to the longitudinal treatment of dually diagnosed patients with PTSD is offered. The needs of special populations such as rape victims and children are emphasized throughout.

Historical Perspectives

Despite a long history of appreciation for the devastating effects of trauma, the diagnosis of stress-related illness has endured generations of misunderstanding, inadequate research, and conceptual struggles. The diagnosis of alcohol-ism shares some of the besieged history that chronicles the diagnosis of PTSD.

The intimate connection between external stressors and severe psychological distress was observed and documented in combat veterans by Grinker and Spiegel in 1945.[2] More recently, Solomon and her colleagues have amassed 10 years' worth of prospective research into the effects of combat stress, recurrent stress, and the individual/family repercussions of trauma to Israeli soldiers.[3]

The National Vietnam Veteran's Readjustment Study (NVVRS)[4] and the Centers for Disease Control (CDC)[5] studies represent two large epidemiological surveys evaluating the effects of trauma on a particularly disabled segment of the population exposed to overwhelming stress. Further epidemiological, preclinical, and clinical data on stress are rapidly accumulating in response to these recent developments, supporting conclusions suggested by the pioneering work initiated by Grinker and Spiegel, albeit with a lapse of approximately 40 years.

PTSD, and alcohol abuse in the past, holds an uncomfortable and somewhat tenuous position in the medical nomenclature. Both disorders were classified as either personality disorders or other forms of neurosis until 1980.[6] Some of the reasons are social, some are political, and others illuminate early theoretical revisions by Freud and the primacy of psychosexual drive-based theories in psychoanalysis.

Alcoholism and other substance disorders have come into their own somewhat, apropos to their separate classification since the *Diagnostic and Statistical Manual of Mental Disorders,* third edition (DSM-III),[6] was published. This separate classification reflects recognition by mainstream psychiatry that substances are pathogenetically, if not etiologically, responsible for substance abuse.

PTSD has not yet been accepted as a pathogenetically based classification. Trauma is an essential component of the definition of the disorder nevertheless, implying acknowledgment of its role in the formation of posttraumatic symptoms at some level. On the other hand, PTSD is classified in the *Diagnostic and Statistical Manual of Mental Disorders,* fourth edition (DSM-IV),[7] as an anxiety disorder. During development of DSM-IV, reclassification of PTSD as either an etiologically based stress disorder or a dissociative disorder was discussed.

Discrete disorders have been classified as personal or moral aberrations through many generations of medical practice, but now emerging is some moderate hope that PTSD *and* addiction can be approached as treatable diseases with known pathophysiology. Although we may never eliminate war or abuse, if there is a reliable connection between *known noxious agents* and *stress response syndromes,* efforts to help a host of affected individuals would be well served. Treatment may become even more specific; in the meantime, moderately effective interventions have been demonstrated and are receiving scientific validation.

Epidemiology

PTSD and addiction also share comparable standing as significant societal health concerns. Nearly one third of the adult population in the United States are believed to suffer from problems of alcohol and illicit substance abuse.

The NVVRS data suggest that 15.2% of the male Vietnam combat veteran population currently suffer from post-traumatic stress disorder, and 8.5% of female veterans also suffer the disabling effects of a full-blown syndrome. The lifetime prevalence of PTSD for era veteran controls are 2.5% and 1.1% for men and women, respectively. Another 350,000, about 10%, of Vietnam veterans are shown to experience symptoms that adversely affect their lives but are insufficient to warrant a diagnosis.

Findings from the NVVRS study suggest a large unmet need for PTSD treatment among Vietnam veterans. Approximately three eighths of male veterans and one quarter of female veterans with combat-related stress sequelae have never consulted a professional about mental health problems. These statistics raise profound questions about the degree of unmet need for PTSD services in other, less well-characterized populations such as victims of rape, child abuse, and other crimes. Civilian controls in the NVVRS study reveal lifetime prevalence rates of 1.2% PTSD for men and 0.3% for women, data that are somewhat but not drastically different from Epidemiological Catchment Area (ECA) data on the general population (0.5% in men and 1.2% in women).[8]

The ECA survey[8] is one of the few large epidemiological studies on the subject of PTSD in civilian samples but is believed to seriously underrepresent the scope of the problem. These data are wholly inconsistent with studies of at-risk groups and may be a reflection of the fact that *physical attack* and *combat* were the only two types of traumatic exposure queried in that sample. Studies that systematically assess a wide range of victimization experiences reveal PTSD prevalence rates of 75% and greater.[9]

A national random sample of adult women, reported by the National Victim Center and Crime Victims Research and Treatment Center, indicates that 12.9% of women (about 12 million) have been raped at least once during their lifetime. Other information, including a longitudinal study on 65 rape victims,[10] leads Foa and Riggs to the conclusion that "it is likely that rape victims constitute the largest group of people with PTSD in this country."[11]

In contradistinction to studies of combat-related stress, threat to life, limb, and property seem relatively unrelated to chronic PTSD symptoms in two studies of natural disaster as compared with premorbid factors.[12, 13] In victims of natural disaster, distress is regarded as a highly personalized reaction within a range of responses ranging from enhanced ability to chronic disability.

Reactions to stress are assumed to be mediated by such factors as vulnerability and secondary gain; however, adequate studies to address these issues have not been conducted to date. The psychological significance of a disaster is likewise presumed to be a significant variable but has not yet been adequately studied. Also in a relatively primordial stage of development is research on mitigating mechanisms during the event.

Work in the area of natural disaster therefore has heuristic value for two specific associations. It supports clinical observations that chronic disorder is more likely to ensue from interpersonal forms of stress, including rape, war, and violent crime, especially if the insults are repeated. It also establishes the vectorial relationship between mitigating mechanisms during an event and the cultivation of symptoms. It points the way toward research on the subject of personal vulnerability to the development of stress response syndromes.

Etiology

Causation as it relates to proposed classifications of disease requires that two essential factors be undisputed. The first factor involves the construct validity, or ability to recognize the disorder as a discrete diagnostic entity. This can be established if the disease prevalence increases after exposure to the proposed etiological agent. Two epidemiological databases exist to support the construct validity of PTSD as a diagnostic entity, with trauma representing the causal association. These two prospective investigations note an increase in PTSD (and only a few other diagnoses) in response to natural disaster and sexual assault. Of note is the fact that PTSD is the only psychiatric diagnosis observed to increase in prevalence in both studies. In the major retrospective studies of Vietnam veterans, preservice variables also contributed somewhat but not completely to the differences observed in prevalence of PTSD between exposure groups.

The second factor, requiring unequivocal endorsement, is the ability to isolate and replicate the proposed causative agent. For example, pneumococcal pneumonia is established as a discrete diagnostic entity with known pathophysiological markers (i.e., sputum, radiology, cultures) and an association with a recognizable agent (the *Streptococcus pneumoniae* isolate). The related question often raised in PTSD is, What constitutes trauma sufficient to incur an etiological designation? Although the complexity of an event such as violence or disaster is great compared with isolation of a microscopic pathogen, a temporal relationship between syndromes and exposures can be identified in both examples. A somewhat uniform and more reliable definition of trauma needs to be developed if it is ever to be ordained as a bona fide cause of disorder.

Despite evidence to the contrary, some researchers continue to suggest that trauma represents a nonspecific trigger for various syndromes, such as major depression, panic disorder, somatic problems, and addiction. These disorders also increase in prevalence after trauma and frequently co-occur with PTSD but not as reliably. Issues such as intensity of the stressor, risk factors in the event, vulnerability of the individual, and subjective appraisal of the event all are still considered as mediating factors in the development of disorder. For example, Kilpatrick and colleagues' study of crime victims looked at event characteristics and their contribution to PTSD symptoms.[14] Indications were that the more *violent* the crime, the more likely the victim was to experience posttraumatic sequelae, with one notable exception: When physical injury and threatened death were controlled for, victims of completed rape experienced long-term PTSD symptoms *independent* of those variables. The rate of PTSD in the completed rape-only group (no injury or threat) was 28.6%, 3.1 times greater than the group of crime victims who experienced none of the three variables (9.2%). Victims who experienced all three variables (completed rape, physical injury, and threatened death) had a PTSD rate of 78.6%

A prospective longitudinal study comparing odds ratios for the development of multiple disorders together or in isolation relevant to specific traumas is needed. Such a study is currently under way to evaluate the effects of the Persian Gulf war on 84 reservists, many of whom experienced symptoms that did not improve in the 6-month follow-up data.[15]

A movement to classify disorders together when they apparently arise after trauma is gaining momentum. Success in this direction may help to resolve some of the etiological uncertainty that remains, but evidence is accumulating that some events are uncommonly distressing. Gatekeeping, the ability to validate disorders causing disability, is an important topic in the discussion of diagnostic classification and cannot be overlooked. However, a more urgent need is to identify and eradicate known human-induced toxicities. Interested readers are referred to Davidson's comprehensive discussion of the topic.[16]

Clinical Characteristics

Diagnostic criteria for PTSD are defined in DSM-IV and are presented in Table 30–1.

Three basic clusters of symptoms can be

Table 30–1. DIAGNOSTIC CRITERIA FOR 309.81 POSTTRAUMATIC STRESS DISORDER

A. The person has been exposed to a traumatic event in which both of the following were present:
   (1) the person experienced, witnessed, or was confronted with an event or events that involved actual or threatened death or serious injury, or a threat to the physical integrity of self or others
   (2) the person's response involved intense fear, helplessness, or horror. **Note:** In children, this may be expressed instead by disorganized or agitated behavior

B. The traumatic event is persistently reexperienced in one (or more) of the following ways:
   (1) recurrent and intrusive distressing recollections of the event, including images, thoughts, or perceptions. **Note:** In young children, repetitive play may occur in which themes or aspects of the trauma are expressed.
   (2) recurrent distressing dreams of the event. **Note:** In children, there may be frightening dreams without recognizable content.
   (3) acting or feeling as if the traumatic event were recurring (includes a sense of reliving the experience, illusions, hallucinations, and dissociative flashback episodes, including those that occur on awakening or when intoxicated). **Note:** In young children, trauma-specific reenactment may occur.
   (4) intense psychological distress at exposure to internal or external cues that symbolize or resemble an aspect of the traumatic event
   (5) physiological reactivity on exposure to internal or external cues that symbolize or resemble an aspect of the traumatic event

C. Persistent avoidance of stimuli associated with the trauma and numbing of general responsiveness (not present before the trauma), as indicated by three (or more) of the following:
   (1) efforts to avoid thoughts, feelings, or conversations associated with the trauma
   (2) efforts to avoid activities, places, or people that arouse recollections of the trauma
   (3) inability to recall an important aspect of the trauma
   (4) markedly diminished interest or participation in significant activities
   (5) feeling of detachment or estrangement from others
   (6) restricted range of affect (e.g., unable to have loving feelings)
   (7) sense of a foreshortened future (e.g., does not expect to have a career, marriage, children, or a normal life span)

D. Persistent symptoms of increased arousal (not present before the trauma), as indicated by two (or more) of the following:
   (1) difficulty falling or staying asleep
   (2) irritability or outbursts of anger
   (3) difficulty concentrating
   (4) hypervigilance
   (5) exaggerated startle response

E. Duration of the disturbance (symptoms in Criteria B, C, and D) is more than 1 month.

F. The disturbance causes clinically significant distress or impairment in social, occupational, or other important areas of functioning.

Specify if:
   Acute: if duration of symptoms is less than 3 months
   Chronic: if duration of symptoms is 3 months or more

Specify if:
   With Delayed Onset: if onset of symptoms is at least 6 months after the stressor

(From American Psychiatric Association Diagnostic and Statistical Manual of Mental Disorders, 4th ed. Washington DC, American Psychiatric Association, 1994.)

manifested in the disorder, and a preponderance of different symptom clusters has been described in response to different stressors.[3] The fixed dominance of symptom clusters is also postulated to develop in the presence of personal vulnerabilities and to depend on the victim's state of mind at the time of the event.

The symptoms of PTSD are delineated along the lines of reexperiencing, avoidance or numbing, and arousal. One or a combination of symptoms can dominate the picture in any individual patient, but various symptoms frequently occur in a phasic fashion, with oscillation between avoidance behaviors/emotional numbing on the one hand and sudden angry discharges on the other hand being the norm. A mental status examination often reveals feelings of anger, guilt, and a preoccupation with the traumatic event. Patients often report that they have no future, that they "died" during the event. A pattern of compulsive repetition predominates the existence of some patients. This motive usually affects more chronically diseased individuals and is characterized by self-destructive behaviors. Pseudohallucinations might also be present but can be distinguished from psychosis on the basis of their internalized nature and the fact that they take place in the absence of other signs of formal thought disorder. These pseudohallucinations often take the form of recollections about particularly stressful material and are often described in terms of "that tape recorder in my head" or "those demons that haunt me."

The clinical picture is often complicated by comorbid conditions such as addiction, major depression, and panic disorder. Associated features include impulsive, sometimes violent behavior, and close relatives and proximal acquaintances are frequent targets.

In DSM-IV, distinctions are made between (1) acute stress reaction, which lasts for less than 1 month, (2) acute PTSD, which lasts more than 1 but less than 3 months, and (3) chronic PTSD, which has a more prolonged course and is the diagnosis most often complicated by addiction. The reason for the distinction between acute stress reaction and PTSD is the observation that many victims of traumatic interpersonal and natural events exhibit symptoms that interfere with functioning but are nevertheless short lived. This is an important development, considering the wealth of opportunities created for research into preventive early treatment and natural history.

The following case demonstrates a typical patient with chronic PTSD and current addiction to cocaine:

Mr. R. is a 43-year-old African-American man who served in heavy combat during his official tour in Vietnam. The patient, 20 years later, vividly recalls several killings and is haunted by visions of mutilated bodies. He remains preoccupied with acts he committed during the war. Mr. R. began using drugs and alcohol in Vietnam, reportedly to "numb" feelings of terror, anger, and despair. The patient's drugs of choice during his service years were alcohol, marijuana, and heroin. He denies any personal or family history of drinking or drug use before his military enlistment.

Mr. R. was raised in an intact family in a suburb of a major urban area. He was an athlete and an honors student in high school. He joined the army because of a stated interest in travel and adventure and was initially stationed in North Carolina. He felt that he was racially discriminated against in boot camp and states that he was somewhat relieved when sent to Vietnam.

After returning home with an honorable discharge, Mr. R. reports a continuation of his drinking, which was rather heavy by that time. The patient reports that he frequently felt "out of control" and nervous and that he experienced frequent nightmares. He reports that alcohol initially provided some relief from those problems. Those problems eventually became more unmanageable, and Mr. R. began making attempts at treatment programs for either PTSD or addiction but was never successful at either. He has a long line of disciplinary discharges from the hospital for inability to uphold behavioral "no-harm" contracts, frequently invoked after he safely recovered from the effects of chemical toxicity/withdrawal. He has likewise been excluded from addiction treatment communities for problems with violence. In his late 30s, he switched to cocaine, which he regards as a "cleaner" addiction, albeit fraught with its own setbacks.

Mr. R. was married briefly but identified angry outbursts toward his wife as a major issue that destroyed the relationship. He maintained custody of his two children, whom he raised with the help of his mother in her home. His work history is sporadic, although he was able to complete vocational training and demonstrates above-average intellect.

Mr. R. is currently trying again to engage in treatment. He is being investigated for child abuse and is very ashamed of the way he's lived. He is also terrified of himself and his propensity for violence; he is looking for advances in symptom management that will afford him the requisite impulse control to remain in treatment this time.

Epidemiology of the Posttraumatic Stress Disorder/Addiction Interface

It is well documented that 60% to 80% of treatment-seeking veterans with PTSD have an increased incidence of addiction. Not quite as clear is the incidence of addiction in the population of PTSD veterans who are not in treatment. Two large epidemiological studies concerning combat-related posttraumatic stress in the Vietnam War generation have already been cited. The NVVRS[4] revealed that approximately three fourths of male Vietnam veterans with PTSD had a lifetime addiction disorder and 22% had a current substance abuse disorder.

The lifetime prevalence of alcohol and drug dependence found in Vietnam combat veterans overall was approximately 40%, equal to the lifetime prevalence of those disorders in Vietnam-era veterans studied. Interestingly, these rates were higher than the civilian control group studied, whose lifetime prevalence of alcohol and drug dependence disorders was about 25% and higher than ECA data on the general population, which estimates the prevalence of addiction in the range of 17%. One plausible methodological reason for the discrepancy involves sampling differences between veterans in the study and civilians. The veterans in the study were recruited using military personnel files. Civilians were contacted using household sampling methods, which are likely to miss certain forms of pathology associated with homelessness and incarceration. Sociocultural influences on behavior that encouraged drinking/drug use and biases affecting military service during the Vietnam era may also account for the difference.

The NVVRS data reveal that for women, Vietnam combat veterans have lifetime and current alcohol rates of 9.1% and 1%, respectively. Lifetime alcohol abuse/dependence is higher in women who served in Vietnam (combatants) than in female veterans stationed in the United States, in Europe, in Korea, or at sea (noncombatant Vietnam veterans, 8%) or in civilian women (2%). Drug disorder prevalence is 1% lifetime and 0% current in this study of female Vietnam veterans, a rate not significantly different from that in noncombatant Vietnam veteran females or civilian women. Only lifetime *alcohol* prevalence in women is significantly affected by co-occurrence of PTSD, with rates almost double those of noncombatant veterans not suffering from PTSD.

The CDC report[5] found no significant difference in rates of addiction between combatant and noncombatant Vietnam veterans. They did, however, report a concentrated increase in the prevalence of anxiety, depression, and alcohol use disorders among Vietnam veterans who also were affected by the *numbing/avoidance* cluster of PTSD symptoms.

Neurochemical Hypotheses for Posttraumatic Stress Disorder

KINDLING

Post and Kopanda pioneered investigation of the biological facts regarding repeated bioelectrical stimulation of certain brain regions in rodents and cats, frequently cited as a *kindling phenomenon*.[17] An excellent review of the subject can be found in Neppe and Tucker's numerous works.[18]

In animal studies, subthreshold stimuli become capable of triggering ictal responses, after repeated intermittent threshold stimulation of analogous brain areas, such as the amygdala, hippocampus, and piriform areas. Behaviors associated with kindling in animals tend to be paroxysmal, repetitive, and physiologically determined.

Indirect clinical evidence supports the application of the animal model of kindling to human behavioral correlates. Indications to support the hypothesis include the following observations:

• Patients with behavioral dyscontrol symptoms exhibit fairly autonomous and unsuppressible drive states. Their impulses appear to supercede cortical inhibition in an episodic fashion. Also, they are emotionally labile and exquisitely sensitive to experiences that mimic the original insult. These features resemble psychomotor seizures in key ways.

• Most syndromes that share these features, with the exception of idiopathic epilepsy and functional psychosis, have a known association with severe physical or psychological trauma.

• Evidence suggests that patients with partial complex seizure disorders experience clinical improvement in *bipolar* and *aggressive* disorders in response to carbamazepine.

Limbic kindling due to repeated neuropsychological trauma and presumed bioelectrical effects thereof has thus been postulated as a mechanism in PTSD, as it has in other forms of traumatic brain injury, including alcohol withdrawal, head injury, and cocaine abuse. An open trial with carbamazepine in combat veterans with PTSD demonstrated efficacy in all symptom clusters, including reexperiencing.[19, 20]

The study of kindling phenomena, so far, is compatible with the major neurobiological models of PTSD. Pretreatment of animals with benzodiazepines and other central nervous system (CNS) depressants suppresses the development of both kindling phenomena and stress-induced analgesia (discussed later). Anticonvulsants, especially carbamazepine, have been shown to effect endpoint stabilization of already kindled tissues. These views suggest and support clinical indications for benzodiazepines or adrenergic antagonists in acute stress reaction and imply that anticonvulsants may alleviate symptoms of reexperiencing in chronic stages of PTSD.

Another possible mechanism to account for the apparent neurophysiological disturbance in patients with PTSD is a chemical alteration sometimes referred to as *chindling* or *sensitization*.[18]

Chindling mechanisms may also point to a model of addiction based on the effects of repeated chemical insults to the CNS. Chindled pathways in the amygdala and hypothalamus, for example, may correlate with the development of an autonomous drive state much like hunger, thirst, and sex. The physiological correlate to these symptoms is believed to be similar to the reverse tolerance found in abusers of cocaine and other stimulants.

If the nature of kindled responses can be elucidated, understanding of the molecular sequelae following trauma can lead us to the development of more effective and safe immediate treatments for acute stress reactions. It may also point to secondary prevention methods to offset development of chronic PTSD.

The development of reasonable pharmacological interventions in addiction that support rehabilitation efforts or reverse the disease process entirely is also possible. More fundamental understanding of these phenomena could render unique opportunities for rational thinking about the neurophysiological correlates of personality. Traumatic events and noxious interpersonal insults may someday be understood not only from a sociological perspective but on the basis of their end effects on tissue systems. G-proteins, second messengers, and corticosteroid alterations may be important mediators, and much current research interest is focused on the psychiatric correlates to observed changes in these substances.

It is possible that kindling or chindling models might account for the intractable nature of PTSD and addiction symptoms and their refractoriness to standard interventions. Controlled clinical trials evaluating the efficacy of anticonvulsants and other antikindling agents are expectantly awaited.

AUTONOMIC AROUSAL

Interest in the neurobiology of PTSD and the conclusions reached has paralleled the evolution of knowledge about alcohol and street drugs. Stress has been shown to activate the locus caeruleus (LC) in a similar fashion to pain and other physiological compromises, resulting in central noradrenergic-mediated alarm behaviors in animals.

It is possible to produce a conditioned emotional response in animals such that if a neutral stimulus (conditioned stimulus [CS]) is coupled with a traumatic stimulus (unconditioned stimulus [US]), the CS eventually elicits an alarm behavior (unconditioned response [UR]). The behaviors in animals subjected to this experiment are correlated with permanent increases in brain metabolites of noradrenaline, suggesting a chronic central noradrenergic hyperactivity in animal stress-response syndromes.

Animal models have also shown that inhibiting the LC with drugs including ethanol, clonidine, and heroin can prevent the conditioned response. These agents lose their efficacy in the prevention of LC alterations over time with repeated exposure. Severity and repetitiveness of the event(s) seem also to mediate development of chronic *per stimulus* startle responses in animals. For example, more intractable neurochemical changes have been correlated with more grievous forms of trauma.

Some observations that suggest alterations in noradrenergic function in human patients with PTSD include the following:

• Patients with PTSD have decreased platelet alpha-2-adrenergic receptor numbers and decreased platelet monoamine oxidase activity.

• Increased methoxyhydroxyphenylglycol, blood pressure, and heart rate responses, in addition to flashbacks, occur when yohimbine is administered to subjects with PTSD compared with controls.[21, 22]

All the evidence taken together suggests central sympathetic hyperactivity in patients with PTSD mediated by a neurobiologically altered LC that is chronically hypersensitive to stimuli. This parallels the clinical observation that patients with chronic PTSD, for years and sometimes a lifetime, experience extreme psychological discomfort over reminders of the event. A rape victim who experiences panic when in the proximity of the crime scene is an example of this phenomenon.

Noradrenergic hyperactivity in response to *alarming stimuli* or *lactate infusion* and the ability of central noradrenergic-blocking agents to suppress these responses in humans lend further credence to the pivotal role of this neurotransmitter in PTSD.

INESCAPABLE SHOCK

Van der Kolk and colleagues applied the animal model of stress-induced analgesia to PTSD,[23] based on several lines of evidence. The model chronicles the ability of animals with inescapable shock ([IS], the experimental condition for learned helplessness) to withstand pain when reexposed to a subsequent stressor within a brief time. For example, IS affords rats the ability to "play dead" in the presence of a cat, even if the rat is being shocked at the moment the cat is presented. Non-IS rats jump away from the shock and into harm's way. It is believed that analgesia in the presence of known stressors is a self-sustaining biological mechanism documented in several species.

Clinically, "negative" symptoms of PTSD resemble learned helplessness in animals. Studies of human surgical stress reveal elevated beta-endorphin levels, and some self-mutilators likewise demonstrate raised metenkephalins. Van der Kolk hypothesizes that the "numbing and catatenoid reactions following trauma in humans correspond to the central nervous system catecholamine depletion that follows inescapable shock in animals."

He further postulates that the human expression of stress-induced analgesia in patients with PTSD leads to a phasic depletion of endogenous opioids. A subsequent addiction to trauma or exogenous opioids is believed to be explained by the desire of these patients to modulate endogenous opioid levels, thereby offsetting a chronic oscillating state of endogenous opioid withdrawal. This model is receiving support in the literature through clinical studies of naloxone-reversible stress-induced analgesia in patients with PTSD.[24, 25]

A UNIFYING THEORY

Neither central noradrenergic hyperactivity nor endogenous opioid depletion by itself would explain cocaine addiction observed in some patients with PTSD, nor the tendency to abuse substances well beyond their ability to achieve a beneficial response. This point is illustrated when one considers the fact that ethanol loses its antianxiety effect with chronic use. Chronic drinking actually causes dysphoria over time. Also, it is not completely clear why patients with autonomic arousal would abuse central stimulants. Both phenomena are observed in patients with chronic PTSD complicated by addiction.

Miller and Gold[26] hypothesized a common neurochemical mechanism for addiction to pharmacologically distinct drugs. Their model may reconcile some of the apparent contradictions that distinguish the dual diagnosis of stress disorders and chemical abuse. For example, a hedonism model has been proposed as an alternative to the self-medication hypothesis of ethanol abuse in PTSD. One may take the view that all addiction is, ultimately, self-medication of the human condition with hedonism

at its core. Some individuals seem to be more physiologically vulnerable to using external sources of pleasure/reward. Patients with PTSD may be among a subset of individuals who are driven to abuse substances on the basis of a biological predisposition. This notion will be supported if further data regarding opioid depletion, linked to IS, are found to be a valid physiological marker in posttraumatic stress.

According to Miller and Gold's model, a reinforcement center at the level of the ventral tegmental area exists and has been tested extensively as such in animals. Enhancement of dopamine concentrations in the ventral tegmental area can be effected by all the major drugs of abuse, including cocaine, nicotine, cannabis, and opioids. Engagement of reward systems, especially in the presence of purported emotional numbing and endogenous opiod depletion, may offer an explanation for both (1) the seemingly paradoxical predilection for patients with PTSD to abuse cocaine and (2) co-occurence of addiction to chemically different drugs in a given individual.

There is at least preliminary evidence[27] that patients with avoidance/numbing symptoms of PTSD have a preference for cocaine. The variance in drugs of choice among PTSD sufferers may be explained, at least partially, with respect to common effects of dissimilar agents on the dopamine reward system. Alternatively, the eventual catecholamine depletion that accompanies chronic cocaine addiction may offer a form of escape from autonomic arousal that is reinforcing in itself.

SUMMARY

To summarize, various neurochemical models have been proposed in PTSD. Most of these models share neurosubstrates with the addictions and may explain the frequent comorbidity observed in clinical populations. Chronic sympathetic nervous system arousal in PTSD is similar in some ways to withdrawal states and may represent a drive state predisposing to CNS depressant abuse. Endogenous opioid depletion on the basis of a vicious cycle of release in response to conditioned traumatic stimuli may account for either opioid addiction or addiction to other reward mechanism-activating substances. Chronic alcohol abuse causes dysphoria, causes alcohol to lose its antianxiety effect, and has not been shown to reverse the physiological alterations noted in animal models of PTSD. It is consequently clear that self-medication with alcohol has severe shortcomings. It is also evident that pharmacological agents to more specifically engage and reverse proposed biological mechanisms in PTSD require development. Preliminary evidence suggests that PTSD is a heterogeneous condition with different neurobiological substrates. Elucidation of the molecular underpinnings of stress response syndromes would pave the way for development of more specifically efficacious interventions. An overview of the prevailing neurochemical theories of PTSD and their relevance to addiction is provided in Table 30–2.

Psychological Theories of Trauma

ANALYTICAL

Freud was perhaps the first psychiatrist to describe psychic distress in response to external trauma. He posited that the traumatic event, as it symbolically converged with internal drive states (libidinal or aggressive), was capable of penetrating a "stimulus barrier," thus provoking guilt and anxiety. Repression, in early Freudian theory, relieves the organism from guilt and anxiety but requires a large expenditure of energy to prevent the memories from transversing the barrier. Freud viewed abreaction as a means of restoring dynamic homeostasis for the organism, thus conserving psychic energy. Freud revised the seduction hypothesis in response to observations that some of his patients' "memories" were unfounded in reality. In the process of revising the seduction hypothesis, Freud deemphasized external factors as the theoretical source of anxiety, such that abreaction became a much less essential focus of his work. Fantasy became the primary theoretical linchpin of psychic conflict, thus crowding out the notion of traumatic antecedents as the archetypes of distress in modern psychoanalytical theory.

Traumatology, the study of trauma as it relates to psychic distress, has its origins in military medicine in World War I and was influenced by Freud's earlier work. It continued to be refined in World War II, but the study of stress remained essentially concerned with the effects of war and was rarely if ever applied to civilian populations. Combat psychiatrists focused heavily on the normative aspects of traumatic reactions to severe stress. Patients were encouraged to acknowledge their devastated feelings about the impact of war and to work toward achieving some healthy though

Table 30–2. NEUROCHEMICAL POSTULATES OF POSTTRAUMATIC STRESS DISORDER

Neurotransmitter	Alterations	Symptoms Cluster	Drugs Abused	Drug Treatment
Norepinephrine, gamma-aminobutyric acid Excitatory amino acids	Kindling	Explosive	Benzodiazepines Opioids	Carbamazepine Valproate
Catecholamines (stimulus activation)	Decreased monoamine oxidase Decreased alpha-2 adrenergic receptors Increased methoxyhydroxy-phenylglycol	Flashbacks Autonomic hyperactivity	Opioids Alcohol	Clonidine Beta blockers
Catecholamines (chronic stimulation)	Depletion Postsynaptic modulation	Depression	Cocaine Opiates	Antidepressants
Opiates (stimulus activation)	Increased endogenous opioids	Analgesia Numbing of responsiveness Flashbacks	Opiates	Naltrexone
Opiates (chronic stimulation)	Decreased endogenous opioids	Hypervigilance	Opiates Alcohol	?Methadone
Dopaminergic	Increased in acute stress in the frontal cortex	Sensory alterations	Cocaine Nicotine Cannabis Opiates	Abstinence ?Antipsychotics Benzodiazepines
Serotonergic	?	Obsessive thoughts Impulse control problems	?Alcohol	Specific serotonin reuptake inhibitors

brief distance from the front lines. Somewhat ironically, this thinking has more recently been incorporated into counseling of rape victims, and whenever possible, stress response syndromes are viewed as normal reactions to abnormal events.[28]

Traumatologists maintain an interest in the need for abreaction as it relates to discharging the overpowering psychic imprints that follow overwhelming stress. Interventions based on this psychodynamic understanding of trauma involve various means of allowing patients to restore psychic energy. Horowitz emphasizes paying particular attention to the character style of a stressed victim and divides treatment approaches into those that address the *numbing* versus the *intrusive/repetitive* phases of symptoms. He separates the work of therapy into three related but distinct systems of change: those that relate to *controlling processes, information processing,* and *emotional processing* functions.[29]

Nadelson, in her work with rape victims, extends this thinking and elaborates some specific alterations in functioning as they relate to traumatized women. For example, one's sense of sexual self, one's identity in various role assignments, and the sense of living in a safe world are all profoundly affected by the extraordinarily traumatic experience of rape. She also notes that questions about complicity in the assault by the victim herself, as well as by society, are particularly acute, although not unique to rape trauma syndrome. These concerns in particular can account for much shame and may impede recovery.[28]

Spiegel observes that dissociation is a frequent form of numbing in response to trauma. The focus of his work involves the discontinuity in experience, at the expense of self-esteem, inherent in the act of compartmentalizing memories. He notes that this phenomenon is particularly common in sexual abuse victims, in whom self-blame and personality fragmentation are extreme. He cites evidence that dissociation shares several features with hypnotizability, that patients with PTSD are highly hypnotizable, and that hypnosis therefore represents a promising means for achieving access to memories. The use of hypnosis to retrieve memories is well recognized, but the use of controlled dissociation as a means of cognitive restructuring is a unique contribution. Association and integration of repressed memories into consciousness is the goal advanced by this model. Spiegel uses hypnotic trance to help patients recover repressed memories, then employs split-screen imagery to allow patients to integrate the memory into consciousness. He likens the approach to a kind of grief work, in which the task is to place painful life experiences into perspective.[30, 31]

Restructuring is also part of the approach favored by Shapiro, the developer of a possible advance in traumatic memory treatment called eye movement desensitization and reprocessing (EMDR).[32] Elements of both behavioral (discussed later) and dynamic approaches exist within EMDR, in that both desensitization and restructuring are posited to occur.

As with all forms of desensitization and many methods of uncovering, traumatic transference to the therapist is possible. This should be anticipated and mitigated through the use of interpretation or choosing another technique, as indicated. An experienced therapist with firm grounding in standard psychotherapeutic technique is the most suitable candidate for carrying out these interventions.

BEHAVIORAL-COGNITIVE

Classical and instrumental conditioning have been proposed as behavioral mechanisms to account for certain PTSD symptoms, especially the startle response and avoidance behaviors. According to two-factor learning theory, a previously neutral stimulus (CS), when paired with an aversive stimulus (US), can eventually evoke alarm behaviors (UR) by itself. Once the startle reaction is set into motion, according to instrumental conditioning, evasion of both US and CS relieves negative emotions, thus negatively reinforcing avoidance behaviors. Instrumental conditioning offers an explanation for the exquisite generalization that occurs in patients with PTSD and distinguishes PTSD from simple phobias, which can become extinguished over time. Startle reactions appear to develop, in animal models, in response to extreme traumatic stress over time. This model therefore represents a reasonable approximation of the development of alarm states in posttraumatic patients. Two-factor learning theory has led to the development of reasonably effective behavioral techniques such as implosion (flooding) and systematic desensitization.[33] Behavioral interventions are especially useful in reducing alarm states but have limited utility with regard to reexperiencing phenomena in PTSD.

COGNITIVE

Foa and colleagues performed the only controlled study of cognitive therapy with PTSD victims to date.[34] Borrowing from Lang's[35] analysis of fear structures, they concluded that three kinds of information are important in processing a traumatic event: *information about the event itself*, data about *one's own responses at the time the trauma occurred*, and an interpretation about the *meaning of the stimulus and response elements*. They propose that reexposure to a feared situation, coupled with reprocessing of the data surrounding the event, could change the fear structure associated with the event. They suggest that this process helps to uncouple the memory from its associated symptoms. For example, a patient who left her abusive husband ended up in a homeless shelter. She was raped while waiting in a doorway for the shelter to open. Shortly after the event, the patient blamed herself and was consumed with guilt for allowing herself to be caught in such a vulnerable position. Reprocessing of the event allowed this patient to be reminded that she was fleeing from a dangerous situation when the rape occurred. Restructured awareness that leaving one's abusive husband is a *self-affirming* act freed this patient from her guilty preoccupation.

Treatment

OVERVIEW

It is interesting and useful to synthesize diverse theories about a single disorder into a meaningful clinical paradigm of the disease spectrum. For example, behavioral theories of operant conditioning in traumatic stress are consistent with neurobiological evidence implicating permanent alterations in norepinephrine

brain systems. Sympathetically mediated activation of the hippocampus and amygdala may serve to encode traumatic memories and enable enhanced startle reactions, even to stimuli that resemble (but are not) the original stressor. Enhanced startle reactions that are adaptive immediately surrounding a traumatic event become maladaptive when generalized to domestic situations. Not surprisingly, a common goal of patients with PTSD is to dampen the heightened physiological arousal they experience. Likewise, the model of IS suggests a central role for the endogenous opioid system in mediation of the original trauma and implicates a neurobiological mechanism for repetition compulsion in stressed populations.

Evidence of behavioral, psychodynamic, and biological mechanisms that integrate the conceptualization of PTSD are proposed. A worthy undertaking, which has received little attention in the psychiatric literature, is integration of the treatment of PTSD/addiction in a way that is consistent with these unifying mechanisms. A combination of parallel, integrated, and sequential treatment is proposed for the specific treatment of PTSD. Sobriety should serve as the fulcrum on which all other treatment strategies are balanced. Figure 30–1 is a graphic representation of this idea.

PHARMACOLOGY

Pharmacological treatment should address as specifically and efficaciously as possible the symptom complex most troubling at any given phase of the illness. The nomogram in Figure 30–2 can serve as a general outline of our recommended approach to the medical management of patients with PTSD.

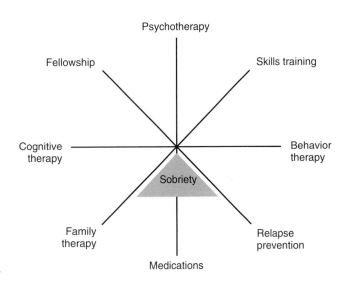

Figure 30–1.

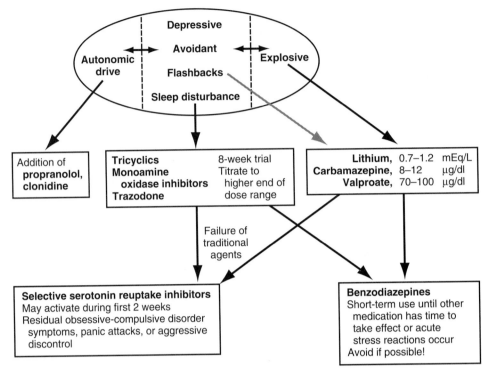

Figure 30–2. Symptoms and treatment of posttraumatic stress disorder.

Antidepressants

As shown in Figure 30–3, tricyclic antidepressants are the mainstay of treatment for patients with PTSD. The majority of the literature is based on case reports, retrospective trials, and open trials. However, there are four placebo-controlled studies of antidepressants (reviewed by Solomon and colleagues[36]). Three of these studies involve tricyclic antidepressants (imipramine hydrochloride, desipramine hydrochloride, and amitriptyline hydrochloride). Overall, they report general improvement, especially in symptoms of depression. Most studies used doses of antidepressants at the higher end of the dose range. Studies that excluded patients with major depression revealed better overall PTSD symptom improvement. Avoidance and intrusive symptoms were not impressively reduced in patients with PTSD subjected to controlled studies of tricyclic antidepressant treatment generally. Limitations of the usefulness of the information include (1) the relatively short duration of the trials (from 4 to 8 weeks maximum), (2) lack of documentation of blood levels, and (3) inconsistency in the use of rating scales. On the other hand, the most powerful medication studies to date involve tricyclic antidepressants and support their central role. An inability to

reduce startle reactions and intrusiveness may be an important limitation to tricyclic antidepressant treatment in PTSD and suggests the need to study other agents or add a second agent to address these problems specifically. There is also a need for longer trials, which would address longitudinal changes.

Phenelzine is the only other antidepressant that has been subjected to double-blind investigation. Efficacy was demonstrated with this agent at doses of 75 mg/day, even on measures of intrusive symptoms, and it was somewhat superior to imipramine in one of the two studies on the subject.[37, 38] The well-chronicled dietary restrictions and requisite compliance limit the utility of this agent, especially in patients addicted to chemicals, who may also exhibit problems with impulsivity. On the other hand, scientific data uphold its use, and it may have a role in highly motivated abstinent patients with refractory or atypical depression, especially if they also suffer from PTSD.

Fluoxetine, a specific serotonin reuptake inhibitor (SSRI), has shown promise in case reports and in one open trial involving 19 combat veterans.[39] Effectiveness was demonstrated in all three PTSD subscales. If these results withstand more rigorous investigation, SSRIs may become especially useful agents in PTSD com-

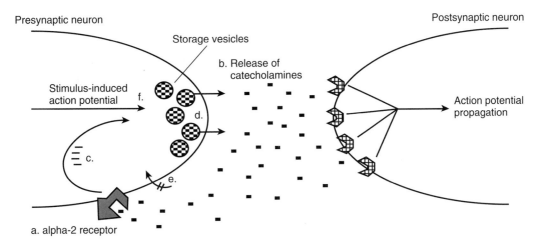

a. A 40% decrease in platelet alpha-2 concentrations has been documented in posttraumatic stress disorder (PTSD).
b. Patients with PTSD have been shown to exhibit an increased catecholamine responsiveness to trauma-related stimuli.
c. The proposed mechanism of deficient autoregulation is alpha-2 activation due to a decreased number of these receptors, allowing a greater outflow of catecholamines per stimulus.
d. During nonstimulus periods, a relative deficiency is created owing to the depletion of catecholamine stores, similiar to the sporadic increase in catecholamines and depletion of catecholinergic stores occurring with chronic cocaine use. This depletion could lead to up-regulation of postsynaptic receptors consistent with the modified biogenic amine theory in depression.
e. Tricyclic antidepressants would essentially block the reuptake of catecholamines, thus providing constant concentrations of catecholamines at the alpha-2 receptor site and constant inhibition of the presynaptic outflow of norepinephrine. Once a trauma stimulus is experienced, the outflow may be modulated by the presence of catecholamines at the alpha-2 site. The clinical outcome may be the reported lag time that patients experience during antidepressant treatment between stimulus and reaction, thus allowing behavior modification by the patient rather than reported explosive behavior discontrol experienced before medication management.
f. Anticonvulsants may help to decrease outflow responsiveness by decreasing kindling and stabilizing neural reactivity.

Figure 30–3.

plicated by addiction. No trials have to date been reported with sertraline or paroxetine in PTSD.

Antianxiety Agents

Benzodiazepines. One controlled study[40] of an antianxiety agent, alprazolam, at a dose of 0.5 to 6 mg/day, exists in the literature so far. Sixteen of 20 patients in this study experienced improvement, especially in symptoms associated with autonomic arousal such as sleeplessness, irritability, and anxiety. Two limitations of benzodiazepine therapy auger against their widespread use in complicated PTSD. These limitations include (1) the well-documented abuse potential, which poses a significant conundrum in the treatment of chemical dependence, and (2) the potential for disinhibition of rage, which is especially prominent in some subgroups of patients with PTSD and which was shown to occur in the controlled investigation of alprazolam. On the other hand, acute stress reaction may benefit from short-term benzodiazepine therapy, in highly reliable patients. These agents may support a return to normalcy, which is a worthwhile objective that can offset development of chronic PTSD. Benzodiazepine use should be limited to a maximum of 4 to 6 weeks; if possible, a shorter duration is recommended.

Adrenergic Blockers

Propranolol. Propranolol has been found effective in controlling residual symptoms of autonomic hyperarousal at doses of 120 to 160 mg/day. Potential benefit has been demonstrated with this agent in combination with tricyclic antidepressants, in clinical settings, and in one controlled open trial.[41, 42] Patients must be monitored hemodynamically with vital signs determinations, including assessment for orthostatic hypotensive changes, at least daily during the initial titration period. Clinicians prescribing propranolol should also take heed of the documented potential for iatrogenic depression with this agent.

Clonidine. Clonidine has been shown to prevent opiate withdrawal at doses ranging from 0.2 to 0.6 mg/day. There is a demonstrated deficiency of alpha-2-adrenergic receptors in platelets of patients with PTSD.[43] Diminution of negative feedback resulting in increased norepinephrine outflow, postulated to result from loss of the regulatory effect of alpha-2 receptors, could at least partially account for increased arousal in PTSD. Alpha-2-receptor agonist activity by clonidine may serve to increase the inhibitory feedback mechanism, thus modulating catecholaminergic outflow in PTSD. This agent in particular may benefit opiate-dependent patients with PTSD. This hypothesis, however, remains untested.

Mood Stabilizers

Carbamazepine has received favorable reviews in clinical and open prospective trials of patients with PTSD.[19, 44] It may be especially useful in treating intrusive recollections in light of its purported antikindling properties, and this expectation was validated in a prospective study by Lipper.[19] However, most studies of patients with bipolar disorder for mood dyscontrol document levels at 8 to 12 μg/ml, whereas levels in Lipper's study range from 7.3 to 9.7 μg/ml. Given that a subgroup of patients with PTSD have abnormal findings on electroencephalography (EEGs) and experience episodic dyscontrol, guidelines for use of carbamazepine in patients with subictal abnormal EEGs should apply to the PTSD population as well.[45] It is interesting to note that patients studied in the PTSD/carbamazepine trial had normal EEG findings but demonstrated diminution in hostile, impulsive behaviors nevertheless. This anticonvulsant and others deserve further investigation as a primary or adjunctive treatment in traumatic stress. Valproic acid, which has its locus of action on the inhibitory gamma-aminobutyric acid (GABA) system, has shown promise in 10 of 16 patients with PTSD at a mean plasma concentration of 70 μg/ml and an evaluation period of 10.6 months (range 2 to 16 months).

Lithium has shown beneficial effects in patients with mood dyscontrol and explosive disorder due to dampening of neuronal response to stimuli and antikindling effects. Open trials have been promising with this agent also, and controlled studies are awaited.

APPROACH TO THE ADDICTION: BIOLOGICAL

Patients with opiate addiction may benefit from adjunctive naltrexone maintenance to discourage addictive behavior during other therapeutic maneuvers. It is possible, although not proved, that naltrexone dampens the ability of the endogenous opioid system to become engaged in an oscillating fashion in response to stress. Patients with alcohol addiction may likewise benefit from disulfiram. Patients should be engaged and motivated for ongoing fellowship treatment to support compliance with either of these agents, and the benefits must be weighed against side effects and potentially life-threatening toxicities. A discussion of prescribing guidelines for naltrexone and disulfiram may be found elsewhere in this textbook. Alcohol and other CNS depressant drug abstinence may uncover other symptoms of PTSD that were unrecognized during the active stage of the addiction. These symptoms should be monitored, and appropriate pharmacological interventions initiated to support ongoing therapies in other modalities.

Considerable interest has been shown in desipramine as it relates to stimulant addiction. Its strong norepinephrinogenic action appears to reverse the down-regulation of postsynaptic norepinephrine receptors that occurs with chronic cocaine use. This agent should be considered first in patients who present with stimulant abuse and PTSD. There is clearly a need for better understanding of this problem and for development of more appropriate intervention strategies. An overview of the various neurochemical systems implicated in PTSD and the locus of action targeted by recommended treatments of the disorder are presented in Figure 30–3. Interventions affecting mechanisms at these loci are believed to afford more effective relief, offsetting the drive to self-medicate often cited by this population.

APPROACH TO THE ADDICTION: PSYCHOSOCIAL

Ample evidence in the literature supports the notion that inadequately treated psychiatric symptoms interfere with addiction treatment.[46] The most rational approach to treatment of addicted patients with PTSD involves treatment of both disorders concurrently.[47] Abundant clinical and some research evidence also shows that an inadequately treated addiction interferes with ongoing psychological treatment of PTSD. We therefore agree with other researchers who recommend that the addiction be treated before commencement of *long-term* PTSD treatment.[48] It is reasonable to approach symptom reduction as an adjunct to other modalities. According to Osher and Kofoed's[49] model of dual-diagnosis treatment, there are four phases of addiction treatment for mentally ill persons. These four stages are discussed next.

Engagement

The engagement phase is characterized by assistance with a patient's immediate concerns. It may involve help with legal difficulties, financial matters, and symptom reduction. The family may require attention and may be the initial stimulus for the patient's motivation to get well. This is best accomplished by direct assessment and intervention of the family's social needs in the early phases of engagement.

During the course of these early supportive interventions, appraisal of the extent of substance ingestion can be made in collaboration with the patient and family. More classical intervention style techniques in which the family has a vital role in confronting a patient about the destructiveness of his or her behavior are recommended against, at least in the early phases. Denial in addiction is in the service of protecting drinking behavior. It *interferes* with functioning[50] and is therefore confronted directly in straightforward chemical dependence interventions. Nace[51] distinguishes the denial-numbing stance of PTSD from the maladaptive gainsaying that characterizes addictive defensiveness. He postulates that much of the denial observed in PTSD may be more accurately described as "hypersuppression," a somewhat adaptive coping strategy that allows *maintenance* of functioning. Nace therefore cautions against confrontational approaches to patients with PTSD early in the course of treatment. He recommends instead that an alliance be developed with the these patients first, but he also advises addiction treatment *before* engagement of these patients in ongoing therapy.

Nace's very thoughtful and relevant discussion unfortunately oversimplifies the possibility that *both types* of denial are extant in an addicted patient with PTSD. In the process of adaptively suppressing memories of the traumatic experience, a patient often concurrently avoids recognition of the consequences of abusive behaviors. Maladaptive behavior is destructive to patients in all phases of treatment and should be gently but firmly confronted.

As stated previously, the engagement stage of integrated treatment is very important in that it prepares patients for consideration of longer-term modalities of intervention. As already pointed out, addiction treatment is less efficacious in patients with inadequate relief

from psychiatric symptoms.[46] Therefore, symptom relief through pharmacological means is very important in the early phase and may represent the agency through which sobriety can be tolerated. Patients may require help with detoxification immediately. They may also possess motivation to be observed for symptoms that surface once the detoxification is completed, especially if there is legal coercion or a financial motive for seeking treatment.

Frequent contact with and availability of the physician are essential to appropriate and timely intervention during this period. Inpatient or day hospital treatment is therefore ideal, if possible, for attaining maximum symptomatic relief; it is also probably the most likely setting to support abstinence during a rather vulnerable period in the treatment.

Persuasion

Persuasion is "the process of convincing engaged patients to accept long-term abstinence-oriented treatment."[49] Again, symptom reduction may be an important prerequisite for treatment at this level.

Once patients are feeling well enough to handle the information in a constructive manner (i.e., denial or hypersuppression has been replaced with more adaptive coping strategies), they may be presented in a clear and direct manner with objective information that suggests a diagnosis of chemical abuse or dependence. This information may include results of physical and laboratory findings but may also include a frank discussion about the types of social and legal difficulties responsible for the engagement. This discussion may also be an opportunity to discuss the observed exacerbation of PTSD symptoms directly resulting from substance abuse.

The persuasion step may immediately follow the engagement phase, and parallel treatment of the addiction may begin while patients are still in the process of engaging. The choice of an inpatient versus an outpatient treatment program to support sobriety depends on the severity of the chemical dependence diagnosis, the presence of concurrent physical health problems or residual psychiatric symptoms, and the adequacy of social supports.[52] Again, an inpatient setting is ideal but is not essential to this type of intervention. Patients are presumably abstinent, and they may be interested in remaining within the protective atmosphere of an inpatient setting. They may be ill equipped to manage the rigors of early recovery without such support. On the other hand, patients who are highly motivated and who have adequate resources may achieve the same goals in an outpatient or day hospital program.

Patients who require inpatient addiction treatment should be expeditiously referred and admitted/transferred to an addiction unit once their commitment to the goal of abstinence and their ability to make such a commitment have been established. Peers and family members should be readily available both to bolster a patient's resolve and to point out, in a nonjudgmental fashion, the problems leading to a conclusion that addiction treatment is necessary and desirable. Appropriate transfer to an addiction treatment program for specific addiction treatment marks the beginning of a step in the sequential treatment of the addiction. Further, more ongoing, treatment of the PTSD may resume once this step is completed. However, clinical wisdom dictates that the behaviors learned and the skills developed to sustain abstinence are essential prerequisites to more long-term work in chronic PTSD. Controlled studies are required to validate this point.

Active (or Primary) Treatment

Active treatment represents the classical form of early rehabilitation treatment and often takes the form of a 21- or 28-day intensive program. The focus in active treatment is on education about the principles of recovery such as the 12 steps. Skills training is also an essential component. Families should have an active role in this phase of recovery as well, to help emphasize the issues that initiated the process and to begin the process of recovery themselves.

Decisions about the next phase in the sequence should be considered and resolved during the active phase of addiction treatment. For example, patients with chronic PTSD may consider a long-term inpatient program specifically designed to address traumatic stress.[53] Outpatient treatment, involving several modalities of integrated treatment, may represent an acceptable alternative. Studies of separate components of outpatient programs involving medications, behavioral techniques, cognitive techniques, and psychodynamic techniques have demonstrated efficacy. Studies of the process of integrated treatment for this population are lacking.

Relapse Prevention

It is well documented that the early period of recovery after active treatment is the most vulnerable. Emotional distress, craving, and inadequate aftercare attendance all are associated with higher relapse rates.[54] Comprehensive relapse prevention efforts are therefore recommended as an ongoing tool to support long-term abstinence. These interventions may take the form of ongoing education about "triggers," or effects and events that lead to drinking/drug-taking behavior. They may also involve solid advice about symptom reduction resources when evidence of disease recurrence becomes apparent.

Relapse prevention typically occurs in a group format and enlists the support of other recovering individuals as well as professionals trained to recognize symptoms and triggers.[55] Relapse prevention may represent a return to parallel or integrated treatment concurrent with primary/ongoing PTSD intervention.

Directions for the Future

The systematic study of trauma has been slow to evolve despite auspicious beginnings. Data are accumulating to unequivocally validate stress response syndromes as distinct diagnostic entities with variable features. Comorbidity is a common occurrence with which efforts to study the natural history of the disorder have been riddled. Addiction is especially prevalent in PTSD and should be routinely assessed. Treatment of stress disorders complicated by substance abuse should be integrated where feasible, and parallel processes should take place when clinically indicated. More broad-based population studies are needed to address the links between PTSD and addiction in other populations of trauma survivors, with special attention to the staggering population of affected women. Women crime victims represent unique subjects for prospective study that should not be overlooked. There is both a humanitarian and a scientific mandate to reverse the neglect that has beleaguered our profession and our patients apropos to this subject.

Development of methods for the study of reactivated trauma in response to recurrent victimization experiences has particular implications for the study of interpersonal violence. Stressors such as child abuse and domestic violence may represent preceding triggers to the development of PTSD-like disorders, and public health approaches to these profound crises deserve urgent attention.

It is possible that heightened sensitivity to the effects of a range of victimization experiences will open floodgates, allowing the traumatic antecedents to behavioral aberrations to attain full recognition. For example, diseases such as borderline personality disorder may someday be conceptualized with a posttraumatic focus. Should this happen, the diagnosis of posttraumatic symptoms will have come full circle.

Reasonably effective treatment is available for known stress response and substance disorders, alone and in combination. However, a high level of motivation and commitment to the modest goals of recovery is essential. Until a simple pathophysiological lesion can be identified and cured with the proverbial "silver bullet," these chronic diseases may continue to be plagued by controversy over what the proper catalyst in recovery should be. Efforts to intervene in the meantime will continue to hinge on caring professionals' appreciation of the nature of personal responsibility. Irrespective of the cause of a disorder, patients who appreciate their own role in the treatment respond best to appropriate rehabilitation efforts. As practitioners, we anticipate that any success—and much can be expected—depends on our ability to understand patients' point of view while we simultaneously engage them in the task. The disease model works very well in the treatment of alcoholism in that respect, and the treatment of PTSD is not far behind.

Several questions remain in the field of traumatology. We have only ascertained the tip of the iceberg with respect to our understanding of effective clinical interventions for addictive *or* stress response disease. Prospective trials to firmly establish the etiological link between trauma and disease states remain a sine qua non. At issue is to what extent vulnerability has a role in the development of PTSD. We must decide amidst sound investigation what constitutes unusual stress. Only then may our society either prevent the reality of trauma or effectively control its aftereffects.

REFERENCES

1. Miller NS, Chappel JN: History of the disease concept. Psychiatr Ann 21:4, 196–205, 1991.
2. Grinker RR, Spiegel JP: Men Under Stress. Philadelphia, Blakiston, 1945.
3. Solomon Z: Combat Stress Reactions: The Enduring Toll of War. New York, Plenum, 1993.
4. Kulka R, et al: Trauma and the Vietnam War Generation: Report of findings from the National Vietnam Veterans Readjustment Study. New York, Brunner-Mazel, 1990.
5. US Dept of Health and Human Services: Health Status of Vietnam Veterans. Centers for Disease Control. Vol IV: Psychological and Neuropsychological Evaluation. Atlanta, US Government Printing Office, 1989.
6. American Psychiatric Association: Diagnostic and Statistical Manual of Mental Disorders, 3rd ed. Washington, DC, American Psychiatric Association, 1980.
7. American Psychiatric Association: Diagnostic and Statistical Manual of Mental Disorders, 4th ed. Washington, DC, American Psychiatric Association, 1994.
8. Helzer J, Robins L, McEvoy L: Posttraumatic stress disorder in the general population: Findings of the Epidemiologic Catchment Area Survey. N Engl J Med 317:1630–1634, 1987.
9. Kilpatrick D, Resnick H: Posttraumatic stress disorder associated with exposure to criminal victimization in clinical and community samples. In Posttraumatic Stress Disorder: DSM-IV and Beyond., Washington, DC, American Psychiatric Association, 1993, pp 113–143.
10. Rothbaum B, Foa EB, Riggs DS, et al: A prospective examination of post-traumatic stress disorder in rape victims. Journal of Traumatic Stress 5:455–475, 1992.
11. Foa E, Riggs D: Posttraumatic stress disorder and rape. In Oldham J, Riba M, Tasman A (eds): American Psychiatric Stress Review of Psychiatry. Washington, DC, American Psychiatric Press, 1993, pp 273–303.
12. McFarlane A: Relationship between psychiatric impairment and a natural disaster: The role of distress. Psychol Med 18:129–139, 1988.
13. McFarlane A: The aetiology of post-traumatic morbidity: Predisposing, precipitating and perpetuating factors. Br J Psychiatry 154:221–228, 1989.
14. Kilpatrick DG, Saunders BE, Amick-McMullan A, et al: Victims and crime factors associated with the development of crime-related posttraumatic stress disorder. Behav Ther 20:199–214, 1989.
15. Southwick S, et al: Trauma-related symptoms in veterans of Operation Desert Storm: A preliminary report. Am J Psychiatry 150(10):1524–1528, 1993.
16. Davidson J: Issues in the diagnosis of posttraumatic stress disorder. In Olaham J, Riba M (eds): American Psychiatry Press Review of Psychiatry. Washington, DC, American Psychiatric Press, 1993, pp 141–156.
17. Post R, Kopanda R: Cocaine, kindling and psychosis. Am J Psychiatry 133:627–634, 1976.
18. Neppe V, Tucker G, Neuropsychiatric aspects of seizure disorders. In Yudofsky S, Hales R (eds): American Psychiatric Press Textbook of Neuropsychiatry. Washington, DC, pp 397–426. American Psychiatric Press, 1992.
19. Lipper S, Davidson JRT, Grady TA, et al: Preliminary study of carbamazepine in post-traumatic stress disorder. Psychosomatics 27:849–854, 1986.
20. Keck E Jr, McElroy S, Friedman L: Valproate and carbamazepine in the treatment of panic and posttraumatic stress disorder, withdrawal states, and behavioral dyscontrol syndromes. J Clin Psychopharmacol 12 (Suppl): 36S–41S, 1992.
21. Bremner J, Davis M, Southwick S: Neurobiology of posttraumatic stress disorder. In Olaham J, Riba M (eds): American Psychiatric Press Review of Psychiatry. Washington, DC, American Psychiatric Press, 1993, pp 183–204.
22. Kosten T, Krystal J: Biological mechanisms in posttraumatic stress disorder: Relevance for substance abuse. Recent Dev Alcohol 6:49–68, 1988.
23. Van der Kolk B, Greenberg M, Boyd H, et al: Inescapable shock, neurotransmitters, and addiction to trauma: Toward a psychobiology of posttraumatic stress. Biol Psychiatry 20:314–325, 1985.
24. Van der Kolk B, Greenberg MS, Orr SP, et al: Endogenous opioids, stress induced analgesia, and posttrau-

matic stress disorder. Psychopharmacol Bull 25:417–421, 1989.

25. Pitman R, Van der Kolk B, Orr SP, et al: Naloxone-reversible analgesic response to combat-related stimuli in posttraumatic stress disorder. Arch Gen Psychiatry 47:541–5544, 1990.

26. Miller N, Gold M: A hypothesis for a common neurochemical basis for alcohol and drug disorders. Psychiatr Clin North Am 16(1):105–117, 1993.

27. McFall M, Mackay P, Donovan D: Combat-related posttraumatic stress disorder and severity of substance abuse in Vietnam veterans. J Stud Alcohol 53:357–363, 1992.

28. Nadelson C, Notman M: Psychodynamics of sexual assault experiences. In Stuart I, Greer J (eds): Victims of Sexual Aggression: Treatment of Children, Women and Men. New York, Van Nostrand Reinhold, 1984, pp 3–17.

29. Horowitz M: Stress response syndromes: Character style and dynamic psychotherapy. Arch Gen Psychiatry 31:764–781, 1974.

30. Spiegel D: Hypnosis in the treatment of victims of sexual abuse. Psychiatr Clin North Am 12(2):295–305, 1989.

31. Spiegel D, Cardenal E: New uses of hypnosis in the treatment of posttraumatic stress disorder. J Clin Psychiatry 51(Suppl)10:39–43, 1990.

32. Shapiro F: Efficacy of the eye movement desensitization procedure in the treatment of traumatic memories. Journal of Traumatic Stress Studies 2:199–223, 1989.

33. Foy D: Treating Post-Traumatic Stress Disorder: Cognitive Behavioral Strategies. New York, Guilford, 1992.

34. Foa E, Rothbaum BO, Riggs D, et al: Treatment of post-traumatic stress disorder in rape victims. J Consult Clin Psychol 59:715–723, 1991.

35. Lang P: Imagery in therapy: An information processing analysis of fear. Behav Ther 8:862–886, 1977.

36. Solomon S, Gerrity E, Alyson M: Efficacy of treatments for posttraumatic stress disorder: An empirical review. JAMA, 268(5):633–638, 1992.

37. Frank J, Giller EL, Kostren TR, et al: A randomized clinical trial of phenelzine and imipramine for posttraumatic stress disorder. Am J Psychiatry 145:1289–1291, 1988.

38. Shestatzky M, Greenberg D, Lerer B: A controlled trial of phenelzine in posttraumatic disorder. Psychiatry Res 24:149–155, 1988.

39. Nagy L, Morgan CA, Southwick SM, Charrey DS: Open prospective trial of fluoxetine for posttraumatic stress disorder. J Clin Psychopharmacol 13(2):107–113, 1993.

40. Braun P, Greenberg D, Dusberg H, Lerer B: Core symptoms of posttraumatic stress disorder unimproved by alprazolam treatment. J Clin Psychiatry 51:236–238, 1990.

41. Kinzie J, Leung P: Clonidine in Cambodian patients with posttraumatic stress disorder. J Nerv Ment Dis 177(9):546–550, 1989.

42. Kolb L, Burris B, and Griffiths S: Propranolol and clonidine in treatment of the chronic posttraumatic stress disorder of war. In Kolk BVD (ed): Post-traumatic Stress Disorder: Psychological and Biological Sequelae. Washington, DC, American Psychiatric Press, 1984.

43. Perry B, Giller E, Southwick S: Altered platelet alpha-2 adrenergic binding sites in posttraumatic stress disorder. Am J Psychiatry 144:1324–1327, 1987.

44. Wolf M, Alavi A, Mosnaim A: Posttraumatic stress disorder in Vietnam veterans: Clinical and EEG findings; possible therapeutic effects of carbamazepine. Biol Psychiatry 23:642–644, 1988.

45. Neppe V, Tucker G, Wilensky A: Fundamentals of carbamazepine use in neuropsychiatry. J Clin Psychiatry 49(Suppl 4):4–6, 1988.

46. McLellan A, Luborsky L, Woody GE, O'Brien CP, Druley KA: Predicting response to alcohol and drug abuse treatments: Role of psychiatric severity. Arch Gen Psychiatry 40:620–625, 1983.

47. Kofoed L, Friedman MJ, Peck R: Alcoholism and drug abuse in patients with PTSD. Psychiatr Q 64(2):151–171, 1993.

48. Marmar C, Foy D, Kagan B, Pynoos RS: An integrated approach for treating posttraumatic stress. In Oldham J, Riba M, Tasman A (eds): American Psychiatric Press Review of Psychiatry. Washington DC, American Psychiatric Press, 1993, p 269.

49. Osher F, Kofoed L: Treatment of patients with psychiatric and psychoactive substance abuse disorders. Hosp Community Psychiatry 40(10):1025–1030, 1989.

50. Vaillant G: Theoretical hierarchy of adaptive ego mechanisms. Arch Gen Psychiatry 24:107–118, 1971.

51. Nace E: Posttraumatic stress disorder and substance abuse: Clinical issues. Recent Dev Alcohol 6:9–26, 1988.

52. Collins G: Contemporary issues in the treatment of alcohol dependence. Psychiatric Clin North Am 16(1):33–48, 1993.

53. Koller P, Marmar C, Kanas N: Psychodynamic group treatment of post-traumatic stress disorder in Vietnam veterans. Int J Group Psychother 42:225–246, 1992.

54. Hoffman N, Miller N: Perspectives of effective treatment for alcohol and drug disorders. Psychiatric Clin North Am 16(1):127–140, 1993.

55. Marlatt G, Gordon J: Relapse Prevention. New York, Guilford, 1985.

Treatment of Addiction in Childbearing Populations*

Valerie D. Raskin, MD

Substance use and substance use disorders during pregnancy appear to be increasingly common and more generally recognized as major social and public health problems. Addiction to alcohol, tobacco, and illicit drugs during pregnancy has been associated with low birth weight, prematurity, fetuses that are small for gestational age, fetal alcohol syndrome, fetal loss, and obstetrical complications including placenta previa and abruptio placentae.[1-5]

Although perinatal addiction to drugs (especially cocaine) has received the greatest notoriety, in theory, any psychoactive substance use during pregnancy may be of concern because safety is not established for any. Long-lasting neurobehavioral sequelae including cognitive, emotional, or behavioral disabilities in infants exposed prenatally to low or moderate levels of psychoactive substances have been described.[4, 6] To the extent that substance use disorders are characterized by continued use despite the consequences, relatively lower levels of substance use during pregnancy may constitute addictive disorders if the user is aware of the potential adverse consequences of such use and is unable to abstain nonetheless.

That illicit drug use is always or even usu-

ally harmful to the fetus as a result of direct drug effect is considered medical truth by the public. Concern about "crack babies" and their irreversible "inability to love" is widely discussed in the popular media.[7] These stereotypes about crack babies appear to influence our scientific judgment. One study documented that reports that showed adverse effects of fetal cocaine exposure were more likely to be accepted for scientific presentation than those that show no adverse effect, despite apparent methodological superiority of the latter.[8] Clinicians are likely also not immune to the influence of the media on their attitudes and their understanding of perinatal addiction.[9] If that is the case, we risk mistakenly overemphasizing cocaine use in childbearing populations and underemphasizing other known teratogens such as cigarette smoke and alcohol.

Without depreciating the potential reproductive hazards of cocaine use in pregnancy, one must also recognize that studies in this area are best characterized as inconsistent or contradictory.[9] However, overwhelming evidence implicates indirect as well as collateral polysubstance effect on adverse neonatal outcome. In other words, a crack baby may be suffering the consequences of poverty, lack of prenatal care, intrauterine sexually transmitted disease, inadequate nutrition, abusive or neglectful parenting, multiple foster placements, or alcohol, to-

*Adapted with permission from Raskin VD: Psychiatric aspects of substance abuse disorders in childbearing populations. Psychiatr Clin North Am 16:157–165, 1993.

bacco, amphetamine, or other drug effect as much as a direct teratogenic effect of cocaine.[10]

Efforts targeted at indirect causes of adverse perinatal outcome (e.g., lack of prenatal care) are effective in reducing adverse maternal and infant outcome even in the presence of continued drug use.[11, 12] For example, women who use cocaine in pregnancy and who made even as few as four obstetrical visits delivered infants with birth weights between 262 and 316 g higher (varying with ethnicity) than their peers who received no prenatal care.[13] Further, even those women who made only one to three prenatal visits delivered infants of greater birth weight, ranging from 22 to 150 g more (again, varying with ethnicity).[13] Attention to maximizing participation in adequate prenatal care must be included in any comprehensive treatment program for pregnant addicts.

Despite the relative overemphasis on the hazards of cocaine use, other psychoactive substances that are less socially condemned are more clearly hazardous to a fetus or more damaging in the aggregate because of widespread use. Any alcohol use at any time in pregnancy may cause fetal damage; the Surgeon General of the United States now recommends complete abstinence from alcohol during all trimesters of pregnancy,[14] yet current estimates indicate that one fifth of pregnant women report drinking alcohol.[15] Low levels of marijuana exposure during the first trimester alone have been linked to abnormal sleep patterns in infants.[16] Approximately one third of pregnant women smoke cigarettes during pregnancy.[15] Although smoking cessation early in pregnancy eliminates the increased risk of low birth weight,[17] treatment for nicotine addiction in pregnancy has been largely disappointing.[18]

These are critical factors to be considered in developing prevention, diagnosis, and treatment for substance use disorders in the childbearing population. It is common to frame discussions of perinatal addiction in terms of the gravid uterus. Such a framework discounts addicted women and is ridiculously simplistic in light of the complex problem of perinatal addiction. First, the childbearing population must be recognized as including women not yet pregnant, pregnant women, and women who have recently delivered. Second, because many of the consequences of substance use disorders in pregnancy are attributable to indirect causes, attention to psychosocial factors and psychiatric morbidity in the substance-dependent pregnant population is necessary for developing treatment targeted to women. Finally, the unique stresses and risks of the postpartum period must be considered in providing meaningful care with any lasting effect.

The Preconception Population

Preconception care refers to health promotion before pregnancy, especially for conditions that might be damaging early in pregnancy.[19] Preconception interventions for substance use disorders in childbearing women are appropriate because (1) substance use disorders are unhealthy for these women at any time and (2) fetal damage may have already occurred before pregnancy is diagnosed or before intervention is successful. Recovery is generally a rocky process marked by relapses and slips from abstinence; fetal well-being is most likely to be guaranteed if recovery occurs before rather than during pregnancy.

In considering the reproductive potential of addicted women of childbearing age, two unique features must be considered. First, addiction treatment programs typically encourage the use of condoms for prevention of human immunodeficiency virus (HIV) infection. Clinicians must keep in mind that although condoms are effective at HIV prevention, they are far less effective in preventing pregnancy than other contraceptives. For some women, combined use of condoms and another method (such as Norplant or oral contraceptives) is an appropriate means of preventing or delaying pregnancy until recovery is better established.

A second overwhelmingly common phenomenon among women is custody loss due to addiction. Women who have lost or surrendered custody or caregiving responsibility for their children are at high risk for subsequent unplanned pregnancy. Markedly persistent grief following custody loss in the setting of substance dependence is common.[20] Pregnancy in general may be unconsciously sought as a way of healing loss, especially loss of a child.[21] A painfully futile cycle of custody loss followed by unplanned subsequent pregnancy and further drug use in pregnancy may ensue.[20] Denial and bargaining for the lost child (i.e., vows to oneself to abstain in a future pregnancy) may lead to fetal drug or alcohol exposure in early pregnancy in a woman who has recently lost custody owing to active addiction. Although both clinician and patient may *consciously* believe that rapid subsequent pregnancy after custody loss would be undesirable, the powerful unconscious attraction of subsequent pregnancy to replace the lost child should alert the clinician that an addicted patient with recent custody loss may soon become pregnant again.

The Pregnant Population

Pregnancy may be a very powerful motivator for abstinence, reduced use, or entry and reentry into treatment for substance use disorders.[22, 23] It may seem "only natural" that pregnancy would enhance motivation for abstinence or treatment. However, the ability to diminish one's substance intake because of pregnancy varies with the presence or absence and extent of addiction. The data on alcohol use in pregnancy (which can reasonably be assumed to generalize to other psychoactive substances) indicate that although heightened public awareness of the risks of alcohol use in pregnancy has resulted in a significant decrease in alcohol consumption during pregnancy, the proportion of heavy drinkers has not decreased.[15] Further, the prevalence of alcohol use in pregnancy remains highest in groups already at risk for poor perinatal outcome: single women and smokers.

Thus, although pregnancy may provide a unique opportunity to intervene in addiction—perhaps not unlike incarceration—it is important to recognize that those who discontinue substance use before conception or on learning of pregnancy may be those with lesser dependence. An addict who presents to treatment *because* of her pregnancy must also be appreciated as one who did not seek or succeed in treatment *in the absence* of pregnancy. Assuming that a pregnant, substance-dependent woman has not been able to (1) quit independently in response to public education efforts, (2) quit before becoming pregnant, or (3) quit on learning that she is pregnant tells us that this person presents for treatment with a very persistent chemical dependence. Fortunately, it appears that among women identified as using drugs during pregnancy, severity of psychosocial distress, psychosocial impairment, and polysubstance use is positively linked with treatment for the addiction during pregnancy (i.e., those most in need of treatment receive it).[24] The severe nature of an addiction that persists into pregnancy enters into complex risk-benefit analyses of pharmacological measures and may justify aggressive methods such as nicotine replacement in pregnant addicts unable to quit smoking by using behavioral and educational methods.

It is extremely important in treating such patients to try to understand what it is about the psychological experience of her pregnancy that enhances entry into treatment. One possibility is the hope for healing the damaged self that pregnancy offers. Like an adolescent or otherwise narcissistically vulnerable pregnant woman, a chemically dependent mother often looks to her fetus to help her feel complete, to organize her fragmented self, and to provide her with a sense of achievement and pride. Pregnancy literally offers the hope of filling an enormous inner emptiness.

Pregnancy also offers a unique opportunity to nurture oneself through identification with one's fetus. If one becomes the idealized parent, one can sample the experience of being cared for by such a parent. A pregnant addict may unconsciously attempt to reparent herself by becoming a better parent. Drug-dependent pregnant women are more likely than a control group to have been beaten and sexually molested as children.[25, 26] Many pregnant addicts are themselves children of addicted parents. Given such harsh realities of being parented, the wish to be cared for by an idealized parent is understandably great.

How does what we know about the maternal-fetal emotional relationship apply in the circumstance of addiction? In general, we know that maternal-fetal emotional attachment is a progressive phenomenon—the love that a mother feels for her fetus grows over time, in part in response to events that increase the sense of reality of the baby, such as quickening (the experience of the baby kicking), "showing," and medical interventions such as fetal ultrasonography. Treatment (e.g., an art therapy group in which group participants create images of themselves and their babies) that enhances the reality of the fetus may also enhance an addict's motivation.

We also know, however, that loss or the threat of loss can be a powerful barrier to attachment—one protects oneself from anticipated loss by attempting to hold back emotional investment or by devaluing the lost object. It is worth noting that past loss of child custody or caregiving responsibility or future threat of the loss of child custody is exceedingly common in perinatal addicts. For example, in a sample of multiparous pregnant heroin addicts who presented at delivery with minimal or no prenatal care, more than 90% had lost custody or caregiving responsibility for one or more children for some period.[20] Almost half had lost children irrevocably to the state child welfare system, with an average number of three children removed from custody. One hundred percent stated that they anticipated the possible loss of custody of their babies after childbirth. Such a patient should not be assumed to have naturally enhanced motivation for abstinence or treatment for the sake of her baby.

Ironically, pregnancy is often a significant obstacle to substance disorder treatment. Pregnancy poses both covert and overt barriers to treatment. Access may be limited on the basis of pregnancy, on the basis of substance abuse (with crack cocaine and opiate addiction especially problematic), on the basis of poverty or Medicaid coverage, or on the basis of comorbid mental illness.[27] Access is most limited to those pregnant women who fall into multiple categories: Finding treatment slots for the pregnant, mentally ill, impoverished heroin addict, for example, is a formidable task.

Access is also limited by the realistic needs of childbearing women who are often single parents. For example, residential programs commonly exclude or limit the number and ages of children who may accompany a mother to treatment. Inpatient programs virtually all exclude her other children. Outpatient programs may be scheduled in a way that allows patients to maintain or begin employment (e.g., beginning in late afternoon or early evening). Such a schedule is the exact opposite of what a caregiving mother with school-aged children can likely manage. For patients with the sole responsibility for preschool-aged children, the need for childcare so that they can participate in treatment is real. To the extent that pregnant substance dependents are especially likely to have chronic addictions, as a group they often have depleted their sources of social support. In other words, surrogate caregivers who might assist a pregnant addict with her childcare needs are typically scarce.

Other barriers to treatment may be less obvious. Insufficient attention to the special programmatic needs of women is another barrier to treatment. Gender-specific issues associated with chemical dependence in pregnancy include the commonly associated past or ongoing interpersonal violence, high comorbidity of depressive disorder, and gender-specific consequences including loss of child custody and its associated maternal bereavement.[20, 28–31]

Several studies have indicated that domestic and other interpersonal violence is more common in both adolescent and adult women who use substances during pregnancy. Pregnant adolescent drug users are three times more likely than their nonuser peers to report being threatened, abused, or in fights during pregnancy.[32, 33] Women hit during pregnancy are more likely to be heavy users of drugs.[34, 35] Ethnic differences have been detected in patterns of drug use in pregnant battered women, with cocaine, marijuana, and tobacco use found at increased rates in white non-Hispanic, African-American, and Hispanic women, respectively, relative to their nonbattered pregnant peers.[35] Possible explanations put forth include self-medication, increased risk of violence in general in the environment of the substance abuser, or diminished ability to leave a coaddicted abusive partner who facilitates the addiction.

Evaluation for posttraumatic stress disorder (PTSD) should be a routine part of the clinical assessment of a pregnant addict. As noted previously, victimization is especially common among drug-dependent women. Routine screening for a history of rape or physical assault in this population will yield answers such as, "Do you mean just this year?" In addition to high frequencies of childhood abuse, because prostitution in order to obtain drugs is common, physical or sexual assault by a pimp or customer is also common. Psychic numbing, occurring in chronic PTSD, may impair maternal-fetal bonding or the development of internal motivation for abstinence, and symptoms such as flashbacks may be used to rationalize continued substance use. Intrusive memories and images of victimization may emerge during detoxification, as one's sensorium clears. Pregnancy itself often mimics or triggers memories of the experience of loss of one's bodily autonomy.

Attention to the woman's partner is especially important in the treatment of chemical dependence in pregnancy. Although the threat of the loss of a substance-dependent partner is often of great concern to chemically dependent women at any time, it is especially so during pregnancy and in the postpartum period, when increased interpersonal dependence is normative.[36] Unless the risks of losing the emotional or financial support of a substance-using partner at the worst possible time as a possible hazard of one's own abstinence is recognized, treatment may fail before it has begun.

Countertransference problems are usually troublesome when treating pregnant substance abusers. Pregnant substance abusers are often the recipients of unconscious and sometimes even conscious negative attitudes toward the "bad mother." Identification with the fetus is quite common in treating pregnant women, regardless of diagnosis. Although identification with the fetus by the treating clinician is probably not entirely avoidable, when especially strong, this may leave the mother feeling that her uterus or her fetus is worthy of treatment—not her. Narcissistically vulnerable pregnant women often experience others as overly or solely concerned with the fetus, at their expense.[37] Clinicians need to be especially sensitive to this and would do well to discuss abstinence in terms of the benefits to the woman. For example, rather than suggesting that abstinence will be good for her baby, one might note that achieving abstinence will help her self-esteem. Conversely, identification with the fetus may lead to excessive rescue fantasies and efforts by the therapist, which might impede a woman's appropriate responsibility for her own recovery.

In a related countertransference phenomenon, a woman's motivation to improve her health for the sake of the baby may be inappropriately accepted at face value. Clinicians must be aware of the almost universal socialization regarding maternal sacrifice and the idealization of motherhood that we share with our addicted pregnant patients. We must challenge our patients to develop genuine internal motivation for recovery. Pregnant addicts should be confronted about seeking treatment for the sake of the baby. As an example, one might say, "I'm glad you want to do it for your baby, but you matter too—you need to want to stay clean for yourself, or both you and the baby are in trouble." Motivation on behalf of the baby alone may be excellent initially. However, if a program accepts this either explicitly or implicitly (e.g., calls itself the Healthy Babies program), treatment is incomplete. A strong emphasis on improvement for the baby's sake carries two risks: disenfranchisement of the mother (a narcissistically vulnerable mother often experiences emphasis on the baby as rejection of herself) and high relapse rates after childbirth.

Paradoxically, programs that give special consideration or special privileges to pregnant women often encounter unique problems that result from that.[36] Accelerated placement due to pregnancy may evoke jealousy or hostility toward those receiving favored status. A special problem arises in the management of pregnant methadone recipients with so-called dirty urines. Most methadone programs rapidly detoxify then discharge patients after a certain number of continued positive urine toxicology test results. If a program does so for everyone but pregnant patients, very negative feelings may arise among both other patients and staff, and these must be addressed openly.

The Postpartum Population

The postpartum period is an especially vulnerable period for psychiatric morbidity under optimal conditions. The birth of a first child is listed in DSM-III-R as an example of a severe stressor, or 4 on a scale of 1 to 6. Stresses associated with childbirth and caring for an infant include the physical stress of delivery or major surgery, chronic sleep deprivation, many new tasks with little opportunity for respite, increased demand for limited space and financial resources, and the demands and resentments of other dependents who feel jealous of the attention the new baby receives. Psychologically, a new mother has to adjust to the fact that her actual baby often compares unfavorably with the hoped-for, idealized baby. If her baby has been expected to fill great deficits in herself, the psychological stress that a woman feels in postpartum period may be great.

In addition to typical postpartum psychosocial stress, chemically dependent women have particular postpartum stressors that may be linked to relapse. First, there is the stress of caring for a child at increased risk for special needs because of prematurity, low birth weight, or irritability, for example.[36] Second, the postpartum period is a high-risk time for exacerbation of affective disorders, which are themselves more common in chemically dependent women than in the general population of women.[28] The role of depressive symptoms in relapse is not known for all substances, but dysphoric affect has been linked to relapse in ex-smokers.[38] Third, temporary or permanent loss of custody may be experienced as a catastrophic event. Fourth, coping with having one's baby test positive for HIV infection or to develop acquired immunodeficiency syndrome as an infant may present a further catastrophe.

Treatment for chemical dependence in pregnancy must attend to the very high risk of postpartum relapse. Chemically dependent women are at special risk for relapse after childbirth for several different reasons. First, relapse is most common after the end of active treatment. In the population of pregnant women who stop smoking during pregnancy, relapse in the postpartum period ranges from 50% to nearly 90%.[39, 40] If the treatment program emphasizes treatment for the sake of the fetus (e.g., diminishes or discontinues treatment after childbirth), the period of highest relapse risk will coincide with the period of greatest psychosocial stress.

The postpartum period is a time in which some childbearing women enter treatment for the first time. Women who delivered infants with a positive urine toxicology screen may be judicially ordered into treatment in order to maintain or regain child custody. Beyond all else, these patients must be understood as having failed to enter treatment or to receive or sustain the benefits of treatment during pregnancy, so that the very great extent of their dependence is recognized.

Conclusion

The use of crack cocaine during pregnancy, although important, should not be overemphasized relative to other known teratogens (e.g., alcohol and tobacco); to indirect psychosocial factors associated with poor pregnancy outcome, such as lack of prenatal care and untreated infection; and to the hazards of substance dependence before and after pregnancy. Although pregnancy may enhance motivation for abstinence, the persistence of addiction that continues despite pregnancy must be appreciated. Psychiatric comorbidity, ongoing interpersonal violence, past and threatened child custody loss, and markedly impaired experiences while being parented are common in pregnant addicts. The postpartum period should be understood to be one of great risk for relapse for addicted women who achieve abstinence during pregnancy.

REFERENCES

1. Finnegan L: Clinical effects of pharmacologic agents on pregnancy, the fetus, and the neonate. Ann N Y Acad Sci 196:28–284, 1989.
2. Benowitz NL: Nicotine replacement therapy during pregnancy. JAMA 266:3174–3177, 1991.
3. Little BB, Snell LM, Klein VR, Gilstrap LC III: Cocaine abuse during pregnancy: Maternal and fetal implications. Obstet Gynecol 73:157–160, 1989.
4. Streissguth AP, Barr HM, Sampson PD: Moderate prenatal alcohol exposure: Effects on child IQ and learning problems at age 7 1/2 years. Alcohol Clin Exp Res 670–673, 1990.
5. Zuckerman B, Frank DA, Hingson R, et al: Effects of maternal marijuana and cocaine use on fetal growth. N Engl J Med 320:762–768, 1989.
6. Fried PA, Watkinson B, Dillon RF, Dulberg CS: Neonatal neurological status in a low-risk population after prenatal exposure to cigarettes, marijuana, and alcohol. Journal of Developmental and Behavioral Pediatrics 8:318–326, 1987.
7. The crack children. Newsweek, February 12, 1990, pp 62–63.
8. Koren G, Graham K, Shear H, et al: Bias against the null hypothesis: The reproductive hazards of cocaine. Lancet 2:1440–1442, 1989.
9. Mayes LC, Granger RH, Bornstein MH, et al: The problem of prenatal cocaine exposure—a rush to judgment. JAMA 267:406–408, 1992.
10. Coles C: Risks to the infant. In Pregnant Drug Abusers, Clinical and Legal Controversies. Presented at the Annual Meeting, American Psychiatric Association, New Orleans, 1991.
11. Allen M: Perinatal outcome after intensive prenatal care for chemically dependent women (abstract). Annual Meeting, American College of Obstetrics and Gynecology, New Orleans, 1991.
12. MacGregor SN, Keith LG, Bachicha JA, Chasnoff IJ: Cocaine abuse during pregnancy: Correlation between prenatal care and perinatal outcome. Obstet Gynecol 74:882–885, 1989.
13. Racine AD, Joyce TJ, Anderson R: The association between prenatal care and birthweight among women exposed to cocaine in New York City: A correction. JAMA 271:1161–1162, 1994.
14. USDHHS: Surgeon General's Advisory on Alcohol and Pregnancy. FDA Drug Bulletin 11:9–10, 1981.
15. Serdula M, Williamson DF, Kendrick JS, Anda RF, Byers T: Trends in alcohol consumption by pregnant women—1985 through 1988. JAMA 265:876–879, 1991.
16. Scher MS, Richardson GA, Coble PA, et al: The effects of prenatal alcohol and marijuana exposure: Disturbances in neonatal sleep cycling and arousal. Pediatr Res 24:101–105, 1988.
17. Wainwright RL: Change in observed birth weight associated with change in maternal cigarette smoking. Am J Epidemiol 11:668–665, 1983.
18. Mayer JP, Hawkins MA, Todd RT: A randomized evaluation of smoking cessation interventions for pregnant women at a WIC clinic. Am J Public Health 80:76–78, 1990.
19. Jack BW, Culpepper L: Preconception care: Risk reduction and health promotion in preparation for pregnancy. JAMA 264:1147–1149, 1990.
20. Raskin V: Maternal bereavement in the perinatal substance abuser. J Subst Abuse Treat 9:149–152, 1992.
21. Swigar ME, Bowers MB, Fleck S: Grieving and unplanned pregnancy. Psychiatry 39:72–80, 1976.
22. Waldorf D: Natural recovery from opiate addiction: Some social-psychological processes of untreated recovery. J Drug Issues 13:237–280, 1983.
23. Tunving K, Nilsson K: Young female drug addicts in treatment: A twelve year perspective. J Drug Issues 15::367–382, 1985.
24. Smith IE, Dent DZ, Coles CD, Falek A: A comparison study of treated and untreated pregnant and postpartum cocaine-abusing women. J Subst Abuse Treat 9:343–348, 1992.
25. Regan DO, Leifer B, Finnegan L: Depression, self-concept, and violent experience in drug abusing women and their influence upon parenting effectiveness. NIDA Res Monogr 49:332, 1984.
26. Miller BA, Downs WR, Testa M: Interrelationships between victimization experiences and women's alcohol use. J Stud Alcohol 11(Suppl):109–117, 1993.
27. Chavkin W: Mandatory treatment for drug use during pregnancy. JAMA 266:1556–1561, 1991.
28. Blume SB: Chemical dependency in women: Important issues. Am J Drug Alcohol Abuse 17:49–60, 1991.
29. Griffin ML, Weiss RD, Mirin SM, et al: A comparison of male and female cocaine abusers. Arch Gen Psychiatry 46:122–126, 1989.
30. Miller LJ: Psychotic denial of pregnancy: Phenomenol-

ogy and clinical management. Hosp Community Psychiatry 41:1233–1237, 1990.

31. Swett C Jr, Cohen C, Surrey J, Compaine A, Chaviz R: High rates of alcohol use and history of physical and sexual abuse among women outpatients. Am J Drug Alcohol Abuse 17:49–60, 1991.

32. Amaro H, Zuckerman B, Cabral H: Drug use among adolescent mothers: Profile of risk. Pediatrics 84:144–151, 1989.

33. Marques PR, McKnight AJ: Drug abuse among pregnant adolescents attending public health clinics. Am J Drug Alcohol Abuse 17:399–413, 1991.

34. Amaro H, Fried LE, Cabral H, Zuckerman B: Violence during pregnancy and substance use. Am J Public Health 80:575–579, 1990.

35. Berenson AB, Stiglich NJ, Wilkinson GS, et al: Drug abuse and other risk factors for physical abuse in pregnancy among white non-Hispanic, black, and hispanic women. Am J Obstet Gynecol 164:1491–1499, 1991.

36. Methadone Treatment: Drugs and Reproductive Health. Rockville, MD: National Institute on Drug Abuse Training Project. Participant Manual, February 1991.

37. Trad PV: A matter of need (infant psychiatry). Psychiatric Times 9:28–29, 1992.

38. Shiffman S: Relapse following smoking cessation: A situational analysis. J Clin Psychol 50:71–86, 1982.

39. McBride CM, Pirie PL: Postpartum smoking relapse. Addict Behav 15:165–168, 1990.

40. Sexton M, Hebel JR, Fox NL: Postpartum smoking. In Rosenberg MJ (ed): Smoking and Reproductive Health. Littleton, MA, PSG Publishing, 1987, pp 222–226.

Treatment of Adolescent Addiction and Behavior Disorders

Catherine A. Nageotte, MD, MS Health Services • David L. Goldberg, MD

Adolescents with psychoactive substance use disorders and disruptive behavior disorders present enormous challenges to clinicians. Lack of consenus on the cause of both substance use disorders and disruptive behavior disorders inhibits development and funding of intervention programs, as well as necessary program evaluation and outcomes research. As a result, the type of assessment and intervention that adolescents with comorbid psychoactive substance use disorder (PSUD) and behavior disorder receive is highly dependent on what part of the services sector they enter. For example, adolescents entering the mental health or juvenile justice system may receive intervention targeted to alter their criminal behavior, but any comorbid addiction disorders, if identified, may be viewed as part of the behavior problem rather than an independent disorder warranting addiction intervention. Conversely, if an adolescent enters an addiction program, assessment and intervention may focus on the addiction and result in underdetection and undertreatment of comorbid disruptive behavior disorders. Psychoactive substance use or intoxication impairs impulse control, judgment, learning, and cognition. When coupled with a disruptive behavior disorder characterized by similar problems, the consequences of underdetection and undertreatment can be devastating.

The disruptive behavior disorders include attention deficit hyperactivity disorder (ADHD), conduct disorder (CD), oppositional defiant disorder (ODD), and disruptive behavior disorder. As a group, these are the most commonly diagnosed disorders of children and adolescents receiving mental health services. ADHD is a syndrome of at least 6 months' duration characterized by three cardinal features: impulse control problems, hyperactivity, and inattention. In addition, the child or adolescent must demonstrate impairment in at least two settings (school, work, or home). At least some of the symptoms should be present before the age of 7 years. The symptoms are not exclusively observed during the course of a pervasive developmental disorder, schizophrenia, or other disorder of anxiety, personality, mood, or reality testing.[1] Long-term consequences include lower IQ score, poor work and social performance, and persistence of symptoms into adulthood.

Although studies have shown increased rates of substance abuse in later life for children diagnosed as having ADHD,[2] others have shown no increased incidence of substance abuse.[3] A literature review examining hyperactivity as a risk factor for development of later alcohol addiction suggested that the critical risk factor is not hyperactivity but CD.[4] Adoption studies suggest that the only significant predictor of adult alcoholism, besides familial alcoholism, is CD.[5]

CD is a repetitive and persistent pattern of behavior in which the basic rights of others or the age-appropriate social norms are violated. Specific behaviors include aggression toward people or animals, vandalism, deceitfulness, theft, and serious rule violations. Three or more problematical behaviors must have occurred in the past 12 months and at least one in the past 6 months. The behavior disturbance causes clinically significant impairment in social, academic, or occupational functioning. The behavior disturbance should not be specific to one particular setting.[1]

Historical information must be obtained from the adolescent, parents, and collateral sources to enhance diagnostic reliability. Many children and adolescents minimize the extent of their negative behavior. On the other hand, many with other neuropsychiatric problems demonstrate the behavioral signs listed in DSM-IV, but their subjective symptoms may include paranoia or psychosis. A psychotic child may run away and destroy property because voices tell him to do so. Clinicians must be careful to use multidimensional assessments of adolescents with suspected CD, either when evaluating research data or when treating individuals.

Psychoactive substance use is extremely common in adolescents with CD. On the other hand, CD is not especially overrepresented among those with addictive disorders in general. In fact, substance abuse was one of the criteria for conduct disorder in DSM-III. In DSM-IV, however, both a substance-related disorder and CD diagnosis should be made if the criteria for both are met, even though certain antisocial acts may be a consequence of the substance-related disorder.

ODD is a recurrent pattern of negativistic, defiant, disobedient, and hostile behavior directed toward authority figures that persists for at least 6 months. Four or more of the following problem behaviors should be present: temper tantrums, noncompliance, deliberately annoying others, blaming others for one's mistakes or misbehavior, irritability, and frequent demonstration of resentful or angry affect. A criterion is met only if the given behavior occurs more frequently than is typical for persons of comparable age and developmental stage. Misbehavior should result in clinically

significant impairment in social, academic, or occupational functioning. The disruptive behavior is not as severe as that in CD. Low self-esteem, mood lability, low frustration tolerance, swearing, and the precocious use of alcohol, tobacco, or illicit drugs are not uncommon.[1]

Child-Adolescent Psychoactive Substance Use Versus Child-Adolescent Psychoactive Substance Use Disorder

The term *child-adolescent psychoactive substance use* (CAPSU) refers to stage I (experimentation) use of psychoactive substances, including alcohol. *Child-adolescent psychoactive substance use disorder* (CAPSUD) refers to stages 2, 3, and 4 (drug seeking, preoccupation with drug/mood swing, and using to feel normal, respectively).

Comorbidity

Comorbidity refers to the coexistence of more than one disorder in the same person at a given point in time,[6] Although the association may reflect a causal relationship between or an underlying vulnerability to both disorders, they may also be unrelated to any common cause or vulnerability.[7] The term *comorbidity* is used here to refer to those adolescents who meet diagnostic criteria for at least one psychoactive substance-related disorder, as well as diagnostic criteria for at least one disruptive behavior disorder, as defined earlier. The term *dual diagnosis* may also be applied to a patient in whom one disorder exists independently of an addictive disorder.

In practice, the concept of comorbidity (in this case, PSUDs and psychopathology) should form a basis for classifying adolescents exhibiting similar presenting phenomenology, treatment course, and treatment outcomes, in addition to facilitating practitioners' diagnostic assessment of and treatment matching for these adolescents.[8] However, erroneous application of the comorbidity concept can also lead to errors in assessment and treatment, because it is often unclear whether apparent psychiatric symptoms are due to the substance abuse itself or to a coexisting psychiatric disorder. Although a clinician may make attempts to determine a temporal sequence of symptom onset relative to the use of psychoactive substances, the information given by the adolescent or collaterals may be inaccurate owing to impaired recall.

A host of methodological problems limits the generation of research evidence to support the concept of comorbidity of behavior disorders and CAPSUDs. First and foremost, data demonstrating the reliability and validity of DSM-IV alcohol- or substance-related disorders criteria in children and adolescents do not yet exist. To date, reliability and stability of comorbid psychiatric disorders and PSUDs are reported in research conducted in adult populations. Studies reporting high rates of comorbidity among child and adolescent subjects have been conducted in clinical settings, where comorbidity rates may be higher than in the general population owing to treatment-seeking bias, known as *Berkson's bias.* Many of the behavioral criteria of ADD, ODD, and CD can also be consequences of alcohol and substance abuse (i.e., ignoring parental prohibitions, school truancy, angry and resentful attitude, impairment in functioning, and presence of symptoms in two or more settings), thus complicating determination of diagnostic specificity and positive predictive value of a given diagnostic criterion or set of criteria. However, a review of longitudinal studies of high-school and college students indicates that many behaviors and psychological symptoms thought to be consequent to drug use may actually predate psychoactive substance use.[9] Similarly, 68% of adolescents with PSUDs reported a combination of depression, anxiety, and CD behavior preceding the regular use of drugs and alcohol.[10]

Clinical differentiation between symptoms and signs of psychoactive substance intoxication, withdrawal, or both and a comorbid behavior disorder is quite difficult.[11] Assessment of CAPSUDs is further complicated by the fact that CAPSU is illegal, increasing the tendency for children or adolescents either to underreport or to flatly deny use, even when confidentiality is assured by those seeking the sensitive information. Kaminer suggests that use of a "best estimate" procedure may be helpful in enhancing the accuracy of the diagnostic process, especially when data from direct interview are either missing or inaccurate owing to the subjects' withholding or providing false information.[12] A clinician makes a best estimate diagnosis by combining information obtained by another clinician's direct interview of a subject, information in the medical record, and collateral reports.

Epidemiology

Early studies conducted in the 1970s with cohorts of adolescents from the general population found a relationship between psychoactive substance use and psychiatric symptoms.[13–15] More recently, 19 (7%) of 275 children and adolescents from a community-based sample received a DSM-III diagnosis of alcohol or substance abuse disorder; 17 of these also received one or more additional diagnoses.[16] Among 57 adolescents consecutively admitted for treatment of PSUDs and concurrent psychiatric disorders, 42% received a diagnosis of CD after administration of a structured clinical interview using DSM-III criteria.[17] In a sample of inpatient adolescents with PSUDs, 62% were diagnosed with CD and 30% with major depression; 28% received triple diagnoses of CD, PSUD, and depression.[18] These more recent findings suggest the following possibilities: (1) Treatment-seeking bias may explain higher rates of comorbidity in clinical versus community-based samples of adolescents; (2) use of different conceptual and diagnostic strategies results in different prevalence estimates; and (3) the high rates of comorbid CAPSUDs and psychopathology, including CD, are real and warrant appropriate treatment considerations.

Comorbid Psychoactive Substance Use Disorders and Implications for Treatment

Assuming that high rates of comorbidity of psychiatric disorders and PSUDs among clinical samples of adolescents accurately reflect reality, effective treatment planning and resource allocation to enhance treatment reimbursement for these adolescents are imperative. Few drug treatment programs are designed specifically to serve adolescents, and fewer are specifically designed to serve adolescents with comorbid PSUDs and disruptive behavior disorders.

The treatment of comorbid CD-PSUD is difficult; poor prognosis appears to be the rule rather than the exception. Prognosis may be improved if clinicians attempt to match adolescents' treatment needs to the treatment modality.[19] The American Society for Addiction Medicine (ASAM) Patient Placement Criteria define four levels of care that, when combined with six treatment dimensions, facilitate a clinicians' matching an adolescent's treatment needs with the appropriate addiction treatment intensity and degree of environmental restriction. The four levels of care are as follows: (1) level I, outpatient treatment; (2) level II, intensive outpatient treatment; (3) level III, medically monitored intensive inpatient treatment; and (4) level IV, medically managed intensive inpatient treatment. The six ASAM dimensions of care are (1) acute intoxication and/or withdrawal potential, (2) biomedical conditions and complications, (3) emotional/behavioral conditions and complications, (4) treatment acceptance/resistance, (5) relapse potential, and (6) recovery environment.[20]

ASAM Patient Placement Criteria indicate that adolescents with comorbid psychiatric disorders, including disruptive behavior disorders, should receive at least intensive outpatient treatment, if not medically monitored or medically managed inpatient treatment. Although adolescents rarely require medical detoxification, intensive inpatient treatment permits medical monitoring of the resolution of psychoactive substance-induced organic mental disorders, as well as early intervention for the emergence of serious psychiatric symptoms such as acute psychosis, with or without affective symptoms, which warrant acute intervention.

After an adolescent is placed in the appropriate level of treatment, matching of treatment elements may further improve retention and outcome. This is particularly germane to adolescents diagnosed with CD-PSUD because CD encompasses a wide array of behaviors that vary in their onset, etiology, and risk factors, for which a single treatment approach is unlikely to be effective. Four treatment elements may be particularly beneficial for adolescents with disruptive behavior disorders and PSUDs: parent management training, functional family therapy, problem-solving skills training, and community-based treatment.[21] The first three have strong cognitive-behavioral components, whereas community-based treatment offers a complementary component for treatment as well as for prevention and relies heavily on the assumption that segregation of deviant youths will lead to increased severity of maladaptive behavior. Consequently, mixing with nonreferred (normal) youths in the community and participation in shared activities may reduce antisocial behavior.[22]

Pharmacotherapy

Children and adolescents with comorbid ADHD-PSUD should continue to be treated with psychostimulants as the first line of pharmacotherapy for their ADHD. Abuse of therapeutic stimulants by patients with ADHD is rare.[23] Use of antidepressants should be considered when a comorbid anxiety or depressive disorder is present, but a clinician must weigh the benefits of antidepressant therapy against the risk for emergence of deleterious side effects if used in combination with alcohol or other psychoactive substances.

No medication has documented efficacy in improving symptoms of CD in children and adolescents. Although clinicians may prescribe neuroleptics, lithium, propranolol, or carbamazepine to decrease aggression or improve impulse control, there is no documented evidence of efficacy and the associated risks far outweigh the benefits of doing so. Similarly, no medication has documented efficacy in improving symptoms of ODD in children and adolescents.

A detailed description and discussion of adolescent addiction treatment is found in Chapter 30.

Conclusion

Comorbid PSUDs and disruptive behavior disorders pose a tremendous threat to the health and well-being of American youth. Prudent clinicians, teachers, and parents should maintain a healthy degree of suspicion that psychoactive substance use is only part of a complex cadre of problems with which many adolescents struggle. Although consensus exists among adolescent addiction treatment experts and among adolescent mental health experts, more attention to consensus development between the two groups is indicated. The very nature of comorbidity implies heterogeneity within the population of adolescents presenting with comorbid addiction and disruptive behavior disorders. As such, matching treatment interventions to the individual needs of each patient (individual treatment planning) is essential. Data gathered from randomized controlled trials incorporating longitudinal follow-up will aid in clinical identification of subgroups sharing risk factors, treatment response, and prognosis and may be used to improve treatment effectiveness.

REFERENCES

1. American Psychiatric Association: Diagnostic and Statistical Manual of Mental Disorders, 4th ed. Washington, DC, American Psychiatric Association, 1994.
2. Gittelman R, Mannuzza S, Shenker R, et al: Hyperactive boys almost grown up, I: Psychiatric status. Arch Gen Psychiatry 42:937–947, 1985.
3. Weiss G, Hechtman L, Milroy T, et al: Psychiatric status of hyperactives as adults: A controlled prospective 15-year follow-up of 63 hyperactive children. J Am Acad Child Psychiatry 24:211–220, 1985.
4. Alterman AI, Tarter RE: An examination of selected typologies: Hyperactivity, familial and antisocial alcoholism. In Galanter M (ed): Recent Developments in Alcoholism, vol. 4. New York, Plenum, 1986.
5. Cadoret RJ, Troughton E, O'Gorman TW, et al: An adoption study of genetic and environmental factors in drug abuse. Arch Gen Psychiatry 43:1131–1136, 1986.
6. Feinstein AR: The pre-therapeutic classification of comorbidity in chronic disease. J Chronic Dis 23:455–468, 1970.
7. American Psychiatric Association: Excerpts from The American Psychiatric Glossary—Appendix 2. In Hales RE, Yudofsky SC, Talbott JA (eds): Textbook of Psychiatry, 2nd ed. Washington, DC, American Psychiatric Association, 1994, p 1584.
8. Bukstein OG, Brent DA, Kaminer Y: Comorbidity of substance abuse and other psychiatric disorders in adolescents. Am J Psychiatry 146(9):1131–1141, 1989.
9. Kandel DB, Kessler RC, Margulies RZ: Antecedents of adolescent initiation into stages of drug use: A developmental analysis. In Kandel DB (ed): Longitudinal Reasearch in Drug Use: Empirical Findings and Methodological Issues. Washington, DC, Hemisphere Publishing Corp, 1978.
10. Stowell RJA, Estroff TW: Psychiatric disorders in substance-abusing adolescent inpatients: A pilot study. J Am Acad Child Adolesc Psychiatry 31:1036–1040, 1992.
11. Mirin SM, Weiss RD, Griffin ML, Michael JL: Psychopathology in drug abusers and their families. Compr Psychiatry 32:36–51, 1991.
12. Kaminer Y: Dual Diagnosis: Adolescent Psychoactive Substance Use Disorders and Psychiatric Comorbidity in Adolescent Substance Abuse: A Comprehensive Guide to Theory and Practice. New York, Plenum, 1994, 87–117.
13. Braucht GN, Brakarsch D, Follingstad D, Berry KL: Deviant drug use in adolescence: A review of psychological correlates. Psychol Bull 79:92–106, 1973.
14. Vener AM, Stewart CS, Hager DL: Depression and the adolescent in middle America. Presented at the 67th Annual Meeting of the American Sociological Association, New Orleans, LA, 1972.
15. Paton S, Kessler R, Kandel D: Depressive mood and adolescent illicit drug use: A longitudinal analysis. J Gen Psychol 131:267–289, 1977.
16. Keller MB, Lavori PW, Beardslee WR, et al: The clinical course and outcome of substance abuse disorders in adolescents. J Subst Abuse Treat 9:9–14, 1992.
17. DeMiio L: Psychiatric syndromes in adolescent substance abusers. Am J Psychiatry 146:1212–1214, 1989.
18. Bukstein OG, Glancy LJ, Kaminer Y: Patterns of affective comorbidity in a clinical population of dually-diagnosed adolescent substance abusers. J Am Acad Child Adolesc Psychiatry 31:1041–1045, 1992.
19. Kaminer Y, Tarter RE, Bukstein OG: Comparison between completers and non-completers among dually diagnosed substance abusing adolescents. J Am Acad Child Adolesc Psychiatry 31:1046–1049, 1992.
20. Hoffman NG, Halikas JA, Mee-Lee D, Weedman RD: Patient Placement Criteria for the Treatment of Psychoactive Substance Use Disorders. Washington, DC, American Society of Addiction Medicine, 1991, pp 60–107.
21. Kazdin AE: Teatment of antisocial behavior in children: Current status and future directions. Psychol Bull 102:187–203, 1987.
22. Offord DR, Jones MB, Graham A, et al: Community Skill-Development Programs for Children: Rationale and Steps in Implementation. Ontario, Canada, Canadian Parks and Recreation Program, 1985.
23. Weiss G, Hechtman LT: Hyperactive Children Grown Up: Empirical Findings and Theoretical Considerations. New York, Guilford Press, 1986.

Addiction Psychiatry and Long-Term Recovery in 12-Step Programs

John N. Chappel, MD

Psychiatric practice is enhanced by knowledge and skill in treating alcohol and other addictive disorders. The data cited elsewhere in this book reflect the ubiquity of addictive disorders in psychiatric practice. Unfortunately, many psychiatrists have had little if any training in addiction psychiatry. Our experience in acute care settings has often led to pessimism about the treatability of addictive disorders and long-term recovery from them.

Long-term recovery from addiction is not well understood. Relapse rates after short-term treatment are high. Follow-up on patients becomes more difficult with each passing year. The 12-step programs have demonstrated an ability to hold a substantial number of recovering addicts in continuing participation and sobriety. As the oldest and largest of these fellowships, Alcoholics Anonymous (AA) can be of great help in understanding long-term recovery from alcoholism. This chapter summarizes the data that have been compiled by AA in its triennial surveys, which began in 1968.*[1]

---

*The information on the triennial surveys conducted by AA was obtained from the General Service Office of AA. The use of these data does not imply agreement by AA, which has no opinion on any conclusions or interpretations made in this chapter.

None of the other 12-step fellowships has undertaken an ongoing study of the size and extent of AA's. We assume that there would be many similarities in Narcotics Anonymous (NA) and the other 12-step programs that help other drug addicts and their families, but confirmatory data are lacking. The 1989 *Review of Psychiatry* describes AA as a "vital adjunct to the management of alcoholics."[2] The authors of this section of the *Review* express the opinion that AA is "the ideal setting for long-term maintenance of sobriety." They outline steps that a psychiatrist can take to enhance the likelihood that the patients they refer will have a constructive experience in AA.

The Membership Survey

Since 1968, the membership of AA has grown at a remarkable rate. In that year, the first membership survey was carried out. This survey was prompted by a physician trustee on the General Service Board of AA. Its purpose was to provide more accurate information about the fellowship of AA to professionals working with alcoholics or in the field of alcoholism. A second major goal was to provide information to AA members to help them work more effectively in helping other suffering alcoholics. The available data indicate that AA has continued to be successful in that mission. Table 33–1 shows the annual growth of membership from 1970 to 1989. The consistency in growth has been remarkable. The largest growth spurt in a single year occurred in 1972, the year after Bill Wilson died, with an increase of 15.6%. The last 6 years listed in the table, from 1983 to 1989, show a consistent 6% to 7% growth annually. The 1992 survey did not include a membership estimate, thus accounting for the absence of more recent information in the table. It should be noted that these membership figures are conservative. Many AA groups do not register with the General Service Office and are therefore not included in the membership estimate.

This steady growth has occurred despite the high dropout rate from AA. In five surveys during the 15-year period from 1977 to 1989, an analysis of the respondents who had been in AA for 1 year or less shows a steady decline (Fig. 33–1). The decline is greatest during the first 3 months. The information from each survey "strongly suggests that *about half those who come to AA are gone within 3 months*."[1] Because the survey is anonymous, without individual follow-up, the reasons for individuals' leaving after their initial exposure to meetings cannot be determined. This loss of people who might benefit from AA's program of recovery is a challenge not only to AA but to all professionals who refer people to AA. Psychiatrists can do much to identify and work with the resistance that so many patients have to working a 12-step program of recovery.

The first survey results in 1968 were viewed with a great deal of caution. Subsequent surveys showed consistent results and trends. During the years, "confidence began to grow that the results were, within limits, representative of the Fellowship as a whole."[1] It should

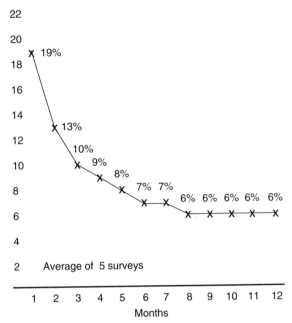

Figure 33–1. Alcoholics Anonymous members who have been in the fellowship for 12 months or less.

be noted that within 12-step programs, such as AA and NA, all the members together are referred to as the *Fellowship*. In 1983, a scientific sampling process was adopted. Questionnaires were sent to a 3% stratified sample of each delegate's area in the United States and Canada. This made it possible to reduce the number of questionnaires, as shown in Table 33–2, but to increase confidence that the results are representative of AA as a whole, although not of any specific group or area.

Stable Aspects of Alcoholics Anonymous

The most challenging stable aspect of AA is the high dropout rate, already noted. The average of five surveys, from 1977 to 1989, is shown

Table 33–1. MEMBERSHIP OF ALCOHOLICS ANONYMOUS (UNITED STATES AND CANADA)

Year	Membership (Thousands)	Year	Membership (Thousands)
1970	193	1980	476
1971	211	1981	520
1972	244	1982	585
1973	261	1983	656
1974	331	1984	702
1975	337	1985	751
1976	369	1986	804
1977	404	1987	853
1978	410	1988	917
1979	445	1989	979

Table 33–2. NUMBER OF COMPLETED QUESTIONNAIRES ON EACH SURVEY

1968	11,355
1971	7,194
1974	13,467
1977	15,163
1980	24,950
1983	7,611
1986	6,977
1989	9,394
1992	6,500

in Figure 33–1. The dropout rate decreases after 3 months and is relatively stable after 6 months. These data indicate that simply attending AA meetings is not enough. Confirmation of this fact is found in Walsh and colleagues' study showing that alcoholics randomly assigned to AA suffered more frequent relapses and were less likely to be abstinent at follow-up than those assigned to treatment that educated them about their disease and helped them learn how to use AA.[3] Although the reasons for this continuing high dropout rate are not known, some of them can be inferred. AA's concern is to make its program more attractive to newcomers without promotion. Although AA wants the hand of every member to be available to any suffering alcoholic, absolutely no pressure is applied to have people join or continue in the program. One reason for this stance is that some of an alcoholic's suffering comes from others in contact with him or her. It has been said that if you look carefully, a footprint can be seen on the posterior of every alcoholic entering treatment. The usual response to such pressure is resistance and resentment. Psychiatrists and other mental health professionals have skills that can be effective in reducing resistance and resentment. If we applied these skills to alcoholics starting to get involved in AA, the dropout rate might be reduced.

Resistance to AA probably comes from three main sources. The first source of resistance is external pressure, whether it comes from loved ones, friends, work, or a judge. Psychiatrists and other mental health professionals, as objective third parties, can help reduce this resistance through cognitive restructuring by emphasizing both the care behind the pressure and especially the benefits of working a program of recovery in AA.

The second source of resistance is denial. An alcoholic or other addicted person is usually the last one to know about her or his alcoholism. Addiction has been said to be the only disease that tells the person that they don't have it. If we keep collecting information and present it to our addicted patients, this evidence will eventually penetrate or wear down the denial. The connection of pain in an addicted person's life to the use of alcohol or other drugs is one of the most effective counters to denial.

The third source of resistance is to AA itself. There is much misinformation about AA, usually based on hearsay or media reports. In a study of 407 professionals in recovery from alcoholism, Bissell and Haberman found the following mistaken beliefs about AA[4]:

1. It is a religious organization that may be fanatic or cultlike.

2. It is a kind of folk medicine with no scientific basis.

3. As a substitute dependence for alcohol, it is an equally unhealthy addiction.

4. The members are of a much lower or different social class, and I will have nothing in common with them.

Psychiatrists and other mental health professionals who are knowledgeable and experienced about AA can do much to dispel or correct these erroneous beliefs by disseminating the following information:

1. AA and other 12-step programs are spiritual programs and not religions. The only requirement for membership in AA is a desire to stop drinking. The internal surrender to a power greater than oneself has been viewed as a useful step in growth and development from a psychoanalytical point of view.[5] AA allows and encourages individuals to have whatever experience they are capable of, including none. There is no dogma, theology, or creed to be learned. There is no record anywhere, in more than 60 years of experience with millions of alcoholics in AA, of anyone's being rejected or asked to leave a meeting because of his or her spiritual beliefs or lack of them, as has happened in many religions.

2. The accumulated experience of chronic alcoholics attaining and maintaining sobriety was a form of field research that worked out an effective system of treatment for alcoholism. AA has been scientifically validated in prospective scientific studies.[6]

3. As a substitute dependence for alcohol, AA makes it possible for alcoholics to stop drinking. Addiction to AA or the other 12-step programs, if it exists, does not remotely resemble the havoc created by addiction to alcohol in an alcoholic's life. Heavy participation in 12-step programs in the early phases of recovery is like dependence on a cast or crutches while a fracture is healing. In the case of a fracture, it would be malpractice for a physician not to provide these substitute dependencies when faced with evidence of damage to the bone. Continued dependence on AA is more analogous to continued dependence on education and exercise. Like the latter, the 12-step programs promote both health and continued growth and development. It is my observation that people who work a continuing 12-step pro-

Table 33–3. OCCUPATION OF ALCOHOLICS ANONYMOUS RESPONDENTS (1992 SURVEY)

Manager/administrator	11%
Educator	3%
Medical profession (M.D.s)	2%
Service worker	6%
Professional/technical	19%
Homemaker	5%
Sales worker	6%
Craft worker	5%
Laborer	10%
Clerical worker	5%
Transportation (equipment operator)	2%
Retired	9%
Unemployed	11%
Disabled	5%
Other	1%

gram of recovery in AA develop the mature ego defense mechanisms of altruism, humor, anticipation, suppression, and sublimation.[7] In addition, they develop personal characteristics of honesty, openness, humility, and gratitude. It would be a great benefit to all of us if the continuing practice of psychiatry had similar effects.

4. All social classes are represented in AA. The survey data indicate that the membership is heterogeneous. The occupations represented in the survey in 1992 are listed in Table 33–3. If anything, professionals are overrepresented in AA. Data from the Epidemiologic Catchment Area (ECA) survey indicate that the lowest rates of alcoholism (4.1%) are found among professionals and managers.[8] The highest rates (13.6%) are found among skilled laborers. AA makes efforts to welcome any alcoholic regardless of sex, race, religion, disability, sexual preference, or any other distinguishing characteristic. Although the groups sampled in the survey are selected in accordance with scientific sampling, there is no assurance that everyone at a meeting of that group responds to the survey questionnaire. Those who are not used to surveys or who have literacy problems are less likely to respond and thus may be underrepresented in the data. At present, the membership survey suggests that lower socioeconomic groups and possibly minorities are underrepresented.

Despite the high dropout rate, many people continue to participate in AA. The proportion of the membership with recent, intermediate, and long-term sobriety has remained relatively stable. In 1992, these proportions were as follows:

35% sober less than 1 year (recent unstable sobriety)
34% sober between 1 and 5 years (intermediate sobriety)
31% sober longer than 5 years (stable sobriety)

During the past 15 years, the average months of sobriety have remained very close to 4 years, with an increase to 5 years in 1992. Thus, at any given meeting of AA, a newcomer or visitor will have a good chance of meeting someone with many years of experience in sobriety.

In analyzing the data, considerable attention has been paid to "survival rates" in AA. This rate describes continued sobriety and activity in the Fellowship. When the data are corrected for proportions and frequency of attendance at meetings, the following statements are made in the analysis of the 1989 survey[1]:

1. Of those sober less than 1 year, about 41% will remain in the Fellowship another year.
2. Of those sober less than 5 years, about 83% will remain in the Fellowship another year.
3. Of those sober 5 years or more, about 91% will remain in the Fellowship another year.

These data, combined with data from the Comprehensive Assessment and Treatment Outcome Research (CATOR) studies, emphasize the importance of the first year of sobriety. During a 10-year period, CATOR collected intake data on more than 50,000 adults from 80 treatment programs and 6000 adolescents from 28 programs.[9] One-year follow-up samples showed total abstinence rates of 63% to 75%. Most relapses occurred during the first 6 months. The strongest relationships to good outcome were attendance at AA or other 12-step meetings and participation in aftercare programs that provide group education and support. These data suggest that a key time for knowledgeable and skilled professional support is in the first year after an alcoholic stops drinking. The researchers report that one of "the most consistent findings in CATOR treatment outcome studies over the past 10 years is the significant relationship between support group involvement after treatment and recovery status."[9] The vast majority of this support group involvement (98%) was in AA.

There has also been stability in several areas central to working a program while in AA. The survey has shown that more than 80% of responding members have a sponsor. This fell to 78% in 1992, but it is too early to indicate a trend. The role of a sponsor or mentor who shares his or her experience and provides guidance for a newcomer in working the steps and other parts of a program of recovery has always been emphasized in AA. Research indicates that having a sponsor significantly reduces the risk of relapse.[10] Some addiction psychiatrists like to have contact with their patient's sponsor during treatment.

A similar proportion of AA members, more than 80%, have a home group, which serves as a symbolic extended family for recovering alcoholics. The home group gives each AA member responsibilities that provide an introduction to service. Service activity in AA is a powerful influence in countering the psychopathology produced by addiction. Activity in service is unlikely to occur if the AA member only attends meetings. An additional benefit of the home group is the help that a recovering alcoholic receives in developing and using a phone list. This activity has been found to reduce significantly the risk of relapse.[10] Men, in particular, are resistant to asking for help. Clinicians can help men overcome this resistance by emphasizing the fact that a troubled alcoholic's call helps the AA member who is called. It was Bill W.'s recognition of the fact that he had to talk to another alcoholic in order to stay sober that started AA in Akron in 1935.

Attendance at AA meetings has also been very stable. The average has been close to three meetings a week, both during the past 15 years and between different lengths of sobriety. For example, in the 1989 survey, the average frequency of attendance for those with less than a year of sobriety was 3.0 meetings a week. The frequency slowly decreased until at 20 to 25 years of sobriety, the average was 2.7 meetings a week. The 1992 data suggest a decrease to 2.5 meetings a week. From a clinical point of view, the problem is in the first year. Treatment programs recommend 90 meetings in 90 days after completion of treatment. Obviously, this is not happening. Psychiatrists and other mental healthcare professionals will serve their newly sober patients well by encouraging more frequent attendance at AA and other 12-step meetings. Vaillant found that stable sobriety in recovering alcoholics was associated with attendance at 300 or more AA meetings.[6]

In 1980, three new questions were added to the survey regarding the AA member's physician. At that time, 71% stated that their doctor knew they were in AA, a figure that has increased slightly (74%) in the subsequent 12 years. More revealing is the fact that 57% did not know whether their physician presented AA as a program of recovery to his or her patients. An even higher percentage (74%) did not know whether their doctor had been to an AA meeting. The survey analyst concluded that "These results suggest a less than candid relationship between AA's and their physicians."[1] Another way of looking at these data is that recovering alcoholics have difficulty being assertive with their physicians. We can help in this area. If our patients can become more assertive in educating their physicians about AA, the number of physician referrals to AA may increase.

Changing Aspects of Alcoholics Anonymous

One of the least dramatic but most significant changes in the composition of AA membership has occurred in the number of women. In 1968, the percentage of women in the survey was 22%. Within 10 years, this percentage had risen to 31%. In 1992, continued slow increase had occurred to a level of 35%. This ratio of 1.9:1.0 for men and women is much lower than the ratio found in the ECA study.[8] The data from that study show a lifetime prevalence of alcoholism in men of 23.8%, compared with 4.6% in women, for a male-to-female ratio of 5.2:1.0. The least difference is in the 18- to 29-year-old group, but even here the 2.9:1.0 ratio is much higher than it is in AA.

One way of interpreting these data is that AA has successfully moved from its early bias against women. In the early days of the Fellowship, many of the members did not believe that women could be alcoholics. As a result, the early AA literature is written as though all the members were men. Some professionals who are not familiar with the program have concluded that women will be deterred by this aspect of AA. It would now appear that AA is more attractive to female alcoholics than to male alcoholics. This difference may reflect a greater willingness on the part of women to accept a treatment that emphasizes growth and development activities such as sharing life experience, service, and becoming open to spiritual experience.

There are no data on minority representation in AA. There is, however, a great deal of interest in AA's reducing the barriers and making the program more attractive to blacks, Hispanics, Native Americans, and people with disabilities. This is in keeping with the singleness of purpose expressed in the intent that the hand of AA should be available to any alcoholic.

The percentage of young people in AA increased from 7.1% who were younger than 31 years in 1968 to almost 20% in 1992. This change reflects the fact that alcoholism is most often a disorder of youthful onset. Almost 40% of alcoholics have their first symptoms between the ages of 15 and 19. The percentage of those younger than 21 years in AA rose sharply from 1% in 1977 to almost 3% in 1983, where it has remained through 1992.

It is hoped that the increase in young people means that alcoholics are seeking and getting help earlier in their disease. However, the change may also reflect a more rapid rate of severity of addiction when drugs are added to alcohol.

Of more concern is the steady decrease in AA members older than 50 years. The proportion has steadily fallen from 37% in 1977 to 24% in 1992. This decrease in older membership has not been accompanied by a decrease in average sobriety, which has remained stable at 4 years and may be increasing. The percentage of the membership with more than 5 years of sobriety has also been stable. Given the increasing number of members in AA, it is not clear whether more older members are dropping out or whether the increasing number of younger members has made the proportion of older ones smaller. There is some concern in the Fellowship that the combination of youth and drugs has been aversive enough to cause older members to drop out.

The most dramatic change in the surveys has been in response to the question "Were you addicted to any drugs other than alcohol?" The increase in those replying "yes" has risen steadily from 18% in 1977 to 46% in 1989. Although they are two different samples, the latter figure from the AA membership is remarkably similar to the 47% of the ECA sample of alcoholics who had a second diagnosis, the majority of which was drug abuse or drug dependence.

The issue of other drug addiction poses a real problem for AA. Early in AA's history, it was decided that alcoholism would be the single focus of the program. The adaptation of the 12 steps and 12 traditions to form the basis of the unaffiliated program of NA was encouraged. However, many people come to AA meetings wanting to talk about drugs other than alcohol. Some of the worst problems have been caused by treatment centers that sent large numbers of newly sober drug addicts and alcoholics to AA meetings. Psychiatrists and other mental health care professionals can help their dually addicted patients by educating them about the differences between AA and NA. AA's singleness of purpose is widely credited with the depth and intensity of recovery attained by many of its members. Patients can engage in this recovery by focusing on their relationship with alcohol when they attend AA meetings. If someone suggests that they belong in other programs, the only response needed is, "I'm here because I want to stop drinking."

There has been a slow but steady change in how people begin to attend AA. The largest number, 34%, enter the program through contact with other AA members. This 12th-step activity has fallen from 44% in 1977. At that time, 19% came through the combination of treatment facilities and counseling. By 1992, 36% entered AA through treatment facilities and counseling agencies. This was a 4% decline from 1989. Slowly declining in importance were "on my own" (33% to 29%) and "doctor" (10% to 7%).

The importance of alcohol and drug treatment programs has been confirmed by Walsh and colleagues' study, which found that treatment combined with AA produced significantly higher rates of abstinence for employed alcoholics than did referral to AA alone.[3] AA does not affiliate in any way with treatment programs. It is, however, very willing to extend its hand to any suffering alcoholic. AA meetings held in treatment programs or other institutional programs are independent of those organizations. Treatment Facilities committees, sometimes called by the old name of Hospital and Institutional committees are available nationally and locally to help alcoholics who are in treatment find and make use of AA. They cooperate with healthcare professionals, as does the Cooperation with the Professional Community (CPC) committee, to help their alcoholic patients in treatment find access to AA meetings.

AA wants to be friends with psychiatrists and other healthcare professionals. Bill W., one of AA's cofounders, articulated this position in an address to the American Psychiatric Association.[11] We psychiatrists need to be friends with AA and other 12-step programs in order to provide our addicted patients with effective long-term treatment. A misconception is that when patients enter AA, they drop out of psychotherapy and other psychiatric treatment. The percentage of AA members who have received professional help while in the program has risen from just over 40% in 1980 to just under 60% in 1992. These figures are just a little lower than the percentages of individuals who received professional help before entering AA. More importantly, 87% of those who received treatment or counseling said it played an important part in their recovery from alcoholism. It is very likely that AA members will seek out psychiatrists and other mental health professionals who are familiar with their program of recovery and supportive of it. It has been my observation during the past 10 years that AA members who are actively working a program of recovery fare very well in medical and psychiatric treatment. The only conflict occurs when dependence-producing medications are prescribed. Most AA members fear these medications, especially benzodiazepines, sedative-hypnotics, and opioids. They experienced so much pain from their former practice of self-medicating symptoms with alcohol or other drugs that they prefer not to repeat the experience.

Discussion

The data described earlier support the clinical use of the recovery status examination, which consists of the following seven questions.[12] Each question (italicized in the following paragraphs) taps into a different aspect of what it means to work a 12-step program of recovery.

1. *What are you currently using?* This question includes tobacco, alcohol, over-the-counter medications, and prescription drugs in addition to other recreational and street drugs. Although few patients are ready to discontinue tobacco or caffeine use, the question raises consciousness about their addicting qualities and the advantages to health in stopping or restricting their use.

2. *What is your program of recovery?* This open-ended question reveals the recovering person's understanding of what it means to work a program of recovery in AA or other 12-step programs. If there is no mention of the fundamentals[6] of substitute dependencies (nonchemical ways of changing brain chemistry), unambivalent social support (a recovery support system), and reminders of the aversive effects of addicting drugs ("keeping the memory green"), then a lot of educational work needs to be done, accompanied by a search for resistances to recovery.

3. *What meetings are you attending?* This central part of any program of recovery has both a quantitative and qualitative component. Early in recovery, frequent attendance may be important in maintaining sobriety. This fact is reflected in the almost universal recommendation that newly sober individuals attend 90 meetings in 90 days. Useful information can be obtained from supplementary questions such as What do you do at meetings? What meetings do you like best? What meetings do you get the most out of?

4. *What are you doing with your home group?* Participation in this basic unit of AA serves many important functions in a recovery support system of accepting and tolerant relationships. It introduces a recovering person to both the group conscience and service. For many, this is where a sense of responsibility begins for their own important role in helping the group function more effectively in its task of helping other alcoholics stay sober.

5. *How do you use your phone list?* The act of reaching out to others for help has been shown to prevent relapse. Professionals can help educate their patients about how this apparently weak and selfish act is not only healthy but actually helps the person who is called.

6. *Where are you in your step work?* Each step has its own purpose, and each contributes both to sobriety and to continued personal growth and development. If a professional is familiar with the utility of each step, useful suggestions can be made to assist psychotherapy. For example, step 3 can help patients manage anxiety over some aspect of their life that they cannot change. Steps 4 and 5 assist the process of self-exploration, which is a basic part of psychotherapy. Steps 8 and 9 can help repair relationships that have been strained or disrupted. Consistent, disciplined step work contributes to continuing growth and development in recovery.

7. *What are you working on with your sponsor and those you sponsor?* This activity has also been shown to prevent relapse. Sponsors serve many roles. The initial choice is usually someone who appears to be a good role model. This person helps greatly with step work. Sponsors are sources of support in times of need and exert caring pressure to help recovering persons continue to work their program. The next step of becoming a sponsor for someone else moves the individual into a creative activity that promotes personal growth and development as she or he generatively passes on what has been learned. Research support for sponsoring was found in a 10-year follow-up of more than 200 alcoholics, where 91% of those who sponsored others were in stable recovery at 10 years.[13]

Conclusions

AA has demonstrated success in producing steadily increasing membership, with no loss of the proportion of those with more than 5 years of sobriety. It has been recognized as effective long-term treatment for alcoholism by healthcare professionals experienced in treatment of addictions.

The triennial membership surveys of AA have shown stability in

1. A 50% dropout rate within the first 3 months of starting AA. Only 41% of those in the first year will remain in the Fellowship for another year.

2. Roughly equal numbers of those with less than 1 year, 1 to 5 years, and more than 5 years of sobriety, with an average length of sobriety of 4 to 5 years.

3. Members having a sponsor and belonging to a home group (about 80%).

4. Attendance by members at 2.5 to 3 AA meetings a week, regardless of duration of sobriety.

5. Members telling their doctor that they are in AA but not helping their doctor learn about the program.

The survey data also indicate that AA is changing in the following ways:

1. The number of women members has increased to more than one third of the total.

2. The number of people younger than 30 years has increased to more than one fifth of the total.

3. The number of people older than 50 years has decreased to just under one fourth of the total.

4. The number of members who were also addicted to other drugs has increased (46%).

Psychiatrists and other mental healthcare professionals can use these data and knowledge of AA to

1. Increase the effectiveness of referrals of addicted patients to AA or other 12-step programs regardless of age, sex, race, or other characteristics. All are welcome and can benefit.

2. Deal with resistance that occurs when patients begin to make contact with AA or other 12-step programs.

3. Help alcoholic and other addicted patients through the difficult first year of sobriety.

4. Encourage their addicted patients to use AA and other 12-step programs as a path for personal growth and development.

5. Help dually addicted patients use AA's singleness of purpose to facilitate their recovery.

6. Work with alcohol and drug treatment programs in helping patients transfer to AA and other 12-step programs so that they can continue to work an effective program of recovery.

7. Cooperate with members of the local AA Treatment Facilities and Cooperation with the Professional Community committees to learn about and to train other healthcare professionals in using AA and the other 12-step programs in treating their addicted patients.

8. Provide psychiatric treatment for AA and other 12-step program members in ways that support and sustain their program of recovery, especially avoiding dependence-producing medications. When these are necessary, they are used in ways that support recovery and do not lead to relapse.

9. Monitor the recovery of their addicted patients and help them learn what it means to work a 12-step program of recovery through use of the recovery status examination.

REFERENCES

1. Alcoholics Anonymous: Comments on AA's Triennial Surveys, 1989 and 1992. Available from AA World Services, Box 459, New York, NY 10163.
2. Tasman A, Hales RE, Frances AJ (eds): Review of Psychiatry, vol 8. Washington, American Psychiatric Association, 1989.
3. Walsh EC, Hingson RW, Merrigan DM, et al: A randomized trial of treatment options for alcohol abusing workers. N Engl J Med 325(11):775–782, 1991.
4. Bissell L, Haberman PW: Alcoholism in the Professions. New York, Oxford University Press, 1984.
5. Khantzian EJ, Mack JE: Alcoholics Anonymous and contemporary psychodynamic theory. Recent Dev Alcohol 7:67–89, 1989.
6. Vaillant GE: The Natural History of Alcoholism. Cambridge, MA, Harvard University Press, 1983.
7. Vaillant GE: Adaptation to Life. Boston, Little, Brown & Co, 1977.
8. Helzer JE, Burnam A: Epidemiology of alcohol addiction: United States. In Miller NS (ed): Comprehensive Handbook of Drug and Alcohol Addiction. New York, Marcel Dekker, 1991, pp 9–38.
9. Harrison PA, Hoffmann NG, Streed SG: Drug and alcohol addiction treatment outcome. In Miller NS (ed): Comprehensive Handbook of Drug and Alcohol Addiction. New York, Marcel Dekker, 1991, pp 1163–1197.
10. Sheeren M: The relationship between relapse and involvement in Alcoholics Anonymous. J Stud Alcohol 49:104–106, 1988.
11. William W: The Society of Alcoholics Anonymous. Am J Psychiatry 106(5):370–375, 1949.
12. Chappel JN: Effective use of Alcoholics Anonymous and Narcotics Anonymous in treating patients. Psychiatr Ann 22(8):409–418, 1992.
13. Cross GM, Morgan CW, Mooney AJ, et al: Alcoholism treatment: A ten year follow-up study. Alcohol Clin Exp Res 14:169–173, 1990.

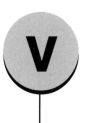

TREATMENT PROCESS

Inpatient and Outpatient Treatment of Alcoholism—Essential Features

Gregory B. Collins, MD

The healthcare industry is in a state of rapid change, and no sector has experienced the brunt of this change more than treatment of chemical dependence. After the initial rapid proliferation of alcoholism treatment centers in the 1970s and 1980s, this sector underwent a painful, cost-driven contraction, and many centers have gone out of business altogether. Those that remain have changed dramatically, from 28-day inpatient Minnesota model programs (often with no aftercare component) to multilevel programs focusing on outpatient services, with minimal inpatient backup for extremely unstable patients only. Patients are assigned by triage to a level of care matching their level of severity and are moved to levels of lesser intensity as their condition improves. The result has been a far lower cost per case, often yielding reductions of 50% to 70%.

This rush to cut costs has forced chemical dependence programs to change dramatically and to challenge old assumptions about the way effective treatment must be provided. The results of these cataclysmic changes are not yet available, and it remains to be seen whether patient outcomes are better, worse, or the same as before. The essentials of treatment—the basic concepts, methods, and goals—have not changed very much, however. The essentials of the healing process, from team building and fundamental philosophy to detoxification and rehabilitation methods, remain much the same and serve as the foundation stones on which the miracles of recovery are wrought.

A Multidisciplinary Team Approach

At first glance, it would seem that the founders of Alcoholics Anonymous (AA), Drs. "Bob" Smith and "Bill" Wilson, did not rely on a multidisciplinary team to find their own sobriety and launch the fellowship of AA. Nonetheless, if one studies the roots of the AA movement, it is clear that the multidisciplinary approach was one of the main strengths of the movement as it gathered in the knowledge of physicians, psychiatrists, clergy, nurses, and recovering individuals, all working together to help alcoholics attain the elusive goal of lasting sobriety.[1]

This early multidisciplinary approach in AA evolved into a highly specialized but nonetheless multidisciplinary method widely used in chemical dependence treatment programs. With assistance from many disciplines, a chemically dependent person is first detoxified and then is restored to physical, emotional, and spiritual health. The effective accomplishment of this broad restorative goal requires the input of people with different skills—a true multidisciplinary group. It would seem obvious that such a group would need to work together in a harmonious fashion to accomplish this goal of total recovery of chemically dependent persons. Because an alcoholic can easily "divide and conquer," factionalizing staff and playing on bias and rivalries to remain entrenched in the addictive cycle, staff coordination and teamwork must be achieved and maintained to facilitate the process of change and recovery.

Ruth Fox, MD, Medical Director of the National Council on Alcoholism, has noted, "treatment of the alcoholic, to be successful, must be multidisciplinary."[2] Because chemical dependence is a physical, emotional, social, and spiritual disease, the skills needed to treat all aspects of this disease process are of such breadth that it is all but impossible for one person to adequately treat the whole person. Brotman, in an attempt to enumerate the disciplines required for the treatment of alcoholism, states, "while only time and extensive research will yield the clue to optimum composition of such a team, I would suggest that it might include the disciplines of medicine, psychiatry, nursing, social case work, community organization and research." Thus, the team would incorporate a broad array of skills addressed to the major areas of functioning in a patient's life.[3]

It is also essential that communication between team members be honest and empathic. Too large a team makes close support and trust difficult and could lead to splitting within the team. Too small a team can lead to enabling of each other, a lack of perspective, or a situation in which new ideas and attitudes are not tolerated. A mature team, as described by Spratley, has six Cs: clarity, congruence of purpose, competence, confidence, continuity, and caring attitudes.[4]

Within this congruence of purpose, a team with diverse skills is needed. Because the goal of treatment is to allow patients their best chance for recovery, a multidisciplinary team affords the best opportunity because the contribution of each member of the team is different as a result of specific training. In all cases, physical health or at least a stable physical condition is an essential aspect of recovery, necessitating the skills of physicians and nurses. Additionally, a psychiatrist may see subtleties of a patient's emotional state that may need specific treatment that others might miss. Likewise, a social worker may see precarious areas in a patient's social network that a psychiatrist might not be attuned to. A psychologist can identify nuances in a patient's cognitive functioning that may not otherwise be discovered. The 12-step component,[5] provided by counselors and AA volunteers, also is essential after discharge, because patients cannot take the treatment team home.

The 12 steps[5] and peer supports are essential in continually reinforcing the changes, attitudes, and perspective for the maintenance of stable, quality sobriety. A true multidisciplinary team approach to treatment allows the widest possible range of modalities in helping a person to regain health physically, emotionally, cognitively, socially, and spiritually.

To accomplish its task of restorative rehabilitation, a multidisciplinary team establishes its own internal culture based on certain assumptions. In general, these assumptions reflect the values, norms, philosophy, rules, climate, and system of organization within which the team functions. In most treatment milieus, these values, norms, and philosophies include the 12 steps[5] and the overarching abstinence-oriented philosophy of AA.

Behind these unifying virtues or principles is the assumption that team members will live by these principles and not merely mouth the words and will, in their individual ways, be living powers of example for role modeling of healthy attitudes and behaviors. It is not necessary that staff members be recovering individuals themselves. Rather, the ability to live by the principles and the ability to empathize and lead others to a better life supersede personal recovery experience. Additional group norms may extend to dress (casual or professional), language (use of profanity by patients or staff), or attitude (competition vs. cooperation). The establishment of these norms is by no means an easy or natural aspect of team evolution. The varied backgrounds and experiences of typical chemical dependence team members yield a diversity of opinions on these subjects, which can lead to rivalry. The fine balance between a fractious diversity and a working consensus around group norms is elusive and fragile. An operating consensus around the disease concept of chemical dependence and the philosophical unity around the 12 steps[5] and philosophy of AA offer a solid conceptual framework that all team members can comfortably accept, thereby buffering differences and interpersonal frictions.

Even within this framework of philosophical unity, the team must exist in a larger system, such as a hospital, social service program, or even a self-help fellowship. The team must be able to respond to the demands and norms of the larger system in which it exists. It cannot merely look inside itself for validation, or a self-serving myopia and complacency will soon result.

For a multidisciplinary team to function well, the members need to know that they are working together for a common purpose. This common purpose may be to provide outstanding patient care. This goal may be defined by the larger system such as a hospital, and although there may be general agreement about this goal and principle, consensus may not be so easily reached about specifics. Quality may not be defined either. Quality goals such as abstinence from mood-altering chemicals, patient satisfaction, high productivity, program solvency, and "caring" may be, to a degree, mutually exclusive. The extent to which component members of the team prioritize these valued goals and the way they go about attaining them constitute the dynamic web of tension that exists in the organizational team. This methodological step can be accomplished by fiat ("this is what we are going to do and this is how we are going to do it") or by a consensus-based approach, using discussion, deliberation, debate, and finally decision making.

A working assumption of any successful team is that all team members are willing to operationalize and "own" a part of that goal. Not only has the larger system mandated that the functional team will contribute to the goal, but each team member must vigorously support the goal and be willing to act with the utmost responsibility to accomplish its achievement. Team members who do not accept or adequately prioritize the goal are soon out of step with group norms and introduce disharmony and friction into the smooth flow or the organizational components. Without these vital and healthy team attitudes, the elusive goal of lasting sobriety in the context of a new, AA-oriented way of life will flounder on the rocks of divisiveness and competition. In a successful team, each member must fully share in the ownership and responsibility for providing high-quality, sobriety-oriented patient care. Thus, an exciting sense of meaningful participation and team spirit permeates the task.

An effective interdisciplinary team incorporates a dynamic, interactive, fluid pattern of interrelating to achieve internal and external goals important for the completion of its task. The team must move from an amorphous state of nondefinition of role to one that incorporates a certain amount of role clarity, without inflaming role-based rivalries and "turf battles." The team must also function within the philosophical framework in which the input of all members is valued and important, balancing the strong influence of core members while at the same time fostering participation and ownership by supportive and temporary team members as well. All of these issues must be dealt with smoothly and imperceptibly in order for certain internal goals to be achieved—that is, fostering the recovery of chemically dependent patients while addressing external pressures as well. These external pressures may come from government funding agencies, hospital administrations, insurance companies, professional reference groups, or even recovered volunteers. Each of these groups may have its own agenda for who should be doing what and how it should be done. The team must address itself to the needs and wants of these constituencies and must negotiate an acceptable modus operandi with these external influences on its functioning. Who is best suited for the job by skill, experience, and interest is a question the group must resolve by its deliberative decision-making process. The team must then support the decision and enthusiastically participate in its implementation with their expertise and energy.

A multidisciplinary team approach to the treatment of chemical dependence is a concept that extends well beyond the mere presence of different disciplines. All of the different disciplines must work together to accomplish the task of restorative rehabilitation, yet the way in which they work together is critically important as well. Team members must overcome their natural reference group loyalties and competitive biases from past training and experiences to work together in a cooperative fashion to facilitate the process of recovery. It is only by setting limits on individual "ownership" and entitlement that real teamwork can emerge. Such individuality, if left unchecked, probably is destructive to team morale and functioning in the long run. Ultimately, the group process or the "group conscience" (as AA puts it) will show that its wisdom is superior to that of any one individual, regardless of discipline, background, or experience.[6]

The Treatment Process

Contemporary treatment, whether provided on an inpatient or an outpatient basis, is rehabilitative, educational, corrective, and restorative for mind, body, and spirit. Treatment is based on an illness model with the goal of overcoming dependence on alcohol and drugs. The dependence is perceived as physiological, with profound effects that serve to perpetuate the acceleration of the disease process in a malignant and eventually fatal fashion. Treatment interrupts this malignant process, physically removes the offending chemical, alters the victim's psychology to promote self-understanding and to prevent relapse, fosters physical restoration and a return to overall health, and assists in the rebuilding of the psychosocial support system that has been damaged by the disease.

The Entry Phase

It is probably true to an extent that those who are dependent on alcohol and drugs enjoy the substances they use and find comfort, relief, narcosis, or euphoria in them. Genetic susceptibility probably plays a part in this powerful interaction between susceptible host and poisonous pathogen. The drug induces its own taking by controlling the victim's attitudes, thinking, and behavior in ways that foster and maintain access to the substance, which is viewed by the victim as evermore beneficial or needed. Outside positive influences are viewed as meddlesome, intrusive, and interfering and are resisted with anger, alibis, deceptions, and a host of other defense mechanisms. The sick process between host and pathogen continues until a crisis forces a reappraisal. The crisis may be an internal one as the person, in more lucid moments, perceives the gradual loss of control in the mounting psychosocial deterioration that ensues. Alternatively, the crisis may be an external one, brought about by concerned others—spouses, children, employers, licensing bodies, or others—who perceive either the intoxication, personality changes, or psychosocial neglect that occurs consequent to the unrelieved dependence. The crisis is most often externally produced, and at least initially, the victim is constructively coerced to seek help. Not atypically, the individual presents (or rather is presented) for an evaluation in an angry, defensive, noninsightful posture, surrounded by angry or tearful supporters. The treatment process begins with an assessment, typically a preliminary one, that obtains identifying data, a comprehensive history of the person's chemical exposure, and at least a cursory review of the biopsychosocial consequences of the substance dependence. Based on the extent and severity of the compulsive dependence and on the ability of the person to work effectively at treatment goals in a particular level of treatment intensity, a treatment plan is formulated. A particular level of care is recommended and decided on, and the victim, willingly or reluctantly, takes the first step in what is hoped will be a lifelong rehabilitative and recovery process. The treatment team may have at its disposal a wide array of levels of care to accommodate the various needs of those affected. These levels of care may include inpatient or intermediate-stage rehabilitation, partial hospitalization, primary intensive outpatient treatment, long-term residential, and long-term support groups. The clinician performing triage can choose one, several, or all of these modalities in devising an individualized treatment plan. All of them will ideally support the goal of abstinence and improvement of physical, emotional, social, and spiritual health.

Inpatient Treatment

Inpatient treatment, which had its roots in AA sobering-up houses in the late 1930s, took on a professional identity in hospital settings in the early 1950s. In a few such hospitals, such as St. Thomas Hospital in Akron, Ohio, St. Vincent Charity Hospital in Cleveland, Ohio, and Willmar State Hospital in Willmar, Minnesota, patients could be admitted to a special unit for detoxification and facilitation into AA for follow-up. Although the rest of the professional, medical, and psychiatric world remained hostile or skeptical about AA, these units embraced the principles of AA and afforded a hospitable milieu in which alcoholics could seek relief and AA members could carry their message. These units became more sophisticated with the passage of time, as the disease concept of alcoholism and drug dependence was progressively elaborated by Jellinek[7] and others. The subsequent elaborations included elucidation of the defense mechanisms of denial, rationalization, and projection of blame; the application of psychological modalities including group therapy and reality therapy in overcoming the resistances and defenses; and family counseling to overcome denial through interventions, to promote family healing, and to eliminate the disease and reinforcing aspects of family psychopathology. Because of the popularization and reputation of Hazelden as a pioneering institution in this regard, the widely used inpatient treatment format came to be known as the Minnesota model.[8] This model incorporated a unit-based concept or one based in a freestanding specialized facility that provided services to address the unique needs of alcoholics and chemically dependent people. These services included a medical examination, laboratory assessments, medications for detoxification, nursing supervision through the detoxification phase, and a high degree of exposure to intensive sobriety-oriented psychotherapy. Residents of such programs could be identified as patients, addicts, alcoholics, students, or even guests, and they typically remained sequestered in such units for 28 to 30 days, although in some places the length of stay was shorter, on the order of 2 weeks. There can be no doubt that such Minnesota model programs helped innumerable people in obtaining a detoxification at the hands of experts and in overcoming their alcoholic resistances so that they became lifelong practicing members of AA. These inpatient units and residential treatment settings spread rapidly because of their initial successes and because of a relatively favorable insurance reimbursement climate that paid for the treatment of alcoholism in such facilities. Eventually, however, such programs came under mounting criticism for inadequate outcome data, relatively high cost (compared with outpatient treatment), and their spiritual basis in the philosophy of AA. As a result of these forces, inpatient treatment on a 30-day Minnesota model has become less the norm. The therapeutic relationship between patients, providers, and insurers has broadened to include fourth parties, insurance intermediaries who manage chemical dependence treatment with an emphasis on assigning an appropriate level of care based on medical necessity and severity. This fourth-party inroad has unquestionably altered the way inpatient chemical dependence treatment is provided in the vast majority of cases. Twenty-eight-day inpatient-based treatment is increasingly rare, except in cases in which self-payment is an option. At this time, inpatient facilities have had to modify their goals owing to these financial and political realities. The main focus at present for inpatient units is stabilization—medical and psychological—and preparation for rehabilitation on an outpatient basis. The large inpatient facilities, often with 100 beds or more, are increasingly being shaped into small crisis stabilization units. Simply put, alcoholism treatment until recently was synonymous with a 30-day inpatient Minnesota model, which was the exclusive treatment. The next step was self-help in AA or a similar group. At present, the inpatient treatment is but *part* of the treatment, that being the initial stabilization phase, with fairly rapid movement to outpatient status or to an inexpensive halfway house, and treatment continues with multiple levels, often in multiple settings.

What has emerged is therefore a shortened and condensed version of the Minnesota model of treatment, if it is provided at all. The fourth-party managed-care insurers often insist that an admission can be authorized only if a patient meets certain criteria. Such criteria vary from company to company and may include medical parameters such as blood pressure exceeding 150/100, pulse greater than 120, or other medical indicators such as internal bleeding or jaundice. Alternative criteria might include psychiatric risks such as stated suicidal ideation with a plan, drug-induced psychosis, or mental status changes consistent with the likelihood of severe withdrawal reaction (hallucinosis, confusion, agitation). Some companies have additional criteria such as a necessity for prior outpatient treatment attempt and failure (perhaps repeatedly) or no evidence of chronicity or recidivism.

Detoxification and Medical Stabilization

The process of detoxification could be said to involve two component parts, both of which are of equal importance in the treatment process. The first component—ostensibly the more physiological of the two—involves assessment and treatment of the acute withdrawal symptoms. Because of the phenomenon of physiological tolerance, a chemically dependent person becomes physiologically "normal" only with repeated and progressively larger amounts of the addicting substance. The body becomes habituated and physiologically dependent on the external supply of mood-altering substance to effect artificially induced relaxation, euphoria, stimulation, or narcosis. While subjectively enjoying or benefitting from these effects, the addict's body is, at the same time, gearing up metabolic enzymes and neurological alterations that tend to neutralize the effects of the external substance. Thus, the subject needs more and more of the addicting substance to effect the desired change. As tolerance becomes even more pronounced over time, the subject at first uses the substance for euphoria, then to feel normal, and finally to avoid withdrawal symptoms. The amounts of substance used can be truly astounding, especially in cases of opiates, barbiturates, and alcohol. Once this stage of advanced tolerance has set in, the person is physiologically "hooked" and experiences the opposite of the drug's beneficial effect in the withdrawal state. The withdrawal state is perceived by the subject as irritating or even excruciating. Subjective suffering can occur on a broad continuum from mild to extreme, with both psychological and physiological distress. Symptoms depend on the drug or substance involved but generally include nervous system rebound overstimulation, anxiety, diaphoresis, elevations of pulse and blood pressure, and a sense of acute physiological distress. Other symptoms, such as nausea, vomiting, and seizures, may occur depending on the offending drug. If acute subjective suffering is extreme, patients can not endure the pain and return to the temporary comfort of the substance, frequently by leaving treatment abruptly or against medical advice, by suffering a relapse or worse, by never achieving complete sobriety.

Detoxification then involves supplanting the addictive substance in the subject, providing enough substitute medication so that physiological signs and symptoms of withdrawal are prevented and so that the subjective sense of suffering is reduced. Long-acting benzodiazepines are frequently used for alcohol and minor tranquilizer dependence, methadone or clonidine is frequently used for opiate dependence, and barbiturate dependence is usually treated with a drug of the same chemical family. In brief, adequate substitute medication is provided so that withdrawal symptoms are prevented or resolved and so that an external source of control over the addictive substance is established (i.e., the hospital staff is in control of administering the drug). Once the initial dose is established, a regimen that tapers off the medication can be implemented. The goal and desired endpoint is achievement and maintenance of a drug-free state. The attainment of this drug-free state may occur quickly—even immediately—in some individuals but may be achieved only slowly and painfully in others. The amount, frequency, pharmaceutical quality of the addictive drug, and individual metabolic factors, probably genetically determined, cause wide variability in the course of withdrawal and detoxification.

The age of the subject and state of overall medical debilitation also are significant determining factors in severity.

Because of the wide range of subject withdrawal reactions, ranging from nonexistent to life threatening, detoxification is frequently initiated with medical or nursing assessment, with the focus on the presence or absence of withdrawal symptoms. If physiological or psychological symptoms are present, ongoing monitoring is usually provided, and inpatient treatment settings are frequently used for this level of detoxification treatment. Once stabilization of vital signs, withdrawal symptoms, and subjective suffering are achieved, the process of rehabilitation treatment can begin.

The second component of the detoxification process is the more psychological one. It involves the suffering individual's subjective sense of wanting or craving the drug. This drug craving is probably not primarily psychological at all but rather is most likely a behavioral-cognitive expression of the physiologically induced withdrawal reaction. Physical withdrawal symptoms may or may not be present, and it is probably a mistake to view psychological craving or drug hunger as evidence of lower acuity in the withdrawal reaction. Both physical and psychological effects are equally debilitating, and both can undermine and frustrate the attainment of long-term sobriety if unattended. Cravings tend to be strongest with stimulants such as cocaine and amphetamine and with opiates. Detoxification must address this psychological component as well. The symptoms of craving typically abate rapidly with abstinence from the addicting drug. Time is generally on the side of the treatment team; the longer a person is in an abstinent environment, the better the reduction of craving symptoms. The endpoint on this process is not necessarily as clear as that which occurs with the resolution of physical symptoms, however. The person may consciously feel that the craving has abated, but it may still remain at a level of marginal awareness. Thus, treatment involves isolation of the individual from the offending drug, it is hoped for a long enough period to allow lessening of the craving and compulsion to use. The staff is often in a better position to judge this endpoint than is the patient, and subjective psychological signs such as the restoration of calm, the resolution of anger and irritability, and the establishment of an attitude of cooperation often signal stabilization. If discharge is effected too quickly, before this state of emotional equanimity is reached, a relapse to substance-induced narcosis is more likely.

The withdrawal process then is highly variable and is to a certain extent unpredictable. If definite symptoms (physical or psychological) are present, the wisest course is also the safest—inpatient treatment with medication and supervision. Treatment must of necessity be individualized, and universally applied treatment plans should be avoided, whether they provide too much or too little treatment.

Medical stabilization usually occurs in parallel with the detoxification process. An assessment of physical and medical history, as well as of current signs and symptoms, should be a part of every chemical dependence intake assessment. An updated medical examination, with blood and urine testing, electrocardiogram, and chest radiograph are invaluable in moderate to advanced cases. Risk of human immunodeficiency virus infection should be assessed and testing performed if appropriate. The presence of medical comorbidity should always be kept in mind, because chemically dependent individuals are susceptible to diverse medical ailments. Virtually any organ system can be affected, and the variety of possible medical comorbidity is too broad to be discussed here. Nonetheless, physicians have an important role in the treatment process by attending to the physical complications of the addiction and by overseeing the intensive treatment and restoration of the physical aspect of these patients. Sickness of the body is indeed part of the sickness of the mind that exists in addictive disease. Simplistically stated, one cannot think properly if the mind (and brain) are sick. Physical stabilization is the platform on which subsequent aspects of cognitive, emotional, behavioral, social, and spiritual restoration are built. The process of rehabilitation and recovery can now begin.

Treatment of Pathological Mental State

An actively addicted person is not in a normal mental or emotional state, nor is the person merely affected by using too much of the offending substance. Instead, the development of tolerance in addiction generally involves profound alterations in the person's thinking, attitudes, emotions, and behavior, generally ways that reinforce and allow access to the offending drug. Negative emotions are preponderant—anger, resentment, guilt, shame, or, alternatively, grandiosity. These negative emotional states are powerful, long-lasting phenomena that provide the emotional justifications for continued drug use. Anger and resentment foster the drug use through inherent spitefulness and entitlement, as well as, more indirectly, by cutting off attempts by others to control the substance use. The user feels no obligation to comply with those who are the hated objects of his or her anger, and those around the user become progressively more helpless, isolated, and impotent in their attempts to provide external controls against the addict's substance use. In fact, their attempts to control only seem to inflame the alcoholic or addict all the more, with the end result of more harmful substance use. Guilt and shame produce a similar result in the acceleration of refuge in the offending chemical. Shame and guilt promote isolation from potentially helpful interveners. The progressive self-loathing fosters an attitude of hopelessness and despair that frustrates the possibility of constructive change. The addictive process continues unabated. Others are given to grandiosity and euphoria, emotions that provide a false and exaggerated sense of self-confidence and self-validation. The opinions and perspectives of others are discounted and scorned. Entitlement soon follows: "I am the greatest, I am entitled to whatever I want." Because craving for the offending drug is the preeminent biological and psychological desire, nothing or no one is allowed to interfere with the person's entitlement to his or her addiction. These pathological mood states serve to perpetuate access to the drug, by promoting a sense of personal entitlement and by limiting the power of outside influences. These pathological states must be attacked vigorously, both initially and subsequently on a long-term basis in the treatment process. They become deeply ingrained by the disease process and are difficult to resolve in treatment. Their persistence is an ominous sign and may indicate that the person has not totally accepted the need for sobriety, or it may indicate a residual, unresolved emotional stumbling block that may continue to frustrate recovery.

These pathological mood states are buttressed by and exist hand in hand with pathological cognitive or thinking states. Better known as *defense mechanisms,* these patterns of cognition reinforce the negative emotions that perpetuate the drinking and offer the avenue for pathological emotional expression. The sick emotions give rise to the sick thinking, and vice versa. An addict's thinking is itself sick. Denial blocks the full appreciation of the extent and severity of the addiction. Control over the substances is not realized, and the gravity of the addictive consequences is denied partially or totally. Chemical excess is seen by the afflicted person as necessary and good, because of exaggerated rationalization in which incongruous and illogical alibis and excuses are offered. Projection of blame, taken to an extreme, reinforces a person's self-justification while mobilizing anger and resentment outwardly. The addictive behaviors are propagated, including drug overuse, concealment, lying, alibiing, and unresponsiveness to direction. Beneath the irritability and anger may lurk the reality of mental confusion, stemming from toxic effects on the brain. Thinking may be dull, judgments may be illogical, and behaviors may be primitive and instinctual. Apathy and mental dullness are eventually evident, with shrinkage of intellectual interest and growing social isolation. The person's behavior may become hermitlike, with the exception of forays to obtain additional substance. The social system and the affected person part company mutually out of embarrassment, frustration, and drug-induced alienation. Job, family, and community fall away, and the alcoholic or addict can have unlimited access to the chemical without outside censorship, responsibilities, or interferences. With nothing to slow it down, the addictive process rapidly accelerates, and the fulminant toxicity and catastrophic consequences will endanger or end the addict's life.

Thus, these two important citadels of pathology—emotional and cognition—are the focal points for the early phase of treatment. Emotions are powerful and defenses are well entrenched at the beginning. Attempts to intervene are perceived as blaming or attacking and are therefore usually futile. For this reason, the treatment process generally begins with nonjudgmental education about the disease process. Movies, lecture sessions, and sharing sessions from recovering addicts instruct patients about the nature of the addictive process and its effects on the mind and body. Education is nonpejorative and therefore nonblaming. However, learning can only occur in the presence of an open and receptive mind, free of anger, defensiveness, and negative emotions. Because this negative state characterizes most addicts at the beginning of treatment, the defensive stance must be softened, especially in severe cases, by the presence of supportive, caring, nonjudgmental people who are sincerely concerned for the best interest of the patient. Milieu therapy can provide the right balance of objective detachment and loving support that addicts require. Once defensive resistances are down, the learning process can begin. Most people know intuitively that alcohol and drugs can be harmful. The disease process itself, however, blocks the realization that the process is actually happening to them and that they are caught in a downward spiral, out of control. The consequences of addiction are seen by an addict as random misfortunes or temporary problems rather than as a result of a fulminant and ever progressive destructive disease process. The education aspect of treatment allows self-recognition and self-diagnosis. Treatment professionals call this all-important phase *step-one work*, based on the first step of the 12 steps of AA.[5] This step focuses on the recognition and acceptance of powerlessness and unmanageability over alcohol and mood-altering drugs. The importance of this step cannot be over-emphasized. The degree and quality of work on this step determine, to an enormous extent, the subsequent treatment course and the outcome of the therapy. Those who "work a good first step" generally have a much smoother progression through the remainder of treatment, which generally adds only qualitatively to a person's recovery.

Many inpatient programs, based on a Minnesota model, emphasize the first five steps of AA.[5] These steps emphasize making a decision to accept outside help, turning one's life over to outside help (including a spiritual higher power), and taking and sharing a moral inventory. Minnesota model programs operate to facilitate this process in every way possible. A number of modalities are used to accomplish this rehabilitative work. Group therapy with other addicted peers, facilitated by at least one and perhaps more rehabilitation professionals, is used to foster identification with and acceptance of the reality of the disease process, the need for corrective action, and the strong endorsement of program principles. Because all the peers are facing the same situation, they have a high level of mutual acceptance and trust, and entrenched defenses can be confronted and, it is hoped, set aside. Group inventory taking, done in the form of inventory sharing or other forms of self-disclosure such as shared biographies, often reveals individual strengths and weaknesses, documents the destructive disease process, and allows access to helpful correction and praise. The result is a corrective emotional experience in which addicts recognize their own powerlessness over the drug, accept the need for ongoing help from this supportive treatment network, and resolve to continue on a path toward rebuilding a new, healthier identity. Once this happy state is achieved, addicts are ready to move on to the next (less intensive) level of care.

Treatment plans are individualized and take into account strengths, weaknesses, and psychosocial realities in building a long-term sobriety program. In the inpatient milieu, great attention is given to detail in altering old (addictive) ways. The staff works incessantly to bring out the patient's better self, with constant emphasis on good grooming, manners, language, attitude, and conduct. A sound preaddictive personality is often discovered, and old strengths and talents, long buried by addictive neglect, are allowed to flourish anew. Patients often rediscover themselves as attractive and competent individuals without the distorting influences of drugs. In other cases, adaptive social skills have never been developed because of the early onset of the disease process, and rehabilitation must involve teaching new social skills and behaviors. Nonetheless, there is a sense of something dramatic happening— the birth or rebirth of a new person. A sense of personal specialness is reinforced by encouraging some reverence for this rebirth process as a unique, remarkable, and almost mystical experience. Patients often feel physically, emotionally, and spiritually transformed.

This transformation is sustained by progression to the aftercare phase of the program, with its emphasis on outpatient group support in the hospital and the community. Twelve-step work (volunteering) is encouraged after discharge, as alumni (with stable sobriety) take newcomers to community AA meetings or to hospital-sponsored self-help groups.[9] Annual reunions bring hundreds of alumni and their family members together with staff to celebrate recovery. The reinforcing potential of these reunions is tremendous. Many patients look to these reunions as milestones in recovery, often staying sober for the next one. These celebrations, volunteer activities, and hospital-based self-help groups give patients a sense of specialness and pride in their recovery.

Family therapy is an important aspect of Minnesota model treatment. Family members of an addict typically are other victims of the disease and are also unwitting accomplices. Family members are victimized by an addict's self-absorption, entitlement, guilt, rage, and erratic behavior. They are frequently the objects of extreme emotional neglect or physical abuse. Their frustration and rage are understandable, especially in view of the addict's persistent denial that such events ever occurred or had any significance.

The family itself plays a part in the propagation of the illness through the family members' own reactions to the addict. Their rage and anger foster in the addict more defensiveness, withdrawal, and resentment or perhaps shame and guilt, with the resultant worsening of negative emotions and with the progression of more substance use. The family members may also be caught up in their own denial and rationalization mechanisms, accepting the addict's alibis and excuses or minimizing the extent and severity of the addictive disease process. They often resist or sabotage the eventual prescription—the need for permanent abstinence and for ongoing support from the treatment network. These lifestyle changes may be resisted out of habit, stigma, misunderstanding, ignorance, or denial. The persistence of these faulty beliefs can eventually erode an alcoholic's resolve and can precipitate relapses. The family members are typically exposed to educational videos, staff discussions, and other family members who have been through the recovery process. In a very real way, they must recover also from their own misconceptions, defenses, and rationalizations. The lifestyle changes that are inherent in a continued recovery program must be supported by them in a wholehearted, grateful, and enthusiastic way. Treatment programs exert strong efforts by staff and volunteers to accomplish this transformation.

This intensive process, as described earlier, has historically been carried out in inpatient hospital units or residential isolated settings for physical stabilization, detoxification, personality transformation, strength, social and family supports, and spiritual cleansing and renewal. The environment is almost hermetically sealed, and the transformation process is aggressively fostered around the clock while old addictive patterns are discouraged and corrected. It is a total immersion form of treatment, and few outside distractions are tolerated. Many programs prohibit newspapers, magazines, or television. Contacts with the outside are usually limited severely.

The power and effectiveness of this treatment approach are impressive. Patients relinquish their well-entrenched addictive defenses, learn the program steps, and conform to the recommended treatment plan for abstinence and continued involvement in a support network, usually AA. Chemical dependence professionals have a high level of confidence in this form of therapy; they have seen its power and know it works. The relatively favorable insurance reimbursement climate, which was present during the 1980s, allowed for the rapid duplication of this treatment method in literally thousands of hospitals and freestanding facilities. The explosion of costs led to a harsh regulatory backlash—the development of managed care companies, whose mission has been to reduce drastically these expenditures. What has emerged is an environment in which patients are, practically speaking, limited to outpatient alternative programming for their chemical-dependence treatment. Hospitalization and residential treatment are used far less frequently at present, and inpatient lengths of stay have dropped precipitously from 28 days to a few days, if hospitalization is used at all. Treatment providers have scrambled to adjust to these new fiscal constraints and have tried to adapt the Minnesota model of treatment to an outpatient or less costly format. Patients now frequently move through a system of levels of care matching their levels of severity or impairment. Also, instead of lengthy hospitalizations, stepdown treatment is frequently provided in long-term halfway houses or three-quarter-way house settings, often for 1 to 12 months or longer. Halfway houses severely limit the amount of outside activity that residents may have, essentially providing a long-term extension of Minnesota model treatment in an inexpensive, shared living environment. Three-quarter-way houses typically offer more freedom, perhaps with opportunities to find outside work, and often provide little or no staff supervision. Both types of facilities emphasize continued abstinence and vigorous involvement in AA. The cost for such facilities, because of the minimal level of staffing and medical sophistication, is very low. Many hospital-based programs are now referring patients after inpatient discharge to such long-term residential facilities for stabilization, for further work on defenses, and for strengthening of treatment principles and recovery behavior.

Outpatient Treatment

Outpatient care may take place as aftercare (after inpatient or residential) or as entry level treatment, complete with detoxification and rehabilitation therapy. Outpatient treatment typically begins with a thorough assessment of medical and detoxification needs. Patients with severe psychiatric comorbidity, severe withdrawal reactions, or severe medical complications are referred for inpatient care. Patients who previously failed structured outpatient treatments are likewise often referred for inpatient therapy.

Evening treatment was designed with employed drug and alcohol addicts in mind. Evening treatment programs are set up to meet their needs for a fairly intensive treatment experience without the disruption of work and personal life from inpatient treatment. According to Cocores,[10] evening program candidates usually are experiencing mild difficulties at work as a result of drug and alcohol addiction. Marital problems, minor legal incidents, and minor psychiatric consequences are common to this group of patients. Cocores describes a common evening intensive program model as follows: Patients attend two group therapy sessions from 6:30 to 10:00 PM each Monday, Tuesday, Thursday, and Friday evening for 6 to 8 weeks. Biweekly, random, supervised, comprehensive urine drug screens are obtained during their first two phases of treatment. Patients are encouraged to attend the self-help meeting on Wednesday evening, Saturday, and Sunday. Patients then attend the evening program twice each week for an additional 2 weeks (phase 2). A patient in phase 3 attends one session per week for about 9 months. Phase 3 reinforces relapse prevention, healthier day-to-day activities, and personal growth with respect to improved communication skills and self-improvement of character defects. Most patients are well integrated into self-help groups and have self-help sponsors during phase 3 of treatment.[10]

Day treatment, or partial hospitalization, is a lower-cost outpatient treatment alternative to inpatient stay. Collins and colleagues[11] described a daycare program in which patients attend a full day of rehabilitation meetings from 9:30 AM to 5:00 PM Monday through Friday. This format provided a close approximation of Minnesota model treatment with its education, group therapy, disease concept emphasis, and incorporation of AA philosophy. Family therapy is also provided in this model. As described by Collins and associates,[11] patients attended a total of 22 sessions per week while in the daycare program. Patients typically left the hospital at 5:00 PM to return home and to attend neighborhood AA meetings, with four AA meetings per week being the minimum required. The researchers also noted a transition to a short-term aftercare phase following 2 weeks of intensive daycare. This aftercare phase consisted of 12 weekly 2-hour sessions with a combined educational and discussion format. Topics focused on maintenance of sobriety issues, such as avoidance of old drinking friends, taking things a day at a time, attendance at AA, or returning to work. Attendance at AA was heavily emphasized for long-term maintenance of sobriety. Al-Anon and Ala-Teen were also strongly encouraged for family members.

Criteria for admission to daycare and intensive outpatient programs, according to Collins, were different from those for inpatients. Daycare patients must be able to remain abstinent without the need for detoxification and without the structure of 24-hour staff supervision. They must have no acute or impending medical crisis and no serious withdrawal complications. Daycare is regarded as less protective treatment, thereby requiring greater patient motivation, transportation capability, and ability to remain abstinent. Patients in daycare modalities typically are transitioning from being inpatient, have financial constraints, are unable to leave work, or are unable to provide childcare during a lengthy hospitalization. The cost of such intensive outpatient programs is substantially less than (generally about half the cost of) inpatient programs. Collins and co-workers noted, in a 7-month retrospective follow-up study, that improvement and a satisfactory level of sobriety were obtained in 41.6% of patients. The dropout rate, however, for daycare program patients totaled 23%, almost double that for inpatients (14%). It remains to be seen whether the lower cost of care for such intensive outpatient and day treatment services is only achieved with a tradeoff in higher rates of dropout and relapse.[11]

Outpatient detoxification has been similarly troublesome. Stinnett described the attempted outpatient treatment of alcohol withdrawal syndrome in 116 patients; 50% were successfully treated, 20% dropped out, and 30% required hospitalization. Stinnett concluded that outpatient treatment for the alcohol withdrawal syndrome was effective for certain alcoholics.[12] Whitfield and colleagues described treatment of 1114 consecutive alcoholic patients in outpatient detoxification centers. Ninety of these patients were subsequently sent to hospital emergency departments for further examination, and 28 were admitted to the hospital. Of the 1024 patients who remained as outpatients, one developed delirium tremens and was hospitalized, 12 had one or more seizures, 6 were hospitalized for two or more seizures, and 38 had hallucinosis but were managed as outpatients. These facilities did not rely on psychoactive drugs or on the presence of nurses or physicians and demonstrated that a large number of select alcoholics

(but not all) could be detoxified in this way, at a very low cost, with hospital and emergency room backup.[13]

These reports demonstrate that although outpatient detoxification can be an acceptable modality for alcoholics, there is a group of patients for whom it is unsuitable and for whom hospitalization is necessary. The level of risk that is acceptable will probably remain a matter of debate and controversy between cost-driven payors and safety-seeking providers.

Aftercare outpatient therapy, usually cognitive and behavioral in nature, aimed at prevention of relapse, has become popular with the emphasis on outpatient modalities. The effectiveness of such outpatient aftercare remains a matter of some debate, however, Pittman and Tate noted a modest improvement in outcome if aftercare was provided on a consistent basis.[14] On the other hand, Armor and colleagues, evaluating 44 alcoholism treatment centers funded by the National Institute on Alcohol Abuse and Alcoholism, found no difference in remission rates of patients receiving inpatient care alone and patients receiving outpatient aftercare, in addition to inpatient care.[15] These researchers concluded that "the prognosis for remission depends more on a client's alcoholic and social conditions at entry to treatment than on any particular treatment characteristics, including amount."[15] Vannicelli, in a complex analysis of aftercare outcomes, noted that it is possible that aftercare has an impact only when it follows an intensive inpatient program and only when caregivers are those who provided the inpatient care. In noting a relatively high success rate in 6 months (81%), she identifies three possible critical elements—intensive inpatient care, long-term aftercare, and well-developed links between the two.[16]

Relapse prevention programs, as part of aftercare, are a newer phenomenon. These are frequently based on a social learning model and emphasize self-control and enhancement of coping skills. In addition, individuals are encouraged to avoid chancy or high-risk situations that could endanger sobriety. Although an association between aftercare attendance and good outcome is clear, it is not entirely clear whether the aftercare support drives the outcome or whether alcoholics with a favorable prognosis continued to be involved in aftercare. It may be that both conditions are operative, because Collins and associates noted that patients who participate in more treatment modalities fare better than those who participate in fewer.[17]

Summary

Despite substantial changes in the healthcare system, the essentials of treatment have not changed drastically. The formulation of a dynamic, adaptable team, capable of providing the treatment in a knowledgeable and caring way and of impacting the philosophy of abstinence-based recovery through word and deed, is the essential starting point. The 12 steps, 12 traditions, and experienced word of AA provide the unifying philosophy that enables staff members, patients, and volunteers to overcome individual differences and bind together into a cohesive, effective team—one in which the whole is greater than the sum of its parts.

The methodolical parameters of treatment continue to change—perhaps more rapidly than in any other branch of the healing arts—as 28-day inpatient residential universal treatment gives way to treatment matched to illness severity in time, amount, and cost. Treatment centers are evolving into treatment systems, aimed at providing a wide range of services from intensive inpatient detoxification in hospitals to ambulatory low-intensity counseling programs. Yet the essentials of treatment remain the source—the process of healing by carrying the message of help and hope for suffering alcoholics through the disease concept and through the accumulated experience of untold thousands of recovering people and professionals who have left such a legacy of wisdom to guide us in our efforts.

REFERENCES

1. Alcoholics Anonymous: Alcoholics Anonymous Comes of Age. New York, Alcoholics Anonymous Publishing, 1957.
2. Fox R: A Multi-disciplinary approach to the treatment of alcoholism. Int J Psychiatry 1:34–44, 1968.
3. Brotman R: Total treatment. Int J Psychiatry 1:45–46, 1968.
4. Spratley TA: The practical business of treatment—1. A Multi-disciplinary and team approach. Br J Addict 84(3):259–266, 1989.
5. Alcoholics Anonymous: Twelve Steps and Twelve Traditions. New York, Alcoholics Anonymous World Services, 1953.
6. Collins GB, Weiss K, Cozzens DT, et al: A multidisciplinary team approach to the treatment of drug and alcohol addiction. In Miller NS (ed): Comprehensive Handbook of Drug and Alcohol Addiction. New York, Marcel-Dekker, 1991, pp 981–999.
7. Jellinek EM: The Disease Concept of Alcoholism. New Haven, College and University Press, 1960.
8. Cook CH: The Minnesota Model in the management of drug and alcohol dependency: Miracle, method, or myth? Part II: Evidence and conclusions. Br J Addict 83:735–748, 1988.
9. Collins GB, Janesz JW, Byerly-Thrope J, Colli J: Hospital sponsored transitional chemical dependency self-help groups. Hosp Community Psychiatry 36:1315–1317, 1985.
10. Cocores J: Outpatient treatment of drug and alcohol addiction. In Miller NS (ed): Comprehensive Handbook of Drug and Alcohol Addiction. New York, Marcel Dekker, 1991, pp 1213–1222.
11. Collins GB, Watson EW, Zrimec GL: A hospital day care program for alcoholics. Gen Hosp Psychiatry 2:20–22, 1980.
12. Stinnett JL: Outpatient detoxification of the alcoholic. Int J Addict 17(6):1031–1046, 1982.
13. Whitfield CL, Thompson G, Lamb A, et al: Detoxification of 1,024 alcoholic patients without psychoactive drugs. JAMA 239(14):1409–1410, 1978.
14. Pittman DJ, Tate RL: A comparison of two treatment programs for alcoholics. Q J Stud Alcohol 30:888–899, 1969.
15. Armor DJ, Polich JM, Stambul HB: Alcoholism and Treatment. Prepared for the National Institute on Alcohol Abuse and Alcoholism. Santa Monica, CA, Rand Corp, 1976.
16. Vannicelli M: Impact of aftercare in the treatment of alcoholics: A cross-lagged panel analysis. J Stud Alcohol 39(11):1875–1886, 1978.
17. Collins GB, Janesz JW, Byerly-Thrope J, et al: The Cleveland Clinic Alcohol Rehabilitation Program: A treatment outcome study. Cleve Clin Q 52:245–251, 1985.

Emerging Concepts of Alcoholism Treatment: Challenges and Controversies

Gregory B. Collins, MD

A number of signals indicate that the alcoholism treatment industry has reached maturity, as all industries eventually do. After the booming expansion of the 1970s and 1980s, when the industry grew from a small handful of facilities to more than 3000 centers nationwide, stabilization and even contraction seem to have occurred, based on very tight reins on reimbursement for care. This tightening no doubt came about as a result of the proliferation of programs, each one of which added cost to the payout side of the insurers' ledger sheets. Rapid escalation of this accumulated cost has forced a harsh retrenchment and consolidation as insurers have switched from indemnity-based (open-ended) payment methods to managed care to control and limit the flow of payout dollars. The newly imposed limits on payout were also based on challenges to fundamental assumptions long held dear by the individuals in the treatment industry. The payors began asking hard questions, seeking data to justify the large payouts for treatment, or seeking ways to reduce cost, sometimes dramatically. These challenges, however nettlesome to the tradition-bound world of Minnesota model treatment, will be the major dynamics in the determination of the future

directions—even the very survival of the alcoholism treatment industry for the rest of the twentieth century. These challenges range from the most basic, such as, What is effective treatment? and Does treatment work? to more subtle issues, such as, Can we compare inpatient and outpatient treatment results? and How important is aftercare? Overall, new emphasis is placed on empiricism—looking for outcome data—rather than on faith or even humanitarianism, to justify the types of treatment that will be available for patients in the future. Let us now examine these challenges and controversies with an eye toward balancing efficacy of treatment and reasonableness of cost.

What Is Effective Treatment of Alcoholism?

Contemporary treatment is a process that fosters a return to physical health initially, generally with a medically supervised detoxification regimen, with or without medications. Hospital-based settings frequently use benzodiazepines for withdrawal management, and comprehensive physical examinations and laboratory studies help in the diagnosis and treatment of alcohol-related medical conditions such as seizures, hepatitis, anemia, malnutrition, gastritis, neuropathies, and many others. Physicians and nurses generally assess and treat this phase of the condition, which may range in severity from benign to catastrophic. As a result, detoxification may be brief or fairly prolonged, lasting mere minutes to weeks, depending on severity. Most inpatient settings have a routine 1- to 3-day detoxification period, perhaps in a specialized location, under close medical-nursing supervision. Once medical stabilization and withdrawal from alcohol, other drugs of abuse, and detoxification medications are achieved, an alcoholic progresses to a phase of psychological-cognitive-behavioral rehabilitation, aimed at strengthening motivation for abstinence through continued treatment in Alcoholics Anonymous (AA). Because treatment incorporates a broad range of goals and methods owing to the complexities presented by alcoholics, a multidisciplinary approach to treatment is widely used.[1] The rehabilitation phase assists in overcoming the disease process with its characteristic denial, minimization, and rationalization. Well-developed staff skills are required in individual and group therapy to change or influence the attitudes and behaviors of such patients. Because brain damage is a frequent concomitant of substance addiction, assessment skills are needed, using psychological testing and other forms of psychiatric/psychological evaluation. Social stabilization and restructuring are very important, because patients who have a severely damaged social support system are at a great disadvantage in developing a new, recovery-oriented support system after leaving the treatment center.

Finally spiritual skills are developed, based on the AA 12-step program to promote aspects of healthy spirituality, placing a strong emphasis on examination of spiritual deficits and needs while enhancing a process of spiritual revitalization.

These widely divergent skills that are needed for treatment of the many facets of the addictive disease process illustrate why it is so important for patients to be treated not by one individual but by a multidisciplinary team in order to ensure the best chance of recovery.[1] Mann[2] describes the treatment process as based on the following principles: (1) Treatment does not "cure" the disease—the expectation is that by instituting an achievable method of abstinence, the disease will be put into remission. (2) All therapeutic efforts are directed at help-ing patients reach a level of motivation that will enable them to commit to this abstinence program. (3) An educational program is developed to assist patients in becoming familiar with the addictive process; to provide insight into compulsive behaviors, medical complications, and emotional aspects; and to promote maintenance of physical, mental, and spiritual health. (4) A patient's family and other significant persons are included in the therapeutic process, with the understanding that recovery does not occur in a vacuum but rather in interpersonal relationships. (5) Patients are indoctrinated into the AA program and instructed about the content and application of the 12 steps of the program. (6) Group and individual therapy is directed at self-understanding and acceptance, with emphasis on how alcohol or drugs has affected patients' lives. (7) Mandatory in treatment is participation in a longitudinal support and follow-up program based on the belief that as in the management of all chronic disease processes, maintenance is critically important to the ultimate outcome of any therapy. This follow-up usually consists of ongoing support provided by the treatment facility as well as participation in community self-help groups such as AA, Narcotics Anonymous, Opiates Anonymous, and so forth.

Mann also notes that the therapy is based around these basic therapeutic goals for patients:

To gain insight into the extent and consequences in their lives of their alcohol and drug use

To become aware of the defense mechanisms used to facilitate their continued alcohol and drug use

To recognize and admit to themselves that they indeed are alcoholic and addicted to drugs

To recognize the extent of their emotional and spiritual impairment

To examine their relationships and see how they have been adversely affected by their use of alcohol and drugs

To develop strategies that will prevent them from returning to the use of alcohol and drugs in the future[2]

Treatment then involves multifaceted goals related to healing in physical, emotional, cognitive, attitudinal, psychosocial, and spiritual parameters. These aims are fostered despite ignorance, stigma, resistance, and support system pathologies, including enabling, rescuing, and other forms of therapeutic sabotage. In many ways, treatment involves a rebirth or remaking of an individual in a very sudden yet profound way, as an individual undergoes a dramatic transformation from a sick, self-destructive pariah to a dramatically revitalized, valuable, contributing member of society. It is no wonder that with their difficulties, complexities, and lofty goals, treatment professionals have opted for specialized units in which to work their miracles in the settings most conducive to this process. Historically, these settings have been hospital inpatient units or freestanding inpatient residential settings.

To What Extent Is Inpatient Treatment Needed?

The explosive growth of inpatient units and residential settings for the treatment of alcoholism gives eloquent testimony to the attractiveness of this method of treatment. Treatment professionals themselves argue that inpatient care provides a safe and secure environment, under close medical-nursing supervision, with around-the-clock psychotherapy through didactic sessions, group therapy, and positive peer pressure. A vigorous introduction to the principles of AA is virtually always a significant component to the treatment. Inpatient care allows a patient's total immersion in the recovering milieu, the best way to overcome the well-entrenched denial system of an alcoholic. The impact of this inpatient experience is generally profound. Many patients report their inpatient stay to be among the most powerful and lasting emotional experiences of their lives.

Nonetheless, inpatient treatment is not without its controversial aspects. Critics would argue that there are few data to show that inpatient treatment produces consistently better outcomes and would argue that there is risk of overdiagnosis and overtreatment and that the trend toward hospital-based care is a reflection of better insurance reimbursement than is available for outpatient treatment. The rhetoric on both sides of the inpatient/outpatient treatment issue can be vehement, and a rational analysis is difficult to achieve.

Moore, in an excellent review of the subject of hospitalization, notes that "a paradox has gradually emerged . . . we used to plead, argue, and use diagnostic subterfuges to gain hospital admission for alcoholic patients. All major medical and hospital associations gave at least formal support to this effort. Then the public demanded that hospitals do their duty, and health insurance coverage for alcoholism (usually covered under psychiatric benefits) im-

proved. On occasion, local hospital empire building has resulted in an excess of beds. With financial security, the alcoholic patient has become popular. We have arrived, but only to discover that we may have oversold ourselves."[3]

"Today we are seriously questioning the proper use of the health dollar in admitting alcoholic patients to acute hospitals. New alternative resources and treatment systems may be as effective and much less costly. As so often happens, rather than a careful consideration of where the acute hospital fits in, there is a growing wave of anti-hospital feeling that, if not properly considered, may shove the pendulum too far back again."[3]

In a meta-analysis of empirical studies supporting the efficacy of specific techniques and practices in the inpatient treatment of alcoholism, Adelman and Weiss noted several findings that were associated with positive outcome: treatment programs that accept and encourage "constructive coercion" by referring parties, such as employers; short waiting lists and rapid flexibility to accommodate new referrals; group intake interviews; group-oriented milieu with group peer support; and counselors with high interpersonal skills. Additionally, they noted favorable outcome characteristics in programs that featured routinely performed medical assessments and used appropriate medications for detoxification. Involvement of patients' employers in the hospitalization also had a positive effect on treatment outcome, suggesting that vocational assessment, liaison, and vocational rehabilitation were of significant value. Several studies in their review supported the finding that alcohol treatment programs that include disulfiram (Antabuse) in their therapeutic armamentarium may have advantages over programs that do not. AA involvement, group therapy involvement, and patient-developed therapy contracts and aftercare were seen as beneficial.[4]

The relationship of length of stay to outcome is another controversial subject. Adelman and Weiss note that the results of research examining the relationship between lengths of stay in inpatient alcoholism programs and treatment outcome are confusing and often contradictory.[4]

Stein and colleagues noted that among 58 alcoholic men provided detoxification and aftercare services with or without intensive psychosocial in-hospital treatment, no significant difference was noted between the groups on any measure at 13 months after admission. The detoxification-only group received 9 days of hospitalization, whereas the rehabilitation group received 30 days of hospital stay in this study.[5] Similar findings were noted by Page and Schaub, who evaluated results in 86 alcoholic male inpatients who were randomly assigned comparable 3-week or 5-week treatment programs. Although both the 3- and 5-week groups demonstrated a significant improvement on both Minnesota Multiphasic Personality Inventory and follow-up data, few differences between the groups were revealed. The researchers concluded that there was little justification for prolonging inpatient treatment beyond 3 weeks and suggested that the inpatient phase of alcohol treatment be brief and oriented to developing a well-structured, extended outpatient program.[6]

On the other hand, Adelman and Weiss found several studies that documented improved outcome correlating with longer inpatient stay.[4] Among these studies were those by Bromet and colleagues, who found that length of stay correlated inversely with the propensity for rehospitalization 6 to 8 months after discharge.[7] Welte and associates noted that alcoholics with low social stability reported better outcome if inpatient stay exceeded 30 days.[8] McClellan and coworkers found that patients who were favorably discharged after 5 to 14 days demonstrated markedly worse outcomes than individuals who spent 15 or more days in treatment.[9]

Methodological problems frequently confound such comparative studies, especially on the basis of randomness or selection criteria used to determine lengths of stay. Adelman and Weiss concluded that some subgroups of alcoholic patients apparently fare better in longer inpatient treatment programs but that length of stay is less important for other patients.[4]

My group's experience at the Cleveland Clinic Foundation suggests that the correlation between the length of stay and the outcome is confounded by the problem that the sickest patients have the longest stay. Their complicating factors of medical illness, psychiatric disability, and gross psychosocial impairment result in longer stays and poorer prognosis than in those with fewer disabilities at the outset. Truly random patient assignments to inpatient or outpatient treatment tracks are difficult to achieve for these reasons, and comparative analyses should be interpreted with caution. It would appear best to deduce that not all patients need hospitalization and that among those who do, some require more and longer inpatient involvement than others to achieve a satisfactory level of safety and stability with a reasonable hope for recovery.

The identification of these sicker patients may depend on the application of well-designed criteria. Even with such criteria in place, the wide spectrum of human variables in the alcoholic population and the differences in professional clinical judgment likely confound any easier resolution of the questions about hospitalization and length of stay. Perhaps individual clinical judgment, with its legal and ethical checks and balances, may prove to be the best determinant of hospital use after all. As Glatt says, "Outpatient clinics for the many who do not require hospitalization is a need which will become progressively more urgent the more public education lessens the stigma attached to the diagnosis of alcoholism and the more medical training teaches doctors to recognize the condition in the early phases, but there will always remain alcoholics who need specialized hospital treatment."[10]

Whitfield notes that hospitalization is appropriate in some situations and should be used in concert with outpatient treatment. He identifies indications for inpatient treatment as danger to self; danger to others; functional impairment, moderate to severe; need for structured environment; unsuccessful recovery by adequate outpatient treatment; support systems weak or unavailable; a patient's desire to be hospitalized; severe alcohol-disulfiram reaction; and medical or psychiatric illness, usually a consequence of the alcoholism, requiring hospitalization. He further estimates that 25% to 40% of alcoholic patients require at least one inpatient treatment for alcoholism during the long course of their outpatient alcoholism treatment.[11]

What Is the Role of Outpatient Treatment Modalities?

Outpatient treatment for alcoholism may be provided as "primary treatment" or as part of the continuum of care that may follow hospitalization. Primary outpatient treatment programs are growing in popularity and are perceived as a less expensive but acceptable alternative to more costly inpatient care. The swing to outpatient treatment, however, has not been without controversy, because only a few years ago some responsible professionals in the alcoholism treatment field would have regarded outpatient treatment as irresponsible and perhaps dangerous. Time has shown, however, that primary outpatient treatment programming has a definite place in the therapeutic armamentarium and that it may be the treatment of choice for a sizable group of alcoholics. The advantages of primary outpatient treatment include not only reduced cost but also much less disruption of family and occupational life due to hospital confinement. Outpatient treatment modalities may have somewhat less stigma and a greater degree of patient acceptance. In a thorough review of outpatient treatment of drug and alcohol addiction, Cocores noted that such outpatient treatment requires careful individualized planning, because various treatment approaches are available and should be applied appropriately to each patient, depending on history and needs.[12] First, a thorough evaluation is conducted, including taking a drug and alcohol history and determining prior treatment attempts, as well as taking a medical history and performing a physical examination to evaluate withdrawal symptoms, psychiatric symptoms, and psychosocial stability. The assessment is often carried out in the hospital emergency room, but freestanding clinics with easy access to hospitals are acceptable. Severe addicts, including those using daily opiates, benzodiazepines, or alcohol, are often referred for inpatient detoxification, because the need for medical detoxification is a major contraindication for involvement in outpatient treatment. After detoxification is completed, a clinical decision is made about the appropriateness of continued inpatient rehabilitation or outpatient treatment. Failed prior outpatient treatment attempts may signal that inpatient care is required, but previously untreated individuals are often assigned to outpatient programs. A history of a major psychiatric illness may signal a requirement for supervised inpatient care, and acute psychosis or ideation regarding suicide or homicide is an exclusionary criterion for outpatient treatment as well.

Cocores describes "recovery-sensitive individual counseling as effective, if provided along with self-help group attendance and regular urine testing." Adult evening treatment programs frequently deal with higher-functioning individuals who are experiencing mild difficulties at work or in marriage because of substance addiction. Cocores describes a common evening treatment model as consisting of two group therapy sessions from 6:30 to 10:00 PM four nights weekly for 6 to 8 weeks, along with self-help meetings and urine testing. Twice-weekly counseling sessions then are held for 2 weeks, and then weekly visits for 9 additional months, during which time patients are well integrated into self-help groups.[12]

Day treatment is yet another effective primary or secondary treatment modality. Collins and colleagues described a daycare program in which patients attend a full day of rehabilitation meetings from 9:30 AM to 5:00 PM, 5 days weekly, then return home to attend AA meetings in the evening. Despite a relatively high dropout rate of 23%, 41% of patients remained abstinent at a 7-month measuring point. The dropout rate was substantially greater than the inpatient dropout rate of 14% in that study. The higher dropout rate was balanced by reduced cost of treatment and by the availability of treatment for patients who are unable to be hospitalized.[13] Cocores notes that daycare patients are often unemployed, lower-functioning individuals, often with dual-diagnosis issues. Therefore, day drug treatment programs must have dual-diagnosis identification and treatment capabilities, as well as intensive vocational counseling with the goal of securing employment.[12] A daycare program established by a large industrial corporation found equivalent treatment outcomes between daycare patients and those who had previously been treated in rehabilitation centers. Bensinger and Pilkington recommend day treatment as a first treatment intervention and in instances of relapse.[14] The preponderance of evidence shows that day treatment is an acceptable and desirable alternative to costly inpatient care for patients with psychosocial stability, active employment, a reasonable level of motivation, and no prior failed outpatient treatments.

Outpatient detoxification has been a hotly debated subject for many years. To what extent can detoxification services be provided on an outpatient basis? Alcoholics, because of their medical and withdrawal syndrome complications, do present some medical risk. Delirium tremens, hypertension, hallucinosis, seizures, and internal bleeding are frequent concomitants of chronic alcoholism. Coexisting but non–alcohol-related medical pathologies such as diabetes, tuberculosis, acquired immunodeficiency syndrome, pneumonia, and other infections are also fairly common in this population. Psychiatric dual-diagnosis difficulties also abound, in the form of suicidal and homicidal ideation, severe depression, anxiety, and personality disorder. Inpatient detoxification certainly offers the benefits of close medical and nursing supervision, with its frequent monitoring of vital signs, behavior, and laboratory results. Medicines are reliably distributed and reliably taken in known, regular amounts. Access to alcohol and other drugs is interdicted. All these advantages are achieved but at a very substantial cost, especially considering the fact that only a small percentage of alcoholics have an absolute need for such services. Balancing risk and cost is a thorny dilemma for today's healthcare planners, providers, and administrators. Whitfield and colleagues reported detoxification of 1024 alcoholic patients without the use of psychoactive drugs in ambulatory, chronic alcoholics at a social detoxification setting. Although the researchers claim success using reassurance, reality orientation, and careful staff monitoring, one case of delirium tremens occurred and 12 patients had seizures. Thirty-eight patients with hallucinosis were treated in the social units without using drugs. Although these patients were self-selected and although presumably sicker patients went to hospital emergency rooms or clinics, Whitfield and associates make a compelling case for the use of nonmedical sobering-up detoxification stations as part of a community-based alcoholism treatment network. In any case, emergency or inpatient hospital backup is always required and in fact was often used in Whitfield's group of patients.[15]

Sausser and coworkers comment that "not all alcoholics who present for detoxification are in need of it. The decision to hospitalize the alcoholic for withdrawal should be based on screening criteria developed to fit each physician's comfort level in dealing with the alcoholic client and the many needs of the alcoholic himself." He notes that the absence of a proper home environment, the presence of medical complications, impending delirium tremens, a lengthy drinking history, a history of past seizures, and withdrawal reactions indicate a need for hospitalization. The use of medications in outpatient detoxification is controversial, but Sausser and colleagues recommend the use of benzodiazepines on a short-term basis, along with phenytoin (100 mg four times daily) for patients with a history of seizures. They recommend chlordiazepoxide and diazepam for patients who are to remain in the home in bed recovery, because of these drugs' sedative effects, and use of clorazepate for patients who intend to continue in employment or who will remain active.[16]

As a whole, these studies suggest that outpatient detoxification services have an appropriate place in a community-based armamentarium of alcoholism services but that their effectiveness or utility should not be overstated, because many patients require more secure and more intensive services for necessary care.

Comparisons of Inpatient and Outpatient Treatment of Alcoholism

Considerable interest has been expressed in comparisons of inpatient versus outpatient treatment. Numerous studies have explored this controversial and economically sensitive issue, frequently with the result that benefit payors are quick to state that "outpatient is just as good as inpatient treatment." A more careful analysis of these comparative studies reveals serious methodological problems in their interpretation and tends to argue against any firm conclusion when comparing these two modalities. In a comprehensive review of outcome for drug and alcohol addiction treatment, Harrison and associates note that "one common error in the interpretation of outcome study results is the comparison of inpatient and outpatient recovery or improvement rates, even though the inpatient and outpatient populations are very dissimilar with respect to characteristics that may influence outcomes . . . unless random assignment of patients is utilized in a study design, a selection bias typically results from the patients' referral or self-selection into inpatient or outpatient modalities. In addition, even if random assignment is made, researchers must restrict which patients are permitted in the study sample; the most severely and the least severely affected are usually excluded. Finally, randomization does not guarantee that no initial differences existed in group assignment."[17] Harrison and coworkers further note that in their review of such research comparisons, "studies that compare intake characteristics of inpatients and outpatients consistently report among inpatients a higher prevalence of factors generally associated with a poorer prognosis. Despite initial differences showing inpatients to be sicker than outpatients, nonrandomized studies consistently show no differences in outcome and follow-up, but similar recovery rates for inpatients and outpatients do not prove that the treatments they received are equally effective."[18] Similar outcomes for the two groups may mean merely that less-impaired drug and alcohol abusers respond to outpatient treatment about as well as more-impaired drug and alcohol addicts respond to inpatient treatment. No conclusions about the relative efficacy of the treatments can be drawn from such studies, unless patient subgroups are matched for intake characteristics and analyses conducted for interactions between patient variables and treatment type. None of the studies reviewed reported such an analysis.[17]

Harrison and coworkers review the Comprehensive Assessment and Treatment Outcome Research (CATOR) data, which evaluated 10 years of intake data on more than 50,000 adults from 80 programs in 29 states and 6000 adolescents from 28 programs in 15 states. The data reveal significant differences between inpatient and outpatient treatment populations. Inpatient programs have a greater proportion of patients older than 50 years, whereas outpatient programs have a greater proportion of patients younger than 30. Inpatients have less formal education and are less likely to be employed. Inpatients are more likely to be daily drinkers and to use drugs on a frequent basis. Inpatients show more signs typically associated with chronic addiction and physical dependence and have had prior chemical dependence treatment. The researchers report that inpatients have more episodes of intoxication at work, more histories of antisocial behavior, and more history of depression and suicidal ideation. Recent use of medical care is also much higher among inpatients, and the differentials are greater than can be accounted for by their older age. The results reveal that of the 6042 patients admitted to treatment into inpatient centers, 84% completed their treatment programs, and of this group of completers, 12% refused to consent to follow-up interviews. These facts introduce contact bias, which serves to create more favorable treatment outcome results because nonresponders have previously been found to fare more poorly than responders. In a selected sample of 1918 inpatient treatment completers who were interviewed at 6 and 12 months after discharge, 72% remained abstinent from alcohol and other drugs for at least 6 months and 63% were abstinent for the entire first year.[17]

Approximately three of four inpatients in the CATOR follow-up sample reported some involvement in a formal aftercare program sponsored by the treatment center. Excluding the nonparticipants, a strong relationship can be noted between length of aftercare involvement and abstinence. Inpatients involved in aftercare for a full year after treatment had an 84% abstinence rate, compared with 72% for those involved for 6 to 11 months and 54% for those involved for less than 6 months.[17] This relationship does not prove directional causality, because patients with a more favorable prognosis may be those who become active in aftercare.

One of the most consistent findings in the CATOR data is the significant relationship between support group involvement after treatment and recovery status. Almost half of the patients in the inpatient follow-up sample attended AA or other support groups every week; their 1-year abstinence rate was much higher than that for monthly attenders, infrequent attenders, those who never attended at all, and those who stopped attending.[17] Again, the question of causality is only partially answered, however.

An analysis of the CATOR data shows that abstinent patients reporting psychosocial difficulties in the first follow-up interval (6 months) were much more likely than those without these problems to suffer a subsequent relapse. Because rates of boredom, craving, and social difficulty are significantly higher among abstinent patients who subsequently suffer a relapse, the association between problems and relapse cannot be dismissed as merely an attempt on the part of these patients to rationalize their return to drug or alcohol use. These results offer strong support for relapse prevention efforts that incorporate comprehensive plans for relapse prevention.[17]

Of the 1918 patients in the follow-up inpatient sample, 63% reported total abstinence for the year after treatment and an additional 24% reported at least 6 months of abstinence out of 12 months. Most relapses occurred during the first 6-month interval; 88% of patients who are abstinent the first 6-months maintained this status for the full year.[17]

The CATOR outpatient follow-up sample, based on 914 patient discharges, shows the treatment completion rate (75%) to be lower than that for inpatients (84%), with younger patients being much more likely to drop out. Dropouts were more likely to be unemployed or to have low income, as well as a history of recent criminal behavior. Harrison and associates point out that the follow-up sample represents only 39% of the original sample of treatment completers, limiting the generalizability of findings. Of this selected sample, 83% remained abstinent from alcohol or other drugs for the first 6 months after treatment and 75% were abstinent for a full year. The higher rate of successful outcomes is consistent with the more favorable prognosis projected for outpatients in terms of their greater social stability and lesser drug involvement and symptom severity.[17] Outpatients had better attendance at

AA and higher rates of aftercare participation than inpatients, perhaps because inpatients are frequently at long distances from their treatment centers. In conclusion, Harrison and colleagues state that the greatest proportion of treatment outcome variance is attributable to patient characteristics rather than program characteristics, but they also state that the possibility that better programs can produce better outcomes cannot be dismissed simply because research has not yet reached the level of sophistication to document such differences.[17] The researchers also note that "since the outcome results were based on only a minority of treatment completers in both inpatient and outpatient samples (approximately 40%), there is obviously a great deal of room for sample bias." They also note problems in extrapolating observed results to entire samples because it cannot be ruled out that noncontacted patients are faring worse than projected and that treatment noncompleters are much more likely to resume drug or alcohol use if they stop at all.[17]

In an important study of inpatient versus outpatient treatments, Walsh and coworkers randomly assigned a series of 227 alcoholic industrial workers to one of three rehabilitation regimens: compulsory inpatient treatment, compulsory attendance at AA meetings, and a choice of options. Inpatient backup was provided if needed. Groups were compared in terms of 12 job performance variables and 12 measures of drinking and drug use during a 2-year follow-up period. Results indicated that all three groups improved, but no differences were found among job-related outcome variables. On drinking and drug use, however, significant differences between groups were found. The hospital group fared best, and that assigned to AA the least well. Those allowed to choose a program had intermediate outcomes. Additional inpatient treatment was required significantly more often by the AA group (63%) and the choice group (38%) than by subjects assigned to the initial treatment in the hospital (23%). The estimated cost of inpatient treatment for the AA and choice groups averaged only 10% less than the cost for the hospital group because of their higher rates of additional treatment. The researchers concluded that even for employed problem drinkers who are not abusing drugs or who have no serious medical problems, an initial referral to AA alone or a choice of programs, although less costly than inpatient care, involves more risk than compulsory inpatient treatment and should be accompanied by close monitoring for signs of incipient relapse.[19]

In a controlled trial of inpatient or outpatient treatment of alcohol dependence, Edwards and Guthrie found similar results for randomized inpatients and outpatients. However, they caution that their results could mask particular subgroups of patients for whom one or the other treatment is more suitable. "There are, in all probability, patients who will benefit from two to three months respite in hospital with forced removal from drinking, and who would not recover if left in the disorganized social setting with which they can no longer cope." The researchers do not believe that their findings undermine the position of the specialist inpatient units but point to a need for alcoholism treatment systems to be expanded so that the units form part of a properly comprehensive service.[20]

Cole and associates, in a review of the literature on inpatient and outpatient treatment of alcohol and drug addicts, find attrition to be a major factor in treatment. They note that "while several hypothesized advantages for both inpatient and outpatient treatment are advanced, it is pointed out that, because of methodological and situational differences among the studies, comparisons are difficult and risky to make. After suggesting that there is little evidence to cause one to tout either inpatient or outpatient treatment based on relative effectiveness, it's proposed that a flexible treatment program utilizing both inpatient and outpatient treatment with a focus on reducing attrition is most likely to maximize effectiveness."[21]

The Role of Aftercare in Treatment

Although involvement in AA and other self-help groups has long been a mainstay of treatment for chronic alcoholism, professionally provided aftercare services are a more recent innovation. Aftercare has typically consisted of four primary components: (1) an emphasis on the importance of aftercare and on a mechanism for increasing the likelihood of contact between the patient and the treatment facility; (2) a means of including both the patient and his or her family in aftercare; (3) a forum for aiding the patient and his or her family in using behavioral problem-solving skills for obtaining solutions to problems that arose; and (4) keeping patients in AA.[22] Aftercare can be provided through individual counseling, specialized group counseling, and hospital-sponsored self-help groups. Studies of aftercare, however, have yielded mixed results. Some investigators noted benefit, others noted none, and studies that did report benefit left unanswered the question of whether aftercare actually influenced positive outcome or whether patients who were faring well were more likely to attend aftercare sessions.[22] Some researchers have suggested that "the prognosis for remission depends more on a client's alcoholic and social conditions at entry to treatment than on any particular treatment characteristics, including amount."[23]

Relapse prevention training, which specifically addresses issues relevant to the maintenance of sobriety, is gaining in popularity. The goal of relapse prevention is to provide individuals with the skills to anticipate, avoid, or cope with high-risk situations that threaten their sense of control and increase the probability of relapse. A related goal is to provide individuals who do "slip" with the ability to overcome the impact of violating the commitment to sobriety and reduce the negative consequences of a drinking episode.[24] Such aftercare and relapse prevention work might best be provided at the work site rather than at a treatment center and should involve a significant role for employee assistance program coordinators. Nontraditional approaches involving extremely vigorous outreach and follow-up may yield improved results, especially in work site programs, but studies are lacking.

What Is the Role of Alcoholics Anonymous in the Treatment Process?

Mann notes that patients who complete primary treatment and follow their aftercare plan are those who fare best in long-term follow-up studies. Those who do not follow through with the aftercare recommendations fare poorly.[2]

AA is a fellowship of individuals whose only commonality is the desire to quit drinking. Participation is entirely voluntary, and members subscribe to a philosophy and behavior code based on 12 steps and 12 traditions. The AA philosophy encompasses mental, emotional, and spiritual aspects, and newcomers look to more senior members as positive role models in the application of program fundamentals. An AA-based recovery program is a spiritual, cognitive, and behavioral way of life that enhances a personal and interpersonal sense of well-being while promoting a value

system based on honesty and humility. Members typically do not consider AA as a "treatment" per se, which they associate with professionalism and a fee-for-service approach. AA philosophy, although emphasizing psychological restructuring, does not rely on traditional psychiatric methods. Treatment programs typically put heavy emphasis on participation in AA, both during and after the acute treatment phase.[25] Despite the near universality of AA as a treatment recommendation, empirical studies of its effectiveness have been few and are severely hampered by philosophical and methodological problems. With indeterminate criteria for membership, no accurate membership list, no formal organization, and traditions of anonymity and nonprofessionalism, tabulation of meaningful results is difficult at best.[26] Nonetheless, because of its dominance philosophically and numerically in the recovery field, investigators persist in asking whether AA really works.[27] Because any treatment method is as good as the amount of effort and energy put into it by a participant, there is some circularity to the answer to this question. AA works if an individual works at it. Active AA participation has frequently been identified by individuals who have a good outcome. Hoffmann and colleagues found that among those individuals who attended AA weekly, 73% were able to achieve 6 months of sobriety. Less frequent attendance correlated with lower rates of sustained sobriety.[28] Collins and associates noted a strong correlation between any AA attendance and improved outcome; 83% of AA attenders fared well after 18 months, compared with 65% without AA.[29] Despite these strong correlations, the issue of causality is problematical. Does AA attendance produce good outcome, or do alcoholics with a more favorable prognosis gravitate to and participate in AA? The answer to this question requires a truly randomized study, which might well be impossible owing to the need for matching for various socioeconomic and demographic variables in a large population.[27] The vast majority of treatment professionals, however, seem convinced that participation in self-help groups such as AA and related programs such as Narcotics Anonymous and Cocaine Anonymous produces the most favorable chance for recovery, in terms of both length of sobriety and quality of life. The challenge remains for empirical scientists to evaluate and measure this philosophical movement and to gain a better understanding of the far-reaching impact of its approach.

Does Treatment Work?

This seemingly simple question is undoubtedly easier to answer in a medical-surgical context than in a psychological-behavioral one. As noted earlier, any psychological treatment works to the extent that an individual invests time and energy in adapting to a new framework of thinking, attitudes, and behavior. Indeed, treatment works for those who work for it—but how many do? Several studies have documented good posttreatment success. Collins and colleagues noted 65.1% of alcohol addicts and 78% of drug addicts achieving favorable outcomes in a sample whose mean length of time after treatment was 8 months. Treatment modalities that correlated with positive outcome included inpatient rehabilitation, outpatient psychotherapy, current activity in AA, and taking disulfiram.[29] A 10-year follow-up study of 200 male and female patients found 61% reporting complete or stable remission of their alcoholism for at least 3 years before the survey and 84% reporting stable psychosocial status. Successful outcome was possible regardless of severity of drinking history or psychosocial status. Involvement in AA was a good predictor of favorable outcome.[30] In another study of 742 patients evaluated at 6 months' follow-up, significant improvement was found in virtually all areas in both alcoholics and drug addicts. Major changes occurred in alcohol and drug use, employment, criminal behavior, and psychological function. Patients undergoing long-term treatment showed greater improvement and better 6-month outcomes than those undergoing short-term therapy on 12 of 18 criteria.[30] Despite these relatively favorable studies showing good outcome, the issue of causality is not easily resolved. Nathan, in a meta-analysis of outcome studies, notes that although abstinence rates 1 year after treatment for favorable treatment prospects may reach or exceed 50%, rates at 1 year for poor treatment prospects may not reach 25%.[31] Outcome differences were more closely related to patient factors, including motivation, chronicity and severity of alcoholism, age and gender, and personal, interpersonal, familial, educational, and vocational resources rather than to treatment factors, including theoretical orientation, content, locus, and intensity of treatment, which generally predicted treatment outcome poorly. Outcome studies support the view that patients with greater external and internal resources and with success experiences tend to fare better than those without. This is reflected, to a degree, in the tendency for better outcomes with higher social class, as measured by educational attainment and occupational status.[29] The possibility that patient variables are a more reliable predictor of outcome than program content does not mean that treatment per se is ineffective. Rather, in a way perhaps analogous to an educational model, those who bring more to the process, even if only in the form of greater motivation, seem to achieve greater success. The challenge for treatment professionals is to enhance the efficacy of treatment by identifying beneficial component parts and perhaps through improved matching of these treatment components with patient socioeconomic and psychological variables.[31]

Is Alcoholism Treatment Cost Effective?

It is generally agreed that the costs of alcoholism in this country and around the world are staggering. An estimate of the dollar value/social cost in the United States alone amounted to approximately $70 billion in 1985,[32] yet treatment is a costly proposition. Perhaps no other form of medical intervention receives as much cost-benefit scrutiny as alcoholism, possibly because of the seemingly voluntary nature of substance addiction and because of uncertainties about treatment outcome. Are dollars spent for treatment returning value to society? Although this same question could well be asked in relation to the treatment of any disease or disability, the answer might be problematical. Should treatment be cost effective in social/economic terms? Is this a valid criterion for evaluating the desirability of providing treatment? Treatment is usually provided in Western societies on the basis of humanitarian rather than cost-effectiveness grounds. Nonetheless, because questions of possible waste or inefficiency are urgent ones in the context of our modern era of medical cost containment, it is reasonable to examine the issue of cost effectiveness for alcoholism treatment. Can our society afford to treat alcoholism—and can it afford not to?[31]

In a benefit-cost analysis conducted on 3034 clients from state-monitored alcoholism treatment programs in Oklahoma, this analysis showed a return to society of $1.98 for every dollar invested in alcoholism treatment.[33] Similarly, a study of alcoholics in a Health Maintenance Organization (HMO) treatment system found that utilization and costs of all forms of inpatient care for both nonalcoholic family members and alcoholic family members dropped after alcoholism treatment began and ultimately reached a level similar to the matched (nonalcoholic) comparison group. Outpatient care also decreased in terms of frequency and cost for all members of an alcoholic's family. Total healthcare cost per family member decreased substantially over time after initiation of treatment of the alcoholic family member.[34] Application of these concepts at the microeconomic level can help in determining healthcare policy. For example, among two groups of HMO participants, one with a full substance addiction benefit and the other with a 50% copayment, it was noted that the full-benefit group tended to have higher utilization rates and made significantly more treatment contacts than the 50% copayment group. Both payment groups improved, but the full-benefit group tended to be somewhat more improved.[35] Finally, in a study of 150 million healthcare claims for more than 5 million privately insured individuals and their dependents, significant support was found for the cost effectiveness of substance addiction treatment. The overall national utilization rate is three admissions per 1000 covered lives, with only 3.4% of persons admitted for substance addiction treatment, compared with circulatory diseases accounting for 10.8%, digestive disorders 9.5%, and psychiatric illness 5.98%. Medical payments for substance addiction treatment constituted only 3.8% of all expenditures. These data document the correlation with length of inpatient stay and favorable outcome, because 48% of those hospitalized for 7 days or less for substance addiction were rehospitalized within a year. When patients stayed between 22 and 30 days, only 21% were readmitted within a year. The authors of the study point out that the cost of the consequences of untreated substance addiction outweighs treatment costs for the causative condition.[36]

Summary

In summary, the hard questions posed to us about treatment, efficacy, and cost must now be continually addressed in the new discourse of the healthcare marketplace. The alcoholism treatment industry must recognize the reality that it has matured from a new phenomenon to a fixed line item on the budget of payors. As such, alcoholism must compete for healthcare dollars with all the other medical and surgical illnesses, in a universe of shrinking healthcare budgets. To compete effectively, the alcoholism treatment field needs to adapt to the shift from humanitarianism and blind faith to a position based on sound reasoning and meaningful empirical data.

The insights and data gathered in this chapter can, I believe, form the framework for a response to critics and pessimistic payors. We have seen that treatment does work, roughly in proportion to the effort people put into it. Treatment has evolved from a "one-size-fits-all" 28-day inpatient model to diverse levels of intensity with differing intensity and cost. All of the levels work to produce favorable results, and comparisons of one level with another are seen to be of doubtful validity because of the near impossibility of achieving random patient assignments or matching groups of patients. Inpatient, outpatient, aftercare, and self-help groups all work for those patients who work well with them and for those who need them. Matching this need (in the form of illness severity) to level of care (lowest feasible cost) forces treatment toward a new emerging concept: one with multiple levels of care, well integrated for seamlessly smooth transition of patients, meeting a broad spectrum of patient needs, and monitoring itself for outcome and cost effectiveness. All these changes must and will come about, but the fundamentals' philosophy of the treatment process will serve as the constant formulation stone of the industry. Treatment providers will continue to emphasize what has worked so well in the past—the illness model; the healing of mind, body, soul, and family; and reliance on one alcoholic to help another—so well perfected in the fellowship of AA.

REFERENCES

1. Collins GB, Weiss K, Cozzens DT, et al: A multidisciplinary team approach to the treatment of drug and alcohol addiction. In Miller NS (ed): Comprehensive Handbook of Drug and Alcohol Addiction. New York, Marcel-Dekker, 1991, pp 981–999.
2. Mann GA: History and theory of a treatment for drug and alcohol addiction. In Miller NS (ed): Comprehensive Handbook of Drug and Alcohol Addiction. New York, Marcel-Dekker, 1991, pp 1201–1212.
3. Moore RA: Ten years of inpatient programs for alcoholic patients. Am J Psychiatry 134(5):542–545, 1977.
4. Adelman SA, Weiss RD: What is therapeutic about inpatient alcoholism treatment? Hosp Community Psychiatry 40(5):515–519, 1989.
5. Stein LI, Newton JR, Bowman RS: Duration of hospitalization for alcoholism. Arch General Psychiatry 32:247–252, 1975.
6. Page RD, Schaub LH: Efficacy of a three- versus a five-week alcohol treatment program. Int J Addict 14(5):697–714, 1979.

7. Bromet E, Moos R, Bliss F, et al: Post treatment functioning of alcoholic patients: Its relationship to program participation. J Consult Clinical Psychol 45:829–842, 1977.

8. Welte J, Hynes G, Sokolow L, et al: Effect of length of stay in inpatient alcoholism treatment on outcome. J Stud Alcohol 42:483–491, 1981.

9. McClellan AT, Luborsky L, O'Brien CP, et al: Is treatment for substance abuse effective? JAMA 247(10):1423–1428, 1982.

10. Glatt MM: Lancet 1(493):791–792, 1967.

11. Whitfield CL: Outpatient management of the alcoholic patient. Psychiatr Ann 12(4):447–458, 1982.

12. Cocores J: Outpatient treatment of drug and alcohol addiction. In Miller NS (ed): Comprehensive Handbook of Drug and Alcohol Addiction. New York, Marcel Dekker, 1991.

13. Collins GB, Watson EW, Zirmec GL: A hospital day care program for alcoholics. Gen Hosp Psychiatry 2:20–22, 1980.

14. Bensinger A, Pilkington CF: An alternative method in the treatment of alcoholism: The United Technologies Corporation Day Treatment Program. J Occup Med 25(4):300–303, 1983.

15. Whitfield CL, Thompson G, Lamb A, et al: Detoxification of 1,024 alcoholic patients without psychoactive drugs. JAMA 239(14):1409–1410, 1978.

16. Sausser GJ, Fishburne SB, Everett VD: Outpatient detoxification of the alcoholic. J Fam Pract 14(5):863–867, 1982.

17. Harrison PA, Hoffmann NG, Streed SG: Drug and alcohol addiction treatment outcome. In Miller NS (ed): Comprehensive Handbook of Drug and Alcohol Addiction. New York, Marcel-Dekker, 1991, pp 1163–1197.

18. Evenson RC, Reese PJ, Holland RA: Measuring the severity of symptoms in outpatient alcoholics. J Stud Alcohol 43:839–842, 1982.

19. Walsh DC, Hingson RW, Merrigan DM, et al: A randomized trial of treatment options for alcohol-abusing workers. N Engl J Med 325(11):775–782, 1991.

20. Edwards G, Guthrie S: A controlled trial of inpatient and outpatient treatment of alcohol dependency. Lancet 1(489):555–559, 1967.

21. Cole SG, Lehman WE, Cole EA, Jones A: Inpatient versus outpatient treatment of alcohol and drug abusers. Am J Drug Alcohol Abuse 8(3):329–345, 1981.

22. Ahles TA, Schlundt DG, Prue DM, Rychtarik RG: Impact of aftercare arrangements on the maintenance of treatment success in abusive drinkers. Addict Behav 8:53–58, 1983.

23. Armor DJ, Polich JM, Stambul HB: Alcoholism and Treatment. Prepared for the National Institute on Alcohol Abuse and Alcoholism. Santa Monica, CA, Rand Corporation, 1976.

24. Ito JR, Donovan DM, Hall JJ: Relapse prevention in alcohol aftercare: Effects on drinking outcome, change process, and aftercare attendance. Br J Addict 83:171–181, 1988.

25. Collins GB, Barth J: Using the resources of AA in treating alcoholics in a general hospital. Hosp Community Psychiatry 30(7):480–482, 1979.

26. Tournier RE: Alcoholics anonymous as treatment and as ideology. J Stud Alcohol 40:230–239, 1979.

27. Glaser FB, Ogborne AC: Does AA really work? Br J Addict 77:123–129, 1982.

28. Hoffmann NG, Harrison PA, Belille CA: Alcoholics Anonymous after treatment: Attendance and abstinence. Int J Addict 18(3):311–318, 1983.

29. Collins GB, Janesz JW, Byerly-Thrope J, et al: The Cleveland Clinic Alcohol Rehabilitation Program: A treatment outcome study. Cleve Clin Q 52:245–251, 1985.

30. Cross GM, Morgan CW, Mooney AJ III, et al: Alcoholism treatment: A 10 year follow-up study. Alcoholism 14(2):169–173, 1990.

31. Nathan PE: Outcomes of treatment for alcoholism: Current data. Ann Behav Med 8(2–3):40–46, 1986.

32. Rice DP, Kelman S, Miller LS, Dunmeyer S: The Economic Costs of Alcohol and Drug Abuse and Mental Illness. 1985. Rockville, MD, National Institute on Drug Abuse, 1990.

33. Rundell OH, Paredes A: Benefit-cost methodology in the evaluation of therapeutic services for alcoholism. Alcohol Clin Exp Res 3(4):324–333, 1979.

34. Holder HD, Hallan JB: Impact of alcoholism treatment on total health care costs: A six year study. Adv Alcohol Subst Abuse 6(1):1–15, 1986.

35. Hayami DE, Freeborn DK: Effective coverage on use of an HMO alcoholism treatment program, outcome, and medical care utilization. Am J Public Health 71(10):1133–1143, 1981.

36. Treatment is the Answer: A White Paper on the Cost Effectiveness of Alcoholism and Drug Dependency Treatment. Laguna Hills, CA, National Association of Addiction Treatment Providers, 1991.

Treatment of Protracted Drug-Induced Syndromes

Richard B. Seymour, MA • David E. Smith, MD

Nonmedical use of hallucinogens, popularly called *psychedelics*, may have had its greatest notoriety during the 1960s and early 1970s, but the use of these drugs, with or without psychiatric comorbidity, continues to be prevalent. A resurgence of psychedelic drug use has been noted. The use of higher-dose lysergic acid diethylamide (LSD) and some of the more exotic hallucinogens has been joined since the 1980s by increasing use of methylenedioxymethamphetamine (MDMA) and its congeners. MDMA use appears frequently at "raves," youth gatherings that reflect the "acid tests" and early rock music gatherings of the 1960s.[1, 2]

Perhaps more markedly than any other drug group, hallucinogens have been associated with protracted psychiatric syndromes. These include the release of suppressed materials during MDMA use, reactions to flashback, exacerbation of underlying psychiatric problems, and the emergence of posthallucinogen perceptual disorder (PHPD). This chapter discusses these and other problems associated with hallucinogens and other drugs.

Hallucinogenic Drugs

The terms *hallucinogen* and *psychedelic* have been loosely applied to substances that are used to achieve so-called altered states of consciousness. These include LSD and the LSD-like drugs: mescaline (peyote), psilocybin, and psilocin; probably LSD-like DMA, DOM, and DMT; and psychedelic stimulants and entactogens such as MDA, MDE, and MDMA. Other drugs that have protracted syndromes include scopolamine, the disassociative anesthetic phencyclidine (PCP), and marijuana's delta-9-tetrahydrocannabinol (THC).

Unlike the LSD-related psychedelics, PCP and THC tend to produce long-term effects by continued action of the drugs. THC is highly lipid soluble, and a complex relationship exists between THC, which can be measured in the blood after self-administration, and rapid transfer into lipid and other areas of the body and brain. Direct correlation between self-reports of euphoria and blood levels have been hindered by this relationship and the metabolism of THC in the liver into 11-hydroxy-THC and 11-nor-COOH THC[3] and tens of other metabolites with psychoactive properties. THC and THC metabolites are primarily excreted in the feces. The slow release of THC and active metabolites from lipid stores and other areas may explain the so-called carryover effects on driving and other reports of behavioral changes over time.[4]

Hallucinogen Toxicity in Street Use

During the clinically supervised stage of LSD's sociopharmacological study, adverse reactions were rare. Cohen,[5] one of the pioneer clinical investigators of LSD, reported that the incidence of psychotic reactions lasting more than 48 hours was 0.8 per 1000 in experimental subjects and 1.8 per 1000 in mental patients. However, by June 1967, when the Haight-Ashbury Free Medical Clinic first opened its doors on the corner of Haight and Clayton Streets in San Francisco, negative LSD experiences, or "bad trips," as the acid culture called them, were frequent.[6]

Although banning LSD in 1966 may have decreased the immediate availability of that drug, it did nothing to diminish young people's increasing appetite for drug experience. A second wave of drug experimentation in the late 1960s produced massive addiction of methamphetamines, barbiturates, and eventually heroin by a less discerning population. The sociocultural impact of these drugs was combined with public perceptions of the psychedelic threat, and the government declared a generic war on drugs. In 1970, when new federal legislation produced a graduated sequence of drug schedules, based on abuse potential versus medical use, all of the known psychedelic drugs were placed in schedule one, as highly dangerous drugs with no potential for medical use.[7]

From Acid Tests to the Era of Raves

In the mid-1960s, the public use of LSD and other psychedelics was initiated at a series of gatherings held in large auditoriums, such as San Francisco's Longshoremen's Hall. These so-called acid tests were characterized by dancing to the electronic music of such underground groups as the Grateful Dead, accompanied by pulsating strobe lights and projected "light shows." LSD was made illegal in 1966, but the use of psychedelics at many rock concerts had become a common practice.

In the late 1980s, a new wave of group psychedelic celebrations came into being. The first of these, appearing overseas in England and Germany, were called "acid houses," even though the primary drug being used was MDMA.[8] These celebrations or so-called raves spread to the United States, and rather than being based at specific venues, as most rock concerts have been, were held at relatively impromptu sites, advertised through "rave shops" and an MDMA underground network, and attended mostly by invitation.[9]

Raves can be seen as a marriage of psyche-

delic and cybernetic, the twin fascinations of a new generation. At these celebrations, the music is intensely rhythmic and starkly electronic, global in its nature, and the young attendees often dance all night. Some events can last for days on end. Attendees often rave throughout weekend cycles on an ongoing basis. The stimulant qualities of MDMA probably serve to support such activity. Attendees often trade off between using MDMA and LSD, usually taken at low, nonpsychospiritual doses, in order to stay awake, a practice they call "candy-flipping."[2]

Severe Toxic Reactions to MDMA

Severe reactions to what users believed to be MDMA have been reported, including prolonged psychotic reactions. As with any consciousness-affecting drug, these psychotic breaks can happen, especially if the user has underlying psychopathology.

Hayner, at the Haight-Ashbury Free Clinics' Rock Medicine Program, and McKinney, at the San Francisco Bay Area Regional Poison Control Center, reported two severe cases involving MDMA. These apparently involved idiosyncratic life-threatening reactions to the drug.[10]

Treatment, Support, and Recovery Options

IMMEDIATE AND CHRONIC PROBLEMS WITH PSYCHEDELIC DRUGS

In 1967, Smith identified the adverse effects of psychedelic drugs as "largely psychological in nature" and classified them as either acute toxicity, effects occurring during the use of the drug, or chronic aftereffects.[11] Although some physiological consequences have occurred, particularly with MDMA, these have been primarily of an idiosyncratic nature, whereas in most cases the adverse effects of these drugs still appear to be psychological in their nature.

The acute toxic effects take many forms. Individuals often knowingly take a hallucinogenic drug and find themselves in a state of anxiety as the powerful psychedelic begins to take effect. They are aware that they took a drug but feel that they cannot control its effects. This condition is similar to that of being unable to awaken from a threatening dream. Some users experiencing a bad trip try to flee the situation physically, potentially endangering themselves. Others may become paranoid and suspicious of their companions or other individuals.

Not all acute toxicity is based on anxiety or loss of control. Some people taking psychedelics display decided changes in cognition and demonstrate poor judgment. They may decide that they can fly and may jump out of a window. Some users are reported to have walked into the sea, feeling that they were "at one with the universe." Such physical mishaps have been described within the acid culture as "being God but tripping over the furniture." Susceptibility to bad trips is not necessarily dose related but can depend on the experience, maturity, and personality of the user as well as set and setting (i.e., the circumstances and the environment in which the trip takes place). An individual sometimes complains of unpleasant symptoms while intoxicated but later speaks in glowing terms of the experience. Negative psychological set and environmental setting are the most significant factors contributing to bad hallucinogenic trips.[6]

TREATMENT OF ACUTE TOXICITY

Techniques originally developed within the psychedelic community and adopted by free clinics and other counterculture-oriented treatment centers, as reported by Smith and Shick,[12] are based on the findings that most psychedelic bad trips are best treated in a supportive, nonpharmacological fashion by restoring a positive, nonthreatening environment. At large rock concerts, emergency talk-down procedures are carried out by Haight-Ashbury staff and volunteers in a quiet space set up specifically for treating acute psychedelic toxicity.

Talk-downs of most acute toxicity reactions can be accomplished without medication or hospitalization. Paraprofessionals with psychedelic drug experience have been particularly effective at such sites as large rock concerts. Amelioration of bad trips has even been accomplished by long-distance telephone calls.[13]

An understanding of the phases generally experienced in a hallucinogenic drug trip is most helpful in treating acute reactions. After orally ingesting an average dose of 100 to 250 μg of LSD, the user experiences sympathomimetic or stimulant responses, including elevated heart rate and respiration. Adverse reactions in this phase are primarily managed by reassuring the patient that these are normal and expected effects of psychedelic drugs. This

reassurance is usually sufficient to override a potentially frightening situation.

From the first to the sixth hour, visual imagery becomes vivid and may take on frightening content. Patients may have forgotten taking the drug and, given acute time distortion, may believe this retinal circus[14] will continue forever. Such fears can be dispelled by reminding the individual that these effects are drug induced, by suggesting alternative images, and by distracting the patient from those images that are frightening.

Wesson and Smith[15] noted that medication may be necessary and should be given either after the talk-down has failed or as a supplement to the talk-down process. During the first phase of intervention, oral administration of a sedative, such as 25 mg of chlordiazepoxide (Librium) or 10 mg of diazepam (Valium), can have an important pharmacological and reassuring effect.

Patients may suffer a toxic psychosis or major break with reality in which one can no longer communicate with the individual. If the patient begins acting in a way that causes an immediate danger, antipsychotic drugs may be administered. Only if an individual refuses oral medication and is out of behavioral control should antipsychotics be administered by injection. Haloperidol (Haldol, 2.0 mg intramuscularly every hour) is the current drug of choice. Any medication, however, should only be given by qualified personnel. If antipsychotic drugs are required, hospitalization is usually indicated. It has been found at the Haight-Ashbury Free Clinics, however, that most bad acid trips can be handled on an outpatient basis by talk-down alone.

As soon as rapport and verbal contact are established, further medication is generally unnecessary. An individual occasionally fails to respond to the foregoing regimen and must be referred to an inpatient psychiatric facility. Such a decision must be weighed carefully, however, because transfer to a hospital may of itself have an aggravating and threatening effect. Hospitalization should be used only as a last resort if all else has failed.

TREATING CHRONIC PSYCHEDELIC DRUG AFTEREFFECTS

Chronic psychedelic drug aftereffects present situations in which a condition that may be attributable to ingestion of a toxic substance occurs or continues long after that substance has been metabolized. With the use of psychedelic drugs, four recognized chronic reactions have been reported[15, 16]: (1) prolonged psychotic reactions, (2) depression sufficiently severe to be life threatening, (3) flashbacks, and (4) exacerbation of preexisting psychiatric illness. A fifth chronic reaction has been listed in the DSM-III-R, PHPD.

PHPD should be differentiated from a prolonged psychotic reaction, because patients with PHPD have persistent perceptual disorder with the development of anxiety, panic, and phobia but do not have a delusional system or a break in reality. From a treatment perspective, patients with PHPD describe a negative reaction to haloperidol, whereas the antipsychotic drug group comprises the drugs of choice in patients with prolonged psychotic reactions. PHPD should also be differentiated from flashbacks, because PHPD is a continuous disorder that does not necessarily occur after bad trips whereas a flashback is an episodic disorder usually associated with a recurrence of the previous bad trip. Flashbacks require reassurance but not pharmacological intervention. The focus with PHPD is abstinence-oriented recovery, and the drug group that appears most beneficial is the specific serotonin reuptake inhibitors, coupled with the benzodiazepines if a patient is experiencing severe panic.[2]

Some people who have taken many hallucinogenic drug trips, especially those who have had acute toxic reactions, show what appears to be serious long-term personality disruptions. These prolonged psychotic reactions have similarities to schizophrenic reactions and appear to occur most often in individuals with preexisting psychological difficulties, such as primarily prepsychotic or psychotic personalities. Psychedelic drug-induced personality disorganizations can be severe and prolonged. Appropriate treatment often requires antipsychotic medication and residential care in a mental health facility, followed by outpatient counseling.

FLASHBACKS

By far the most ubiquitous chronic reaction to psychedelics is flashbacks. Flashbacks are transient spontaneous occurrences of some aspect of the hallucinogenic drug effect occurring after a period of normalcy that follows the original intoxication. This period of normalcy distinguishes flashbacks from prolonged psychotic reactions. Flashbacks may occur after a single ingestion of a psychedelic drug but more commonly occur after multiple psychedelic drug ingestions.

Flashbacks are a symptom, not a specific disease entity. They may well have multiple causes, and many cases called flashbacks may have occurred although the individual had never ingested a psychedelic drug. Some investigators have suggested that flashbacks may be due to a residue of the drug retained in the body and released into the brain at a later time. Although this is known to happen with PCP and drugs similar to it, there is no direct evidence of retention or prolonged storage of such psychedelics as LSD.

Individuals who have used psychedelic drugs several times a month have indicated that fleeting flashes of light and afterimage prolongation occurring in the periphery of vision commonly occur for days or weeks after ingestion. Active and chronic psychedelic drug users tend to accept these occurrences as part of the psychedelic experience, are unlikely to seek medical or psychiatric treatment, and frequently view them as "free trips." It is inexperienced users and individuals who attach a negative interpretation to these visual phenomena who are likely to be disturbed by them and to seek medical or psychiatric help. Although emotional reactions to a flashback are generally contained within the period of the flashback itself, prolonged anxiety states or psychotic breaks have occurred after a frightening flashback. There is no record of flashback activity specifically attributable to psychedelic drug use occurring more than a year after the individual's last use of a psychedelic drug.[12]

LONG-TERM CONSEQUENCES OF PSYCHEDELIC DRUG USE

Long-term study of adverse psychedelic drug reactions has revealed the existence of low prevalence but quite disabling chronic consequences of LSD use. Of particular concern is PHPD.[17] Individuals with PHPD have a persistent perceptual disorder that they describe as being like living in a bubble under water. They also describe trails of light and images following movement of their hands and often talk of living in a purple haze. This perceptual disorder is aggravated by use of any psychoactive drug, including alcohol and marijuana, and is distinguished from flashbacks, which are episodic rather than chronic phenomena. Patients with PHPD often feel anxiety, even panic, and become phobic and depressed. Our experience has been that PHPD sufferers do not have a disturbed psychiatric history before the onset of psychedelic drug use and that PHPD can occur even after a single dose.

With more severe, prolonged LSD reactions, such as an LSD-precipitated schizophrenic reaction or severe depressive disorder, individuals almost always have a premorbid psychiatric history and require inpatient treatment. With prolonged psychotic reactions, antipsychotic medication is required, and with the prolonged depressive reactions, antidepressant medication is required. A major concern is that adolescents with depressive reactions to psychedelic use may suffer severe depression culminating in suicide.

With PHPD, drug-free recovery with supportive counseling is often adequate treatment, although recovery may take several months and antianxiety medication may be needed to treat the secondary anxiety and panic disorder that develop when individuals feel that they are irreversibly brain damaged and will never see normally again.

TREATMENT ISSUES WITH MDMA

On May 17 and 18, 1986, the Haight-Ashbury Free Medical Clinics' Training and Education Project and the Merritt Peralta Chemical Dependency Recovery Hospital's Institute for Addiction studies cosponsored a national conference on MDMA. Cochaired by Smith and Seymour, the conference focused on all aspects of the MDMA controversy, including chemistry, pharmacology, therapeutics, addiction treatment, and enforcement. Seymour's book *MDMA*[18] was used as the syllabus, and selected proceedings were published as the October-December 1986 issue of *Journal of Psychoactive Drugs*.

Since that time, the Training and Education Project has become an informational clearinghouse for clinical information on MDMA and related substances. The following information is based on data from (1) client visits and telephone inquiries at the Haight-Ashbury Free Medical Clinics' Drug Detoxification Project; (2) telephone inquiries and subsequent interviews with MDMA users at the Training and Education Project; (3) inquiries received from and subsequent interviews with drug addiction treatment professionals throughout the country encountering MDMA as a drug of addiction; (4) consultations with psychotherapists who used MDMA in their clinical practice; and (5) the collective experience of the Haight-Ashbury Free Medical Clinics with MDMA, MDE, and 2-CB; amphetamines, including the methoxylated amphetamines such as MMDA and

DOM (STP); and such psychedelics as mescaline, DMT, LSD-25, and psilocybin during the past 20 years.

MDMA AND RELATED DRUG TOXICITY

Acute MDMA toxicity is essentially the result of taking too much MDMA in too short a time. This results in some physical or psychological dysfunction. The symptoms appear to be time and dose related. These symptoms range from a mild caffeinelike toxicity to potentially life-threatening stimulant overdoses.

Prolonged MDMA toxicity is a result of chronic or regular ingestion of MDMA. The symptoms range in severity from mild dysphoria to frank paranoid psychosis and relate to acute toxicity, chronicity of use, and secondary drug effects such as sleep and appetite suppression.

MDMA-induced anxiety syndromes are problems related to MDMA's ability to bring unconscious material to consciousness. We have hypothesized that these anxiety syndromes are primarily caused by the lack of resolution and integration of now-conscious and often emotionally potent materials. These anxiety syndromes appear to be psychodynamic in nature and not purely toxicological. They last beyond the period of actual drug intoxication.

Low-Dose Toxicity

Greer and Tolbert[19] described some of the low-dose therapeutic-range toxic reactions such as jitteryness, mild anxiety, mild apprehension, and jaw clenching. Because many MDMA users view MDMA use as a relatively important event and many users even formally ritualize such use, an anticipation and apprehension of the events to come may blend with the sympathomimetic properties of MDMA to further heighten apprehension and perhaps even produce fear in predisposed people. Generally, most of the sympathomimetic reactions are dose related and are typically mild. Nonmedicinal approaches, such as support, quiet surroundings, and reassurance that the symptoms will fade over time, should be successful in reducing this apprehension. In most cases, individuals taking MDMA at the doses used in therapy (i.e., 50 to 150 mg) are aware that problems they may be experiencing are drug related.

Medium-Dose Toxicity

At somewhat higher doses (i.e., 250 to 300 mg MDMA), dose- and setting-related psychopathology may develop. In persons with low tolerance to stimulants, a medium-dose acute toxicity may result from ingestion of this amount.

Visual distortions have been reported, such as viewing an object that appears to be shimmering, shiny, or perhaps moving in a jittery fashion or with geometric embellishments. MDMA users are aware that these distortions are drug induced, and they do not appear to carry any particularly positive or negative content. Also, they do not typically interfere with the therapeutic goals of insight and empathy for most individuals. Some users have reported that they desire to be alone, and some report that they become slightly concerned about others' noticing their behavior and knowing that they are intoxicated. A slightly paranoid sense or self-conscious tendency appears to be dose related. These feelings of self-consciousness may only occur while inside a building or in crowds, and users may have a tendency to move outdoors.

Many MDMA users may suffer fairly distressing depression, which may emerge rapidly, especially if there is a sudden shift in consciousness away from the particularly empathic or euphoric stage of the MDMA experience. The subjective aspect of this depression may have to do with returning to fairly normal consciousness after having experienced often significantly beautiful or meaningful feelings.

High-Dose Toxicity

The most obvious and most clinically important acute toxicological problem involves high-dose MDMA toxic reaction. Depending on personal variables such as prior drug experience (especially with stimulants, hallucinogens, and PCP), tolerance to the effects of the drug, and the setting, the toxic range for MDMA may be as low as 300 mg for some people but 400 mg or more for others. Toxic symptoms follow a continuum ranging from anxiety and panic with or without tachycardia to psychotic reactions with paranoia and violence. Hypertensive crises and even cerebrovascular accidents and cardiac arrhythmias can theoretically occur, as with cocaine and the amphetamines.

Some MDMA users may use MDMA in combination with other drugs, such as MDA or marijuana. Other drugs that may have similar properties and effects to those of MDMA include 2-CB, 4-bromo-2,5-dimethoxyphenethylamine, MDE (Eve), and N-ethyl-3,4-methylenedioxymethamphetamine.

Treatment Considerations. The medical management of MDMA toxicity follows a continuum. At the lower doses or at the least severe reactions, appropriate medical treatment may simply be a supportive, reassuring interaction with patients, moving them to a perceived safe environment and reducing stimuli. Patients should be told that the distressing symptoms will fade over time. It would be optimal if someone with psychotherapeutic skills were to spend time with the individual, given that potent psychodynamic issues may come forth. It is best for patients not to be left alone but to remain with someone who is capable of providing psychological support.

For moderately dysfunctional anxiety symptoms that increase with severity, 5 to 10 mg of diazepam may be given orally. For patients who also experience tachycardia, propranolol, 10 to 20 mg, can be given orally. If propranolol is given intravenously, administer from 0.5 to 1 mg very slowly at a maximum of 1 mg/minute, up to a total of 6 mg.

If the symptoms are more severe, consideration should be given to containment if (1) anxiety merges into aggressive behavior, (2) patients show evidence of stimulant psychosis with violence to themselves or to others, or (3) patients demonstrate suicidal verbalizations or behaviors. If a patient has a stimulant psychosis and is markedly anxious, either (1) give haloperidol, 5 mg twice daily, and assess remaining anxiety; or (2) give 5 to 10 mg of diazepam orally. If anxiety is effectively treated, give diazepam every 4 to 6 hours for a maximum of about 40 mg/24-hour period. If stimulant psychosis remains and seems to carry a risk of violence or danger to the patient or others, give haloperidol, 5 mg orally twice daily. Gay, of the Haight-Ashbury Free Clinics' Rock Medicine Program, treats severe adverse psychedelic drug reactions with 2 and 2 (i.e., 2 mg lorazepam and 2 mg haloperidol) and has found that this technique greatly reduces both emergency hospital admissions and prolonged toxicity.[20]

For persistent adrenergic crisis, give propranolol orally in doses of 40 to 60 mg at 4- to 6-hour intervals for the duration of the crisis. A pulse of 90 or less is the goal. Many patients suffering from stimulant psychosis are resistant to haloperidol and may in fact request a sedative-hypnotic to reduce anxiety. Some of these patients may be able to handle the stimulant psychosis if anxiolytic therapy is given. The important diagnosis criterion is, Does the psychotic break represent a clear danger to the patient or to others? Also note that because both the amphetamines and haloperidol lower seizure threshold, caution should be used. Also, some patients may be very sensitive to the sedative-hypnotics and may proceed into coma with even lower doses than recommended; thus, caution is urged. The treatment of stimulant-related problems and treatment concerns is discussed in depth in Wesson and Smith's book *Amphetamine Use, Misuse and Abuse*.[21]

Prolonged High-Dose MDMA Toxicity

Persons who use high doses of MDMA (or any mood-altering drug) on a daily basis are likely to have a substance addiction disorder. Most people who use MDMA for its psychotherapeutic benefits dislike the stimulant properties of MDMA, but some people actively seek out this experience. Clearly, society's present problems with cocaine speak to the fact that stimulant addiction is commonplace. In interviews with MDMA users, it was revealed that some cocaine dealers also sold MDMA as an adjunct to their normal trade, and many cocaine addicts were introduced to MDMA in this setting. Also, amphetamine addicts who have had access to MDMA may have used MDMA as an alternative to amphetamine or turned to MDMA as a supplement to their amphetamine use. Because drug switching is a regular part of drug addiction, a regular stimulant addict might have a tendency to use MDMA at higher doses and for longer periods and to use this drug for its stimulant rather than its empathogenic qualities. These individuals might also exhibit cross-tolerance to MDMA and might thus be able to ingest fairly large quantities of the drug.

Daily or chronic use of a central nervous system stimulant can exhaust a person's physical and psychological strength. In chronic high-dose users, mood swings, emotional lability, and anxiety can increase, alternating with depression in times of abstinence. In time, stimulant psychosis, paranoia, and violence can emerge.

Prolonged Low-Dose MDMA Toxicity

Although high-dose chronic use of MDMA suggests stimulant addiction, extended use of lower doses may suggest a different type of drug use. Stimulant addicts understand and desire the stimulant effects of amphetamines and cocaine. That is not the case with a number of people we have interviewed. These individuals most often are engaged in generalized

drug experimentation, and their chronic use is usually over a finite period, usually a week or two.

The effects of this prolonged MDMA use at lower doses include mild psychopathology. Interviewees describe a lack of mental clarity, being "out of sorts," and having mild mental confusion and slight memory impairment. Some mention a lack of motivation, mild disorientation, and forgetfulness. They may have some sleep dysfunction, and some nutritional needs may not be met if the pattern continues. They did not report anxiety or hyperactivity, however, possibly because of titrating or controlling their doses during the day. They also state that cessation of MDMA use returns them to their normal emotions and psychological state.

Treatment Considerations. It is important that the possibility of addictive disease be assessed. The chronicity of use, as opposed to event-specific use or very rare use, may be a signal of addictive illness. Appropriate treatment for addiction includes inpatient or outpatient chemical dependence treatment based on an abstinence model of supported recovery. Appropriate referral should be made to such 12-step programs as Alcoholics Anonymous or Narcotics Anonymous.

MDMA-Induced Anxiety Syndromes

Although it is atypical for a drug user to contact a drug treatment facility to report *positive* drug experiences, we do receive reports of unsupervised, positive psychodynamic facilitation in MDMA users who call, write, or visit the clinics for literature or questions about MDMA. However, the opposite is also true. For some users, MDMA brings to the surface unconscious material that may be manifested in various negative ways.

These problems seem unrelated to volume, dose, or duration of MDMA use. We have identified such problems as a delayed anxiety disorder secondary to MDMA ingestion. In these cases, MDMA users report one or more symptoms of anxiety, typically emerging shortly after their initial MDMA experience. These symptoms range from mild anxiety or concentration difficulties to a full-blown disorder such as panic attack with hyperventilation and tachycardia, phobic disorders, paresthesias, or other anxiety states.

In some cases, patients are particularly concerned about a certain part of their body. They may perceive that their hand is shaking or that their extremities are cold and clammy.

Subjective reactions to these concerns can range from mildly annoying to highly inhibiting. The dysfunction may require psychiatric or psychological intervention.

These clients reported that they took MDMA for therapeutic reasons, although not as an adjunct to therapy. When asked what specific therapeutic goals they had in mind, patients responded that they were dealing with family problems, relational difficulties, and high-stress patterns in their lives.

Conclusion

Although other drugs may have protracted physical sequelae, the hallucinogens and similar drugs are most likely to produce protracted psychiatric syndromes. LSD and MDMA are currently the prototypical drugs in this group. MDMA, used in group settings at raves, is becoming the center of a resurgence of psychedelic drug use. LSD remains a frequent component for older users and is increasingly used by younger patients. In the 1960s, psychedelic drugs were thought of as a means of achieving cosmic insight and spirituality. Today, the trend among those users is to seek spirituality and to follow the various 12-step approaches to abstinence.

REFERENCES

1. Seymour RB, Smith DE: Hallucinogens. In Miller NS (ed): Comprehensive Handbook of Drug and Alcohol Addiction. New York, Marcel Dekker, 1991.
2. Seymour RB, Smith DE: The Psychedelic Resurgence: Treatment, Support, and Recovery Options. Center City, Hazelden, MN, 1993.
3. Wall ME, Sader BM, Brine D, et al: Metabolism, disposition and kinetics of delta-9-tetrahydrocannabinol in men and women. Clin Pharmacol Ther 34:352–363, 1983.
4. Gold MS: Marijuana. In Miller NS (ed): Principles of Addiction Medicine. Washington, DC, American Society of Addiction Medicine, 1994.
5. Cohen S: Lysergic acid diethylamide: Side effects and complications. J Nerv Ment Dis 130:30–40, 1992.
6. Smith DE, Seymour RB: Dream becomes nightmare: Adverse reactions to LSD. J Psychoactive Drugs 17(4):297–303, 1985.
7. Seymour RB: MDMA: Another view of ecstasy. PharmChem Newsletter 14(3):1–3, 1985.
8. Saunders N: E for Ecstasy. London, Nicholas Saunders, 1993.
9. Beck J, Rosenbaum M: Pursuit of Ecstasy: The MDMA Experience. New York, State University of New York Press, 1994.
10. Hayner GN, McKinney HE: MDMA: The dark side of ecstasy. In Seymour RB, Wesson DR, Smith DE (eds): MDMA: Proceedings of the Conference. J Psychoactive Drugs 18(4):341–348, 1986.
11. Smith DE: Editor's note. J Psychedelic Drugs 1(1):1–5, 1967.
12. Smith DE, Shick JFE: Analysis of the LSD flashback. J Psychedelic Drugs 3(1):13–19, 1970.
13. Alpert R: Psychedelic drugs and the law. J Psychedelic Drugs 1(1):7–26, 1967.
14. Michaux H: Miserable Miracle. San Francisco, City Lights Books, 1963.
15. Wesson DR, Smith DE: Psychedelics. In Schecter A (ed): Treatment Aspects of Drug Dependence. West Palm Beach, CRC Press, 1978.
16. Seymour RB, Smith DE: Drugfree: A Unique, Positive Approach to Staying Off Alcohol and Other Drugs. New York, Facts on File Publications, 1987.
17. American Psychiatric Association: Diagnostic and Statistical Manual of Mental Disorders, 3rd ed. Washington, DC, American Psychiatric Association, 1987.
18. Seymour RB: MDMA. San Francisco, Partisan Press, 1986.
19. Greer G, Tolbert R: Subjective reports of the effects of MDMA in a clinical setting. In Seymour RB, Wesson DR, Smith DE (eds): MDMA: Proceedings of the Conference. J Psychoactive Drugs 18(4):319–328, 1986.
20. Miller PL, Gay GR, Ferris KC, et al: Treatment of acute adverse psychedelic reactions: I've tripped and I can't get down. J Psychoactive Drugs 24(3):277–279, 1992.
21. Wesson DR, Smith DE: Amphetamine Use, Misuse and Abuse, New York, GK Hall & Co, 1979.

Abstinence-Based Treatment and Depression

Norman S. Miller, MD •
Debra L. Klamen, MD •
Norman G. Hoffmann, PhD

Major Depression and Addictive Disorders

Previous studies with large cohorts of more than 10,000 subjects have demonstrated that abstinence-based treatment approaches for alcohol and drug disorders are effective. Rates for continuous abstinence of 70% to 80% are achieved at 1 year after continuing treatment and are greater when combined with attendance at Alcoholics Anonymous (AA).[1, 2]

The Epidemiological Catchment Area (ECA) study found high rates of comorbidity in treatment settings, between 30% and 50% for major depression in alcohol and drug dependence. The prevalence of depression in association with alcohol and drug disorders is high, according to epidemiological and clinical studies.[3] The prevalence of depression as a consequence of alcohol and drug use or as an independent comorbid disorder has been reported as frequent in cross-sectional and retrospective studies (30% to 50%).[4, 5]

Depression is generally assumed to have a negative or unfavorable impact on treatment outcome. One current approach in clinical practice is to provide additional treatment for antecedent or concurrent depression whether or not it has been determined to have a sig-

nificant effect on the response to addiction treatment.[6] Studies suggest that the presence of a history of lifetime diagnosis of major depression, whether it is primary depression (that which occurs before the onset of alcoholism) or secondary depression (that which occurs after the onset of alcoholism), has a significant impact on the prognosis of alcoholism.[4, 5]

Abstinence-Based Treatment

PROGRAM CHARACTERISTICS

The abstinence-based method of addiction treatment is of particular interest because more than 98% of centers for addiction treatment use it. The characteristics of abstinence-based treatment were examined in a national study of 125 private, hospital-based, and free-standing alcohol and drug inpatient treatment centers.[7] Data were collected by independent evaluators in on-site interviews.[7]

To a highly significant degree, treatment center ideology is based on a belief in the disease concept of alcoholism. Treatment programs are based on the 12-step program of AA. In more than 90% of the programs, a treatment goal

351

other than complete abstinence is not acceptable for any patient in recovery.[7]

Additionally, a dominant form of long-term support for alcoholics throughout the world is offered by attendance at AA. In a stratified random sample of 10,000 members of AA collected in 1989, 44% were abstinent at 1 year, 83% between 1 and 5 years, and 91% for more than 5 years in AA.[8] The abstinence-based method is derived from an integration of principles of AA and professional services focused on behavior change. These principles have evolved during the past 40 years. Successful referral to AA is a major emphasis of the treatment, and the relationship between treatment and AA has been steady and mutually reinforcing. Thirty-seven percent of the membership of AA comes from these abstinence-based treatment programs.[8] Clinicians and researchers who treat and study alcoholics/drug addicts are encouraged to become familiar with this method of treatment.[8]

The majority of abstinence-based programs studied were inpatient, although a significant number were outpatient. The abstinence model is based on an integration of professional services and 12-step support systems. The model of treatment is structured in form and content and involves both group and individual therapies. The primary or intensive phase provides daily group and individual sessions for inpatients and at least 9 hours of sessions per week for outpatients. The primary phase is followed by a less intensive and tapered continuing care consisting of weekly outpatient services for a period of months to a year or two. Educational and family components are part of the typical content. In addition, services for other physical and psychiatric conditions may be included in some programs for those who suffer from more than just the addictions and their consequences.

CONTROLLED STUDIES

Controlled studies find significant treatment outcomes in abstinence-based programs, particularly when combined with referral to continuing care and AA.[9, 10] The first randomized clinical trial on abstinence-based treatment of 141 subjects showed significant improvement in drinking behavior as compared with a more traditional form of treatment. The dropout rate was 7.9% for the abstinence-based program and 25.9% for traditional treatment. In addition, participation in outpatient treatment was significantly better after abstinence-based care.[9]

In a second controlled study, 227 workers newly identified as alcoholics were randomly assigned to three treatment regimens: compulsory inpatient treatment, compulsory attendance at AA meetings, and a choice of options. Inpatient backup was provided if needed. The hospital programs for inpatient treatment were abstinence based, with referral to AA at discharge.[10] On seven measures of drinking and drug use, the hospital group fared best and that population assigned to AA alone fared the least well; those allowed to choose a program had intermediate results. The estimated costs of inpatient treatment for the AA and choice groups averaged only 10% less than the costs for the hospital group because of their higher rates of additional treatment. The conclusion was that although less costly than inpatient care, an initial referral to AA alone or choice of programs involved more risk than compulsory inpatient treatment.

Evaluation studies of large populations (> 10,000 subjects) are available for the abstinence-based methods that report abstinence rates at 1 year of greater than 90% when combined with continuing care and attendance at AA after discharge. Favorable outcomes on other parameters such as improved psychosocial functioning, employment, and legal histories also have been reported in these studies.[1, 2]

EVALUATION STUDIES

The data on the subjects from evaluation studies of abstinence-based treatment were derived from voluntary admissions in 38 inpatient and 19 outpatient programs in a version of the general registry system of Comprehensive Assessment and Treatment Outcome Research (CATOR). The treatment providers were representative of the universe of for-profit treatment centers in the United States as defined and elaborated upon in the national survey.[7] CATOR is an independent evaluator for the addiction treatment programs that pay for the services. CATOR is not government supported through grant funding, is not a government agency, and is not owned by a treatment provider. The function of CATOR is to act as an external clinical auditor in evaluating the efficacy of the programs for achieving recovery from addiction and documenting correlates in recovery for the subjects as defined by the evaluation service.

The subjects selected consisted of a sample of 6355 from inpatient, outpatient evening, outpatient day, day hospital, and inpatient/evening programs from 41 sites. The subjects received a structured interview by evaluators employed by CATOR for data documentation of treatment outcome reflecting abstinence, psychosocial adjustment, psychiatric and medical use, employment status, and legal complications. The selection and evaluation of subjects were conducted prospectively in a structured personal interview on initial admission (383 questions) to the treatment program and by a structured telephone interview (110 questions) in the subsequent acquisition of data in follow-up at 6 and 12 months. The data were generated by experienced technicians whose full-time responsibility was to collect and enter data. The data analyses were conducted by statisticians. The personal and telephone interviews for data collection have been tested for validity and reliability in other studies.[1, 2]

The general descriptions and results of treatment outcome for the population have been reported elsewhere.[1, 2] Comparison of inpatient and outpatient programs for demographic and outcome characteristics has been reported elsewhere.[1, 2] Similar comparisons were used to determine the effects of continuum of care and the impact of treatment in this study.

For inclusion in the evaluation studies, the subjects required (1) a DSM-III-R diagnosis of substance use disorder and an evaluation specifically for (2) a DSM-III-R diagnosis of major depression. Excluded from the study were those who were not able to comprehend and cooperate with the structured evaluation (represented 3% of the total population). The completion rate for treatment stay was 5548 (87.3%): 263 (4.1%) were transferred, 348 (5.5%) left against medical advice, and 196 (3.1%) were discharged for noncompliance.

The majority of the treatment programs monitored were variations of the Minnesota abstinence-based 12-step principles with professional counseling services. The 12-step model adheres to the DSM-III-R recommendations that substance use disorders be independent and further stipulates that they require specific treatment. Most programs regularly refer the majority of patients to AA and encourage attendance at continuing care provided by the treatment program. Our subjects were selected from programs providing the predominant mode of treatment for addictive disorders nationally.

Sociodemographic Characteristics

The majority of the patients attended an inpatient treatment site (78.4%) followed by an outpatient structured program (16.9%). The population most represented was middle aged (35.7), male (70.6%), white (88.9%), high-school educated (84.6%), married (43.3%), employed (73.3%) (income $10,000 to $50,000), and living alone (55.7%). However, there was considerable variability on many of the demographic characteristics. Females (29.4%), blacks (7.9%), singles (56.7%), unemployed (16.4%), high (13.7%) and low education (15.4%) and incomes (<$10,000 [29.9%] and >$50,000 [5.9%]), and living with others were also represented. A substantial minority had received previous psychiatric treatments (31%), including treatment specifically for depression (24.2%).

The age of first use of alcohol was 16.8 years and of marijuana was 17.4 years.

DIAGNOSTIC CHARACTERISTICS OF MAJOR DEPRESSION

The rate of lifetime diagnosis of major depression was 43.7% and of subclinical depression was 9.6% in the total sample examined (6248). More than half of the patients had two or more symptoms of depression, and 35.9% had five or more symptoms of major depression. The most common diagnosis of a substance use disorder was of alcohol (51.3%), followed by cocaine (19.7%) and marijuana (12.3%) dependence. Most of the patients completed the program (87.3%).

Treatment Outcome Based on Abstinence Rates

The abstinence rate at 6 months was 74.2% for the overall sample was 67.7% for the second 6 months. The overall abstinence rate for one continuous year was 55.4% (Table 37–1). There were no significant differences in abstinence rates between those without a lifetime diagnosis of major depression and those with such a diag-

Table 37–1. Abstinence Rates

Abstinence and Relapse in First 6 Months		
	Frequency	*Percent*
Abstinent 6 months	4077	74.2
Relapse	1421	25.8
Abstinence and Relapse in Second 6 Months		
	Frequency	*Percent*
Abstinent 6 months	4249	67.7
Relapse	2025	32.3
Abstinence and Relapse for 1 Year		
	Frequency	*Percent*
Abstinent all year	3522	55.4
Abstinent past 6 months	238	3.7
Relapse	2595	40.8

nosis for either men (54.4% vs. 54.4%) or women (58.0% vs. 56.0%). In other words, the percent of those who suffered a relapse during the first year after addiction treatment was the same whether or not a diagnosis of major depression was present in their histories (Table 37–2).

In general, there were no significant differences between abstinence rates between non-depressed and depressed patients within drug diagnoses except for cocaine dependence in men (38.7% vs. 45.2%). The abstinence rates for alcohol, prescription drugs, cannabis, stimulant, cocaine (females), stimulant, and opiate disorders in men and women were the same. A diagnosis of major depression was not predictive of treatment outcome in any of the substance use disorders except for cocaine dependence in men, for which the abstinence rate was significantly less (see Table 37–2).

Predictors of Treatment Outcome in Those With and Without a Diagnosis of Major Depression

1. Major depression had an effect on continuing care/self-help attendance and treatment outcome. Depressed patients were significantly more likely to be regular attenders (49.2% vs. 45.4%) at self-help meetings or continuing care offered by the treatment provider (Table 37–3).

2. Greater abstinence occurred among regular attenders. Correspondingly, significantly greater abstinence rates for 1 year after discharge were found among those who were regular attenders at self-help meetings and continuing care. Abstinence rates were progressively greater with increasing attendance at self-help and continuing care services, ranging from no attendance, to occasional, to regular attendance. Those who regularly used these treatment opportunities achieved the greatest 1-year abstinence rate (72.2%), compared with occasional attenders (45.5%) and those who did not attend (38.6%) (see Table 37–3).

3. Diagnosis of major depression was not related to treatment outcome when self-help and continuing care were considered. When attendance at self-help groups and continuing care was considered, the presence of a diagnosis of major depression did not pre-

Table 37–2. Treatment Outcomes for Depressed Versus Nondepressed Patients

Treatment Outcome (1 Year) by Diagnosis of Major Depression

Treatment Outcome	No Depression History		Major Depression History	
	Males	Females	Males	Females
Abstinent all year	1492	464	919	584
	54.9%	58.0%	54.4%	56.0%
Abstinent only past 6 months	96	27	74	40
	3.5%	3.4%	4.4%	3.8%
Relapse	1130	309	695	418
	41.6%	38.6%	41.2%	40.1%

(Pearson chi-square $P = 0.36102$ for males, Pearson chi-square $P = 0.66169$ for females)

Treatment Outcome for Major Depression by Drug Type

	Abstinent 1 Year				Relapsed			
	No Depression		Depression		No Depression		Depression	
	M	F	M	F	M	F	M	F
Ungrouped*	115	35	54	40	68	27	27	16
$P = 0.550$†	62.8	56.5	66.7	71.4	37.2	43.5	33.3	28.6
Alcohol	954	288	426	266	643	157	303	179
$P = 0.553$†	59.7	64.7	58.4	59.8	40.3	35.3	41.6	40.2
Prescription drugs	28	26	44	77	17	11	30	40
$P = 0.764$†	62.2	70.3	59.5	65.8	37.8	29.6	40.5	34.2
Cannabis	181	24	125	9	175	35	134	49
$P = 0.527$†	50.8	40.7	48.3	50.0	49.2	59.3	51.7	50.0
Stimulant	28	11	55	39	26	10	28	40
$P = 0.092$†	51.9	52.4	66.3	49.4	48.1	47.6	33.7	50.6
Cocaine	172	68	84	91	278	91	222	119
$P = 0.035$†	38.2	42.8	45.2	43.3	61.8	57.2	54.7	56.7
Opiate	14	12	31	22	19	5	25	15
$P = 0.234$†	42.4	70.3	55.4	59.5	57.6	29.4	44.6	40.5

*Fewer than three criteria for substance use disorder.
†Pearson chi-square (in percentages).

Table 37–3. Abstinence Rates by Treatment Attendance

Continuing Care and Self-Help Attendance—Depressed Patients Were More Likely to Be Regular Attenders at Self-Help and/or Continuing Care

	No Depression	Major Depression
Never attended	609 (19.8%)	390 (16.5%)
Occasional attendance	1072 (34.8%)	808 (34.3%)
Regular attendance	1400 (45.4%)	1161 (49.2%)
(Pearson chi-square $P = 0.00278$)		

Greater Abstinence Among Regular Attenders

	No Attendance	Occasional	Regular
Abstinent all year	394 (38.6%)	868 (45.5%)	1877 (72.2%)
Relapse	626 (61.4%)	1039 (54.5%)	721 (27.8%)
(Pearson chi-square $P = 0.00001$)			

Diagnosis of Major Depression Is Not Related to Outcome When Support Group/Continuing Care Is Considered

	No Depression	Major Depression
No attendance		
Abstinent all year	243 (39.9%)	144 (36.9%)
Relapse	366 (60.1%)	246 (63.1%)
(Pearson chi-square $P = 0.34583$)		
Occasional attendance		
Abstinent all year	489 (45.6%)	366 (45.3%)
Relapse	583 (54.4%)	442 (54.7%)
(Pearson chi-square $P = 0.89075$)		
Regular attendance		
Abstinent all year	1019 (72.8%)	828 (71.3%)
Relapse	381 (27.2%)	333 (28.7%)
(Pearson chi-square $P = 0.40954$)		

Support Groups/Continuing Care and Not Depression Related to Treatment Outcome

	No Attendance	Occasional	Regular
Abstinent all year			
No depression	243 (39.9%)	489 (45.6%)	1019 (72.8%)
Major depression	144 (36.9%)	366 (45.3%)	828 (71.3%)
(Pearson chi-square $P = 0.00001$)			
Relapse			
No depression	366 (60.1%)	583 (54.4%)	381 (27.2%)
Major depression	246 (63.1%)	442 (54.7%)	333 (28.7%)
(Pearson chi-square $P = 0.00001$)			

Diagnosis of Major Depression Is Not Related to Recovery Status at 1 Year

	No Depression	Major Depression
Abstinent all year	1956 (55.6%)	1503 (55.1%)
Relapse	1562 (44.4%)	1227 (44.9%)
(Pearson chi-square $P = 0.66742$)		

dict abstinence rates at 1 year. There were no significant differences between nondepressed and depressed patients in treatment outcome for 1 year according to levels of attendance during postdischarge treatment. Nondepressed and depressed patients had the same abstinence rates within groups—no attendance (39.9% vs. 36.9%), occasional (45.6% vs. 45.3%), and regular attendance (72.8% vs. 71.3%) (see Table 37–3).

4. Support groups and continuing care but not depression were related to treatment outcome. There were no significant differences in abstinence rates for 1 year between nondepressed and depressed patients within

groups—no attendance (39.9% vs. 36.9%), occasional (45.6% vs. 45.3%), or regular attendance (72.8% vs. 71.3%). Greater attendance at postdischarge treatments significantly predicted the abstinence rates, but a diagnosis of major depression did not. Correspondingly, the abstinence rates increased with greater levels of attendance, from none, to occasional, to regular (see Table 37–3).

5. A diagnosis of major depression was not related to recovery status at 1-year follow-up. In comparing abstinence rates at 1 year between nondepressed (55.5%) and depressed (55.1%) patients, there were no significant differences at 1 year. A diagnosis of

major depression did not predict the recovery rate at 1 year (see Table 37–3).

Interpretation

The results are strongly suggestive that a lifetime diagnosis of major depression has little negative impact on the response to the abstinence-based method of addiction treatment for alcohol/drug disorders. Despite relatively high rates of a history of a diagnosis of major depression, its overall effect on treatment outcome for addictive disorders was not significant. The abstinence rates achieved by the nondepressed and depressed subjects who received the abstinence-based approach were not significantly different. The factors associated with a favorable outcome in nondepressed and depressed subjects were similar to those reported previously—namely, continuing care and participation in AA.

Contrary to assumptions made in clinical practice that depression is a prognosticator of a poor response to addiction treatment, depressed patients in this study were significantly more likely to attend continuing care and meetings of AA. It is known that those with a greater severity of illness are more likely to seek treatment, but it is less accepted that a history of depression continues to be associated with participation in long-term management with a favorable outcome. Depression was found to be a positive indicator of compliance with addiction treatment, continuing care, and attendance at AA. More recognized was the finding of significantly greater abstinence among those who were regular attenders at aftercare and AA, whether they were depressed or not. Those who achieved the greatest abstinence rates were those who were the most regular attenders. A dose-response relationship was observed, in that increasing abstinence was associated with greater participation in treatment after discharge—that is, 1-year abstinence was 72.2% for those who regularly attended aftercare and AA versus 38.6% for those who did not.

Of primary interest was that when continuing care and AA were controlled statistically, the lifetime diagnosis of major depression had no significant effect on treatment outcome. Moreover, there was no significant difference between depressed and nondepressed subjects in terms of treatment outcome at 1 year at any intensity of postdischarge treatments, regular versus occasional versus no attendance.

The demographic characteristics were those most closely resembling an educated, married, employed individual. The racial representation was disproportionately greater for whites than minorities, however. Blacks did represent nearly 8% of the sample. The gender ratio was similar to most treatment populations reported (three males to one female). The type of drug diagnosis did not predict treatment outcome except in the case of cocaine addiction in men. The better treatment outcome in depressed male cocaine addicts may reflect the overall finding that depressed addicts were more likely to be greater attenders at treatment and continuing care services and AA. The age of onset of alcohol and cannabis use was found to be consistent with findings of other studies that adolescence is a common period for initiation of alcohol and drug use, particularly among those who progress to addictive use.[1, 11]

The severity of the depression was sufficient for 25% of the total sample to have sought prior treatment for depression. The overall rate of depression was close to 50%; thus, it might be assumed that only half of those who were depressed received treatment for their depression in the past. The high rate of major depression in this sample is consistent with other studies that find depression and addictive disorders to be highly associated.

In many of these studies, the severity of the depression in subjects either before or during active alcohol/drug use or after withdrawal qualified as major depression according to the diagnostic criteria. What was not clear in the cross-sectional and retrospective studies was the actual rate of independent major depression because of the lack of control of the depression symptoms arising from the addictive disorder. The sources of the depression were multiple and poorly delineated in studies. Symptoms of depression may have been due to the consequences of the addictive disorder or independent of it. Longitudinal studies show lower rates of persistent depression after the detoxification period (5% to 15%).[12–14]

The clinical and etiological importance of the relationship between depression and alcohol/drug disorders has often been assumed in studies and clinical practice. Despite popular belief, little evidence shows that depression has a causal role in alcohol consumption, particularly addictive use, as suggested by the interpretations in the ECA studies.[4, 5] Moreover, studies show that alcoholics continue to drink despite alcohol-induced depression, and although nonalcoholic depressives experienced the greatest benefit in enhanced mood as a result of drinking alcohol, they did not drink when depressed.[4, 5] Rather, studies have shown depression to be negatively correlated with drinking in nonalcoholic manic-depressives.[15] The importance of treating the addictive disorder becomes clearer. Continued depression in the presence of drinking is more likely to be caused by the drinking.[16–18]

Conclusions

1. The prevalence rate of a lifetime diagnosis of major depression was high in treatment populations (43.7%) and was similar to the ECA findings.

2. A diagnosis of major depression was not a predictor of treatment outcome in response to specific abstinence-based forms of addiction treatment for substance use disorders.

3. Regular attendance at continuing care and AA meetings was associated with better abstinence rates at 1 year.

4. Persons with comorbid illnesses were more likely to be regular attenders at continuing care and AA meetings.

5. Abstinence rates exceeding 72.3% can be achieved in subjects with a lifetime history of major depression *and* substance use disorders when abstinence-based treatment is combined with continuing care and attendance at AA meetings after discharge.

REFERENCES

1. Hoffman NG, Miller NS: Treatment outcomes for abstinence based programs. Psychiatr Ann 22(8):402–408, 1992.
2. Harrison PA, Hoffmann NG, Streed SG: Drug and Alcohol Addiction Treatment Outcome. In Miller NS (ed): Comprehensive Handbook of Drug and Alcohol Addiction. New York, Marcel Dekker, 1991, pp 1163–1200.
3. Hesselbrock MN, Meyer RE, Keener JJ: Psychopathology in hospitalized alcoholics. Arch Gen Psychiatry 42:1050–1055, 1985.
4. Regier DA, Farmer ME, Rae DS, et al: Comorbidity of mental disorders with alcohol and other drug abuse. JAMA 264(19):2511–2518, 1990.
5. Helzer JE, Pryzbeck TR: The co-occurrence of alcoholism with other psychiatric disorders in the general population and its impact on treatment. J Stud Alcohol 49:219–224, 1988.
6. McClelland AT, Luborsky L, Woody GE: Predicting response to alcohol and drug abuse treatments: Role of psychiatric severity. Arch Gen Psychiatry 40:620–625, 1983.
7. Roman PM: Inpatient alcohol and drug treatment: A national study of treatment centers. Executive Report. NIAAA. Athens, GA, University of Georgia, Institute for Behavioral Research, 1989, pp 1–22.
8. Chappel JN: Long-term recovery from alcoholism. Psychiatr Clin North Am 16(1):430–435, 1993.
9. Keso L, Salaspuro M: Inpatient treatment of employed alcoholics: A randomized clinical trial on Hazelden-type and traditional treatment. Alcohol Clin Exp Res 14(4):584–589, 1990.
10. Walsh DC, Hingson RW, Merrigan DM, et al: A randomized trial of treatment options for alcohol-abusing workers. N Engl J Med 325(11):775–782, 1991.
11. Miller NS, Millman RB, Keskinen S: Outcome at six and twelve months post inpatient treatment for cocaine and alcohol dependence. Adv Alcohol Subst Abuse 9(3/4):101–120, 1990.
12. Schuckit MA: Alcoholism and other psychiatric disorders. Hosp Community Psychiatry 34:1022–1027, 1983.
13. Dorus W, Kennedy J, Gibbons RD, Ravi S: Symptoms and diagnosis for depression in alcoholics. Alcohol Clin Exp Res 11:150–154, 1987.
14. Blankfield A: Psychiatric symptoms in alcohol dependence: Diagnostic and treatment implications. J Subst Abuse Treat 3:275–278, 1986.
15. Mayfield DG, Allen D: Alcohol and affect: A psychopharmacological study. Am J Psychiatry 123:1346–1351, 1967.
16. Tamerin JS, Mendelson JH: The psychodynamics of chronic inebriation. Observations of alcoholics during the process of drinking in an experimental group setting. Am J Psychiatry 125:886–899, 1969.
17. Kosten TR, Kleber HD: Differential diagnosis of psychiatric comorbidity in substance abusers. J Subst Abuse Treat 5:201–206, 1988.
18. Dackis CA, Gold MS, Pottash ALC, Sweeney DR: Evaluating depression in alcoholics. Psychiatry Res 17:105–109, 1986.

New and Experimental Psychosocial Therapies in Alcoholism and Addiction

Joseph Westermeyer, MD, PhD •
Carl Isenhart, PsyD

The literature describing the outcome of alcohol dependence treatment does not recognize any single treatment approach as uniformly effective for all patients. Because all therapeutic techniques have various degrees of empirical support for their efficacy, the challenge for treatment professionals is to match patients with the most effective, safest, least expensive, and most rapidly acting intervention. This approach is based on the premise that treatment can be optimized through patient/treatment matching.[1, 2]

In undertaking an analysis of new and experimental psychosocial therapies, we begin by first defining these therapies. Then we identify critical factors (e.g., demographical variables, clinical characteristics, and longitudinal outcome considerations) that should compose a proper treatment evaluation. It is evident that many research studies in this field do not provide us with information that is useful in many clinical settings. Finally, we categorize these experimental or new therapies as follows: individual psychotherapies, group psychotherapies, social therapies, combinations of psychosocial therapies, and combined pharmacotherapies and psychosocial therapies.

Definitions

New and experimental psychosocial therapies, for purposes of this chapter, include both new psychosocial therapies that have not been evaluated (which are therefore experimental) and old psychosocial therapies that have not been evaluated (i.e., which are therefore also experimental). In other words, this chapter addresses the following groups of psychosocial therapies: (1) older therapies whose efficacy has not been demonstrated; (2) older therapies whose efficacy has been shown to be fair to good, but the appropriate target patient group has not been identified; and (3) new therapies that have not yet been evaluated. Although the focus of this review is on isolated psychosocial therapies, also included are combined psychosocial-somatotherapies (mostly pharmacotherapies), which in many respects are greater than the sum of their parts.

Of interest, some of the therapeutic modalities with the most careful scientific assessments are regarded as experimental. Examples include high-dose methadone maintenance for opiate dependence, Azrin's community reinforcement for alcoholism, aversion therapies for alcoholism, and Outward Bound for adolescent substance addiction. The low value placed on some of these modalities by the treatment community (e.g., high-dose methadone maintenance, aversion therapy) or the cost of setting up these modalities that involve nontraditional approaches (e.g., community reinforcement, Outward Bound) could explain why they are considered only experimental.

Conversely, other treatments with minimal data to support their clinical application remain unevaluated yet solidly within the mainstream of treatment. We know that Alcoholics Anonymous (AA) helps a percentage of patients, but we know little about selecting those likely to fare best with this approach. Some patients improve with minimal interventions, yet we do not know what distinguishes these patients; thus, we tend to provide lengthy, intensive, and extensive treatment as often as we can.

Criteria for Clinical Investigations

What are the elements of an adequate clinical evaluation for treatment of alcoholism/addictions? Unless we can show otherwise, these criteria should be those used in assessing any chronic or recurrent disease or disorder, from cancer to mood disorder. In other words, we should be able to distinguish treatment responders by their demographical characteristics and by their clinical characteristics (e.g., duration, severity, staging). Then we should observe them sufficiently long to be able to discern short-term placebo effects from long-term treatment success.

Demographical Considerations. In order for a therapy to be applied in an effective and economical fashion, clinicians must be able to identify those psychosocial therapies most useful for a particular age, sex, and socioeconomic level (i.e., education, occupation, residence, social status, resources). For most behavioral-neurotransmitter disorders, we do not apply the same therapeutic approaches for 10-, 30-, 50-, and 70-year-olds. However, in the alcoholism/addictions field, most therapeutic approaches have evolved from treatment with middle-class married men in the 30- to 50-year age range. These results have been extrapolated, on faith, to other groups. To apply psychosocial therapies efficiently, we must have information about their efficacy in various demographic groups.

Clinical Characteristics. Severity, duration, symptom patterns, and comorbidity of disorders have major roles in deciding on treatment alternatives. For example, the treatment of a major depression, mild severity, of 2 weeks' duration, with no comorbidity is likely to differ greatly from the treatment of a major depression, with psychotic features, present for 1 year, and associated with panic and agoraphobia. Similarly, in the alcoholism/addictions field, treatment outcome studies must include greater pathological description before treatments can be efficiently and effectively applied. Otherwise, every patient tends to receive every therapy.

Longitudinal Outcome Considerations. To assess psychosocial therapies, adequate periods of time must elapse. Short-term follow-up studies lasting less than several months are confounded by the following factors:

- All therapies, especially psychosocial therapies, have a placebo effect that persists for a few months and then wanes over time.
- Recurrence of alcoholism and the addictions is greatest during the first several weeks to several months after treatment, with stable recovery occurring mostly in those who are abstinent and improved at 6 to 12 months.[1]
- Truly effective therapies are most likely to demonstrate their actual efficacy if compared with a placebo (i.e., as part of a controlled study) for a period lasting 6 months or longer.

Individual Therapies

AVERSION THERAPIES

Aversion therapies are based on *counterconditioning,* the goal of which is to associate alcohol with unpleasant reactions by pairing alcohol with negative images or experiences. A number of procedures have been used to create aversive circumstances.[1] Emetic drugs have been most commonly used to associate nausea and vomiting with alcohol. Electrical and apneic techniques, once used and even closely studied, have fallen into disfavor.

Aversive therapies are controversial because of (1) the potential risk involved, (2) the ethical dilemma of exposing alcohol-dependent individuals to alcohol, and (3) mixed results regarding outcome efficacy. Despite some reports of high abstinence rates (especially in high socioeconomic groups), other studies have shown no increased efficacy of aversive treatment as an addition to standard treatment.

One alternative to the usual chemical-physical aversion techniques is so-called covert sensitization. This technique involves pairing aversive imagery (e.g., mental images of oneself becoming ill and vomiting) with mental images of consuming alcohol. The images may be enhanced by providing whiffs of putrid odors (e.g., valeric acid). Because a patient has control over the process and is an active agent in this approach, covert sensitization has ethical advantages over former aversive interventions. It is also safer. Moreover, it has been found to affect treatment outcome, is less noxious to patients, and can be performed on an outpatient basis.

MOTIVATIONAL INTERVIEWING

Motivational interviewing[3] is an intervention that is particularly suited for individuals who are ambivalent about changing their addictive behavior. It is a patient-centered, nondirective attitude or approach to interacting with patients and moving them toward behavioral changes. Motivational interviewing differs from traditional approaches in that the latter assume that patients have already decided to change. Traditional methods then simply assist patients in accomplishing changes that they want to achieve. Motivational interviewing, on the other hand, facilitates ambivalent individuals in deciding whether they want to change. Responsibility for change is put on the patients.

The clinician's style in motivational interviewing is persuasive, educational, and supportive rather than suggestive, directive, or interpretive. The clinician avoids coercive and argumentative approaches. Patients are not pushed to label themselves as alcoholics. This method views resistance as an interpersonal phenomenon that is partially influenced by the therapist rather than due entirely to the patient. Patient and clinician carefully negotiate and renegotiate treatment goals as they proceed rather than assume that each shares the other's goals. In this therapeutic approach, clinicians may seem both more detached (in that they accept patients' motivation as primary and they accept patients' goals as the goals of treatment) and more involved (in that they persuade, support, and inform patients) than in traditional approaches.

Motivational interviewing has five guiding principles. The first principle is accepting a patient's opinions and perspectives instead of challenging or correcting them. This does not necessarily mean blanket approval of a patient's opinions but rather respectful consideration of a patient's perspective. The second principle is creating and exploiting discrepancies between a patient's ideal self and reality. This process creates cognitive dissonance by having patients detail the ways in which their addictive behavior conflicts with their goals. For example, a man might state as a goal his intent to be a good father but then spend more time in the tavern than with the family. Raising this discrepancy to a conscious level cuts through the denial or minimization often present in such cases. The third principle is to avoid arguments. Arguments frequently elicit resistance. They also stimulate many recovering patients to do the opposite of what was requested, in an attempt to demonstrate their freedom of choice and independence. As a recovering person seeks to achieve freedom from dependence on psychoactive substances, this drive for independence can produce therapeutic results. The fourth principle consists of accepting resistance as a normal and natural part of the change process. In fact, the absence of resistance can be viewed as antitherapeutic because nonresisting patients seldom make behavioral changes. Instead, the resistance plus the distress of cognitive dissonance appears critical to undertaking important changes. The fifth principle is supporting self-efficacy. This involves the clinician's viewing a patient as a person who is able to make changes. Further, the clinician supports a patient's self-perception of being able to change by providing a patient with options and alternatives, which a patient may then choose or refuse.

CUE EXTINCTION

Cue extinction is based on learning theory. As applied to drug use, this theory holds that cues trigger cravings for drugs through classical or pavlovian conditioning.[4] Its application to drug addiction has been based largely on the work of O'Brien and colleagues.[5, 6] The goal of a cue extinction program is to extinguish the association between triggers and cravings by exposing the patient (through imagery) to the craving-arousing cues in a protective environment where drugs are not available. Through a process of desensitization, cues lose their association with drug use. As a result, the cues then lose their ability to elicit urges and cravings.

The process of cue extinction first involves identifying those cues or triggers that elicit an urge to use. Such triggers can be external (e.g., certain people or places or drug paraphernalia) or internal (e.g., thoughts or feelings). A patient then assesses the intensity of the cues on a rating scale, rank ordering them or giving them an arbitrary score (e.g., based on a score of 100 for the strongest cue). A cue extinction program or tool is then devised. After implementation of this program to reduce the intensity of the craving, the rating scale is used again to reassess the craving's intensity.

Several cue extinction tools are commonly used to disassociate the cue from the cravings. Relaxation, one of these tools, is based on reciprocal inhibition. That is, a person cannot experience emotional arousal (i.e., cravings and urges) and relaxation simultaneously. Therefore, relaxation inhibits the experience of cravings. Delay involves the postponement of using to allow the craving to fade. Distraction, often used along with delay, consists of imagining a distracting activity to draw attention away from the craving. Examining the positive and negative consequences of using and not using is another tool. This technique attempts to tilt the balance from wanting to use to not using. Mastery imagery involves patients' imagining themselves in a position of power in which they overcome the craving. Finally, straight thinking has patients identify and change thoughts that may precipitate using. For example, a patient may change the thought "I can handle just one" to the thought "I can't handle just one, because I sometimes end up relapsing."

This approach can also be combined with naltrexone (discussed later).

COGNITIVE THERAPIES

Cognitive therapies are based on the theory that emotional distress is produced or exacerbated by irrational or distorted thoughts or beliefs about events and circumstances. The goal is to help people become more aware of their distorted thinking and to replace those thoughts with more rational thoughts, thereby reducing emotional distress. The basis for applying this approach to substance addicts lies in the theory that they use alcohol or drugs to manage and cope with emotional distress and problems. Consequently, they can use cognitive therapy strategies as alternatives to using addictive substances.[7, 8]

The goal is not to eliminate feelings. Rather, the first goal is recognize feelings, which are then reframed as normal and natural consequences of distressful situations. Patients learn that feelings, if properly managed, can be used to help cope with problems. The second goal is to reduce the intensity, frequency, and duration of the emotional distress and to keep the affect from escalating to the point where the individual makes a bad situation even worse—for example, a woman who, after a disagreement with her husband, goes out drinking and is arrested for driving while intoxicated. In this case, the woman first learns to recognize her feelings toward her husband and then the thoughts that bolster these feelings (e.g., "He hates me" or "He does not respect me"). Through changing the distorted nature of these thoughts (e.g., "He does love me; we simply disagree over this one issue and must negotiate a resolution"), she can then reduce her overwhelming feelings to manageable proportions.

Cognitive and behavioral techniques can be used to challenge and change irrational beliefs. Cognitive strategies include questioning the evidence for the validity of the thoughts, looking at the disadvantages of the thinking patterns, using imagery, and reframing the event into something positive or constructive despite the distress and turmoil. Behavioral strategies include daily thought records, relaxation training, stimulus control, and engaging in graded and risk-taking activities (e.g., performing a feared or stressful activity).

Ellis and coworkers[8] characterized addictive irrational thoughts as being automatic, inflexible, overlearned, dichotomous, overgeneralized, and nonempirical. They also identified common types of irrational beliefs that are prevalent among people who have alcohol/drug problems. These irrational beliefs focus on the following conceptual areas:

1. Ideas about their alcohol/drug use (e.g., "I'm doomed to frustration with alcohol")
2. Ideas about their capacity to deal with emotional distress (e.g., "I can't stand these feelings")
3. Ideas about themselves and their self-worth (e.g., "I'm a worthless person because of my addiction")

These three types of thoughts lead to negative feelings and behaviors. Accordingly, they need to be disputed and replaced by more constructive thoughts.

Beck and coworkers[7] likewise identified certain core addictive beliefs that are important to dispute. Their work has suggested that patients have incorrect or dysfunctional ideas about the psychoactive substance(s) that they are using. These beliefs about the psychoactive substance are as follows:

1. The person needs the substance to function and to feel normal.

2. The substance improves the person's mental or social functioning.

3. The substance creates positive feelings and stimulation.

4. The substance increases the person's sense of power.

5. The substance reduces negative affect.

6. The substance is soothing.

7. The substance is the only thing that reduces urges and cravings.

These researchers also identified permission-giving beliefs that may serve to encourage continued substance addiction. Some permission-giving beliefs may be classified as justification beliefs (e.g., "Who could blame me for using the substance under these circumstances?") and as entitlement beliefs (e.g., "I deserve to use after working on my sobriety for 3 months.").

RELAPSE PREVENTION

The concept of relapse prevention received a great deal of attention after the work of Marlatt and Gordon.[9] It aims at maintaining behavior change after cessation of substance abuse.

Although many types of programs have been instituted since Marlatt and Gordon's original publication, relapse prevention typically involves the following:

1. Anticipating and identifying high-risk situations

2. Generating alternative ways to manage these situations

3. Practicing strategies to prevent relapse from occurring

Strategies for preventing relapse include cognitive and behavioral interventions, lifestyle changes, and reframing the relapse. The last concept of reframing has been particularly important. A distinction is made between a lapse (initial substance use) and a relapse (a continuation of substance addiction to preabstinence levels). Although the main goal is to prevent a relapse, emphasis is also placed on preventing a lapse from becoming a relapse. A major component of this process is to think differently (i.e., reframe the lapse). This consists of changing a patient's view of the lapse as a sign of permanent treatment failure or an indication of hopeless addiction and helping the patient gain a more rational perspective. Patients are urged to view the lapse as a temporary slip, which has occurred in response to a specific set of circumstances and which does not necessarily predict continued use.

The concept of relapse prevention applies to all habitual behaviors. Although adjustments are made to accommodate specific habitual behaviors, the processes of identifying high-risk situations (whether for drinking, smoking, gambling, or overeating) and developing strategies to manage them are similar.

Relapse prevention can be readily integrated into other therapeutic interventions. For example, it may be a component in couples counseling, social skills training, and cognitive interventions. Its independent or additive effect vis-à-vis other modalities is not well understood, although early efforts have begun to assess its utility in association with naltrexone and contingency contracting.[10]

Couples Therapy

Marital stability at entering treatment augurs a favorable treatment outcome.[11] Moreover, marital conflict may contribute to substance addiction, and substance addiction may precipitate marital conflict. Thus, it seems reasonable to assume that couples counseling might improve the chances of a positive outcome in addictive disorders.

The work of O'Farrell and colleagues[12-14] exemplifies the types of interventions available for substance addicts and their partners. O'Farrell and coworkers conceptualize couples counseling as having three phases:

1. Obtaining commitment of the substance addict and the partner to change: The spouse and family members motivate the substance addict to change his or her drinking, and the therapist must obtain the partner's commitment to change

2. Making changes: stopping or reducing substance addiction and changing the interpersonal patterns to create an environment more conducive to sobriety

3. Maintaining changes: preventing relapse and dealing with interpersonal issues associated with sobriety

O'Farrell also described the types of patients most likely to benefit from couples counseling and identified some common obstacles. Substance addiction–related crises, violence, and blaming portend poor outcomes unless they can be rapidly brought under control.

Once a couple's commitment is obtained, several strategies are available to obtain short-term change, as follows:

1. Establishing and clarifying expectations (e.g., Is alcohol kept in the house? Can the nondependent spouse consume alcohol?)

2. Behavioral contracting

3. Disulfiram contracts (discussed later)

4. Identifying and eliminating a spouse's behaviors that may precipitate substance addiction (e.g., nagging, starting arguments over minor matters)

5. Increasing positive encounters and reducing negative encounters

Positive encounters can be increased through arranging caring behaviors (ways to show caring toward the spouse), engaging in shared leisure and recreational activities, and identifying and using core symbols (places, objects, or activities that have special meaning for the couple). Partners who have lost civility, love, and respect for each other can benefit by going through a period of courting in which they date each other. During such a period, they can ascertain whether they can restore the common interests and attractions that once brought them together or establish new themes and venues for a renewed relationship. Negative encounters can be reduced through communication and problem-solving training and by making change agreements. An example of a change agreement would be learning to negotiate requests of each other in lieu of unilateral demands or unspoken (and often disappointed) expectations.

These initial changes can be maintained by preparing for the maintenance stage before the end of the initial change period. This consists, first, in identifying potential high-risk situations. Then the couple rehearses ways to prevent the event. Last, they practice ways to cope with the relapse when or if it occurs. These principles of relapse prevention, drawn from individual patient therapy, apply just as well to couples counseling.

O'Farrell and Cowles[14] described several research projects that support the effectiveness of couples counseling on treatment outcome. In addition, couples counseling can take place in a group format,[15] can help families with more than one substance addict,[13] and has been shown to increase compliance with disulfiram treatment.[12]

Alternative Self-Help Groups

Substance addicts are commonly referred to AA. However, no referral guidelines have been set up to identify those patients likely to benefit from AA, those patients not likely to benefit, and (as with most modes of therapy) those patients likely to be made worse by AA. The effectiveness of AA lacks empirical support, because controlled studies are few and effectiveness relies strongly on compliance for a prolonged period. Studies of AA have shown a high dropout rate, in the range of 85%. Consequently, alternative self-help groups have been receiving more evaluation.

Rational Recovery (RR).[16] RR has a basis in cognitive therapy. It deemphasizes the lifelong commitment to a self-help group and discourages labeling participants as alcoholics. Moreover, it does not use the concepts of powerlessness, loss of control, or a Higher Power. Rather, interventions are based on the concepts of cognitive therapy. Patients use group support and feedback to find rational ways of thinking about their experiences and of managing negative affect to be less dependent on substances. Galanter and colleagues reported positive outcomes with RR.[17]

Women for Sobriety (WFS).[18] WFS was developed to provide women with an alternative to AA. Those who started WFS perceived AA as too negative (because it dwells on past misdeeds, focuses on character defects, and encourages dependence on outside support) and as placing too much emphasis on "drunkalogues" and past mistakes. In contrast, WFS emphasizes rebuilding a woman's self-confidence, thinking in a more positive way, becoming more spiritual, and growing emotionally. Women perceive WFS, compared with AA, as being more supportive, a safer place to discuss women's issues, more positive, and a better way to build self-esteem.

Alcoholics Victorious (AV). AV was begun in 1948 for middle-aged Christian male alcoholics. AV emphasizes that substance addiction is a sin and that developing a relationship with Christ through the "Seven Steps to Victory" is the only way to sobriety. These steps provide guidance for spiritual growth and are based on references to the Bible. The goal is not just to stop using addicting substances but to replace these "sinful" habits with more righteous behaviors through learning God's word and letting Christ fill the void that was previously filled by the use of chemicals.

Social Therapies

SOCIAL SKILLS TRAINING

Social skills training is based on social learning theory.[19] It suggests that people learn to use substances in a habitual and maladaptive way to cope with stress and problems through combinations of the following mechanisms: operant conditioning (i.e., positive and negative reinforcement), modeling, classical (pavlovian) conditioning, and expectancies that develop through interactions with culture, family, and peers. These psychobehavioral-social mechanisms, combined with biological and genetic factors, predispose an individual to be substance dependent.

The goal of social skills training is to teach and enhance interpersonal and intrapersonal functioning as more constructive ways to manage problems. Monti and colleagues[20] developed a comprehensive treatment program based on social learning theory and using social skills training as the major intervention. Deficits in interpersonal functioning include lack of social supports and relationships, social skills deficits, and impaired interpersonal functioning. Intrapersonal dysfunction includes problematical moods, cognitions, and expectations.

Both interpersonal and intrapersonal interventions address general skills deficits as well as those specifically related to substance addiction. For example, general interpersonal interventions include improving listening skills and assertiveness. Specific interpersonal interventions include acquiring drink refusal skills and managing criticism about drinking. General intrapersonal interventions include stress and anger management and relaxation. Specific intrapersonal interventions include managing thoughts about using alcohol or drugs as well as identifying and coping with seemingly irrelevant decisions (i.e., those decisions that, in hindsight, eventually lead up to a relapse). Monti and associates[20] provided empirical support for these types of approaches.

COMMUNITY REINFORCEMENT APPROACH

A community reinforcement approach consists of various social components that suppress alcohol use and provide a wide range of interventions that address problems of living.[21] Overall, these techniques provide an alternative to traditional treatment approaches. The interventions typically last for 4 to 6 weeks. They emphasize rapid integration of patients into the program and involvement of a significant other person committed to a patient's recovery. The significant other person is particularly important because of the need to verify a patient's self-report and the importance of monitoring a patient's disulfiram use.

The community reinforcement approach consists of the following core components:
1. Sobriety sampling (negotiating a period of abstinence to sample the experience)

2. Disulfiram administration (although the research has demonstrated the effectiveness of the community reinforcement approach without the use of disulfiram)
3. Functional analysis of high-risk situations
4. Problem solving and social skills training
5. Social counseling (to develop hobbies and other recreational activities)
6. Mood monitoring

Additional interventions may be available if needed by a patient—for example, counseling, marital therapy, reinforcer access counseling (learning to use common sources of information such as television or the newspaper), relaxation training, and drink refusal training.

Azrin developed the community reinforcement approach in 1973. He and coworkers demonstrated it to be more effective than traditional inpatient and outpatient treatments.[21–24] However, validation studies by other investigators have been lacking.

CIVIL COMMITMENT

The civil commitment process is a procedure by which individuals are involuntarily required to participate in treatment as a result of chronic substance addiction that has resulted in medical, social, or economical impairment. According to Chavkin,[25] three commitment models are typically used:
1. General commitment for mental disorders (where substance addiction is considered a mental disorder)
2. Commitment statutes specific for substance addiction (which may require that an individual be charged with or convicted of a crime)
3. Commitment statutes specific to pregnant substance addicts

Civil commitment for substance addiction problems is not a new concept.[25] Such a process was originally proposed after the passage of the Harrison Act of 1914. Later, in 1919, narcotics farms were established to treat and incarcerate heroin addicts. In 1962, the California Civil Addict Program incarcerated narcotic addicts for as long as 7 years without their being charged with a crime. The Narcotic Addict Rehabilitation Act, enacted by Congress in 1966, committed convicted offender-addicts as well as narcotic users charged with (but not yet convicted of) nonviolent federal crimes. Finally, in 1972, the Nixon administration formed the Special Action Office for Drug Abuse Prevention, which involved compulsory community-based treatment.

The civil commitment process begins with

the courts' being petitioned for a commitment hearing. This petition can be requested by the family or significant other persons, healthcare providers, social service agencies, or law enforcement or other government agencies.[26] The subject of the petition is evaluated by a mental health professional and can have his or her own counsel and independent experts. If the individual is committable, a course of treatment for a specific period is ordered by the court. Treatment interventions include a wide range of options such as inpatient, outpatient, or residential care and aftercare and case management. If an individual is compliant and progress is assessed at the end of the commitment period, the commitment can be lifted. However, if an individual is noncompliant or progress is not noted, the commitment may be extended.

Other options are also available. For example, a continuance may be granted. That is, there is no formal commitment because the patient has agreed to go to treatment and to comply with recommendations. However, the individual is reevaluated at a later date (e.g., in 30 to 60 days) and, depending on his or her status, may have to return to court for another hearing. The commitment can be stayed. In this case, the patient agrees to go to treatment and comply with treatment. As long as the patient is compliant, the commitment is never enacted; however, if the patient is noncompliant, the stay is revoked and the patient is committed.

Outcome research in this area has produced variable results. Dunham and Mauss[27] found that coerced patients had a greater likelihood of positive treatment outcome than noncoerced patients. However, Anglin and colleagues[28] found no difference between voluntary and involuntary patients receiving methadone maintenance.

Combined Pharmacotherapy and Psychosocial Therapy

CONTINGENCY CONTRACTING AND DISULFIRAM

Considerable research has been directed at evaluating disulfiram therapy, usually in association with regular counseling visits, individual psychotherapy, or supervision. Results of studies in which the alcoholic subjects decided whether or not to take disulfiram were variable; one study showed good results in association with disulfiram,[29] and another study demonstrated no benefit.[30] Controlled studies, with random assignment of subjects to disulfiram or placebo, have shown more diverse outcomes: Some have shown modest but definite improvement,[31–33] whereas others have shown limited or no discernible benefit.[34]

In light of these mixed results, other therapeutic approaches have been attempted in combination with disulfiram. One of these is contingency contracting, in which patients agree to take disulfiram on a regular, often supervised basis. In return, alcoholic patients obtain something of value. Unfortunately, we have few studies of this combined approach, and these studies typically have few subjects. Moreover, these studies are either controlled or involve comparison of the pre–contingency contracting course with the post–contingency contracting course. Thus, the results of this combined approach are tentative.

An early contingency contracting–disulfiram study involved the use of money in a security deposit. Failure to make a clinic visit resulted in loss of some of the funds; the remaining amount was returned to the patient at the end of the study. Among 20 subjects, 80% achieved long abstinence in the post–contingency contracting condition as compared with the pre–contingency contracting condition.[35] In a later study, habitual offenders obtained probation as an alternative to incarceration in return for taking disulfiram. This group also fared well in the post–contingency contracting period as compared with the pre–contingency contracting period.[36] Other contingencies widely used by clinicians include return to the family home and continued employment. Despite the widespread use of this technique by many clinicians, it has thus far not received careful research evaluation.

CONTINGENCY CONTRACTING AND NALTREXONE

Naltrexone is an opioid antagonist that blocks the action of opioid drugs.[37] In addition to its role in blocking exogenous opioids in opioid addiction,[38] it has also been used for other disorders (i.e., alcoholism, bulimia) to block endogenous opioids, albeit with equivocal to nil results.[39] Several special populations have taken naltrexone, including addicted physicians, other healthcare workers exposed to opioids in their work, business executives, other middle-class addicts, and incarcerated addicts.[40–43]

Two studies have addressed the combination of contingency contracting and naltrexone. Despite the suggestions of efficacy in both studies, both have their limitations. In the first study involving incarcerated addicts, the contingency was work release from prison.[40] Although the sample size was large, a control group and careful quantitative outcome data were absent. Kosten and Kleber reported data on contingency payments and behavioral modification techniques in a group of naltrexone-treated patients.[10] It appears from their data that use of payments as a contingency improved the retention rate of addicts in treatment by as much as 25% of subjects (grouping the data from several different cells). Moreover, the combination of other behavioral modification techniques (i.e., thought stopping, relaxation techniques) further augmented the effect of contingency contracting in keeping patients in treatment.

MULTIPLE FAMILY THERAPY AND NALTREXONE

Kosten and Kleber have also assessed the interactive effect of naltrexone and multiple family therapy on retention of addicts in treatment.[44] The control group received naltrexone plus routine case management. At 8 months, more than 25% of the patients receiving naltrexone and family therapy were retained in treatment, whereas virtually none of the patients receiving naltrexone and case management remained in treatment. Although this is only one study at one facility in one sample of patients, further studies certainly are warranted. The combination of this blocking agent with a particular psychosocial therapy may be greater than the sum of its parts.

Unfortunately, the Kosten-Kleber study provided no data on family therapy plus case management (without naltrexone) to assess the effect of family therapy in this study. This points up the difficulty (as well as the added expense) of conducting such research on combined therapies. In such studies, one needs not simply one control group but two groups. If A and B are the therapies under study, the investigator must include an A/non-B control group as well as a B/non-A control group to assess the effect of the combined A/B treatment intervention.

In addition to release from incarceration and payments, other contingencies can be used in association with naltrexone. We have used some of the following contingencies:

- For physicians, dentists, nurses, and pharmacists: return to clinical employment in oc-

cupations that involve repeated exposure to opioid drugs; retention of licensure
- For patients with homes and jobs: return to their jobs or homes

Summary

Many older psychosocial therapies have not been adequately evaluated, for various historical, political, and economical reasons. Numerous evaluations conducted in the past are flawed for diverse methodological reasons (i.e., overly small samples, narrow or biased samples, absence of appropriate control group or groups, overly brief follow-up periods, inadequate research instruments, poor descriptions of patients and their outcomes). Thus, many traditional therapies in this field are in fact experimental.

A number of new psychosocial therapies have been developed. These should properly be considered experimental unless adequate research findings document their efficacy. Many of these therapies are elaborations of previous modalities used in the alcoholism/addictions field or of older modalities used for other psychiatric and psychosocial problems. Examples include the following:

- New and safer methods of aversion therapy (using imagery)
- More specific methods of counseling and therapy adapted to patients with alcoholism and addictions (e.g., motivational counseling)
- Cue extinction (a combination of relapse prevention and behavioral modification to address the problem of craving)
- Aspects of cognitive therapy adapted to specific issues of recovery from alcoholism and addiction
- Relapse prevention, especially in combination with other modalities
- Inclusion of new approaches and concepts for couples/marital therapy of alcoholism and the addictions
- New forms of self-help groups (with different compositions, assumptions, values, and goals)
- Social skills training designed specifically for recovering alcoholic/addicted persons
- Community reinforcement (an approach that was studied two decades ago but not replicated in other settings and not widely applied)
- Innovative and therapeutic use of civil commitment designed for the support and

monitoring of recovering persons, with timely intervention in the event of relapse

Especially new are the studies of combined therapies, an area that is both traditional (because many programs involve a shotgun approach using many modalities) and experimental (because the combined effect of even well-researched modalities may be either greater or less than the sum of their independent effects). These combinations may involve two psychosocial therapies, such as contingency contracting and relapse prevention. They may also include combinations of somatotherapies and psychosocial therapies, such as combined disulfiram and contingency contracting or combined naltrexone and family therapy. Few studies have been conducted in this important area. The design of these few studies leaves unanswered questions, pointing up the need for new methods of undertaking such studies (such as the use of more than one control group).

REFERENCES

1. Institute of Medicine: Broadening the Base of Treatment for Alcohol Problems. Washington, DC, National Academy Press, 1990.
2. Miller WR: Matching individuals with interventions. In Hester RK, Miller WR (eds): Handbook of Alcoholism Treatment Approaches. New York, Pergamon Press, 1989, pp 261–272.
3. Miller WR, Rollnick S: Motivational Interviewing: Preparing People to Change Addictive Behavior. New York, Guilford Press, 1991.
4. National Institute of Drug Abuse: Cue Extinction: Handbook for Program Administrators. Rockville, MD, US Dept of Health and Human Services, 1993.
5. O'Brien CP, Childress AR, McLellan T: Pharmacological and behavioral treatments of cocaine dependence: Controlled studies. J Clin Psychiatry 49:17–22, 1988.
6. O'Brien CP, Childress AR, McLellan T: Integrating systematic cue exposure with standard treatment in recovering drug dependent cases. Addict Behav 15:355–365, 1990.
7. Beck AT, Wright FD, Newman CF, Liese BS: Cognitive Therapy of Substance Abuse. New York, Guilford Press, 1993.
8. Ellis A, McInerny JF, DiGiuseppe R, Yeager RJ: Rational-Emotive Therapy with Alcoholics and Substance Abusers. New York, Pergamon Press, 1988.
9. Marlatt GA, Gordon JR: Relapse Prevention: Maintenance Strategies in the Treatment of Addictive Behaviors. New York, Guilford Press, 1985.
10. Kosten TR, Kleber HD: The clinical use of naltrexone: Strategies to improve compliance. Substance Abuse Bulletin 1(3):1–4, 1994.
11. Moos RH, Finney JW, Cronkite RC: Alcoholism Treatment: Context, Process, and Outcome. New York, Oxford University Press, 1990.
12. O'Farrell TJ, Bayog RD: Antabuse contracts for married alcoholics and their spouses: A method to maintain Antabuse ingestion and decrease conflict about drinking. J Subst Abuse Treat 3:1–8, 1986.
13. O'Farrell TJ: Marital and family therapy for alcohol problems. In Cox WM (ed): Treatment and Prevention of Alcohol Problems: A Resource Manual. New York, Academic Press, 1987, pp 205–234.
14. O'Farrell TJ, Cowles KS: Marital and family therapy. In Hester R, Miller WR (eds): Handbook of Alcoholism Treatment Approaches. New York, Pergamon Press, 1989, pp 183–205.
15. O'Farrell TJ: Couples group interventions with alcoholism problems: A behavioral approach. In Zinberg NE, Shaffer HS (eds): Group Approaches to Intoxicant Problems. New York, International Universities Press (in press).
16. Trimby J: Rational Recovery from Alcoholism: The Small Book. Lotus, CA, Lotus Press, 1989.
17. Galanter M, Egelko S, Edwards H: Rational Recovery: Alternative to AA for addiction? Am J Drug Alcohol Abuse 19:499–510, 1993.
18. Kaskutas LA: What do women get out of self help? J Subst Abuse Treat (in press).
19. Abrams DB, Niaura RS: Social learning theory. In Blane HT, Leonard KE (eds): Psychological Theories of Drinking and Alcoholism. New York, Guilford Press, 1987, pp 131–178.
20. Monti PM, Abrams DB, Kadden RM, Cooney NL: Treating Alcohol Dependence: A Coping Skills Training Guide. New York, Guilford Press, 1989.
21. Hunt GM, Azrin NH: A community-reinforcement approach to alcoholism. Behav Res Ther 11:91–104, 1973.
22. Azrin NH: Improvements in the community-reinforcement approach to alcoholism. Behav Res Ther 14:339–348, 1976.
23. Azrin NH, Sisson RW, Meyers R, Godley M: Alcoholism treatment by disulfiram and community reinforcement therapy. J Behav Ther Exp Psychiatry 13:105–112, 1982.
24. Miller WR, Meyers RF, Tonigan JS, Hester RK, (eds): Effectiveness of the Community Reinforcement Approach. Albuquerque, NM, Center on Alcoholism, Substance Abuse, and Addictions, 1992.
25. Chavkin DF: For their own good: Civil commitment of alcohol and drug-dependent women. South Dakota Law Review 37:224–228, 1992.
26. Brown BS: Civil Commitment: International Issues. NIDA Res Monogr 86:192–208, 1988.
27. Dunham RG, Mauss AL: Reluctant referrals: The effectiveness of legal coercion in outpatient treatment for problem drinkers. J Drug Issues 12(1):5–20, 1982.
28. Anglin MD, Brecht ML, Maddahian E: Pretreatment characteristics and treatment performance of legally coerced versus voluntary methadone maintenance admissions. Criminology 27(3):537, 1989.
29. Sereny G, Sharma V, Holt J, Gordis E: Mandatory supervised Antabuse therapy in an outpatient alcoholism program: A pilot study. Alcohol Clin Exp Res 10(3):290–292, 1986.
30. Schuckit MA: A one-year follow-up of men alcoholics given disulfiram. J Stud Alcohol 46(3):191–195, 1985.
31. Gerrein JR, Rosenberg CM, Manohar V: Disulfiram maintenance in outpatient treatment of alcoholism. Arch Gen Psychiatry 28:798–802, 1973.
32. Fuller RK, Williford WO: Life-table analysis of abstinence in a study evaluating the efficacy of disulfiram. Alcohol Clin Exp Res 4(3):298–301, 1980.
33. Chick J, Gough K, Falkowski W, et al: Disulfiram treatment of alcoholism. Br J Psychiatry 161:84–89, 1992.
34. Fuller RK, Branchey L, Brightwell DR, et al: Disulfiram treatment of alcoholism: A Veterans Administration cooperative study. JAMA 256(11):1449–1455, 1986.
35. Bigelow G, Strickler D, Liebson I, Griffiths R: Maintaining disulfiram ingestion among outpatient alcohol-

ics: A security contingency contracting procedure. Behav Res Ther 14:378–381, 1976.

36. Brewer C, Smith J: Probation linked supervised disulfiram in the treatment of habitual drunken offenders: Results of a pilot study. Br Med J 287:1282–1283, 1983.

37. Resnick RB, Volavka J, Freedman AM, Thomas M: Studies of EN-1639A (naltrexone): A new narcotic antagonist. Am J Psychiatry 131(6):646–650, 1974.

38. Greenstein RA, Resnick RB, Resnick E: Methadone and naltrexone in the treatment of heroin dependence. Psychiatr Clin North Am 7(4):671–679, 1984.

39. Mitchell J, Morley JE, Levine AS, et al: High-dose naltrexone therapy and dietary counseling for obesity. Biol Psychiatry 22:35–42, 1987.

40. Brahen LS, Henderson RK, Capone T, Kordal N: Nal-trexone treatment in a jail work-release program. J Clin Psychiatry 45(9):49–52, 1984.

41. Ling W, Wesson DR: Naltrexone treatment for addicted health-care professionals: A collaborative private practice experience. J Clin Psychiatry 45(9):46–48, 1984.

42. Tennant FS, Rawson RA, Cohen AJ, Mann A: Clinical experience with naltrexone in suburban opioid addicts. J Clin Psychiatry 45(9):42–45, 1984.

43. Washton AM, Pottash AC, Gold MS: Naltrexone in addicted business executives and physicians. J Clin Psychiatry 45(9):39–41, 1984.

44. Kosten TR, Kleber HD: Strategies to improve compliance with narcotic antagonists. Am J Drug Alcohol Abuse 10:257, 1994.

Psychotherapy in Addictive Disorders

Robert L. DuPont, MD

Psychotherapy is almost as varied and complex as addictive disease. It may appear that any verbal communication can be described as counseling or psychotherapy, just as many behaviors can be defined as addictive. Hidden behind this definitional haze are core realities of great importance for mental health professionals who help people addicted to alcohol and other drugs.

Both *counseling* and *psychotherapy* are descriptive names for the talking cure that takes place when one person, who is paid for the work, attempts to help another person in a professional relationship. The term *counseling* describes this process when it is conducted by professionals who do not possess a doctor's degree, whereas *psychotherapy* is used by Ph.D.s and M.D.s. The recipients of this treatment are called *clients* by nonmedical professionals and *patients* by medical professionals. I use the terms *psychotherapy* and *patients* to keep the language simple and because of my own background as a physician. This chapter is written by a clinician for other clinicians, with a deep respect for both the serious work of psychotherapy and for the life-and-death struggles of addicted people and their families.

Clearly different from psychotherapy are the 12-step fellowships, which do not involve paid mental health professionals, and psychopharmacology, in which medicine is the major treatment. On the other hand, both mutual aid

and psychopharmacology can be combined with psychotherapy in the treatment of addicted patients.[1,2] Within this definition of psychotherapy are insight-oriented therapies, the cognitive-behavioral therapies (CBT) and other professionally led efforts at skill building such as relapse prevention.[3]

Addiction is the use of alcohol and other intoxicating drugs in ways that involve loss of control, including continued use despite harm and despite efforts (however ambivalent) to stop use, as well as denial and dishonesty.[4,5] Addiction to alcohol and other drugs is a disorder of the brain's reward system that manages pleasure and pain.[6] An addicted person seeks pleasure and the relief of distress by using addicting substances, but the disease inevitably leads to terrible suffering of the addicted person and of the people who care about the addicted person.[7]

Psychotherapy for addiction takes place when mental health professionals work to help addicted patients solve their problems and live better lives in the context of paid professional relationships. When mental health professionals participate as members of 12-step fellowships or as friends or family members of addicted individuals, this is not psychotherapy because it is not part of a professional relationship. When mental health professionals work as unpaid volunteers in addiction treatment programs, their work may or may not be psychotherapy, depending on the roles they assume.

Psychotherapy treats an addicted patient as a whole person who has a unique history and specific needs that include but are not limited to addiction. Psychotherapy also involves the therapist as a person in this process. Psychotherapy is a person-to-person, humanistic way to help patients get well from addictive disease. Psychotherapy enables patients to tell their personal stories and to know that they have been heard by someone who cares about them. The literature on the efficacy of psychotherapy has been reviewed.[8]

The place of psychotherapy in the treatment of drug addiction was reviewed in a comprehensive monograph by the National Institute on Drug Abuse (NIDA).[9] The dominant models of psychotherapy in the treatment of alcoholism have been defined in an extraordinary series of monographs from the National Institute on Alcohol Abuse and Alcoholism (NIAAA) in their Project MATCH Monograph Series.[10-12] These monographs cover the 12-step model, the motivational enhancement model, and the cognitive-behavioral model of psychotherapy for addictive disease. Not addressed are the various forms of dynamic or insight-oriented psychotherapy.

Goals of Psychotherapy for Addictions

At one time, psychotherapists saw their job as helping addicted patients gain insight into the underlying psychological causes of their addictions. Addiction was believed to be a symptom of—and secondary to—a patient's underlying emotional disorders. The guiding idea behind the psychoanalytical approach to psychotherapy for addicted patients was that by working through the underlying psychic conflicts, the symptoms of the addiction would disappear. Along with this approach came the idea that addicted patients who quit using alcohol or other drugs without resolving their underlying emotional conflicts could expect not only a recurrence of their addictive disease but the substitution of other symptoms in place of the addictive behavior. This approach to the psychotherapy for addiction did not lack for courage. It took on the problem of addiction and promised a permanent and complete solution through psychotherapy.

The psychoanalytical model of psychotherapy for addicts now has been abandoned by most mental health professionals who seek to help addicted patients, because therapists who worked with addicted patients for long periods learned that it did not work. Nevertheless, this psychoanalytical model is still promoted by some psychotherapists as treatment for addicted patients, especially those who rarely work with alcoholics and drug addicts. The psychoanalytical view of psychotherapy for addicts remains common in the public discussion of addiction, where the disease of addiction is seen to be secondary to an underlying mental problem and where psychotherapists are assumed to be able to solve addicts' underlying emotional problems.

Setting New Goals

The contemporary approach to the psychotherapy for addiction establishes the goal of psychotherapy as helping addicted persons to understand what is wrong and to learn what to do about it, not to help addicted persons resolve an underlying and usually unconscious psychological conflict. In this more practical approach, the psychotherapist is a guide, a coach, and a teacher who works in partnership with an addicted person to achieve shared goals, including overcoming the addiction. The psychotherapeutic contract for addicted persons is based on the expressed belief of the psychotherapist that "I have some experience and knowledge that may be helpful to you in your efforts to regain control of your life. Take what is useful to you and leave the rest behind."

This model for psychotherapy for addiction is different from the earlier, more theoretical and passive stance of psychodynamic therapists, whose primary goal was to provide a safe place for their patients to explore their own inner mental lives. Although a small percentage of addicted individuals who are in secure recovery even now choose traditional insight-oriented psychotherapy and psychoanalysis, this approach is rarely targeted at the addiction itself. Instead, it focuses on addicted individuals' problem-generating emotional lives, which are separate from but which commonly reinforce their addictive disease. Dynamic psychotherapy can be directed usefully at reducing the character defects of addicted persons.

Because psychoanalytical psychotherapy for addiction has been discredited by its failure to produce good clinical results, it has become common in the addiction field to hear addicted individuals make disparaging comments about all types of psychotherapy. Certainly all healthcare professionals who work with alcoholics and drug addicts are exposed to negative reports from their patients about the high cost and lack of effectiveness of traditional psychotherapy in the lives of addicts.

At first glance, it might appear that psychotherapy has become irrelevant in the treatment of addictive disease. The everyday reality of addiction treatment is dramatically different from this common negative stereotype. It is impossible to find any form of organized treatment for addicts that does not put psychotherapy—the talking cure—at the center of the treatment. Psychotherapy is as important for addiction treatments based on the 12-step model as it is for addiction treatments that rely on the cognitive-behavioral approach. Today in North America, the talking cure for addiction is prospering even as it is being continuously reinvented.

The most important change in psychotherapy for addiction during the past two decades, when addiction treatment became commonplace as a result of the huge drug abuse and addiction epidemic and the resulting increased public concern about addiction, has been the change from a passive psychoanalytical model of psychotherapy to an active educational, directive model of psychotherapy. Along with this change of strategy has come a change of goals. Psychotherapy for addiction is no longer aimed at resolution of a hypothesized underlying emotional conflict but toward teaching skills to cope successfully with addictive disease. Particularly important is introducing addicted individuals and their families to the 12-step fellowships.[13] This new approach has benefited from the contributions of many traditionally trained psychoanalysts who have helped to integrate a dynamic understanding of the mental lives of addicts into this new model of psychotherapy for addiction.[14]

Today in North America, psychotherapy is delivered in all settings where addiction treatment occurs: inpatient, residential, and outpatient. Individual, group, and family psychotherapy are now found in most treatments of addicted patients. Psychotherapy is available in short-term and open-ended formats. It is packaged in comprehensive, highly structured addiction treatment programs, and it is delivered in an unstructured format in the offices of individual mental health practitioners.

Addicted patients are increasingly finding their way to psychotherapy and to organized addiction treatment programs, through referrals provided by employee assistance programs, driving while impaired programs, and a large variety of other bridging programs linking social institutions and addiction treatment, including the new student assistance programs in many high schools and colleges.[15] These programs have an important role in psychotherapy for addictive disorders. They offer substantial expertise and experience about options in the community and about which referrals work best to help addicted individuals.

The Techniques of Psychotherapy for Addiction

Three statements describe the current state of clinical practice of psychotherapy for persons addicted to alcohol and other drugs:

1. Addicts are as varied as any other large group of human beings. Accordingly, they have varied needs. Not only does one approach to psychotherapy not fit all addicted people, but one approach to psychotherapy is unlikely to meet all the needs of even one single addicted person over a long period. Varied approaches are needed to maximize the benefits of psychotherapy.
2. Addiction is a lifelong disease. Psychotherapy for addicted individuals needs to be patient and persistent. It needs to offer hope for a lasting recovery. Beyond all other characteristics, it needs to be based on a realistic respect for addicted patients and for their families. No form of psychotherapy, however brief and structured it is, can hope to succeed if the help is not useful for the course of a lifetime in dealing with the problems of addiction. Short-term interventions help patients build skills and develop strategies that work throughout their life. Recovery requires portable techniques that are adaptable to changing needs for long periods.
3. No form of psychotherapy has been demonstrated in controlled studies to be effective over the long term for any substantial group of addicted people. Support for psychotherapy is not based on controlled clinical trials, but it is based on a large body of clinical experience. The efficacy of psychotherapy for addiction is validated by the choices made by addicted individuals, many of whom are free to choose their own therapists

in the increasingly varied psychotherapy marketplace.

With these three statements in mind, here is a short review of the dominant forms of psychotherapy now being provided to addicted patients in North America:

EDUCATION

One of the most important innovations of the modern abstinence-based model of residential treatment for addiction, the Minnesota model of treatment, is the role of education in the treatment process.[16] The educational approach has been adopted by intensive outpatient addiction treatment programs and even by many solo psychotherapy practitioners. New patients and their families are educated about the disease concept of addiction and introduced to a common language to describe the features of this disease and the process of getting well. Concepts flowing from this educational approach, rooted in the 12-step model, such as *hitting bottom, enabling, denial,* and *recovery,* have become essential tools to understand and to communicate about the experience of addiction. Humor, perspective, and reinforcement are provided by films and videos as well as by lectures. Books are another part of the new educational process. Books dealing with addiction have become so widely used that entire stores and publishing houses are now devoted to the expanding recovery literature, much of it written by people who are professional psychotherapists, who are themselves in recovery, or both.

TWELVE-STEP FACILITATION

Closely related to the role of education about the disease of addiction is the introduction of patients and their families to the 12-step programs through psychotherapy. One of the most important roads to long-term recovery from addiction and to the participation in the 12-step fellowships is formal addiction treatment. In residential addiction treatment, addicted patients have an opportunity to think more clearly with their brains free from the influences of alcohol and other drugs. Patients in residential addiction treatment also have an opportunity to work with their physicians, therapists, and others on the program staff to develop an individualized treatment plan that addresses their needs after the completion of residential treatment. This individual treatment plan may include long-term individual and group psychotherapy as part of an ad-

dicted person's aftercare program. The research on the efficacy of the 12-step fellowships and the integration of 12-step programs into the treatment of patients with dual disorders has been reviewed.[17, 18]

A significant new development in the psychotherapy for addiction has been the important role of therapists who are themselves recovering from addiction. Recovering persons who have specific professional skills in psychotherapy are major contributors to the new approach to psychotherapy for addiction. However, merely being a former alcoholic or a former addict is insufficient qualification to deliver psychotherapy. Having counselors tell their stories of recovery, however heroic they may be, is seldom helpful in the treatment of addicted people. Some early treatment programs simply hired any available recovering alcoholics or addicts to be therapists. The results of this approach were predictably unsatisfactory, ranging from relapses to active addiction to grossly incompetent performance in treatment programs and in the psychotherapy process.

Individuals who deliver psychotherapy to addicted people, whether they are recovering or not, need significant and sustained training in the methods of psychotherapy, and they need to work in the long-term apprenticeships that are at the heart of modern psychotherapy training for all mental health workers. By the same token, even the most skilled professional psychotherapists need a working knowledge of the 12-step programs and of the disease concept of addiction to be effective in helping addicted patients. This knowledge and experience are best achieved by personal attendance at open meetings and by work with professional colleagues who are active in their own recoveries from addiction.

Professionally sophisticated psychotherapists who lack an active understanding of the specific process of recovery from addiction are as unhelpful for addicted patients as are untrained ex-addict counselors. Even the most sophisticated psychotherapists are poorly equipped to treat addicted individuals unless they have spent time working with addicted patients and learning from other mental health professionals who have this experience. Most valuable is the experience of working with addicted persons over the course of many years, because only this long-term experience can give a psychotherapist the perspective needed to see the natural history of addictive disease and the ways people get well and stay well. Particularly valuable in gaining this long-term perspective is attendance at several open meetings of the 12-step fellowships, one of the few places it is possible to find addicted people who have been clean and sober for long periods. Without this specific experience, psychotherapists easily can conclude that addicted persons will respond to the therapist's own particular approach to psychotherapy and that treating addicted patients is fairly easy. As experience is gained and failures accumulate, therapists are likely to conclude that addicts are hopeless. Addicted patients are neither easy nor hopeless. They do get well, and they are often rewarding patients, but they require specific techniques and skills to benefit from psychotherapy.

COGNITIVE-BEHAVIORAL TREATMENT

One of the most hopeful types of psychotherapy for addiction is CBT for addiction. The CBT approach has been especially fruitful in relapse prevention. Cognitive psychotherapies have been reviewed.[19]

CBT of addiction is based on the assumption that addicts benefit from the acquisition of coping skills, including identifying the cues that trigger relapses to addiction and ways to handle urges to use alcohol and other drugs. The CBT approach has become dominant in the treatment of conditions from depression to anxiety and from obesity to cigarette smoking. Psychologists have been in the forefront of these efforts. Even addiction treatment programs that rely on the 12-step fellowships and the more traditional medical programs are benefiting today from a rich infusion of CBT techniques.

INSIGHT-ORIENTED THERAPY

The old warhorse of psychotherapy is the much-maligned insight-oriented, or dynamic, psychotherapy. When it dealt with the problems of addiction, dynamic therapy was a disappointment, but today, as part of a comprehensive effort that includes education, the 12-step programs, and CBT, insight-oriented psychotherapy is making a modest but important comeback. Insight-oriented psychotherapists are now less ambitious and more comfortable in a supporting role. In this role, dynamic psychotherapy is especially helpful for addicted patients who are psychologically minded, for persons with special needs such as victims of childhood abuse, or for those with other psychiatric disorders such as clinically significant anxiety and depression. The efficacy

of brief dynamic psychotherapy has been reviewed.[20–22]

All four of these forms of psychotherapy for addiction have constructive roles in the treatment of the varied population of addicted patients. The different psychotherapeutic approaches are often combined or used in a sequential fashion in both organized addiction treatment programs and in the more flexible long-term treatment of addicted patients. Recognizing addiction to be a lifelong disease rather than a simple bad habit is a big step to understanding both addiction and the roles of psychotherapy in the treatment of addiction.

Suggestions for Psychotherapists Dealing with Addictive Disease

Having offered psychotherapy to addicted patients throughout my professional life, I have developed a healthy skepticism about the value of my own skills and those of my psychotherapy colleagues when it comes to helping addicted patients get well and stay well. I have also acquired a deep respect for the power and elusiveness of the disease of addiction. Nonetheless, I have seen the joys of individuals who confront and overcome active addiction and who go on to live alcohol- and drug-free lives.

I recall working with a 50-year-old patient who was herself a skilled and experienced psychiatrist. She was seeing me for a severe obsessive-compulsive disorder. Her much-loved husband of 25 years died suddenly of cancer. In dealing with her grief, she turned for help to a friend who was a recovering alcoholic active in Alcoholics Anonymous. My patient explained to me that her friend and other people she had known who had successfully dealt with addiction "seem to live on a higher spiritual plane and to have better tools for coping with loss and other problems than most of the rest of us." I knew what she meant. Getting well from addiction involves much more than not using alcohol or other drugs. Recovery requires better ways of living a good life based on sound values such as humility, persistence, honesty, and resilience. To stay sober, addicted individuals have learned that they have to pass on their recovery to others. That is why the 12-step programs are called, by members of the fellowships, "selfish" programs.

The disease of addiction is a disease of the entire self that has a spiritual dimension. The most fundamental aspect of the disease of addiction is dishonesty, and the most fundamental value needed to get well is honesty. I have come to the conclusion that *honesty* is the one-word antidote for all forms of addiction. Psychotherapy can help addicts find and use individualized paths to recovery. Psychotherapy can also help addicted patients cope with their emotional needs that are separate from their addiction.

Addicted individuals who continue to use alcohol and other drugs can be enormously frustrating to psychotherapists as they continue their desperate personal research into addiction in their own lives. Like others who care about addicted people, therapists are often heartbroken by the defeat of their efforts to help their addicted patients. I have learned never to give up and that recovery from addiction is always possible, even in the most hopeless cases. Recovery often comes when it is least expected. Getting well from addiction is, in any event, an inside job, one that only the addicted person can do.

Here are seven simple principles that I have found helpful in my work as a psychotherapist with addicted patients and their families:

1. Give your efforts at psychotherapy the best you have got to give. Addicted patients deserve your best.

2. Stay with your game. Whatever form of psychotherapy you know and feel confident with is right for you. Use it for those addicted patients it can help and admit, to them and to yourself, that your approach to psychotherapy is not right for all addicted patients. Encourage those for whom your form of psychotherapy is not right to search for other routes to the inner peace they seek.

3. Respect but do not fear the disease of addiction, which is a powerful and pitiless teacher for patients and therapists alike.

4. Honor your patients and their personal struggles to solve their terribly difficult problems. Your patients deserve your respect whether or not they stop using alcohol and other drugs. They have been caught in a deadly trap that requires all the skill and strength they can muster if they are to survive.

5. Be humble. Addiction to alcohol and other drugs is a serious, potentially fatal problem. What you have to offer in psychotherapy is of real but limited value to addicted patients. Do not oversell psychotherapy.

6. Accept the financial, administrative, and other limits under which you work and find ways to meet the human needs of your patients, one person at a time, as best you can.

7. Learn what you can from your successes in psychotherapy with addicted patients but treasure your failures, because they are your most powerful and inspiring teachers. As people and as psychotherapists, our failures force us to grow, to learn new skills, and to find better ways to help our patients. Our failures are our best instructors, if we are open to learning from them.

Results of Psychotherapy Research

Psychotherapy is available in 99% of the drug-free, methadone maintenance and multiple-modality drug addiction treatment units in the country and in 97% of the detoxification units.[23] Two barriers to more sophisticated research into the psychotherapy for addiction were identified by Onken and Blaine in their review: (1) The delivery of psychotherapy to addicted patients today is complex, poorly defined, and rapidly changing, and (2) research strategies for psychotherapy research in general do not easily fit the short-term double-blind model used successfully in most pharmacotherapy research, making studies of psychotherapy relatively "messy."[24] NIDA sponsored a technical review of this issue in 1989, leading to the publication of their monograph.[9] The chapters of this important book fall into three categories: review of research findings, methodological considerations, and priorities and conclusions for future research.

Project MATCH from NIAAA attempts to resolve these methodological problems by defining model psychotherapy treatment interventions for alcoholics as a first step to controlled studies of efficacy in their ambitious long-term research project. The multisite clinical trial of NIAAA is based on the common belief of clinicians that when it comes to psychotherapy for addictions, "one size does not fit all." In other words, it is assumed that some psychotherapy is more helpful to particular patients and other forms of psychotherapy are better for other alcoholic patients. This attractive hypothesis, matching particular patients to particular forms of psychotherapy based on research, was not tested in a rigorous fashion before the Project MATCH effort.

The Future of Psychotherapy for Addictions

Predictions of the death of psychotherapy in the treatment of addictive disease were clearly premature. Psychotherapy for addiction has proved to be more adaptable than anticipated by its critics. Today it is difficult to imagine delivering addiction treatment without talking with patients about who they are, how they got where they are, and where they are going as individuals. That personal connection with the meaning of patients' unique lives is the heart of all forms of psychotherapy in addictive disorders.

Psychotherapy will continue to evolve in complex and unpredictable ways to meet the varied needs of addicts using the equally varied talents of dedicated psychotherapists. It is unlikely, based on past experience, that any one form of psychotherapy for addictive disorders will prove dominant or that controlled research studies will have more than a minor role in what is, at heart, a clinical enterprise. Psychotherapy is now offered to addicted patients in a rich and rapidly growing variety. The cost of psychotherapy to patients is governed in part by the extent to which the services are covered by health insurance. Addicted persons and those who refer them for psychotherapy, such as driving while impaired and employee assistance programs, are making increasingly sophisticated decisions about cost as the healthcare market is restricted by managed care and other forces. Whatever happens to the reimbursement levels for psychiatry for addicted individuals, recent experience leaves no room for doubt that there will continue to be a large demand for psychotherapy for addicted persons and their families, both when the disease is active and during recovery.

Twelve-step fellowship meetings offer consumers' views of the local psychotherapy marketplace. Addicts swap opinions about psychotherapists at Alcoholics Anonymous and Narcotics Anonymous meetings, and family members do the same at Al-Anon meetings. Although success with one addicted person or one family does not guarantee success with someone else, addicted individuals and their families are in a good position to compare their particular needs with other members of their mutual-aid fellowships. They can then make their own judgments about which forms of psychotherapy are most likely to help them. No other psychotherapy consumers have such an efficient window on the psychotherapy marketplace as do addicted individuals and their families. The efficiency of this psychotherapy market is leading to rapid improvements in the psychotherapy for addictive disorders as techniques that meet with approval prosper and those that do not wither away.

Summary

Psychotherapy in addictive disease is an all but universal component of the treatment of addictions to alcohol and other drugs. Despite the neglect it has received in both the clinical and the research literature, psychotherapy for addiction is both irrepressible and valuable. Psychotherapy practice is not waiting for the results of research studies. The broad and deep support for psychotherapy for addiction grows out of a shared vision that addiction is rooted in the individual addicted person and that helping addicts one person at a time with talking treatments is necessary for each addicted person to understand what is wrong and what to do about the addiction. The psychotherapeutic approach to addiction is widely recognized to benefit both the patients who receive it and the society that supports it.

REFERENCES

1. Klerman GL, Weissman MM, Markowitz J, et al: Medication and psychotherapy. In Bergin AE, Garfield SL (eds): Handbook of Psychotherapy and Behavior Change, 4th ed. New York, John Wiley & Sons, 1994.
2. Wood EA: Combining psychotherapy with 12-step recovery programs. Psychiatric Times, IX:56–58, 1992.
3. Gorski TT: Relapse prevention and behavioral managed care. Behavioral Health Management 14(3):55–56, 1994.
4. Morse RM, Flavin DK, Joint Committee of the National Council on Alcoholism and Drug Dependence and the American Society of Addiction Medicine to Study the Definition and Criteria for the Diagnosis of Alcoholism: The definition of alcoholism. JAMA 268(8):1012–1014, 1992.
5. American Psychiatric Association: Diagnostic and Statistical Manual of Mental Disorders, 4th ed. Washington, DC, American Psychiatric Association, 1994.
6. DuPont RL: The Selfish Brain: Learning from Addiction. Washington, DC, American Psychiatric Association (in press).
7. DuPont RL, McGovern JP: Suffering in addiction: Alcoholism and drug dependence. In Starck PL, McGovern JP (eds): The Invisible Dimension of Illness: Human Suffering. New York, National League for Nursing Press, 1992, pp 155–201.
8. Literature review shows value of psychotherapy. Psychiatric News XXIX(13):2,24, 1994.
9. Onken LS, Blaine JD (eds): Psychotherapy and Counseling in the Treatment of Drug Abuse. NIDA Res Monogr 104:1990.
10. Nowinski J, Baker S, Carroll K: Twelve Step Facilitation Therapy Manual. National Institute on Alcohol Abuse and Alcoholism Project MATCH Monograph Series, vol 1, NIH Publication 94-3722. Rockville, MD, National Institute on Alcohol Abuse and Alcoholism, 1994.
11. Miller WR, Zweben A, DiClemente CC, et al: Motivational Enhancement Therapy Manual. National Institute on Alcohol Abuse and Alcoholism Project MATCH Monograph Series, vol 2, NIH Publication

94-3723. Rockville, MD, National Institute on Alcohol Abuse and Alcoholism, 1994.

12. Kadden R, Carroll K, Donovan D, et al: Cognitive-Behavioral Coping Skills Therapy Manual. National Institute on Alcohol Abuse and Alcoholism Project MATCH Monograph Series, vol 3, NIH Publication 94-3724. Rockville, MD, National Institute on Alcohol Abuse and Alcoholism, 1994.

13. DuPont RL, McGovern JP: A Bridge to Recovery—An Introduction to 12-Step Programs. Washington, DC, American Psychiatric Association, 1994.

14. Khantzian EJ, Mack JE: Alcoholics Anonymous and contemporary psychodynamic theory. In Galanter M (ed): Recent Developments in Alcoholism, vol 7. New York, Plenum, 1989.

15. McGovern JP, DuPont RL: Student assistance programs: An important approach to drug abuse prevention. Journal of School Health 61(6):260–264, 1991.

16. Office of National Drug Control Policy: Understanding Drug Treatment, White Paper. Washington, DC, Executive Office of the President, June 1990.

17. DuPont RL, Shiraki, S: Recent research in 12-step programs. In Wilford BB (ed): Principles of Addiction Medicine. Washington, DC, American Society of Addiction Medicine, 1994, pp 1–9.

18. DuPont RL: The twelve step approach. In Miller NS (ed): Treating Coexisting Psychiatric and Addictive Disorders. Center City, MN, Hazelden Publishing Group, 1994, pp 177–197.

19. Elliott CH (ed): Cognitive therapy. Psychiatr Ann 22(9):447–492, 1992.

20. MacKenzie KR (ed): Brief psychotherapies. Psychiatr Ann 21(7):395–443, 1991.

21. Crits-Christoph P: The efficacy of brief dynamic psychotherapy: A meta-analysis. Am J Psychiatry 149(2):151–158, 1992.

22. Krupnick JL, Pincus HA: The cost-effectiveness of psychotherapy: A plan for research. Am J Psychiatry 149(10):1295–1305, 1992.

23. U.S. Department of Health and Human Services: National Drug and Alcoholism Treatment Unit Survey. DHHS Publication (ADM) 89-1626. Rockville, MD, U.S. Dept of Health and Human Services, 1982.

24. Onken LS, Blaine JD: Psychotherapy and counseling research in drug abuse treatment: Questions, problems, and solutions. NIDA Res Monogr 104:1–5, 1990.

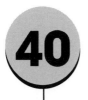

Network Therapy: A Practical Approach to the Office Treatment of Addiction

Marc Galanter, MD

Addiction professionals are regularly confronted by the problem of engaging and retaining patients in treatment. We must therefore consider the effective ways to improve patients' care in the presence of the denial and rationalization that so often lead to relapse and early dropout. This chapter offers an approach to helping with this thorny problem. In order to do this, we consider how family and friends can be engaged in parallel with individual therapy as a therapeutic aide.

A supportive group of individuals close to a patient can provide an effective vehicle for rehabilitation of addictive illness in network therapy, an innovative and pragmatic format for treatment. By means of the network approach to social support, we can take concrete steps to overcome the destructive forces that are so compromising to the continuity of care for substance addicts. An operational definition of network therapy is important here.[1, 2] It is an approach to rehabilitation in which specific family members and friends are enlisted to provide ongoing support and to promote attitude change. Network members are part of a therapist's working team and are not subjects of treatment themselves. The goals of this approach are prompt achievement of abstinence, relapse prevention, and the development of a drug-free adaptation.

Network therapy confronts the confounding problem that therapists have only a marginal ability to influence patients' behavior outside the office. If patients have a slip into drug addiction, their therapists may not be apprised, and even if their therapists know, they can bring little influence to bear. Therapists on their own are limited in the degree to which they can make demands on a patient's life, and patients are free to walk away from the therapeutic situation if it is uncomfortable for them—that is to say, if it challenges a potential relapse into addiction. All these factors make the engagement and orchestration of family and friends into the therapy with a substance-addicted patient an invaluable resource, one that offers remarkable opportunity for the modification of traditional psychotherapeutic techniques to treat substance addiction.

Patient Selection

A broad range of addicted patients, characterized by the following clinical hallmarks of addictive illness, can be treated. They are substance-dependent patients who, on initiating consumption of their addictive agent—be it alcohol, cocaine, opiates, or depressant drugs—frequently cannot limit that consumption to a reasonable and predictable level. This phenomenon has been termed *loss of control* by clinicians who treat alcohol- or drug-dependent persons.[3, 4] Also included are patients who consistently demonstrate relapse to the agent of addiction—that is, they have attempted to stop using the drug for various periods of time but return to it despite a specific intent to avoid it.

This treatment approach is not necessary for those addicted who can, in fact, learn to set limits on their alcohol use; their addiction may be treated as a behavioral symptom in a more traditional psychotherapeutic fashion. Nor is it directed at those patients for whom the addictive pattern is most unmanageable, such as alcoholics with unusual destabilizing circumstances such as homelessness, severe character pathology, or psychosis. These patients may need special supportive care such as inpatient detoxification or long-term residential treatment. What therefore differentiates patients in terms of their suitability for treatment? Factors that are relevant are the intensity of the addiction, the drug to which the individual is addicted, and the severity of a patient's social disability.

Abstinence Orientation

The weight of clinical experience supports the view that abstinence is the most practical goal to propose to addicted persons for their rehabilitation,[5, 6] although patients may sometimes achieve an outcome of limited drinking. For abstinence to be expected, however, a therapist should ensure the provision of necessary social supports for the patient.

This example illustrates how network supports can be useful. If there is a question about a patient's ability to sustain abstinence during the period between sessions, the network members can be enlisted to work with them to provide practical support. The network members are to understand that they are to contact the therapist if they are concerned about the patient's possible use of alcohol or drugs and that the therapist is to contact the network members if concerned about a potential relapse. The overriding commitment of therapists is that they and the network members support patients in maintaining the alcohol- or drug-free state. Open communication on matters regarding substance use should be maintained among the network, the patient, and the therapist. The therapist must set the proper tone of mutual trust and understanding so that the patient's right to privacy not otherwise be compromised. On the other hand, it is made explicit that confidentiality applies to all communications with the therapist that do not directly relate to alcohol or drug problems.

Averting Relapse

Various techniques have been used to minimize the likelihood of substance use in the course of addiction treatment, to avoid a patient's relapse into heavy drug use. In general, this approach is based on the need to avoid the compelling effects of the conditioned abstinence syndrome in addiction.[7] This syndrome serves to explain the vulnerability of addicted individuals to return to drug use whenever they are exposed to cues that have previously been associated with exposure to the drug. Cues to drug or alcohol seeking can be intrinsic, such as specific moods, or they can be extrinsic, such as certain situations or encounters with certain individuals. Any of these could have previously been associated with drug ingestion[8, 9] and should be the focus of attempts at relapse prevention.

The emergence of craving precipitated by such cues can be examined with a patient in both individual and network sessions, in order to clarify the cues that produce a vulnerability to relapse for that person. Because patients may exercise denial in avoiding the awareness of some of these cues, the availability of persons in the network who are well acquainted with patients' patterns of addictive behavior may present a unique opportunity to gain access to relevant information that would otherwise be unavailable. Once these cues have been defined, plans to avoid them can also be made at sessions held with network members. Patients can be given social support to avoid the cues and can receive practical assistance from network members in an attempt to avoid these cues if it is necessary.

In both individual and network sessions, matters of first priority are associated with maintaining abstinence. These include cues encountered by patients that provoke craving. When these arise, they are examined with regard to the circumstances precipitating conditioned drug seeking so that the patient and therapist are prepared to address them. In network sessions, the resources of the group are mobilized to help patients address these issues.

For example, a network member may help patients explore the circumstances that lead them to become involved in a peer group in which social cues for drug use have led to craving.

Use of self-help modalities is desirable whenever possible. For alcoholics, participation in Alcoholics Anonymous (AA) is strongly encouraged. (Groups such as Narcotics Anonymous, Pills Anonymous, and Cocaine Anonymous are modeled after AA and have a similarly useful role for drug addicts.) One approach is to tell patients that they are expected to attend at least two AA meetings a week for at least 1 month to familiarize themselves with the program. If after a month they are quite reluctant to continue and other aspects of the treatment are going well, their nonparticipation may have to be accepted.

Disulfiram can also be a useful tool when taken daily to avert relapse in alcoholic patients. In order for the regimen to be effective, however, patients must continue taking disulfiram every day. By having someone observe that the patient takes disulfiram each morning, the patient cannot inadvertently forget the medication for a day or two, and the possibility of losing the intended effect of this medication is avoided. An observation regimen can be established with a person in the network close to the patient, generally the spouse, because this plan is easily adapted to a couple's morning regimen. Thus, although disulfiram may be of marginal use in a traditional counseling context,[10] it becomes much more valuable when carefully integrated into work with a patient and network.

It is a good idea to use the initial telephone contact to engage a patient's agreement to be abstinent from alcohol for the day immediately before the first session. The therapist then has the option of prescribing or administering disulfiram at that time. For a patient who is earnestly seeking assistance for alcoholism, this is often not difficult if some time is spent on the phone making plans to avoid a drinking context during that period. If it is not feasible to undertake this on the phone, it may be addressed in the first session. Such planning with a patient almost always involves organizing time with significant others and therefore serves as a basis for developing a patient's support network.

Administration of disulfiram under observation is a treatment option that is easily adapted to work with social networks. A patient who takes disulfiram cannot drink; a patient who agrees to be observed by a responsible individual while taking disulfiram will not miss his or her dose without the observer's knowing. This may take a measure of persuasion and, above all, the therapist's commitment that such an approach can be reasonable and helpful. A similar perspective applies to the use of naltrexone for opiate addiction. In this case, the patient takes the medication three times a week (e.g., two 50-mg pills on Monday and Wednesday and three pills on Friday). Observation is organized as with disulfiram.

Network Therapy: A Summary of the Procedures

The network therapy approach is meant to be straightforward and uncomplicated by theoretical bias—for the patient, for the network member, and for the therapist. In this light, the main points to be observed in treatment by the network therapist are reviewed next.

SELECT PATIENTS CAREFULLY

1. Network therapy is appropriate for individuals who cannot reliably control their intake of alcohol or drugs once they have taken their first dose; those who have tried to stop and relapsed; and those who have not been willing or able to stop.
2. Patients whose problems are too severe for the network approach include those who cannot stop their drug use even for a day or cannot comply with outpatient detoxification and those whose associated problems make cooperation unlikely, such as homeless or psychotic persons. Such patients generally need hospitalization.
3. Patients who can be treated with conventional therapy and without a network include those who have demonstrated the ability to moderate their consumption without problems for extended periods and those who have had only a brief addiction.

START A NETWORK AS SOON AS POSSIBLE

1. It is important to see the alcohol or drug abuser promptly, because the window of opportunity for openness to treatment is generally brief. A week's delay can result in a person's reverting to drunkenness or losing motivation.
2. If the person is married, engage the spouse early in treatment, preferably at the time of the first phone call. Point out that addiction is a family problem. For most

drugs, you can enlist the spouse in ensuring that the patient arrives at your office with a day's sobriety.

3. In the initial interview, frame the exchange so that a strong case is built for the grave consequences of the patient's addiction, and do this before the patient can introduce his or her system of denial. That way you are not putting the spouse or other network members in the awkward position of having to contradict a close relation.

4. Make clear that the patient needs to be abstinent, starting now. (Tapered detoxification may be necessary sometimes, as with depressant pills.)

5. When seeing an alcoholic patient for the first time, begin disulfiram treatment as soon as possible, in the office if you can. Have the patient continue taking disulfiram under observation of a network member.

6. Start arranging for a network to be assembled at the first session, generally involving the patient's family and close friends.

7. From the first meeting, you should consider how to ensure sobriety until the next meeting, and plan that with the network. Initially, their immediate company, a plan for daily AA attendance, and planned activities all may be necessary.

MAKE SURE THE NETWORK ATMOSPHERE IS SUPPORTIVE

1. Include people who are close to the patient, have a long-standing relationship with him or her, and are trusted. Avoid members with substance addiction problems, because they will undermine the plan when you need their unbiased support. Avoid superiors and subordinates at work, because they have an overriding relationship with the patient independent of friendship.

2. Get a balanced group. Avoid a network composed solely of the parental generation, or of younger people, or of people of the opposite sex. A nascent network sometimes selects itself for a consultation if the patient is reluctant to address his or her own problem. Such a group will later supportively engage the patient in the network, with your careful guidance.

3. Make sure that the mood of meetings is trusting and free of recrimination. Avoid letting the patient or the network members be made to feel guilty or angry in meetings. Explain issues of conflict in terms of the problems presented by addiction. Do not get into personality conflicts.

4. The tone should be directive. That is to say, give explicit instructions to support and ensure abstinence. A feeling of teamwork should be promoted, with no psychologizing or impugning members' motives.

5. Meet as frequently as necessary to ensure abstinence, perhaps once a week for a month, every other week for the next few months, and every month or two by the end of a year.

6. The network should have no agenda other than to support the patient's abstinence. As abstinence is stabilized, the network can help the patient plan for a new drug-free adaptation. The network is not there to work on family relations or to help other members with their problems, although it may do this indirectly.

KEEP THE NETWORK'S AGENDA FOCUSED

1. *Maintaining abstinence.* At the outset of each session, the patient and the network members should report any exposure of the patient to alcohol or drugs. The patient and network members should be instructed on the nature of relapse and should plan with the therapist how to sustain abstinence. Cues to conditioned drug seeking should be examined.

2. *Supporting the network's integrity.* Everyone has a role in this. The patient is expected to make sure that network members keep their meeting appointments and stay involved with the treatment. The therapist sets meeting times and summons the network for any emergency, such as a relapse; the therapist does whatever is necessary to secure stability of the membership if the patient is having trouble doing so. Network members' responsibility is to attend network sessions, although they may be asked to undertake other supportive activity with the patient.

3. *Securing future behavior.* The therapist should combine any and all modalities necessary to ensure the patient's stability, such as a stable, drug-free residence; the avoidance of substance-addicted friends; attendance at 12-step meetings; medications such as disulfiram or blocking agents; observed urinalyses; and ancillary psychiatric care. Written agreements may be handy, such as a mutually acceptable contingency contract with penalties for the violation of understandings.

INCORPORATE INDIVIDUAL THERAPY INTO THE TREATMENT

1. The patient is seen in individual therapy once or twice a week, and abstinence is the first priority for individual therapy as well as for network sessions. Insight and expressiveness are important, but they must be subordinate to making sure that abstinence is unthreatened.

2. A search for conditioned cues for drug seeking can be used to understand the potential for relapse and to investigate areas of conflict. It is important to explore the emotional, circumstantial, or substance-related events that bring substance use to mind.

3. Ultimately, individual therapy must be directed at the patient's adopting a new and drug-free lifestyle in which abstinence is embedded. Long-term recovery is only as stable as the patient's new adaptation to family, friends, and work. Group or family therapy might be used instead of individual therapy or in addition to it, but only if abstinence is emphasized.

MAKE USE OF ALCOHOLICS ANONYMOUS AND OTHER SELF-HELP GROUPS

1. Patients should be expected to attend meetings of AA or related groups at least two or three times, with follow-up discussion in therapy.

2. If patients have reservations about these meetings, try to help them understand how to deal with them. Issues such as social anxiety should be explored if they make a patient reluctant to participate. Resistance to AA can generally be related to other areas of inhibition in a person's life, as well as to the denial of addiction.

3. As with other spiritual involvements, do not probe patients' motivation or commitment to AA once engaged. Allow them to work out things on their own, but be prepared to listen.

TERMINATE THE NETWORK THERAPY AT THE APPROPRIATE TIME

1. Network sessions can be terminated after the patient has been stably abstinent for at least 6 months to a year, after group discussion of the patient's readiness for handling sobriety without a network.

2. Establish an understanding with the network members that they will contact the therapist at any point in the future if the patient is vulnerable to relapse. They can be summoned by the therapist as well. This should be made clear in a network session before termination.

Two Case Illustrations

ASSEMBLING A NETWORK

Various issues must be addressed to ensure that network members will exert meaningful influence, free from undue tension. For this reason, the therapist must pay careful attention to the patient's social context from the beginning. The following case illustrates how a network is constructed.

A patient was referred because of his excessive and chronic cocaine use. He did not have nearby family or long-standing friends where he now lived, except for his girlfriend, whom he had been seeing for a year. He was at a loss to provide a roster of potential network members but agreed with the therapist that it would be suitable for his girlfriend to join in the next session.

The patients' younger brother, for whom he felt considerable affection, lived 90 miles away. The patient was reluctant to inconvenience him, but his girlfriend became an ally in the therapy in pointing out that his brother would undoubtedly want to help. Her contribution allowed him to make use of assistance that he might otherwise have been reluctant to accept.

Whenever a new member is introduced into the network, the patient should be asked to review relevant aspects of the addiction to date. This recounting is essential to undercut denial; patients cannot fully convey the nature of their problem in the initial months of treatment because they need to protect their denial and to avoid compromising their image in the eyes of those close to them. Furthermore, network members themselves are rarely aware of the full scope of the problems that they will be addressing as they become collaborators in treatment. In the girlfriend's case, this recounting was important because she was exposed to the patient's use of cocaine to enhance their sexual relations. She had no awareness of the extent of the damage to his nasal septum, and she was unaware that his addiction had spread to daytime hours, leading him to frequent binges that compromised his studies.

This case illustrates as well the vigilance necessary in avoiding tension among potential network recruits. Early in treatment, the patient mentioned the availability of a woman friend of his for the network. There was little discussion of the topic, but it was clear that his relationship with the woman left his girlfriend uncomfortable. The therapist curtailed the discussion of the participation of the other woman without going into detail, realizing that his girlfriend's role in the group was vital and that her comfort in participating had to be protected.

THE VALUE OF MULTIPLE RELATIONSHIPS

Various network members can yield the leverage that one particular member alone cannot. Thus, a friend may often make constructive demands on a patient when the therapist and spouse cannot. For example, patients dependent on central nervous system depressants generally experience considerable difficulty in terminating their use because of the anxiety they feel on reducing their dose to zero.

This was evident with one woman who had been consuming large quantities of opiate-based cough syrup (containing hydrocodone) for some years. It was clear that the actual termination of her drug use would be very difficult for her. Although she insisted she could "handle stopping herself," the therapist asked that at least one member be added to the network in addition to her husband. When it came time for her to stop the cough syrup, she developed an elaborate rationale for deferring the termination, and it was clear that the therapist alone could not have circumvented this defense. In addition, she and her husband, who was in the network, had a rather tense relationship, and his influence was limited, as well. Fortu-

nately, her next-door neighbor, a close friend of hers, was also a network member, and she was able to gently join in with the therapist and husband, asking the patient to stop medication, as had been agreed. The friend insisted that deferring the termination would only produce more difficulties later on; she represented an accountability to common sense and a relationship of trust that neither the husband nor therapist could achieve.

ACKNOWLEDGMENTS

The material in this chapter is adapted from the orientation presented in references 1 and 2.

REFERENCES

1. Galanter M: Network therapy for addiction: A model for office practice. Am J Psychiatry 150:28–36, 1993.
2. Galanter M: Network Therapy for Alcohol and Drug Abuse. New York, Basic Books, 1993.
3. Ludwig AM, Bendfeldt F, Wikler A, Cair RB: "Loss of control" in alcoholics. Arch Gen Psychiatry 35:370–373, 1978.
4. Galanter M: Psychotherapy for alcohol and drug abuse: An approach based on learning theory. Journal of Psychiatric Treatment and Evaluation 5:551–556, 1983.
5. Gitlow SE, Peyser HS (eds): Alcoholism: A Practical Treatment Guide. Grune & Stratton, New York, 1980.
6. Helzer JE, Robins LN, Taylor JR: The extent of long-term drinking among alcoholics discharged from medical and psychiatric facilities. N Engl J Med 312:1678–1682, 1985.
7. Wikler A: Dynamics of drug dependence. Arch Gen Psychiatry 28:611–616, 1973.
8. Marlatt GA, Gordon JR: Relapse Prevention. New York, Guilford Press, 1985.
9. Annis HM: A relapse prevention model for treatment of alcoholics. In Miller WE, Heather N (eds): Treating Addictive Behaviors: Processes of Change. New York, Plenum, 1986, pp 407–421.
10. Fuller R, Branchey L, Brightwell DR, et al: Disulfiram treatment of alcoholism. A Veterans Administration cooperative study. JAMA 256:1449–1455, 1986.

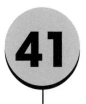

41

Group Therapy in Addictive and Psychiatric Disorders

Michael Levy, PhD

Group therapeutic approaches have long been recognized as having high efficacy for the treatment of chemical dependence.[1] In fact, most inpatient substance addiction treatment programs primarily use a group therapy approach. In addition, outpatient substance addiction programs including intensive day and evening treatment programs generally consist of a structured group therapy program. Clinical work with substance-dependent individuals has naturally been carried over into the treatment of individuals who experience concurrent substance addiction and psychiatric difficulties. Some modifications in technique have been required to take into account the specialized needs of these patients with a dual diagnosis. However, much of the treatment is perfectly appropriate for patients with a dual diagnosis, and group therapy modalities remain an important form of treatment for these patients.

A number of different kinds of group therapeutic approaches are used to treat patients with a dual diagnosis. This chapter outlines the various models of group therapy that are typically used with this patient population. It also discusses some specific types of groups that are often used. The first step, however, is to analyze why group therapy in particular is such an important component in the treatment of patients with a dual diagnosis.

The Advantages of Group Therapy

Compared with individual psychotherapy, group therapy has a number of distinct advantages as a treatment modality for alcohol/drug-addicted and dual-diagnosis patients in particular. Some of these advantages were articulated by Yalom,[2] when he discussed the curative factors of group therapy in general.

INSTILLATION OF HOPE

By the time individuals with a substance addiction problem enter treatment, their lives in large part have probably fallen apart as they have suffered from the consequences of their drug use. The potential losses of significant relationships, housing, and employment, along with possible legal entanglements, can erode one's sense of self and create a feeling of hopelessness. Addicts often enter treatment during times of extreme psychosocial distress, when feelings of despair can be most intense.

Group therapy can provide such patients with an opportunity to hear from others who have been in similar circumstances before and who have moved on from a point of hopelessness. Patients can learn from others whose lives had fallen apart that there is hope for the future. In fact, in Alcoholics Anonymous meetings (AA), an important component of these meetings is a member's "drunkalogue," which outlines the member's downward journey and eventual salvation through the benefits of abstinence. Although the drunkalogue has important treatment efficacy for the member, another key facet is letting others know that there is hope for them as well.

UNIVERSALITY

The ravages that a lifestyle centered around the compulsive use of chemicals can inflict on an individual are tremendous. In addition, to obtain chemicals, substance addicts often involve themselves in activities that they otherwise would not have participated in. These can include illegal activities, stealing from friends and family, and prostitution. When individuals finally enter treatment, they may be overwhelmed with guilt and shame. In fact, they may feel alone in their despair.

A group therapy experience with other individuals who have shared these same difficulties can counter feelings of guilt and worthlessness. Members can hear that other patients have done similar things to obtain drugs. What one has done is accepted by the other group members, and this acceptance can help to diminish a negative self-concept. The sense that they are not alone in the world with their problems is important and can be obtained from group therapy.

SOCIAL ISOLATION

Individuals who are addicted to chemicals often become extremely isolated and withdrawn. Drugs typically become their most important interest, and their social connectedness to the world becomes eroded. They may have lost their families and other significant relationships. What friends they do have all are using chemicals, and these individuals must be avoided if abstinence is to be achieved.

Thus, alienation, social isolation, and loneliness are often huge concerns for newly recovering substance addicts.

A group therapy experience can help to counter these feelings and provide individuals with a group of people with whom to begin to establish relationships. Rather than having only one therapist as a source of support, patients can establish supportive relationships with the group itself and with the other members of the group as well.

THE SHARED COMMON GOAL OF SOBRIETY

Giving up a lifestyle centered around the use and abuse of chemicals is often one of the hardest tasks a substance addict will ever have to accomplish. It demands a major lifestyle change and an entirely new way of coping in the world. In addition, a totally different social support system may have to be developed.

An expression in AA states, "You alone can do it, but you can't do it alone." What this means is that although alcoholics need to take sole responsibility and maintain abstinence on their own, outside support is both crucial and needed. For many alcoholics, the feeling that they are alone in the world maintaining abstinence (me against the world) is often a setup for failure. Instead, the feeling that others share the problem and that they all are working together on the problem can be very relieving and can ease the burden of the lifestyle change. Being in a group where everyone is sharing together in the common goal of maintaining abstinence can provide enormous solace and strength to all members. Yalom[2] notes that a cohesiveness that typically develops is a key curative variable in group therapy.

IMPARTING AND SHARING INFORMATION

If individuals are to learn how to live their lives without chemicals, they must acquire the basic tools to accomplish this. How to deal with urges, how to combat peer pressure, whether or not to attend a social function where chemicals of addiction might be available, or even how to get through a day without using the substance, to name just a few issues, must be learned. Group therapy can provide patients with such information in ways that individual therapy cannot.

In a group therapy experience, patients can hear from other patients and learn from each other what has and what has not worked. Suggestions and advice can be passed from one patient to another, and all patients can brainstorm to address a particular situation that a patient may experience. This opportunity can be invaluable to patients and is one that cannot be duplicated in individual psychotherapy. Other individuals who struggle with the same problem can be a wonderful source of information.

Such suggestions are not meant to tell others what to do with their lives; rather, the suggestions are directed at helping patients to maintain abstinence. All patients who struggle with a chemical dependence problem need advice about how to stop using and how to maintain abstinence. If patients knew how to stop using chemicals, they would not need treatment. Although giving advice is generally contraindicated in more traditional psychotherapy, imparting suggestions to patients about how to maintain abstinence is clearly indicated when treating substance addicts.[3]

As discussed later in this chapter, an important type of group therapy for the treatment of substance addiction is psychoeducational groups. In these groups, important information about various aspects of substance addiction is presented in a largely didactic manner, although interaction among group members is fostered and encouraged. For example, topics can include the medical aspects of addiction, family dynamics, the psychological process of addiction, or assertiveness training. It is generally more advantageous to present such information in a group setting, because questions may be asked and discussion generated in a way that would not occur if the subject matter were presented to one individual only. Presenting the information in a group format also makes much better use of staff time.

HELPING OTHERS

Features common to both psychiatric patients and substance addicts and particularly to those patients who experience both psychiatric and substance addiction problems are negative self-concepts and the feeling that they have nothing to offer anyone. Legal problems, disruption of familial relationships, and general traumas to the self all can erode one's identity and shatter one's self-esteem. As has just been discussed, group therapy can become a place where patients attempt to help one another by giving advice and suggestions. By imparting information and giving support to one another, patients can begin to develop a positive self-concept and a source of pride in themselves.

This potential curative factor inherent in group therapy has been incorporated into the structure of AA. The 12th step in AA states, "Having had a spiritual awakening as the result of these steps, we tried to carry this message to alcoholics, and to practice these principles in all our affairs."[4] Although carrying the message to alcoholics is a way for alcoholics to help others, it also has important treatment implications for the carriers. Participating in 12-step work is also a source of pride and esteem for recovering alcoholics. Additionally, self-esteem can be established and enhanced by becoming a sponsor and helping others with their addiction.

INTERPERSONAL LEARNING

Most individuals first begin using alcohol and drugs during their teenage years. For those individuals who develop an addiction, social relationships have often been conducted under the influence of drugs, and they thus have not interacted with other people in a drug-free state. In fact, Khantzian and colleagues[5] suggest that a core vulnerability to addiction may be difficulties in managing and regulating interpersonal relationships. This is especially true of those patients who experience a comorbid psychiatric illness along with their addiction problem. Furthermore, regardless of premorbid functioning, during the development of a substance dependence problem, addicts tend to become more isolated, and their relationships with others become marked by superficiality, mistrust, and manipulativeness.[6] If addicts are to recover from their addiction, they must move beyond their isolation and learn how to develop healthier relationships with others.

Group therapy provides an excellent means for patients to learn how to establish honest and open relationships with others. Taking risks by sharing one's feelings in a group can begin to diminish patients' isolation and can serve as a building block to establishing connections with others. Feedback about one's own behavior can also be received and can facilitate learning about oneself and one's presentation to others. Group therapy is obviously the treatment of choice to facilitate this process.

TO COMBAT DENIAL

A typical problem among substance addicts is the denial of their substance addiction problems. Patients frequently do not acknowledge that their use of substances is a problem, or even if they do, they often do not believe that resumption of drug use will again result in difficulties. In fact, broaching a patient's denial is often a central goal of treatment. Denial of psychiatric illness by dual diagnosis is also quite common. The result is poor compliance with prescribed medications and with general aftercare plans.

Group therapy as a mechanism to broach denial has certain advantages over individual psychotherapy. For example, if a patient reports that although drug use is sometimes excessive it is typically controlled and thus is not a problem, in a group setting with other individuals who have experienced similar problems, the person can hear from others who "have been there" that they, too, at one time had believed this, only to find out that they were wrong. Hearing from others who have learned the hard way often has more of an impact on patients than hearing from one's therapist. As Nace[7] noted, "Alcoholics can talk to each other in a way that is difficult for the nonalcoholic to do."

Group therapy can also help to decrease the chances that a substance addict will resume using substances again after a period of sobriety, typically resulting in a full-blown relapse. One of the most frequent reasons why substance addicts suffer a relapse is that after a period of sobriety, they begin to think that they can probably drink or take drugs in a controlled fashion without a resulting relapse. Although evidence suggests that some patients can return to moderate, asymptomatic drinking,[8–10] most patients find that this is not feasible because of the greater difficulties with frustration tolerance, affect regulation, self-esteem, and interpersonal skills that patients with a dual diagnosis experience. Alcohol and drugs can also interact with prescribed medication in synergistic ways or can decrease the efficacy of prescribed medication.[11] Even for the majority of patients who experience addiction difficulties without significant comorbid psychiatric difficulties, an attempt to control drug use will in all likelihood result in a full-blown relapse. In a group setting, patients discover from others who have attempted to control their drug use that this approach has inevitably been unsuccessful. Patients who begin to entertain this idea and talk about it in the group have the opportunity to receive feedback about the dangers of attempting this from others who have tried this and failed. Hearing this again and again helps substance addicts not to forget this important fact. Members of AA often report that they continue to go to meetings just so that they never forget that they have a problem for which the only solution is not to have one drink.

TWO CAVEATS

Although group therapy has distinct advantages over individual therapy for the treatment of addiction, it must be stated that group therapy may not be the appropriate method of treatment for all patients who experience a substance addiction problem. Some patients, as a result of their psychiatric difficulties, may be too uncomfortable in groups to obtain benefit from them. Mistrustful, socially phobic, agoraphobic, or paranoid patients, for example, may resist being in a group, and their resistance must be respected. I have also worked with extremely depressed patients who felt unable to participate in group therapy. We must always carefully listen to a patient's resistance, and when indicated, we must work with the patient to develop alternative treatment strategies. It is also possible that patients might feel able to attend certain types of groups but not others. Whatever treatment plan is worked out, treatment must always be individualized to the patient,[8] taking the patient's unique needs into account.

Second, although group therapy is an efficacious treatment modality for the treatment of substance addiction, this should not be interpreted to mean that individual therapy, either in place of or in conjunction with group therapy, should not occur. Patients often may need or desire individual psychotherapy to address issues that either need the intensity of individual therapy or that they do not feel comfortable discussing in a group. It is also possible that some patients may simply connect better to an individual psychotherapist than to a group. Patients who experience cognitive or neuropsychological difficulties, which may be either secondary to alcoholic drinking or which may have a separate autonomous role, may need a more focused, structured, and repetitive approach, which could be better provided by an individual therapist rather than through a group format. Whatever the case, the wishes and needs of our patients must be carefully assessed, and treatment must be individually tailored to them.

Models of Group Therapy

PSYCHOEDUCATIONAL GROUPS

Psychoeducational groups use primarily a lecture-discussion format in which selected topics about various aspects of chemical addiction and the overall recovery process from it are presented to patients. For patients with a dual diagnosis, information presented could also include information about psychiatric illness, the relationships between psychiatric illness and addiction, and the appropriate use of medication, including the potential interaction between prescribed medication and chemicals of addiction. Such groups are critically important, especially for new patients, because they provide patients with essential information about addiction and psychiatric illness and help to teach patients the skills that they need to remain abstinent. These groups attempt to build the basic foundation that will underlie patients' recovery process. Because patients can either remain silent or speak up as their comfort level increases, such groups serve as a good introduction to the process of therapy in general.[6] Written assignments to be completed either during the group meeting or afterward are also a common feature.

These types of groups typically are part of inpatient substance addiction or dual-diagnosis programs and are also an important treatment modality in outpatient day or evening treatment programs designed for the treatment of chemical dependence. The number of patients in these types of groups can range from a small handful to as many as 20. Membership in these groups is usually open owing to the setting in which they occur and the need to treat all the patients who seek treatment in an expeditious fashion. In addition, the clinical effectiveness of psychoeducational groups is less dependent on a closed membership than are more traditional psychotherapy groups (discussed later). However, even in these groups, some stability in membership is helpful because it aids in the development of group cohesiveness. Homogeneity in membership within these types of groups is obvious, because all members have problems with substance dependence. Although patients may not be completely ready to stop using chemicals or ready for treatment in general, they should at least be willing to learn about the process of chemical addiction and the skills that are needed to stop using addictive substances (see Miller and Rollnick[12] and Proschaska and DiClemente[13] for a discussion of motivation for treatment with substance addicts).

Topics generally covered by psychoeducational groups can include the process of addiction, why people use drugs, medical aspects of addiction, addiction as a family illness, leisure activities, stress management, causes of relapse and relapse prevention, assertiveness training and dealing with conflict, anger management, how to say no to alcohol/drugs, sexually transmitted diseases, the need for aftercare and ongoing treatment, and introduction to self-help groups. In addition to these groups, patients with a dual diagnosis should also receive education about psychiatric illnesses, the relationships between psychiatric illness and substance addiction, and the importance of medication compliance and the interaction of prescribed medication with alcohol and other chemicals of addiction. Some specialized groups are also frequently offered, including a men's group, a women's group, or a group for victims of trauma. The trauma group should focus on ascertaining an accurate diagnosis, providing education and support, and helping patients to obtain some measure of control and safety, which obviously includes refraining from chemical use.[14]

Although a psychoeducational group is in some ways like a course, how the information is presented and what themes are highlighted are dependent on the particular subgroup of patients in the group and should be individualized. In addition, although a lecture format is used, group participation and interaction are fostered and encouraged.

SELF-HELP GROUPS

Self-help groups are an extremely important treatment modality for patients who experience substance addiction problems. The most well-known self-help group program is AA. It is estimated that AA has more than a million and a half members worldwide and in the United States alone more than 775,000 members. Other self-help groups modeled after AA include Cocaine Anonymous, Narcotics Anonymous, and Pills Anonymous. Self-help groups have also been developed to help patients who experience other types of addictions such as to gambling and food (Gamblers Anonymous and Overeaters Anonymous).

All self-groups modeled after AA that are designed to help substance addicts encourage complete abstinence from drugs. In addition, the philosophy underlying the program is that addiction to chemicals is a disease and that recovery is a lifelong process. It is suggested that recovery from drug addiction can be accomplished one day at a time and by following the 12 steps of AA, the first of which is to admit powerlessness over the drug.[4] Emphasis is also placed on a Higher Power (however this is understood) outside of oneself to help the person attain abstinence. Various types of meetings include speaker meetings, discussion meetings, beginner meetings, and step meetings. Meetings can also be open to anyone or closed to everyone other than members of AA. Specialized groups have been formed for women, men, gays, and young addicts. Groups can vary tremendously in size from a few members to hundreds.

In speaker meetings, several members who have maintained abstinence tell their story from when they first used drugs to when drugs became destructive and finally to their salvation through abstinence and their involvement in the program. The other members of the group typically identify with aspects of these stories, which can provide a model for one's own recovery. Discussion meetings generally focus on a particular aspect of the recovery process. Step meetings discuss particular steps in the program.

Another important aspect of the program is the use of a sponsor, who is someone chosen by a member to provide guidance and who is readily available to talk by telephone when the need arises. Sponsors should be solidly in recovery as they offer assistance to newer members. (For a more thorough discussion of the philosophy and workings of AA and other similar programs, see Alcoholics Anonymous,[4, 15] Alibrandi,[16] Khantzian and Mack,[17] Mack,[18] Nace,[7] and Zimberg.[1])

Although attempting to evaluate the efficacy of any treatment modality poses major methodological problems, evidence suggests that AA can be a very effective treatment modality to enable patients to achieve abstinence.[19] Certainly, many patients report that without the use of the program, they never would have been able to achieve abstinence. In addition, the sheer numbers of people involved in AA speak for themselves. AA-oriented groups are powerful group therapy experiences, because built into the structure of such groups are all of the advantages that group therapy has over individual therapy, as previously outlined in this chapter. Mack[18] has theorized how the alcohol-controlling capacity of the other members of AA aids alcoholics in self-governance and in taking charge of themselves. Unconditional acceptance of all members incorporated into the program is also a powerful curative factor.

However they work, AA-oriented groups must be considered when working with this patient population. It must be remembered, however, that although patients should be encouraged to at least try AA or other similar groups (to attend at least three meetings per week for 1 month in order to determine whether or not AA is for them), some patients may resist this recommendation. Resistance should be explored because it often concerns the person's inability to acknowledge drug use as a problem. Some patients' resistance is well founded, however, and such patients should not be encouraged to attend meetings.[20] For example, based on life experience and character structure, some patients may find the concept of powerlessness distasteful. For others, the religious overtones of the program or the philosophy that "this is the only way to recovery" may prevent them from connecting to it. Agoraphobic, extremely self-conscious, and paranoid patients obviously may not feel comfortable in such groups. I have also worked with some depressed patients who, despite abstinence and antidepressant medication, continued to be plagued by intense depression. Attending meetings and hearing from others how abstinence improved their lives can lead to increased despair and hopelessness. All therapists who work with drug-involved patients should have some familiarity with such groups. Attending some meetings is a wonderful way to gain knowledge of the program and is strongly encouraged.

Clinicians also need to be aware that patients who have a dual diagnosis and who are being prescribed psychotropic medications may occasionally encounter AA members who tell them that they should stop taking their medication, although this view is not endorsed by AA. Although this advice is not given with malevolent intention, taking it could have disastrous consequences. Treatment providers need to be sensitive to this issue both when referring such patients to this program and throughout treatment.

Rational Recovery (RR) is another self-help group that has been developed to help individuals who suffer from chemical dependence. RR is founded on the principles of Ellis' rational-emotive behavior therapy. It is strikingly different from AA in philosophy. For example, RR eschews the concepts of powerlessness and that of a Higher Power. It also does not believe that chemical addiction is a disease. Although RR is a much smaller program than AA, it is growing and now has more than 500 groups in the United States. RR should be considered for patients who find the philosophy of AA distasteful or who could better connect to this program because of its orientation. (For a more thorough discussion of RR, see Ellis and colleagues,[21] Galanter and associates,[22] and Trimpey.[23])

GROUP PSYCHOTHERAPY

Traditional group therapy has historically not been thought to be useful for the treatment of alcoholism or other substance addiction problems. Indeed, even individual therapy has often been discouraged for this patient population. Although the reasons for this bias are not certain, there a number of possible explanations.

It is possible that individuals afflicted with substance addiction problems are often seen in crisis, are intoxicated and demanding, and thus may be viewed as poor therapy candidates. Or perhaps more traditional therapeutic endeavors have not focused on a patient's chemical use as a problem in and of itself, and consequently, throughout therapy, the patient's substance addiction was not made an important focus of treatment. The result of this was a poor outcome, in large part due to the patient's continued use of substances. It is also believed that therapy could increase a patient's denial of having a problem with chemical use. Specifically, a patient's substance addiction could be viewed as a symptom of some underlying difficulty that needs to be addressed before the patient could be expected to stop the drug use. Consequently, strong encouragement to stop chemical use may not occur, and the clinician inadvertently may collude with the patient's denial.

Whatever the reasons, with some modifications, traditional group therapy can be an effective form of treatment for patients who experience problems with chemical addiction. Within these groups, although remaining abstinent from chemicals is an important focus of treatment, exploration of patients' other intrapsychic and interpersonal problems is also undertaken. How individuals' psychiatric difficulties played a part in their becoming addicted to chemicals is explored. In addition, helping patients to work through particular issues, to learn healthier ways to cope, and to improve relationship conflicts remains an important focus of treatment. Especially with patients with a dual diagnosis, the message that must be imparted is that although stopping chemical use will not make everything better all at once, it is a necessary first step. At all times, the importance of remaining abstinent and of learning other ways to manage discomfort and dysphoric feelings is conveyed to all patients.

Particularly in early recovery, such groups should be homogeneous in terms of all patients in the group having a substance addiction/dependence problem. This is very important because a major focus of the group must be on remaining abstinent. If patients in early recovery are placed in general psychotherapy groups, the focus on abstinence may be lost, which would not be in the patients' best interest. Patients may often request a more general therapy group as a defense against examining their own addiction. This should be explored with patients, and in general, patients should be referred to an addiction psychotherapy group. For a patient who is solidly in recovery and who requests a group therapy experience for other concerns, a referral to a more general psychotherapy group would not be contraindicated.

All patients in the group should be motivated to stop chemical use or at least be willing to look honestly at their drug use to determine whether or not it is a problem. Khantzian and colleagues[5] and Vannicelli[24] suggest that patients should be abstinent before beginning the therapy group. This can be accomplished if patients first participate in psychoeducational groups designed to teach them the essentials about achieving abstinence and avoiding relapses. However, many chronically impaired patients with a dual diagnosis may lack motivation to stop drug use and may not be abstinent. Despite continued drug use, if patients can at least report an interest in learning about how drugs could be affecting them, referring them to a group in which they can meet other patients in various stages of recovery can help to engage them into treatment and eventually into a process of recovery. Within the group, denial can often be broached with the other patients' assistance. Continued substance use, in and of itself, should not be an exclusionary criterion because abstinence is the treatment goal. If a patient continues over time to use substances, remains in denial, or demonstrates no wish to stop, termination from the group needs to be considered because this patient could become a destructive force in the group.

A number of group therapy approaches have been developed for substance addicts.[5, 24–26] All approaches address an addict's characterological difficulties as they become manifested in the group. At the same time, however, with structure and support, abstinence and relapse prevention remain an important focus of treatment. Khantzian and colleagues[5] have developed a modified dynamic group therapy (MDGT) for cocaine addicts. MDGT also has applicability for other substance addicts. These researchers see addicts as having core difficulties in four areas: accessing, tolerating, and regulating feelings; problems with relationships; self-care failures; and self-esteem deficits. MDGT addresses these vulnerabilities as they are manifested with other group members. MDGT uses both supportive and expressive interventions with an active rather than neutral therapist. MDGT is more structured and directed than traditional psychodynamic therapy. It meets twice a week for 26 weeks.

The model described by Vanicelli[24] also pays careful attention to containing substance addiction through the use of negotiated stepwise contracts that can support abstinence (such as AA, disulfiram, naltrexone, or relapse prevention training). In addition, within a dynamically oriented group, the substance addict's characterological difficulties are addressed. Whatever group theoretical orientation is used, the important point is that although an addict's life problems and characterological difficulties are addressed, emphasis is simultaneously placed on abstinence and helping the substance addict to learn other ways to cope with his or her problems. A patient's problem with chemical addiction must at all times remain in the therapeutic field.

Summary

Group therapy is an important treatment modality for patients who experience substance addiction difficulties and for those patients who suffer from substance addiction problems and comorbid psychiatric difficulties. Why group therapy is a highly effective form of treatment for this challenging patient population has been articulated in this chapter. In addition, specific models of groups used with such patients have been discussed. These include psychoeducational groups, self-help groups, and more traditional psychotherapy groups.

REFERENCES

1. Zimberg S: The Clinical Management of Alcoholism. New York, Brunner/Mazel, 1982.
2. Yalom ID: The Theory and Practice of Group Psychotherapy, 2nd ed. New York, Basic Books, 1975.
3. Levy M: A change in orientation: Therapeutic Strategies for the treatment of alcoholism. Psychotherapy 24(4):786–793, 1987.
4. Alcoholics Anonymous: Twelve Steps and Twelve Traditions. New York, Alcoholics Anonymous World Services, 1952.
5. Khantzian EJ, Halliday KS, McAuliffe WE: Addiction and the Vulnerable Self. Modified Dynamic Group Therapy for Substance Abusers. New York, Guilford Press, 1990.
6. Blume SB: Group psychotherapy in the treatment of alcoholism. In Zimberg S, Wallace J, Blume SB (eds): Practical Approaches to Alcoholism Psychotherapy, 2nd ed. New York, Plenum, 1985, pp 73–86.
7. Nace EP: The Treatment of Alcoholism. New York, Brunner/Mazel, 1987, p 174.
8. Levy MS: Individualized care for the treatment of alcoholism. J Subst Abuse Treat 7(4):245–254, 1990.
9. Polich JM, Armor DJ, Braiker HB: The Course of Alcoholism. New York, John Wiley & Sons, 1981.
10. Vaillant GE: The Natural History of Alcoholism. Causes, Patterns, and Paths to Recovery. Cambridge, MA, Harvard University Press, 1983.
11. Johnson M, Ellison JM: Interactions of alcohol, street drugs, and prescribed medications. In Ellison JM (ed): The Psychotherapist's Guide to Pharmacotherapy. Chicago, Year Book, 1989.
12. Miller W, Rollnick S: Motivational Interviewing, Preparing People to Change Addictive Behavior. New York, Guilford Press, 1992.
13. Proschaska JO, DiClemente CC: Toward a comprehensive model of change. In Miller WR, Hester RK (eds): Treating Addictive Behaviors: Process of Change. New York, Plenum, 1986, pp 3–27.
14. Herman JL: Trauma and Recovery. New York, Basic Books, 1992.
15. Alcoholics Anonymous, 3rd ed. New York, Alcoholics Anonymous World Services, 1976.
16. Alibrandi LA: The fellowship of Alcoholics Anonymous. In Pattison EM, Kaufman E (eds): Encyclopedic Handbook of Alcoholism. New York, Gardner Press, 1982, pp 979–986.
17. Khantzian EJ, Mack JE: How AA works and why it's important for clinicians to understand. J Subst Abuse Treat 11(2):77–92, 1994.
18. Mack JE: Alcoholism, AA, and the governance of the self. In Bean MH, Zinberg NE (eds): Dynamic Approaches to the Understanding and Treatment of Alcoholism. New York, The Free Press, 1981, pp 128–162.
19. Leach B, Norris JL: Factors in the development of Alcoholics Anonymous (AA). In Kissin B, Begleiter H (eds): The Biology of Alcoholism, vol 5. New York, Plenum, 1977, pp 441–543.
20. Levy M: Alcohol and addictions (letter to the editor). Am J Psychiatry 149(8):1117–1118, 1992.
21. Ellis A, McInery JF, DiGiuseppe R, Yeager RJ: Rational-Emotive Therapy with Alcoholics and Substance Abusers. Elmsford, NY, Pergamon, 1988.
22. Galanter M, Egelko S, Edwards H: Rational Recovery: Alternative to AA for addiction. Am J Drug Alcohol Abuse 14:499–510, 1993.
23. Trimpley J: Rational Recovery from Alcoholism: The Small Book. New York, Delacorte, 1984.
24. Vannicelli M: Removing the Roadblocks. Group Psychotherapy with Substance Abusers and Family Members. New York, Guilford Press, 1992.
25. Brown S, Yalom ID: Interactional group therapy with alcoholics. J Stud Alcohol 38(3):426–456, 1974.
26. Yalom ID: Group therapy and alcoholism. Ann N Y Acad Sci 233:85–103, 1974.

The Elements of Contemporary Treatment

R. Jeffrey Goldsmith, MD

Treatment for alcoholism and the addictions is a complex fabric woven from the threads of four basic components: patient characteristics, program composition, 12-step groups, and staff talent. Each component, in turn, has its own dynamics and qualities, which must be understood to master the elements of treatment. Although research in addiction medicine has been carried out for half a century, we still understand these components incompletely. Although research has clarified many elements through the years, we must start in our quest for mastery over alcoholism and the addictions with knowledge of these elements.

When evaluating outcome and constructing a program for treatment, it is important to decide whether or not abstinence will be the main measure or the only measure of success. This decision hinges on the concept of loss of control as a biologically based phenomenon, involving cellular changes (sensitization) or unique chemical interactions. If loss of control is biological and permanent and depends on internal variables, then prolonged controlled drinking/drug use is impossible. On the other hand, if loss of control is a psychosocial phenomenon, based on family crisis or individual personality dynamics, then controlled use depends on the patient. These beliefs about loss of control often determine the focus of treatment and influence the design of treatment elements.

From an outside observer's point of view, reduced drinking and drug use by a patient translates into fewer family and personal problems. The Rand Corporation conducted a 4-year outcome study involving nearly 1000 alcoholics, observing them through a course of treatment.[1] Some remained abstinent the entire 4 years, and nearly 20% had 3 years or more of abstinence. They found that the longer a person remained abstinent, the fewer alcohol-related problems he or she had. From a researcher's point of view, this observation suggests that reduced consumption is a legitimate goal of treatment. Furthermore, the Rand Report found that 12% of the subjects reported continued drinking without any symptoms of alcohol dependence at the 4-year follow-up.

In order to understand the full import of these findings, the details of the study must be explored. The Rand researchers decided that they should gather data about the month before the interview. Using sound methodological reasoning, they decided that memory becomes too vague when evaluators ask about experiences more distant than a month. Collecting data for less than a month misses many psychosocial events that are essential to a comprehensive outcome study. Therefore, the treatment outcomes were derived from the month before the follow-up interviews. The initial evaluation at 18 months reported that as many as 40% of the subjects reported controlled drinking. The change from 40% at 18 months to 12% at 48 months suggests that alcoholics may drink in a controlled fashion for brief periods of time but cannot sustain this pattern indefinitely.

Researchers have debated for years whether or not self-report is reliable, generally concluding that the vast majority of the histories are valid and useful.[2] The Rand researchers came to the same conclusion, using their own test for internal validity. They took a history of drinking for the week before the interview and then gave the subjects, unannounced, a breath test for alcohol. About 20% of the subjects denied or minimized drinking when compared with the breath test results. Furthermore, because alcohol is quickly metabolized, only very recent drinking would be discovered by this method. Others could have minimized their drinking and may not have been caught. Thus, 20% is a conservative measure of invalid histories. How does this group of deniers relate to the controlled drinkers? Perhaps the 12% is an artifact.

In addition, the Rand Report found that the mortality rate for drinkers was two and one-half times that of the normal population. Further analysis showed that the group of drinkers younger than 40 years had a mortality rate 4.4 times the expected rate. As the amount of drinking increased, the death rate increased. Is this drinking benign?

In 1978, the Sobells[3] published a report that claimed to have taught alcohol addicts how to drink in a controlled, socially acceptable manner. Pendery and colleagues[4] conducted independent follow-up of this research cohort a few years later and found no controlled drinking, only abstinence, alcoholic drinking, and death. Helzer and associates[5] studied more than 1600 subjects up to 7 years after treatment and found that fewer than 2% of the subjects were drinking in a controlled fashion. These studies suggest that controlled drinking is neither a legitimate nor safe treatment goal for alcohol-dependent patients.

It is also an error to assume that abstinence resolves all problems. People come to treatment with various problems that involve the body, mind, family, and lifestyle in general. McLellan and coworkers,[6] measuring seven domains with the addiction severity index, found that some but not all domains improved when veterans with alcoholism and addictions significantly decreased their use. Medical and family problems (as well as alcohol and drug problems) did respond favorably to a marked reduction in alcohol/drug consumption. The other domains—employment, legal, and psychiatric—did not improve during the 6-month follow-up period, causing the researchers to say that reduced use was "necessary but not sufficient for improvement in these other areas."

Abstinence then becomes a necessary but not sufficient goal for treatment. Large outcome studies with alcoholics report that abstinence is a major factor.[7] Programs that are drug free in orientation produce more abstinence.[8] On the other hand, the dropout rates are higher among addicts when the treatment program has a drug-free orientation compared with the methadone maintenance programs. The proper balance may be to work toward abstinence yet stay empathically in tune with an alcoholic/drug addict to avoid premature termination as a result of rigid insistence on complete abstinence. Increasing the treatment intensity may also support the attainment of abstinence by environmentally supporting an addict.

Patient Characteristics

To be effective, treatment must be individualized for each patient. For years, the treatment community has been program oriented and, on the surface, acted as if one program was suited to various patients. Therapists have for years considered ways to individualize the programs to meet the needs of their patients. The patient mix clearly becomes a critical factor for any therapist or program: the number of women and men, the number of minority patients, which drugs they are using, the presence of comorbid medical or psychiatric illnesses, whether they are employed, and whether they have families who will participate.

Some of these patient characteristics determine whether or not a patient can even enter a treatment program. Treatment effectiveness is irrelevant if a patient cannot remain in treatment. Remaining in treatment has been a problem for women, especially pregnant women, medically ill patients (severe liver disease or chronic pain), and psychiatrically ill patients (acutely psychotic, suicidal, and the very anxious/depressed). In response to this problem, specialized programs have evolved to incorporate interventions necessary for the treatment of these patients, allowing them to participate. Perinatal programs are now available but still uncommon. As liver transplantation becomes more common among alcoholics and drug addicts, treatment programs will evolve collaborative techniques that allow these patients to participate in less-intensive, flexible therapy. Dual-diagnosis programs for mentally ill alcoholics and drug addicts are more common than they used to be.

Some patient characteristics influence treatment effectiveness through patient retention. Minority patients often drop out of treatment that is traditionally oriented toward middle-class European-Americans.[9] Cultural sensitivity technology has burgeoned in the past decade and is now available to therapists and programs. Called *cultural competence*, these strategies and techniques reduced dropout rates and give the essential elements of treatment a chance to have an impact. In addition to minorities, women have been underserved through the years. Research has shown that women are better served in all women's groups[10] and that they have different needs from men.[11] Many programs have a preponderance of male patients, and women patients are often outnumbered by two to one. Research in male-dominated programs has discovered that women prefer individual sessions to group therapy.[7] Adelman and Weiss[12] found that when therapists negotiated with their patients and developed an individualized treatment plan, both retention and treatment outcome were improved. In light of the many crises and multiple life problems that alcoholics and addicts bring to treatment, this is not surprising.

Program Elements

Several treatment paradigms have been used in clinical programs for alcoholism and the addictions.[13] Three main paradigms are popular today. The abstinence-based 12-step paradigm is based on the disease concept of alcoholism and uses the wisdom inherent in the 12 steps of Alcoholics Anonymous (AA).[14] It includes cognitive, behavioral, and motivational techniques.[13] The cognitive-behavioral approach is based on work by Beck and associates and it draws on the idea that behaviors follow from maladaptive cognitive beliefs and assumptions, which can be altered in a systematic therapy.[15] Motivational interviewing is a third technique, which has been developed by Miller and Rollnick[16] and the Sobells.[17] This technique focuses on a patient's motivation to change and strives to increase whatever motivation a patient has, drawing out the desire and commitment to improve one's situation. A fourth paradigm, popular among mental health professionals, is the self-medication hy-

pothesis, which rests on a psychodynamic understanding. It assumes that motivation to use alcohol and drugs is based on a desire to feel better, to medicate some unpleasant feelings.[18]

In the United States today, about 95% of the treatment centers use the abstinence-based 12-step model derived from the disease concept of alcoholism.[19] It is based on the idea that alcoholics have a unique, inherited biology in response to alcohol and that this biology makes it impossible to drink socially.[20] The disease concept recognizes common signs and symptoms that emerge in a chronic, progressive, predictable fashion.[13] These programs hold that complete abstinence is essential to combat loss of control, which can occur with any addictive drug because of the cross-tolerance and common biology. The similarities in drug reinforcement, loss of control, progression of family dysfunction, legal problems, and job problems make alcoholism and the addictions related illnesses.

The emphasis on the biological reinforcement that alcoholics and addicts experience does not mean that the disease concept ignores the influence of psychosocial factors. Research has documented that life stresses are often associated with increased alcohol and drug use.[13] The disease concept, however, emphasizes that this is not to be construed as an etiological relationship. Stress influences patients' desire to use a drug and, to a certain extent, the amount, but stress does not alter tolerance or the loss of control that can occur as a result of use. Furthermore, proponents of other models sometimes attack the disease concept as a way of excusing patients from taking responsibilities for their actions. The disease concept does not provide patients with an excuse, however: Individuals are responsible for any behaviors that occur under the influence and are responsible for taking action to recover from their illness. The only things for which a patient is not responsible are causing the illness in the first place and losing control, which are functions of the biology of the disease. For abstinence-based 12-step–oriented programs, the goals are to persuade or convince patients to commit to a lifetime of abstinence, accept the loss of control, and forgive the behaviors that accompany such loss of control. Programs include education about the disease concept and therapy that encourages discussion of guilt and shame resulting from intoxicated behaviors. Relapse prevention plays an important part because the possibility of relapse is always present.

ENGAGEMENT AND RETENTION

If treatment is to be effective, engagement and retention are critical. Without engagement and retention there can be no dosing of treatment, nor can there be any individualizing of the treatment that is provided. Studies have shown that more treatment sessions result in more abstinence[21] and fewer psychosocial problems.[6] Although this observation suggests that treatment has a dose-response effectiveness, it does not rule out the possibility that people who stay in treatment are already more receptive than those who drop out of treatment. However, coercion has been shown through the years to be an effective way to keep people in treatment and to bring improvement to unmotivated patients.[22, 23] Welte and colleagues[24] found that program completion, not just the total number of sessions, was significantly related to a more favorable outcome. All of these studies suggest that both the total number of sessions *and* patients' receptiveness to treatment are important factors.

Engaging a patient who is markedly ambivalent about quitting alcohol or drugs through the management of motivation and denial becomes critical. Miller and Rollnick[16] and the Sobells[17] have developed techniques for enhancing motivation through a particular interviewing approach. Goldsmith and Green[25] developed the denial rating scale, which has been used to focus psychotherapy on the management of denial. Increased awareness and less denial, as rated by the denial rating scale, have been associated with improved program completion.[25, 26] The three techniques—use of coercion, motivation enhancement, and denial-focused therapy—are important techniques in the treatment of ambivalent patients in the early stages of treatment.

Dropout rates in the first month of treatment in an outpatient setting approach 50%,[27] giving treatment programs considerable room for improvement. Earlier research demonstrated that continuity of care between the intake assessment and the counseling session is associated with higher retention rates.[28] Furthermore, when counselors call their clients or send them letters immediately after a missed appointment, the retention rates are also increased.[29]

Other factors associated with improved engagement and retention include the treatment of psychiatric comorbidity[30] and the inclusion of family members.[31] When addicted patients have comorbid psychiatric illness, the retention is enhanced and their recovery from both illnesses improved when the mental illness and the addiction are treated concurrently. The inclusion of family members, significant others, or employers improved retention rates in both outpatient and inpatient programs. This network therapy has been so successful that Galanter[32] has incorporated it into a new outpatient psychotherapy strategy as a way to enhance motivation and encourage commitment and follow-through with the treatment plan.

GROUP INTERVENTIONS

Group therapy is almost always included as part of a comprehensive program in addition to individual and family therapy. Many studies have found group therapy effective with both alcoholics and drug addicts[33]; moreover, groups focusing on social skills, coping styles, education about the disease, interpersonal dynamics, and treatment of self-deficits all have proved to be effective under research conditions.[7, 34, 35] The focus of a particular group can vary considerably, making it a versatile format. When packaged with other components of treatment, groups contribute significantly, meeting many of the needs of the different patients. Social skills groups, assertiveness training, and interpersonal groups all address the maladaptive interpersonal styles usually noted in this patient population. Such group therapy can be essential in establishing effective communication, decreasing social isolation through social networking, and improving economic functioning by improving on-the-job behaviors. Education groups sometimes seem superficial to a skillful psychotherapist; however, they are important in correcting popular myths about alcohol and drug dependence, as well as in suggesting helpful hints for the early and middle stages of recovery. Psychotherapy groups can facilitate the expression of affect, tension, and fear, allowing an opportunity to discuss the implications of traumatic events. Yalom[36] describes a number of ways in which group therapy promotes healing among group members through the group interactions. Expressive arts therapy groups (art, music, and psychodrama) are important because they offer alternative ways to discover/uncover core issues and express unconscious material that may be difficult or impossible to discuss initially.

Group composition is important to consider when conducting groups. As mentioned earlier, group therapy research has found that women fare better in all-women groups whereas men fare better in groups comprising both sexes.[10] It appears that men talk more about feelings with women present, whereas women are somewhat inhibited and avoid certain topics when men are present. Freedom of self-expression may depend on the style of the group leaders, who can facilitate the discussion of issues, can interpret the resistance to discussing intimate issues, or can avoid the group process altogether by focusing on individuals. How long the group continues, whether or not the members have individual therapists, and how stable the group composition is will affect both the style of the group leader and the group dynamics.[37, 38]

Focusing on group dynamics encourages interpersonal feedback, evoking issues of confrontation, understanding, compassion, trust, and support. Leadership styles also determine how effectively the members deal with those issues that inevitably arise during the group process. Brown[34] discovered that group therapy focused on interpersonal dynamics during the early phases of recovery may actually clash with the focus in AA on staying sober, leaving patients feeling uncomfortable and unwilling to participate in both processes concurrently.

FAMILY INTERVENTIONS

Interventions using family members have been an important part of alcoholism and drug dependence treatment. Family therapy has been essential to change maladaptive patterns, to reduce the likelihood of a family's contributing to a relapse, and to promote the healthy development of all family members. Steinglass and colleagues[39] described two maladaptive or dysfunctional patterns of family dynamics that occur during the active (wet) phase of use and the dry (abstinent) phase of use. Family therapy becomes important to promote healthy change, because abstinence is not sufficient to restore optimal functioning. The exact form of family intervention is not precisely identified. Gliedman and associates[40] developed a technique in which the spouse was treated at the same time for codependence but in a separate group, followed later in the course of treatment with conjoint sessions. McCrady[31] demonstrated that including the spouse in conjoint sessions was important in minimizing the number of separations that occurred in the first year of recovery. Spouse participation in this study also improved the alcoholics' commitment to abstinence. The Johnson Institute developed a technique of family confrontation as a way to engage alcoholics in denial into treatment.[41] This technique involves family rehearsals to help the family through their own denial and ambivalence, not to mention anger and frustration, before they confront the alcoholic and encourage him or her to enter treatment.

INDIVIDUAL THERAPY

Individual counseling is an important and basic element of treatment programs. It has been shown to be helpful with alcoholics and addicts.[7] Individual psychotherapy provided by psychiatrists or psychologists is less common than counseling provided by a counselor. A number of studies with methadone maintenance have shown that psychotherapy provides additional improvement in the treatment outcome beyond basic counseling.[30] Furthermore, treatment of psychiatric comorbidity with a psychiatric collaborator also improves outcome, especially depression.[30] A growing consensus is that psychotherapy must begin with abstinence or a focus on abstinence as a major goal.[35, 42, 43]

12-Step Groups and Aftercare

AA began in 1935 when Bill W. joined with Dr. Bob S. to form a group where alcoholics could find support for their desire to quit drinking. AA was founded on the ideas adopted from the Oxford group, a religious community, and developed the 12 steps, which outline a disciplined, introspective exploration that leads to recovery from the disease of alcoholism.[44] Although AA is not designed as a treatment program, it does help people stay sober. Vaillant[45] found that AA attendance explained 28% of the clinical outcome, compared with 7% for stable adjustment, married, employed, and never detoxified. Because of its effectiveness, AA has grown, both within the United States and beyond. Its principles have been adapted for Narcotics Anonymous, Gamblers Anonymous, Nicotine Anonymous, and others.

Psychotherapists need to understand how AA works and how to use it.[44] When combined with interpersonal group psychotherapy, where the focus was on the interactions between group members, AA did not naturally fit.[34] AA's focus on sobriety and recovery created tension within the group and its focus on interpersonal styles. Only when the group shifted to a recovery-oriented focus did the combination appear useful.

Hoffman and the Comprehensive Assessment and Treatment Outcome Research (CATOR) studies[19] have gathered treatment outcome data on thousands of patients. CATOR found that patients who completed inpatient or outpatient treatment for alcoholism and who attended AA weekly had a 50% greater abstinence rate than those who did not. In a similar analysis, a dose response to aftercare treatment was noted after inpatient treatment. This analysis showed that 12 months of aftercare produced 84% abstinence, compared with 72% for those who had 6 to 11 months and 54% for those involved less than 6 months.

Vaillant[45] reported that recovery needs to be conceptualized as a long-term phenomenon. He found that patients who were abstinent less than 3 years showed psychological adjustments that were similar to those of actively drinking patients. In contrast, Vaillant found that patients with abstinence for 10 years or more had a psychosocial adjustment that was comparable to that of nondrinkers.

AA includes certain practices as part of its routine activities and precludes others.[44] It does not solicit members, charge dues, follow up on members, provide professional care, join councils or social agencies, or provide housing, meals, or transportation. It does provide a number of meetings on a regular basis (some for everyone, some for special populations), focused on the welfare of alcoholics. The membership is open to those alcoholics who have a desire to stop drinking. The services are nonprofessional, accepting contributions from members only. Anonymity is the spiritual foundation of the traditions. Because of the way AA works, it has been pointed out that AA instills hope through contact with other alcoholics who are recovering, encourages self-disclosure and self-exploration, continually emphasizes abstinence as the only path, insists that recovery cannot occur in isolation, and promotes spirituality of a nonsectarian type to steer alcoholics from self-centeredness toward humility, love, and growth. Many professionals who attend open meetings are impressed by the humility, altruistic caring, and gratitude that are characteristic of AA members in action.

Psychotherapists who are familiar with AA and the 12 steps can assess how involved their patients are. Are they going to meetings regularly, even daily? Do they have sponsors, and are they working steps? Which steps are they working, and what is being stirred up by this process? Are they stuck—where? Are they related to an alcoholic, and do they need Al-Anon (for persons concerned about an alcoholic)? Through familiarity with the process of AA, therapists can encourage involvement in the healing powers of AA and lend credibility to the 12 steps, even as they gain credibility through their knowledge of AA and how it works.

Staff Skills

Treatment outcome research has provided some insight into the importance of staff skills. Crits-Cristoph and colleagues[46] developed a statistical method to analyze the impact of the therapist in various treatment outcome studies. In some studies they found no special impact, but in others they found that as much as 29% of the variance was attributable to therapist effects. This suggests that a therapist's skills may be as critical or more so than the type of therapy used.

Graduate training is not an issue here, because M.D.s and Ph.D.s participated in some of these studies. The issue is more likely the capacity to make a connection with patients and to keep the connection while making the necessary confrontations/interventions. Many techniques can be used to become disconnected from alcoholics and addicts. Some staff do not want to work with this patient population. One study[47] found three factors associated with staff retention problems: (1) reluctance to work with drug addicts, (2) the location of the work site, and (3) fear of acquired immunodeficiency syndrome. Some do not have the skills to make the nonjudgmental interventions necessary. Others do not understand patients' experience and fail to make an empathic connection.

Staff codependence has been suggested as a major factor in suboptimal treatment.[48] Secondary codependence includes maladaptive responses to the disconnecting behaviors of an addict (anger, demands, drug use, and failure to show) as well as to the connecting behaviors of an addict (calling in a crisis, drug seeking, and asking for special favors). Primary codependence encompasses the transference reactions of a *therapist* who grew up in a dysfunctional/alcoholic family. Physician training in medical school and residency can make a significant difference in minimizing secondary codependence. Bergen and colleagues[49] demonstrated that students come to medical school with pessimistic attitudes about the treatability of alcoholics and addicts. After a brief, intensive, and well-supervised experience, the students were much more optimistic and interested. Chappel and Schnoll[50] documented that residency training actually generated *increasingly* negative attitudes about the worth of treatment as the training progressed.

Few studies have investigated staff skills. One such study[51] examined the patient retention rate in an outpatient clinic. After establishing a baseline, the researchers were able to increase retention simply by providing supervisory monthly feedback to the counselors about their caseload. This study points out that the administrative system can also have a significant impact.

Conclusions

Many treatment techniques and strategies are effective in bringing relief or change in a focal way. Family tension and miscommunication can be improved as long as the family is included in treatment for a minimum number of sessions. Psychiatric illness can be treated if psychiatric treatment is included as an intervention. The concept of multicomponent programming is important. First made popular in the area of nicotine dependence,[52] multicomponent programming refers to the idea of packaging together various effective interventions to create a treatment program. Each intervention is a component, and the whole is more effective than each component.

Although multicomponent programming has been popular for years, it has not been identified as such. The Minnesota model, a multicomponent program in its own right, was at one time the only recognized program. More recently, specialized programs for mentally ill patients, women, and minority addicts have been developed, making changes in the original program. The idea of multicomponent programming validates this process. As research into clinical effectiveness uncovers key elements to recovery, these elements must be integrated into existing treatment. Clearly this is a basic principle of quality assurance.

The challenge for multicomponent programming is not how many *different* programs can we design but how many *effective* programs can we design. Ideally, each patient should have his or her own program designed according to an individualized treatment plan. Not all programs have a comprehensive assortment of services. The challenge is to discover how to network and to contract for services that provide the critical elements. At some point, *more* services is not the answer. Patients can engage with only a finite number of interventions in a brief period. That we have effective treatment is no longer in doubt. That we have room for improvement is also clear. What to package with what, in what sequence, and which elements should wait until later? This is the challenge.

REFERENCES

1. Polich JM, Armor DJ, Braiker HB: The Course of Alcoholism: Four Years After Treatment. New York, John Wiley & Sons, 1980.
2. Hesselbrock M, Babor TF, Hesselbrock V: Never believe an alcoholic? On the validity of self report measures of alcohol dependence and related constructs. Int J Addict 18:593–609, 1983.
3. Sobell MB, Sobell LC: Behavioral Treatment of Alcohol Problems. New York, Plenum, 1978.
4. Pendery ML, Maltzman IM, West LJ: Controlled drinking by alcoholics? New findings and a re-evaluation of a major affirmative study. Science 217:169–175, 1982.
5. Helzer JE, Robins LN, Taylor JR, et al: The extent of long-term moderate drinking among alcoholics discharged from medical and psychiatric treatment facilities. N Engl J Med 312:1678–1682, 1985.
6. McLellan AT, Luborsky L, Woody GE, et al: Are the "addiction-related" problems of substance abuse really related? J Nerv Ment Dis 169:232–239, 1981.
7. Moos RH, Finney JW, Cronkite RD: Alcoholism Treatment: Context, Process, and Outcome. New York, Oxford University Press, 1990.
8. Price RH, Burke AC, D'Aunno TA, et al: Outpatient drug abuse treatment services, 1988: Results of a national survey. In Pickens RW, Leukefeld CG, Schuster CR (eds): Improving Drug Abuse Treatment. Rockville, MD, US Dept of Health and Human Services, 1991, pp 63–91.
9. Butler JP: Of kindred minds: The ties that bind. In Orlandi MA, Weston R, Epstein LG (eds): Cultural Competence for Evaluation: A Guide for Alcohol and Other Drug Abuse Prevention Practitioners Working with Ethnic/Racial Communities. Rockville, MD, US Dept of Health and Human Services, 1992, pp 23–54.
10. Aries E: Interaction patterns and themes of male, female and mixed groups. Small Group Behavior 7:7–18, 1976.
11. Blume SB: Women, alcohol, and drugs. In Miller NS (ed): Comprehensive Handbook of Drug and Alcohol Addiction. New York, Marcel Dekker, 1991, pp 147–177.
12. Adelman SA, Weiss RD: What is therapeutic about inpatient alcoholic treatment? Hosp Community Psychiatry 40:515–519, 1989.
13. Meyer RE, Babor TF: Explanatory models of alcoholism. In Tasman A, Hales RE, Frances AJ (eds): Review of Psychiatry, vol VIII. Washington, DC, American Psychiatric Press, 1989, pp 273–292.
14. Nowinski J, Baker S, Carroll K: Twelve Step Facilitation Therapy Manual. Rockville, MD, US Dept of Health and Human Services, 1992.
15. Kadden R, Carroll K, Donovan D, et al: Cognitive-Behavioral Coping Skills Therapy Manual. Rockville, MD, US Dept of Health and Human Services, 1992.
16. Miller WR, Rollnick S: Motivational Interviewing: Preparing People to Change Addictive Behavior. New York, Guilford Press, 1991.
17. Sobell MB, Sobell LC: Problem Drinkers: Guided Self-Change Treatment. New York, Guilford Press, 1993.

18. Khantzian EJ: Self-regulation and self-medication factors in alcoholism and the addictions: Similarities and differences. In Galanter M (ed): Recent Developments in Alcoholism, vol VIII. New York, Plenum, 1990, pp 255–271.
19. Hoffman NG, Miller NS: Treatment outcomes for abstinence-based programs. Psychiatr Ann 22:402–408, 1992.
20. Jellinek EM: The Disease Concept of Alcoholism. New Haven, College and University Press, 1960.
21. DeLeon G: Retention in drug-free therapeutic communities. In Pickens RW, Leukefeld CG, Schuster CR (eds): Improving Drug Abuse Treatment. Rockville, MD, US Dept of Health and Human Services, 1991, pp 218–244.
22. Brandsma JM: Outpatient Treatment of Alcoholism. Baltimore, University Park Press, 1980.
23. Ninonuevo F, Hoffman NG: DUI arrestees versus other outpatients in chemical dependency treatment: Initial status and one-year outcome. Int J Offender Therapy Comp Criminology 37(2):177–185, 1993.
24. Welte JW, Hynes G, Sokolow L, et al: Comparison of clients completing inpatient alcoholism treatment with clients who left prematurely. Alcohol Clin Exp Res 5:393–399, 1981.
25. Goldsmith RJ, Green BL: A rating scale for alcoholic denial. J Nerv Ment Dis 176:614–620, 1988.
26. Newsome RD, Ditzler T: Assessing alcoholic denial: Further examination of the Denial Rating Scale. J Nerv Ment Dis 181(11):689–694, 1993.
27. Baekeland F, Lundwall L, Shanahan TJ: Correlates of patient attrition in the outpatient treatment of alcoholism. J Nerv Ment Dis 157(2):99–107, 1973.
28. Nirenberg TD, Sobell LC, Sobell MB: Expensive and inexpensive procedures for decreasing client attrition in an outpatient alcohol treatment program. Am J Drug Alcohol Abuse 7:73–82, 1980.
29. Koumans AJR, Miller JJ, Miller CF: Use of telephone calls to increase motivation for treatment in alcoholics. Psychol Rep 21:327–328, 1967.
30. Woody GE, McLellan AT, O'Brien CP, et al: Addressing psychiatric comorbidity. In Pickens RW, Leukefeld CG, Schuster CR (eds): Improving Drug Abuse Treatment. Rockville, MD, US Dept of Health and Human Services, 1991, pp 152–166.
31. McCrady B: Relative effectiveness of differing components of spouse-involved alcoholism treatment. Subst Abuse 6:12–15, 1984–1985.
32. Galanter M: Network Therapy for Alcohol and Drug Abuse. New York, Basic Books, 1993.
33. Brandsma JM, Pattison EM: The outcome of group psychotherapy with alcoholics: An empirical review. Am J Drug Alcohol Abuse 11:151–162, 1985.
34. Brown S: Treating the Alcoholic: A Developmental Model of Recovery. New York, John Wiley & Sons, 1985.
35. Khantzian EJ, Halliday KS, McAuliffe WG: Addiction and the Vulnerable Self: Modified Dynamic Group Therapy for Substance Abusers. New York, Guilford Press, 1990.
36. Yalom ID: The Theory and Practice of Group Psychotherapy, 2nd ed. New York, Basic Books, 1975.
37. MacKenzie KR: Introduction to Time-Limited Group Psychotherapy. Washington, DC, American Psychiatric Press, 1990.
38. Vannicelli M: Removing the Roadblocks: Group Psychotherapy with Substance Abusers and Family Members. New York, Guilford Press, 1992.
39. Steinglass P, Bennett LA, Wolin SJ, et al: The Alcoholic Family. New York, Basic Books, 1987.
40. Gliedman LH, Rosenthal D, Frank JD, et al: Group therapy of alcoholics with concurrent group meetings with their wives. Q J Stud Alcohol 17:655–670, 1956.
41. Johnson VE: Intervention: How to Help Someone Who Doesn't Want Help. Minneapolis, Johnson Institute Books, 1986.
42. Kaufman E, Reoux J: Guidelines for the successful psychotherapy of substance abusers. Am J Drug Alcohol Abuse 14:199–209, 1988.
43. Zweben JG: Recovery oriented psychotherapy. J Subst Abuse Treat 3:255–262, 1986.
44. Chappel JN: Effective use of Alcoholics Anonymous and Narcotics Anonymous in treating patients. Psychiatr Ann 22:409–418, 1992.
45. Vaillant GE: The Natural History of Alcoholism: Causes, Patterns and Paths to Recovery. Cambridge, MA, Harvard University Press, 1983.
46. Crits-Cristoph P, Beebe KL, Connolly MB: Therapist effects in the treatment of drug dependence: Implications for conducting comparative treatment studies. In Onken LS, Blaine JD (eds): Psychotherapy and Counseling in the Treatment of Drug Abuse. Washington, DC, US Dept of Health and Human Services, 1990, pp 39–48.
47. Decker N, Fann WE, Girardin P, et al: Alcoholism in a general hospital population. In Galanter M (ed): Currents in Alcoholism, vol VI. New York, Grune & Stratton, 1979, pp 33–39.
48. Imhof JE: Countertransference issues in the treatment of drug and alcohol addictions. In Miller NS (ed): Comprehensive Handbook of Drug and Alcohol Addiction. New York, Marcel Dekker, 1991, pp 931–946.
49. Bergen BJ, Price RP, Kinney J: Medical students' conflicting perceptions of alcoholic patients. Journal of Medical Education 55:954–956, 1980.
50. Chappel JN, Schnoll SH: Physician attitudes: Effects on the treatment of chemically dependent patients. JAMA 237:2318–2319. 1977.
51. McCaul ME, Svikis DS: Improving client compliance in outpatient treatment: Counselor-targeted interventions. In Pickens RW, Leukefeld CG, Schuster CR (eds): Improving Drug Abuse Treatment. Rockville, MD, US Dept of Health and Human Services, 1991, pp 204–217.
52. The Health Consequences of Smoking: Nicotine Addiction, a report of the Surgeon General. Rockville, MD, US Dept of Health and Human Services, 1988.

Managed Care for Psychiatric and Addictive Disorders

Joseph A. Flaherty, MD • Kathleen Kim, MD

The dramatic increase in the percentage of the U.S. population covered under any system of managed care has been greeted by physicians as a shocking piece of bad news. Medicine in general and mental health professionals in particular are still experiencing the early stages of mourning (e.g., denial, anger) and mobilizing considerable resources in reaction to this new reality. This reaction, although understandable, is overly simplistic and ignores the social forces that underpin the current economics of medical practice. During the past 30 years, the costs of medical care have burgeoned, with little incentive to either insured patients or their providers to curtail these costs. Both business and government have already realized significant savings by imposing some form of management on their healthcare dollars. Within mental health specifically, we have widely sold our services (i.e., decided what our treatments should be and promoted them) with very little marketing (e.g., conducting medication assessment and consumer surveying to determine what types of treatment people want or will accept). By failing to recognize these realities, we have been blinded to the tremendous opportunities to provide more comprehensive and integrated care to our patients and communities as well as concurrent opportunities for education and for clinical and services research.

Addiction psychiatry is in an ideal position to both thrive and find new models and programs for patients because of a number of factors converging in U.S. society today. Data from the participating Epidemiological Catchment Area (ECA) project sites have raised estimates of the prevalence of addictive disorders in the population to between 11% and 17%, up from the commonly quoted figure of 5% to 10% before the ECA. The public stigma associated with addictive disorders has decreased in the past decade, partly because the prevalence has cut across demographic groups and has affected most American families and communities. Employers, colleagues, educators, and family members have recognized the need for addiction treatments. These groups are aware of the clear benefits of treatments in terms of social, occupational, and educational productivity; direct and indirect economic costs savings; and relief from the burdens of working or living with addicted people.

Additionally, inherent elements particular to addiction treatment are closely aligned with the general paradigm operative in managed care treatment, including

1. Use of less costly but qualified health professionals, such as addiction counselors and case managers
2. Employment of a group model that em-

phasizes psychoeducation in connection with peer group processes

3. A strong reliance on protocol-driven treatment plans that are tailored to different patient populations and individuals

4. A long history of evaluations/outcome research

Although addiction psychiatry must make modifications and continue to evolve its protocols to meet the wide variety of patients requiring services, we should not lose sight of these strong assets. To understand more clearly the direction that addiction psychiatry should go in the era of managed care, it is useful to provide a brief review of the place of addictions in the history of managed care development.

Historical Perspective

Managed behavioral healthcare has been operationally defined by Goodman and colleagues[1] as "any patient care that's not determined solely by the provider." Using this definition, we can exclude the staff model health maintenance models (HMOs) that developed in post–World War II California and Minnesota. During the 1970s, local and national psychiatric societies, such as the American Psychiatric Association (APA), started standardizing peer review methods as well as criteria for specific disorders and particular decision points (e.g., decision to admit). Peer review started out in a retrospective nature, and many organizations routinely had small group peer review of any patients admitted to the hospital. Although the standards were well conceived, it appeared that psychiatric as well as general medical professionals had little appetite for more than perfunctory critiquing or being reviewed by their peers. By the early 1980s, utilization review firms developed to review cases and compared them with norms for lengths of stay in the hospital for other patients with the same diagnosis. The failure of diagnoses to strongly predict lengths of stay for psychiatric disorders was a major impediment to the success of this model in mental health treatment.[2] By the late 1980s, specific speciality-oriented behavioral managed care companies emerged. Insurance companies gave these behavioral managed care companies the responsibility for populations of patients and the authority to examine appropriateness of care decisions based on a model of a continuum of intensities of care (e.g., inpatient, partial, intensive outpatient, medication visits,

and so forth). These managed care companies ushered in features such as inpatient and outpatient precertification, concurrent review of treatment planning, units of care, protocols for specific disorders, and a development of networks of managed care providers, credentialed by these managed care companies. Despite the psychiatric profession's outrage at this threat over autonomy and intrusion on our patients, several positive features emerged from this development:

1. The proportion of mental healthcare spent on patients with major psychiatric and addictive disorders increased as the percentage provided to relatively healthier people decreased.

2. The mental health industry was pressured to consider the concept of differential therapeutics and to make quick and efficient decisions about both the type and level of intensity of care when a patient was first seen by a mental health professional.

3. Long waiting lists and complicated intake processes were eliminated and replaced by movement toward telephone triage and efficient placement of patients either into definitive treatment programs or with clinicians. Financial as well as organizational shortcomings have prevented managed care from attaining a broader goal of trying to deliver population-based care and including potentially mental health–promoting processes such as psychoeducation, stress reduction, and early identification and screening.

The current era of managed care is witnessing several new developments. First, physician groups along with other mental health professionals are developing their own administrative service organizations (ASOs) and competing with managed care companies (or sometimes working in conjunction with them) to take full or partial risk for populations by making bids directly to the corporations, employer groups, or government agencies. This development significantly shifts clinicians' anger away from the managed care companies to their peers and departments as the responsible parties. Potentially strong ethical issues arise when organizations have the power to increase their profits by limiting the amount of care they deliver.[3] Also, future directions in managed mental healthcare are likely to witness movement away from the traditional "carve-out" market (by which mental health and addictions are contracted for separately) to a "carve-in" market in which mental health and addictions are integrated into general medical care under a single capitated risk system.

What has been the effect of these developments in managed care on addiction psychiatry? The 1980s witnessed a dramatic increase in the development of private and not-for-profit hospitals' investment in inpatient substance addiction treatments, capitalizing on the decline of certificate of need legislation as well as the increased inclusion of substance addiction treatment benefits into the standard package of employer- and government-provided insurance. Admissions to private psychiatric hospitals for treatments of substance addiction increased by 64% between 1980 and 1986.[4] This treatment was highly standardized and consisted of a standardized inpatient and outpatient rehabilitation program. Despite lack of sufficient outcome evaluation, the 28-day inpatient stay became a clinical commandment in the abstinence-based residential treatment model in conjunction with the 12-step programs of Alcoholics Anonymous (AA). This so-called Minnesota model was based on the success of excellent treatment programs primarily designed for white, married, and employed men from 20 to 50 years of age. In essence, this inpatient treatment was an ideal target for managed care companies. From 1991 to 1993, inpatient treatment for anything but immediate detoxification was phased out by most payors. In its place, equally standardized outpatient treatment models were quickly formed; these also need to be tested by empirical research that examines which treatment elements for what type of populations are most effective.

The gray zone in addiction managed care is in the area of dual diagnosis. Clearly, many individuals with severe mental illnesses such as schizophrenia and manic-depressive illness and concurrent addictive disorders need specialized treatment programs. The future success of addiction managed care may well rest with the capacity and willingness of large institutions to examine thoughtfully and carefully their data in order to determine the effectiveness of treatments with different populations and avoid attempts to "game" the system by attaching secondary diagnoses to addicted patients for the purposes of inpatient admissions. We are currently experiencing significant change in both the basic benefit package that government and private industry is offering in the area of addiction treatment, and where the public payment for addiction treatment is covered by multiple state and federal agencies (e.g., Medicaid, Medicare, state departments of public aid, mental health, and alcohol and substance abuse, and so on). In addition, the risk is being shifted to employers, managed care companies and providers, and patients (copayments). We are in a transition period in which most addiction programs are treating both public and private patients with various coverage packages, with fee-for-service, reduced fee-for-service, and capitated patient populations in the same programs. It is highly advisable that we collect the kind of data and examine those factors that might shed light on our treatment approaches and then examine the practical exigencies of optimizing what care can be provided to what populations, at what point in their illness, and at what onset and benefit.

Treatment Implications

In the United States, the predominant (90%) form of addiction treatment is abstinence based, which means based on the principles of AA.[5] The fundamental principle of AA is that alcoholism is an addiction to alcohol. The first treatment center to use these principles was started in the 1950s in Center City, Minnesota, and this form of treatment has become known as the Minnesota model.[6] This model requires a fixed length of inpatient treatment (typically 28 days), and it is a highly structured and intensive treatment modality. Two controlled studies[7, 8] have found significant treatment outcomes for abstinence-based programs, particularly when the programs were combined with referral to AA. Treatment outcome evaluation research has confirmed that only abstinence-based treatment combined with regular attendance at AA appears to be effective and to work consistently over time.[5]

The intersection of modern addiction treatment with current medical economics raises two fundamental questions:

1. What treatment modifications of the standard Minnesota model are needed to work with the various patients and populations now entering addiction treatment?

2. How can the results of empirical data on service research be used to inform the process of compromising between the economic realities and quality treatment?

First, it is clear that modern treatment programs have to reach some compromise between the desire to have very structured protocol-driven programs and to tailor the programs to the needs of specific patient populations (at different points in the illness process) and address the push by managed care for the least intensive form of treatment. Taken to its extreme, this would result in a special individualized program for each patient and would reduce the benefits of group processes and protocols. What is emerging, however, is a number of different tracks in addiction treatment, with various levels of intensity, and to some extent the employment of a menu of services. The standards for admission to detoxification before outpatient treatment are being revised and evaluated. Similarly, the type of dual-diagnosis patients who can benefit from addiction treatment is being evaluated, as is the concept of medical necessity for an inpatient stay. It is highly likely that inpatient treatment will not follow standardized protocols with regard to time but with regard to discharge criteria. Outpatient settings may have programs that vary from 2 to 5 days per week in the intensive phase and may vary from 1 to 5 hours per day. In 1990, the Institute of Medicine recommended treatment matching "to ensure that each individual receives the kind of treatment most likely to produce a positive outcome."[9] The type of treatment that patients require (e.g., number of inpatient days or numbers of outpatient hours) is dependent on their clinical condition, previous treatment, concurrent treatment in other psychiatric services, and severity of addiction, as well as careful assessment of support, coping skills, and environmental issues relevant to the possibility of relapse. Treatment matching currently is an underused concept.[10]

Second, case management will have a critical increasing role in monitoring patients' progress through different levels of intensity and into a much longer outpatient surveillance. Much of this case management activity had been initiated by employee assistance programs (EAPs) that took responsibility for the ongoing monitoring of patients in the workplace after they had been through a treatment program. With time, the line between EAPs, case management, and treatment programs will become blurred because employers will desire one organization to perform all these functions. These case managers will require various psychological, social, and medical evaluation skills; will maintain contact with patients as they move geographically as well as throughout the treatment systems; and will have to make community liaison and home visits. The skills of the case manager will have to match the severity of the patients' addictions as well as other characteristics. Case managers working with addicted patients with severe mental disorders need a particular set of skills, those working with adolescents another set of skills, and those working with the medically ill a third set of skills. One of the essential tasks of addiction psychiatry is to collaborate effectively with departments of social work to develop case managers with sufficient general knowledge and skill in counseling and addiction, as well as added competencies with particular patient populations. We also need to avoid the temptation to use individuals with multiple advanced degrees, because that would increase the costs of care dramatically and would lead to a cadre of case managers who feel dissatisfied with their positions and who would seek more administrative posts.

Third, we need to pay more attention to individuals with dual diagnoses and other specific populations. Particular programs need to be designed for dually diagnosed individuals to use extensive community outreach, assertive community training, family psychoeducation, and strong case management. It is likely that the traditional split of the basic psychiatric disorder being treated by one clinician and the addiction disorder treated by a second will prove to be less effective than integrating treatment in a single program, making this a subspecialty area within addiction psychiatry. Similarly, adolescent populations require special program elements such as liaison with school systems, specialized recovery group models, and the recruitment of successful recovered adolescent addicts. In addition, adolescent treatment programs have to pay special attention to the forensic issues of informed consent and parental involvement. Likewise, treatment programs have not been particularly well designed to meet the needs of women. Women often enter addiction treatment later in the course of the illness, ostensibly because of less recognition by primary care providers as well as increased stigma. Additionally, women in poor urban areas have been reluctant to enter treatment programs or AA groups that meet in the evening, and women with young children often have difficulty arranging child care so that they can enter into treatment programs.

Fourth, new, brief forms of treatment intervention are being explored in psychiatry in general, and particular applications for alcohol treatment have been reviewed by Bien and colleagues.[11] They found that brief interventions were significantly more effective than no intervention, commonly had an impact similar to that of more extensive interventions, and could enhance the effectiveness of subsequent treatment. The brief interventions were usually one to three sessions. Common elements of effective brief interventions included (1) feedback of assessment results; (2) an emphasis on personal responsibility for changing one's behavior; (3) explicit advice to reduce or stop drinking; (4) a menu of strategies for reducing drinking; (5) a warm, empathic, and understanding counseling approach, and (6) encouragement of client self-efficacy for change. Bien and colleagues also noted the value of ongoing follow-up as well as the motivational impact of making individuals aware of the discrepancy between their current status and desired goals.

In 13 controlled studies of brief intervention in treatment contexts, brief intervention was compared with more extensive treatment (cognitive-behavioral therapies, marital therapy, standard inpatient and outpatient treatment). Eleven studies[12–22] showed that brief intervention had an overall impact comparable to that of more extensive treatment. Outcome measures included reduction in alcohol consumption and duration of abstinence; follow-up periods ranged from 1 to 10 years. Two controlled studies reported extended treatment to be significantly more effective than brief counseling.[23, 24]

It is important to note that most of these studies have focused on people with minimal to moderately severe alcohol problems. Very few brief intervention trials have studied more severely impaired drinkers or patients with a dual diagnosis. In addition, some evidence suggests a gender difference; brief intervention was found to be more effective than no treatment in men but not in women.[25, 26] In another study, women seemed to benefit more from extended treatment than from brief intervention.[23] At this point, we do not have enough information on client characteristics to identify optimal responders to brief treatment. As discussed earlier, specific patient populations must be matched with appropriate tracks in addiction treatment. Finally, few substantive outcome evaluation studies have addressed brief intervention; thus, its long-term effectiveness is unknown.

Brief intervention seems to be a promising alternative to the standard Minnesota model for clients with less severe alcohol problems. Clearly, if brief intervention proves to be effective, it will be an attractive option to managed care because it potentially repairs the problem without removing an individual from society (and without the costs associated with a 28-day inpatient stay). However, we must examine the efficacy of brief treatment separately from the

costs, or we will confuse our desired outcome measures. Ideally, we would have the data to identify patients for particular tracks in addiction treatment, and we would be able to predict the amount of treatment necessary to achieve the desired discharge criteria. Future research should explore issues such as severity of addiction, gender, dual diagnosis, and costs of treatment to determine how best to compromise between the economic realities and high-quality treatment.

Practical Issues

As change becomes a permanent characteristic in the medical profession, physicians working in addiction programs will need to be actively involved in formulating policy and in contracting from the national level down to the level of their individual programs. It will be useful for addiction psychiatry to develop and refine treatment criteria and standards that can be accepted by larger medical societies (e.g., American Medical Association, APA) as professional endorsement of specific standards of treatment (e.g., APA's standards for treatment of bipolar patients) make it difficult for economic forces to further reduce treatment components in their benefit package.

At the level of group practices, it is important that at least one individual keep abreast of the local, state, and national developments in managed care. For many clinicians, immersion in the world of business of healthcare is frightening and disorienting. The use of such terminology such as *products* and *book of business* are disturbing and offend our sense of a higher purpose in healthcare. Nonetheless, it is critical that we learn to live in this world to be of greater service to our patients and our institutions. Clinicians will be hearing various discussions, formulating treatment protocols, and responding to requests for proposal (RFP's) with packaged plans. A list of certain strategies that may be useful follows:

1. Maintain high-quality services even though quality is not currently considered a priority when companies choose a treatment program. Over time, quality will become an issue as outcome data become more standardized and available for comparison.[27]

2. Make your services user friendly and patient oriented. Review how a patient accessed treatment with you, the entire process from his or her initial phone call through to the follow-up. In addition to the clinical importance of these surveys, big business

and insurance companies will use patients' satisfaction surveys in selecting addiction treatment programs.

3. Although patients are your most important customers, they are not your only customers. Peers, managed care companies, employers, and government are also your customers, and they also have important interests in costs and post-treatment productivity.

4. Gatekeeper satisfaction (e.g., primary care physician, EAP, triage worker) is also critical. Gatekeepers are also our customers. We have to understand their perspective and rectify whatever problems they have with our services. We need to see what type of patients they have difficulty treating, and we need to educate them about the benefits that can be derived from early interventions and treatment.

5. In the area of case management, it is important not to be penny-wise and pound-foolish. In the long run, solid and competent case management is going to save money and result in better treatment.[3]

6. A good information system is critical to the success of addiction programs. Only with strong data (e.g., information about demographics, diagnoses, symptoms, treatments, and outcomes) will we be able to look at what works well for a particular type of patient. Even though we will all be informed by national data, we need to know how well those models generalize to the population of patients whom we see.

7. We have to move away from a standardized one-size-fits-all model into individual menu-driven programs.

8. Diversify services and contracts: Establish ties with EAPs, negotiate for managed care discounted fee for service, expand the range of standard insurance, and develop contracts with business and the public sector.

9. Establish a network with quality providers. Few programs can deliver treatment to all types of their patients. Each program will be lacking in certain kinds of services (e.g., residential treatment, specialized women's programs). In part, you will be judged by the quality of programs you contract with and the ease of patient flow among network modes.

10. In multispecialty group practice, it is crucial to see that addiction treatment is represented well when large capitated contracts are being negotiated.

REFERENCES

1. Goodman M, Brow J, Deitz P: Managing Managed Care. Washington, DC, American Psychiatric Association, 1992.
2. Bartlett J: The emergence of managed care and its impact on psychiatry. New Direct Ment Health Serv 63:25–34, 1994.
3. Kassirer JP: Managed care and the morality of the marketplace. N Engl J Med 333(1):50–52, 1995.
4. Wilson CV: Substance abuse and managed care. New Direct Ment Health Serv 59:99–105, 1993.
5. Miller NS: Treatment of the Addictions: Applications of Outcome Research. In Miller NS (ed): Treatment of the Addictions: Applications of Outcome Research for Clinical Management. Binghamton, NY, Haworth Press, 1995, pp 1–22.
6. Laundergan JC: Easy Does It: Alcoholism Treatment Outcomes, Hazelden and the Minnesota Model. Center City, MN, Hazelden Foundation, 1982.
7. Keso L, Salaspuro M: Inpatient treatment of employed alcoholics: A randomized clinical trial on Hazelden-type and traditional treatment. Alcohol Clin Exp Res 14(4):584–589, 1990.
8. Walsh DC, Hingson RW, Merrigan DM: A randomized trial of treatment options for alcohol abusing workers. N Engl J Med 325(11):752–757, 1991.
9. Institute of Medicine: Broadening the Base of Treatment for Alcohol Problems. Washington, DC, National Academy Press, 1990.
10. Mee-Lee D: Matching in addictions treatment: How do we get there from here? In Miller NS (ed): Treatment of the Addictions: Applications of Outcome Research for Clinical Management. Binghamton, NY, Haworth Press, 1995, pp 113–128.
11. Bien TH, Miller WR, Tonigan JS: Brief interventions for alcohol problems: A review. Addictions 88:315–356, 1993.
12. Edwards G, Orford J, Egert S, et al: Alcoholism: A controlled trial of 'treatment' and 'advice.' J Stud Alcohol 38:1004–1031, 1977.
13. Chapman PI, Huygens I: An evaluation of three treatment programmes for alcoholism: An experimental study with 6- and 18-month follow-up. Br J Addict 83:67–81, 1968.
14. Drummond DC, Thom B, Brown C, et al: Specialist versus general practitioner treatment of problem drinkers. Lancet 336:915–918, 1990.
15. Miller WR, Gribskov CJ, Mortell RL: Effectiveness of self-control manual for problem drinkers with and without therapist contact. Int J Addict 16:1247–1254, 1981.
16. Miller WR, Munoz RF: How to Control Your Drinking, rev ed. Albuquerque, University of New Mexico Press, 1982.
17. Miller WR, Taylor CA: Relative effectiveness of bibliotherapy, individual and group self-control training in the treatment of problem drinkers. Addict Behav 5:13–24, 1980.
18. Skutle A, Berg G: Training in controlled drinking for early-stage problem drinkers. Br J Addict 82:493–501, 1987.
19. Carpenter RA, Lyons CA, Miller WR: Peer-managed self-control program for prevention of alcohol abuse in American Indian high school students: A pilot evaluation study. Int J Addict 20:299–310, 1985.
20. Harris KB, Miller WR: Behavioral self-control training for problem drinkers: Components of efficacy. Psychol Addict Behav 4:82–90, 1990.

21. Sannibale C: The differential effect of a set of brief interventions on the functioning of a group of 'early-stage' problem drinkers. Aust Drug Alcohol Rev 7:147–155, 1988.

22. Zweben A, Pearlman S, Li S: A comparison of brief advice and conjoint therapy in the treatment of alcohol abuse: The results of the marital systems study. Br J Addict 83:899–916, 1988.

23. Robertson I, Heather N, Dzialdowski A, et al: A comparison of minimal versus intensive controlled drinking treatment interventions for problem drinkers. Br J Clin Psychol 22:185–194, 1986.

24. Chick J, Ritson B, Connaughton J, et al: Advice versus extended treatment for alcoholism: A controlled study. Br J Addict 83:159–170, 1988.

25. Anderson P, Scott E: The effect of general practitioners' advice to heavy drinking men. Br J Addict 87:891–900, 1992.

26. Babor TF, Grant M (eds): Project on Identification and Management of Alcohol-Related Problems. Report on Phase II: A Randomized Clinical Trial of Brief Interventions in Primary Health Care. Geneva, World Health Organization, 1992.

27. Grantham JJ: Performance reports on quality—prototypes, problems, and prospects. N Engl J Med 333(1):57–61, 1995.

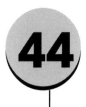

Treatment Outcomes for Addictive Disorders in Psychiatric Settings

Michael S. Easton, MD •
Jan Fawcett, MD

Psychiatric and comorbid addictive illnesses are receiving increasing attention in the literature. Delineation of the problem and recognition of its importance are expanding. Based on our clinical experience and empirical data, it appears that patients with chronic psychiatric disorders and addictions exhibit a more complicated course, use greater treatment resources, and tend to have a worse prognosis. As a result, increasing emphasis has been placed on developing programs in which both the psychiatric and addiction components of these disorders are addressed (hybrid models) in hopes of improving patients' outcome.

We have searched the literature to address a number of pertinent issues concerning this topic. To achieve a better understanding of the relationship between comorbidity and treatment outcome, we have asked the following questions: (1) When treated in a traditional psychiatric setting, do patients with substance-related disorders have poorer outcomes than those without these illnesses? (2) Are specialized dual-diagnosis programs (hybrids) more effective in this patient population? and (3) How do individuals with only substance-related disorders respond to treatment in traditional psychiatric facilities?

Outcome of Comorbid Psychiatric Illness When Treated in a Psychiatric Setting

The majority of studies in this area have been conducted with chronically mentally ill patients in psychiatric inpatient settings and in outpatient clinics (in community mental health centers or Veterans Administration [VA] settings). In our review, we found a wide variety of research designs evaluating course and outcome of individuals with comorbid substance addiction compared with those without. When one looks at large outcome studies regarding the chronic mentally ill, the co-occurrence of substance disorder diagnosis is infrequently evaluated as a specific factor in relationship to outcome. Studies have suggested that these individuals exhibit higher rates of relapse and rehospitalizations, more frequent emergency room visits, and poorer treatment compliance.[1-3] One of the few studies that reported on the differential outcome of these patients receiving standard treatment was by Drake.[3] He reported on the 1-year course of 187 chronic mentally ill patients living in the community.

Patients were monitored by a mobile outreach program. All patients were given a DSM-III-R diagnosis, and psychiatric symptoms were monitored by the modified brief psychiatric rating scale and Andreasen's negative symptoms scale. Psychosocial variables were measured using clinician rating scales. They reported that subjects with comorbid substance addiction diagnosis were younger, were more often male, were less able to manage their lives, were more hostile and disruptive, had poorer medication compliance, and were nearly twice as likely to be rehospitalized during the follow-up year.

Treatment outcome for these disorders has not been adequately evaluated in traditional psychiatric settings, much less in newer dual-diagnosis programs. Finally, little recent research has addressed the response of individuals with only addiction when treated with a traditional psychiatric model (in contrast to an addiction model). This last issue is important because most of these patients will be treated in psychiatric settings, and even in hybrid programs a psychiatric model is the predominant approach.

We were able to find a handful of studies investigating differential outcomes for individuals with substance-related disorders and comorbid depression, bipolar disorder, or schizophrenia. Although most reports agree that comorbid personality disorders (specifically antisocial and borderline personality disorder) and a substance addiction diagnosis hold a poor treatment prognosis, we could find little that adequately addressed this issue. We also discuss here a handful of studies looking at the effectiveness of specialized treatment programs for patients with a dual diagnosis. Finally, we review a small body of old literature discussing the treatment of alcoholism in a traditional psychiatric setting.

MANIC-DEPRESSIVE ILLNESS

It is clear that substance-related disorders occur frequently in this patient population. Unfortunately, the studies investigating outcome for manic-depressive illness with comorbid substance addiction are limited. One publication (Winokur and colleagues, 1994),[4] from the National Institute of Mental Health (NIMH) collaborative program on psychobiology of depression, monitored 131 bipolar patients over 10 years (every 6 months for the first 5 years and yearly for the second 5 years). Diagnosis and symptoms were evaluated using structured rating scales administered by trained

personnel. They found that alcoholism was common in these individuals and spontaneously decreased at the end of 10 years (this has also been described in primary alcoholics[5]). Patients whose alcoholism predated the onset of their affective illness were less likely to have episodes in the follow-up period than patients in whom the affective illness predated the onset of the alcoholism.

The available anecdotal information in the literature points to a few important issues. Alcohol and drug addiction, when present, tend to modify the course and expression of manic-depressive illness, make its diagnosis and treatment more complicated, and produce a poorer prognosis. Himmelhoch and colleagues[6] suggested that substance use may especially complicate the course of illness and prognosis of individuals with rapid cycling or mixed states. It also has been observed that one more commonly encounters substance use when these individuals are manic than when they are depressed.[7] These researchers also suggested that patients with bipolar mixed states and alcohol use have impaired response to traditional pharmacotherapy and poorer courses.[8] Morrison[9] reported that the average duration of illness before first admission to a hospital was substantially higher for patients with bipolar disorder and alcoholism than for nonalcoholic patients with bipolar disorder (203 vs. 37 days, respectively). They suggested this may be due to masking of their symptoms by alcohol. It could also be secondary to these individuals' being more difficult and less apt to seek treatment because of their drinking. There is little doubt that these individuals have somewhat higher rates of suicide and morbidity owing to the effects of both of these disorders.

DEPRESSION

As with manic-depressive illness, few studies have investigated the effect of comorbid substance use on the long-term outcome of depression. Nor have studies looked at the outcome of the substance-related disorder in a depressed population being treated primarily in a psychiatric setting. The NIMH collaborative Study on the Psychobiology of Depression is one of the few long-term studies that has adequately monitored individuals with depression for a number of years. In addition, the investigators have been able to research some issues in this patient population with comorbid substance-related disorders. Two reports pertinent to this topic have been published from this patient sample. Hassin and colleagues[10] reported on the 2-year course of 127 patients with depression and alcoholism. They found that in a significant number, their drinking remitted during the first several weeks of the study and that subjects' drinking continued to improve throughout the 2 years. The cumulative probability of remission of drinking increased every 3 months to 67% by year two. Once in remission, the cumulative probability of relapse by the 2-year point was 29%. Only a portion of the patients actually participated in some form of alcoholism treatment or self-help groups. Diagnosis of schizoaffective disorder was a poor prognostic indicator. Of the patients in whom drinking did not remit, approximately 8% committed suicide. Muller and associates[11] reported on a 10-year follow-up from this sample of 146 patients with major depression and alcoholism. They were compared with 412 patients with major depressive disorder only. The investigators found that individuals without active alcoholism had twice the likelihood of recovery from a major depressive disorder as did actively alcohol-drinking depressed individuals. Once patients had recovered, the presence or lack of an alcoholism diagnosis did not have any predictive value for recurrence of a major depressive episode.

SCHIZOPHRENIA

It is increasingly clear that substance-related disorder is a significant problem among schizophrenic patients. The actual prevalence of addiction is not well delineated, and the research on the impact of substance use on the course and outcome of schizophrenia is contradictory. Studies have suggested that schizophrenic individuals with substance-related disorders have higher relapse rates, more rehospitalizations, longer hospitalizations, more severe symptoms, poorer attitude toward treatment, a higher rate of noncompliance, more complicated discharge dispositions, and an increased rate of homelessness.[13–15]

Comorbidity in this patient population is very pertinent, given that these individuals exhibit poor psychosocial functioning and do not respond well to traditional addiction treatment techniques (confrontational or exploratory group experiences). We are aware of three studies that have attempted to look at the treatment outcome of dually diagnosed schizophrenics treated in specialized psychiatric services.

Kivlahan and colleagues[16] retrospectively evaluated 60 schizophrenic patients who had a history of repeated failure in previous outpatient programs. These patients were treated with aggressive case management addressing both their psychiatric and substance-related illness. Those with a history of substance-related disorder had a higher level of service utilization and achieved smaller increments of improvement than did patients without substance use problems. The investigators concluded that treatment of schizophrenic patients with concurrent substance-related disorder is disproportionately more costly than that of patients without dual diagnoses but that it can be effective. Hellerstein and Meehan[17] studied 10 schizophrenics with comorbid substance disorders who were monitored for 1 year in a weekly supportive group that addressed both their substance disorder and psychiatric diagnosis. Half of the patients remained in the group at 1 year. Patients demonstrated a significant decrease of inpatient days during their year of participation in the group. The researchers concluded that engaging addicted schizophrenic patients in outpatient treatment that supportively addressed both illnesses can decrease hospitalization. Drake and colleagues[18] monitored 18 individuals in a specialized program for 4 years. They reported significant improvement in the sample, 61% of whom achieved stable remission for alcoholism. This percentage is higher than is usually reported in this patient population and compares with longer-term outcomes in individuals without psychiatric illness treated for alcoholism only.

Although these are small open and uncontrolled studies, they begin to look at the issue of specialized services for schizophrenic patients with comorbid substance addiction or dependence. They suggest that this problem can be addressed with some success. As a result of patients' impaired social skills and limited capacity to maintain normal relationships, alternative treatment interventions and long-term treatment strategies need to be evaluated in this patient population.

Dual-Diagnosis (Hybrid) Programs

A small number of studies have attempted to evaluate the effectiveness of specialized treatment services for patients with a dual diagnosis. These studies have investigated both inpatient and ambulatory services models for chronically mentally ill patients.

A number of inpatient studies have tried to evaluate whether the use of dual-diagnosis groups increases the recognition of these problems (by staff and patients), helps individuals begin to address their substance use, and most importantly increases the likelihood that they will receive and follow up with appropriate outpatient treatment recommendations. Kofoed and Keys[19] investigated the use of a twice-weekly group to help patients acknowledge their addiction and seek continued substance abuse treatment. They compared the treatment plans of 119 patients with dual diagnosis on a VA inpatient psychiatric unit with 116 patients on another unit that did not have such groups. They found that the patients who were more frequently exposed to these groups received and accepted treatment plans that incorporated addiction treatment. They also had higher rates of follow-up, which therefore should translate into improved outcomes. In this study, the researchers did not elaborate on patient diagnoses or how information was obtained. Ries and Ellingson[20] reported on a small prospective open study investigating factors leading to improved outcome for dual diagnoses in patients participating in a substance addiction track while hospitalized. Psychiatric diagnoses were determined by DSM-III-R and 1 month follow-ups were obtained through face-to-face structured interviews. They found that definite discharge plans for addiction treatment related to better outcome. Hoffman and coworkers[21] reported on a retrospective chart review of 28 random patients treated in a state hospital inpatient psychiatric–substance addiction unit. The program ran a two-track system for severe or chronically and nonchronically mentally ill individuals with comorbid substance addiction. The chronically mentally ill (psychotic or schizophrenic) track was less confrontational, smaller, and used a more concrete treatment approach. The nonchronically mentally ill track was for higher-functioning individuals. At 3 months, the researchers found similar outcomes between the two groups in terms of abstinence, employment, compliance with treatment, and the occurrence of major untoward events. They concluded that this indicated that more severely mentally ill individuals can have outcomes compatible with the less severely ill when treated in these hybrid programs. They also concluded that patients should be treated separately, based on the severity and chronicity of their psychiatric condition.

These studies, although small, illustrate that specialized treatments can be initiated for these patients in psychiatric settings. They also suggest that doing so will stimulate greater recognition of these issues by the staff and patients. Treatment recommendations will be more inclusive, and patients may have a higher probability of following up with more comprehensive outpatient care.

The treatment efficacy and outcome of ambulatory dual-diagnosis hybrid programs have also been evaluated in a number of studies.

Kofoed and colleagues[22] reported on an open outpatient study of 32 patients. These patients were in a VA population that had chronic psychiatric illness and comorbid substance addiction and were viewed as treatment failures by the traditional programs. They all participated in a hybrid program that used techniques from both psychiatric and addiction medicine. DSM-III-R diagnoses were used, and symptoms were rated using the addiction severity index. Sixty-six percent of the patients dropped out by 3 months, and only 21% of the patients completed a year of treatment. Treatment retention was associated with reduced hospital use. Hanson and coworkers[23] reported on a retrospective chart review of 118 outpatients placed in a specialized program focusing on both psychiatric and substance-related disorders. Most patients attended this clinic 5 days a week for approximately 5 hours a day. By 6 months, one third of the patients remained in treatment, and of these, one third were abstinent for 3 or more months and three fourths stayed in treatment as long as 1 year. Patients who participated and those who remained in treatment longer were more likely to have better outcomes. The major conclusion of this study was that these patients tend to respond favorably to treatment designed to meet their specific needs. Alfs and McClellan[24] described a naturalistic study of 145 patients treated in a specialized dual-diagnosis day program. Their program used nonconfrontational supportive therapy, and abstinence was not a requirement for treatment but was a goal. Sixty-six percent of these chronic patients completed the program, and one third continued in an aftercare group. Diagnoses were not elaborated, nor did they report on various outcome variables. They concluded that these specialized programs improved treatment outcome for this complicated patient population. Lehman and colleagues[25] reported on a 1-year prospective follow-up of

54 schizophrenic patients or patients with an affective disorder with comorbid substance addiction disorder. All the patients were being treated in a community mental health center. One half of the patients were randomly assigned to an experimental track consisting of 5 hours a week of substance addiction treatment (geared toward this population) and intensive case management. Structured Clinical Interview for Diagnosis–derived DSM-III-R were used, and symptoms were evaluated using the alcohol severity index and the quality of life index (QOLI) general life satisfaction scale. At 1 year, there was no difference between groups and a notable lack of change on most outcome measures for the sample. The researchers noted that although there were no group differences in attendance at the standard community mental health center, there were difficulties engaging the patients in the experimental track (many patients failed to participate in these sessions). Obviously, one explanation for the lack of treatment effect is noncompliance. Still, it does point out the difficulty of running these types of programs and engaging chronic mentally ill patients.

Again, these studies are few, of small sample size, and uncontrolled. Considering this, one cannot draw strong conclusions from any individual report. Together the results of these studies appear to suggest that by identifying these individuals, addressing their addictions as primary problems, using various treatment techniques (psychiatric and 12 step), and linking an individual to appropriate long-term aftercare may help improve follow-up and outcomes. They also demonstrate that even in hybrid programs, patient engagement and retention are difficult. Clearly, well-designed random assignment studies need to be carried out to elucidate more adequately the overall efficacy of these programs.

Outcome of Alcoholism Treated in Traditional Psychodynamic-Oriented Treatment Programs

The older literature is interesting in that there are a small number of studies that have specifically investigated the outcome of individuals with alcoholism treated in psychiatric, psychodynamic-oriented treatment programs. Seelye[26] reported on 100 alcoholic patients treated in a traditional psychiatric setting for 2.5 to 5 years (the alcoholism was not viewed as a disease but as a result of underlying psychopathology). The method of follow-up was not described in this report. The patients were predominantly of the upper socioeconomic class. Although patients participated in Alcoholics Anonymous (AA), the therapy was psychodynamically oriented. The researchers reported that 65% of the group had improved (abstinent or significantly decreased drinking-related problems) at follow-up. Harper and Hickson[27] published a 2- to 5-year follow-up of 84 alcoholics treated in a psychiatric inpatient facility (average stay 3 months). The follow-up was conducted by corresponding with the primary care physician or a family member. They reported that at follow-up, 20% were abstaining, 30% were improved, and 26% were unimproved (one third of whom were diagnosed as sociopathic). Eighteen percent died (two of suicide) during the follow-up period, and the remaining were unavailable for follow-up. An early study by Emrick[28] reviewed outcomes in 271 studies published between 1951 and 1972. These studies reported on a wide variety of treatment modalities, settings, and intensities (behavior therapy, disulfiram, psychological-oriented programs, disease model 12-step programs). He reported that approximately 33% were abstinent at follow-up and 83% were controlled drinkers. Sixty-seven percent were considered somewhat or much improved and only 32% were unimproved.

This small number of older studies gives us some interesting insights. Because these are older studies, modern diagnostic or symptom-rating scales were not in use. The means of follow-up in these studies were infrequently described, as were the times of follow-up, and they tended to be retrospective, open, and uncontrolled. They do, however, support data that alcoholics do improve with treatment. Interestingly, the outcomes of these early studies are similar to those reported in more recent literature focusing on addiction programs.[29]

WHAT ONE CAN CONCLUDE FROM THESE STUDIES

It becomes obvious when reviewing the body of literature devoted to this area that it is substantially lacking. All the studies reviewed have significant methodological limitations. Controlled studies are often limited. They frequently investigated populations with heterogeneous psychiatric and/or substance-related disorders. Outcomes were reported using various criteria, and diagnosis and outcome variables were infrequently measured using standardized structured tools. In general, these studies provide some insight into the treatment response of this population in various treatment settings. They all suggest that treatment in psychiatric settings has therapeutic effects on addictive disorders, yet they do not demonstrate preferential or superior treatment efficacy of any specific intervention. Although it is our clinical impression and some empirical data point to the fact that individuals with a dual diagnosis have poorer outcomes, this does not necessarily mean that present treatments are not therapeutic. These poorer outcomes may also be due to lack of recognition, intervention, or compliance with currently available treatments.

Improving Outcome by Initiating Specialized Treatment Models

As previously stated, evidence suggests that increasing the specificity of treatment for these patients may improve outcome. A number of hybrid treatment models have been described in the literature. The models most commonly referred to are serial, parallel, and integrated treatment systems.[31-35] Each has its strength and may be needed in various clinical situations.

TREATING COMORBID CONDITIONS IN A PSYCHIATRIC INPATIENT/OUTPATIENT CLINIC SETTING

Although a dedicated unit to treat patients with a dual diagnosis would be optimal, it is not logistically feasible in many institutions. In such situations, the inpatient facilities would be best served by an addiction track. This track should be able to provide multiple levels of care and a range of services to address the various problems experienced by these individuals (just as is done for psychiatric illness). These services should be interdisciplinary, available daily, and composed of education, group, family, and individual therapy based on patients' needs and matched to individual levels of functioning. In addition, self-help groups (e.g., AA) should be available to those individuals for whom it is appropriate. Not all individuals are willing and ready to deal with their substance addiction problem; therefore, a

subtrack may be necessary to slowly introduce individuals to their chemical dependency problem and gradually help motivate them to accept treatment.

The staff should have the expertise to handle all forms of drug and alcohol detoxification and to evaluate the severity of patients' psychiatric problems and substance addiction. They should also be involved in creating comprehensive treatment plans during the inpatient stay, with linkage to the appropriate outpatient programs. The staff must be well versed in the pharmacological effects of all drugs of addiction, their potential effects on an individual's mental status, and how they may affect various mental illnesses. They must also be adept at differentiating (1) patients with primarily psychiatric disorders who are abusing substances but who do not have a dependence; (2) patients who have primarily substance dependence with psychoactive substance use–induced psychiatric symptoms but no primary psychiatric disorder; and (3) those individuals with primary psychiatric and primary substance abuse/dependence disorders. The treatment recommendations for each of these three groups may vary significantly and are discussed in greater detail in other areas of this text.

OFFICE PRACTICE

Although much emphasis has been placed on inpatient and hospital clinic treatment, continual long-term treatment of these individuals is frequently administered in an office practice (public or private) by a single practitioner. This may occur before, during, or after treatment in a hospital setting or as an individual's only form of treatment. In fact, in 1991, 81% of individuals with addiction problems were treated in settings other than inpatient, residential, or intensive outpatient programs.[36] Comorbidity of these disorders is so common that a significant number of any mental health practitioner's patient population have a substance addiction/dependence disorder at some time during the course of their treatment. For this reason, practitioners must become more aware of how to screen for them so that they can make early treatment interventions. It has frequently been recommended that these individuals be referred to specialized addiction treatment programs, yet studies in primary care medicine have demonstrated increasing evidence that simple interventions by a clinician can produce a treatment response in a significant subgroup of these individuals (primarily alcohol addiction without severe drug addiction/dependence).[37] These same treatment approaches can be used by psychiatrists or other therapists in their office practices. These intervention strategies consist first of a high index of suspicion and, next, familiarity with diagnosis of substance addiction or dependence. After this, patients are educated about addiction and why abstinence is the treatment of choice. They are given advice on how to achieve this goal (e.g., don't keep alcohol in the house, don't associate with people who drink, increase healthy daily activities, and so forth) and given support in whatever means they choose to use. The support of family or significant others is elicited to help individuals in their attempt to abstain, and patients are given referrals to participate in self-help groups (AA and others). Individuals are then seen regularly to monitor their success at achieving and maintaining abstinence.

Individual psychotherapy also needs to be modified into a more structured format in which the initial goal focuses on a means of achieving abstinence and changing behaviors involved in maintaining substance use. These simple interventions have been evaluated in primary care settings in individuals who have alcohol addiction but have not developed dependence. It has also been our clinical experience that these types of interventions are effective for a subgroup of individuals with alcohol dependence syndromes (patients who do not have severe comorbid drug addiction, who are employed, and who have a stable family environment). Whether such interventions are effective for various drug addictions (especially cocaine or narcotic dependence) has not been evaluated. For those individuals for whom such a strategy does not work, the therapist may begin to function as a case manager or treatment coordinator, referring patients to specialized addiction treatment programs and following up with them once they are finished. An important fact to appreciate is that both substance addiction/dependence and psychiatric illnesses tend to be chronic conditions for which individuals need varying levels of care throughout their lives. At different times, either of the illnesses can have different degrees of symptom intensity independent of each other.

FLEXIBLE TREATMENT SERVICE MODEL FOR DUAL-DIAGNOSIS PATIENTS IN A TERTIARY CARE SETTING

At Rush-Presbyterian-St. Lukes Medical Center, a large tertiary care center in urban Chicago, the substance addiction staff consists of a multidisciplinary team (psychiatrist, psychologists, social workers, registered nurses, occupational therapists, and other mental health professionals and trainees), all of whom are well trained in both psychiatric and addiction treatment models. The primary clinical philosophy is that dual-diagnosis individuals have complex problems that result from various causes and that their psychiatric and addictive disorders are co-occurring illnesses that are intertwined in a complicated manner. A wide variety of treatment models are thus adapted to the various individuals based on their needs. Experience has demonstrated that to improve patient outcome, we cannot rigidly adhere to any one model and must be flexible in our treatment approach and goals.

Services for both inpatient and outpatient populations are coordinated by the same team of individuals. The substance addiction program provides a full range of detoxification services for the entire medical center. Because of the changing economic times, many hospitals no longer have dedicated inpatient substance addiction or dual-diagnosis programs but instead have units with various treatment tracks that address the diverse needs of the patients. On the *inpatient units*, the dual-diagnosis and substance addiction tracks closely coordinate with attending physicians and other treatment staff in identifying patients with addictions, intervening, and initiating treatment. Coordinating with the regular staff, the team conducts frequent inpatient groups to educate patients and to help motivate them to attempt abstinence, early recovery, and relapse prevention. The team also focuses on discharge planning and linking individuals to appropriate outpatient programs. In addition, the program has an important role in aiding the staff in increasing their skills in dealing with this patient population. The main goals of inpatient treatment are to identify, diagnose, and stabilize patients so that they can be transitioned into appropriate outpatient programs.

The *outpatient program* comprises numerous services to accommodate the diversity of this patient population. The more severely affected individuals are frequently referred to a psychiatric day hospital (with a specific substance addiction track) so that a wide variety of treatments can be administered in a more structured setting.

Patients who do not need a full day program participate in various outpatient eclectic treatments for 1 to 10 hours a week. In general, patients follow a step-down model in which they start off in the day hospital program (30 to 40 hours per week) or a partial day program (10 hours per week) and step down to less-intensive treatments when ready. The intensive phase of the program tends to be time limited (1 to 3 months), followed by extended long-term care (1 to 2 hours per week for 1 or more years). Because of the chronic nature of these illnesses, long-term continued care may be the most important aspect in sustaining a treatment response. In addition, the long-term treatment groups are stratified on the basis of level of functioning and treatment motivation. After initial treatment, those individuals highly motivated to sustain abstinence (with few if any relapses) are separated from those individuals who are minimally motivated or who have many relapses. Some may argue that this deprives patients with poorer outcome of good role models and of possible help from healthier patients, but our experience has been that less-motivated or sicker individuals take up most of the group time and focus and healthier patients receive less attention, become frustrated, and tend to drop out. Groups are also stratified on the basis of severity of psychiatric illness. Patients who have chronic psychotic symptoms are treated separately from individuals without such problems. Specialized groups for the cognitively impaired (usually as a result of their drug or alcohol use) or individuals with very low intellectual functioning are also available. These individuals may or may not have other psychiatric symptoms, tend to fare poorly in programs geared to a higher-functioning population, and often become unavailable for follow-up. These groups tend to be less intensive and confrontational. More emphasis is placed on environmental changes, and treatment is more behaviorally oriented.

In a tertiary care hospital, another unique population that frequently is underserved requires specialized services: individuals with severe comorbid medical problems, psychiatric symptoms, and substance addiction (such as organ transplant candidates, chronic pain suffers with complicated medical problems, and other individuals with serious medical disability). Specialized services are available for these individuals who, because of their severe medical conditions, are not capable of participating in regular addiction or psychiatric programs. Their treatment at times requires creative approaches. In that they have very specialized needs, their therapy needs to be closely coordinated with their medical care. In lieu of this, the program has incorporated its staff members into many of the subspecialty teams in the hospital.

Conclusion

Only in the past 10 years have epidemiological data and various studies begun to demonstrate the high degree of comorbidity between psychiatric and substance-related disorders. A common clinical belief is that patients with comorbid addiction are more difficult to treat, have poorer outcomes in traditional programs, and require specialized services. Few studies have investigated specific psychiatric syndromes and evaluated differential outcomes for individuals with and without substance addiction. More research is needed in psychiatric settings to evaluate the role of substance addiction in the poor responders or in difficult-to-treat patients. In our treatment centers, we all see complicated cases of comorbid substance addiction/dependence, yet many difficult patients are not thus affected. One must ask the question, Is it just as likely that many of these individuals will fare as well in standard psychiatric treatments and that we should focus our attention on the smaller number of non-compliant patients or nonresponders? Does comorbid addiction raise an individual's risk of becoming a treatment failure, or is it just our lack of recognition of the problem and intervention that diminishes treatment outcome? (In other words, they do poorly because their illness is not being treated, not because the treatment is not effective.) These issues are difficult to address in the currently available studies in that these patients tend to receive a multitude of treatments in different settings (psychiatric or addiction) during the course of their illness. This makes it almost impossible to distinguish particular treatment effects. Studies strongly suggest that the acute phase of treatment is complicated when active psychiatric and substance addiction syndromes co-occur. Still, it is prudent for clinicians to keep in mind that the consequences of comorbid addiction in the long-term course of various psychiatric illnesses have not been adequately evaluated.

REFERENCES

1. Lyons JS, McGovern MP: Use of mental health services by dual diagnosed patients. Hosp Community Psychiatry 40(10):1067–1069, 1989.
2. Solomon P: Receipt of aftercare services by problem types: Psychiatric, psychiatric/substance abuse and substance abuse. Psychiatr Q 58(3):272–276, 1987.
3. Drake RE, Wallach MA: Substance abuse among the

chronic mentally ill. Hosp Community Psychiatry 40(10):1041–1046, 1989.

4. Winokur G, Coryell W, Akiskal HS, et al: Manic depressive (bipolar) disorder: The course in light of a prospective ten-year follow-up of 131 patients. US National Institute of Mental Health collaborative program on psychobiology of depression, Bethesda, Maryland. Acta Psychiatr Scand 89(2):102–110, 1994.

5. Vaillant G: Patterns of recovery. In Vaillant G. The Natural History of Alcoholism. Cambridge, MA, Harvard University Press, 1983, pp 107–211.

6. Himmelhoch J, Mulla D, Neil JF, et al: Incidence and significance of mixed affective states in a bipolar population. Arch Gen Psychiatry 133:765–771, 1976.

7. Liskow B, Mayfield S, Thiele J: Alcohol and affective disorder: Assessment and treatment. J Clin Psychiatry 43(4):144–147, 1982.

8. Himmelhoch JM: Mixed states, manic depressive illness, and the nature of mood. Psychiatr Clin North Am 2:449–459, 1979.

9. Morrison JR: Bipolar affective disorder and alcoholism. Am J Psychiatry 131:1130–1133, 1974.

10. Hassin DS, Endicott J, Keller MR: RDC Alcoholism in patients with major affective syndromes: Two-year course. Am J Psychiatry 146:318–232, 1989.

11. Muller TI, Lavori PW, Keller MB, et al: Prognostic effect of the variable course of alcoholism on the 10-year course of depression. Am J Psychiatry 151:(5):701–706, 1994.

12. Turner WM, Tsuang MT: Impact of substance abuse on the course and outcome of schizophrenia. Schizophr Bull 16(1):87–95, 1990.

13. Cleghorn JM, Kaplan RD, Szechtman B, et al: Substance abuse and schizophrenia: Effects on symptoms but not on neurocognitive function. J Clin Psychiatry 52(1):26–30, 1991.

14. Soni SD, Brownlee M: Alcohol abuse in chronic schizophrenics: Implications for management in the community. Acta Psychiatr Scand 84(3):272–276, 1991.

15. Drake RE, Osher FC, Noordsy DL, et al: Diagnosis of alcohol use disorders in schizophrenia. Schizophr Bull 16(1):57–67, 1990.

16. Kivlahan DR, Heiman JR, Wright RC, et al: Treatment cost and rehospitalization rate in schizophrenic outpatients with a history of substance abuse. Hosp Community Psychiatry 42(6):609–614, 1991.

17. Hellerstein DJ, Meehan B: Outpatient group therapy for schizophrenic substance abusers. Am J Psychiatry 144:1337–1339, 1987.

18. Drake RE, McHugo J, Noordsy DL: Treatment of alcoholism among schizophrenic outpatients: 4-year outcomes. Am J Psychiatry 150:328–329, 1993.

19. Kofoed L, Keys A: Using group therapy to persuade dual diagnosis patients to seek substance abuse treatment. Hosp Community Psychiatry 39(11):1209–1221, 1988.

20. Ries R, Ellingson T: A pilot assessment at one month of 17 dual diagnosis patients. Hosp Community Psychiatry 41(11):1230–1232, 1990.

21. Hoffman GW, DiRito DC, McGill EC: Three month follow up of 28 dual diagnoses in patients. Am J Drug Alcohol Abuse 19(1):79–88, 1993.

22. Kofoed L, Kania J, Walsh T, Atkinson M: Outpatient treatment of patients with substance abuse and coexisting psychiatric disorders. Am J Psychiatry 143:867–872, 1986.

23. Hanson M, Kramer T, Gross W: Outpatient treatment of adults with coexisting substance use and mental disorders. J Subst Abuse Treat 7:109–116, 1990.

24. Alfs DS, McClellan TA: A day hospital program for dual diagnosis patients in a VA medical center. Hosp Community Psychiatry 43(3):241–244, 1992.

25. Lehman AF, Derron JD, Schwartz RP, Myers PC: Rehabilitation for adults with severe mental illness and substance use disorders: A clinical trial. J Nerv Ment Dis 181:86–90, 1993.

26. Seelye EE: Relationship of socioeconomic status, psychiatric diagnosis and sex to outcome of alcoholism treatment. J Stud Alcohol 40(1):57–62, 1979.

27. Harper J, Hickson BV: The results of hospital treatment of chronic alcoholism. Lancet 2:1057–1059, 1951.

28. Emrick CD: A review of psychological oriented treatment of alcoholism: I. The use of interrelationships of outcome criteria and drinking behavior following treatment. Q J Stud Alcohol 35:523–549, 1974.

29. Hofman GH, Miller HS: Treatment outcomes for abstinence-based programs. Psychiatr Ann 22(8):402–408, 1992.

30. Ries R: Clinical treatment matching models for dually diagnosed patients. Psychiatr Clin North Am 16(1):167–175, 1993.

31. Minkoff K, Drake R: Dual Diagnosis of Major Mental Illness and Substance Disorder. San Francisco, Jossey-Bass, 1991.

32. Drake RE, Antosca LM, Noordsy DL, et al: New Hampshire's specialized services for the dual diagnosed. In Minkoff K, Reeds D (eds): Dual Diagnosis of Major Mental Illness and Substance Disorders. San Francisco, Jossey-Bass, 1991, pp 57–67.

33. Kofoed L, Kania J, Walsh T, et al: Outpatient treatment of patients with substance abuse and coexisting psychiatric disorders. Am J Psychiatry 143(7):867–872, 1986.

34. Levy MS, Mann DW: The special treatment team: An inpatient approach to the mentally ill alcoholic patient. J Subst Abuse Treat 5(4):219–227, 1988.

35. Sciaca K: An integrated treatment approach for severely mentally ill individuals with substance disorders. In Minkoff K, Reeds D (eds): Dual Diagnosis of Major Mental Illness and Substance Disorders. San Francisco, Jossey-Bass, 1991, pp 69–88.

36. US Substance Abuse and Mental Health Services Administration, Office of Applied Studies. National Drug and Alcoholism Treatment Unit Survey.

37. Secretary of Health and Human Services: Screening and brief intervention. In Eighth Special Report to the US Congress on Alcohol and Health. Alexandria, VA, US Dept of Health and Human Services, 1993, pp 297–311. Editorial Experts, Inc.

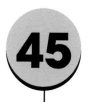

Spirituality and Addiction Psychiatry

John N. Chappel, MD

"The social process is a theme running through all the work on healing. The social fabric is reflected in an individual's health. People without close contact with others have higher morbidity and mortality from many causes than people with intimacy. . . . There is no disease that kills people at the rate loneliness does."

ORNSTEIN AND SWENCIONIS[1]

It may seem strange to open a chapter on spirituality with a comment on our need for social support. Although the available data are sparse, there appears to be a relationship between spiritual health and a capacity to relate intimately with others. This is reflected in the Alcoholics Anonymous (AA) saying that "spirituality is the ability to get our minds off ourselves."[2] At least one study has found a much closer relationship between measures of spiritual health and mental health than between spiritual health and physical health.[3] This close relationship reflects the fact that most people develop their spiritual experiences through contact with other people.

Medical undergraduate and specialty training virtually ignores religious and spiritual issues.[4] Even psychiatry offers little or no instruction in this area that can so often have a profound effect on patients' lives.[5] The reasons for this omission are rooted in two important influences. The first and perhaps most important is that modern medical ethics demand that physicians provide equal care regardless of their patients' or their own religious beliefs.[6] The second is the explosion in medical technology and the resulting emphasis on biomedical issues in medical education and practice.

Changes in psychiatric education and practice are beginning to occur. As of January 1995, all psychiatry residency programs are required to include religious/spiritual factors in their didactic curriculum. The focus of this training is to be on influences on growth and development as well as cultural diversity. DSM-IV-R, for the first time, contains a category V62.61 Religious or Spiritual Problem.[7] "Examples include distressing experiences that involve loss or questioning of faith, problems associated with conversion to a new faith, or questioning of other spiritual values which may not necessarily be related to an organized church or religious institution."

The loss of psychosocial knowledge and skill in medical education led Engel[8] to develop the biopsychosocial model, which now is taught in most medical schools and which has had some impact on medical practice, particularly in family medicine. Hiatt[9] and Kuhn[10] augmented Engel's work by proposing an expansion to a biopsychosocial/spiritual model, on the grounds that adding spiritual approaches could help unify the technical aspects of medicine with such diverse matters as medical ethics and attitudinal influences in healing. There is little evidence that this suggestion has had any influence on medical education or practice.

Addiction psychiatry and addiction medicine, however, cannot ignore spiritual issues. If former patients are asked about factors leading to long-term recovery from alcohol or other drug addictions, a large number mention spiritual experiences or motivation. The most important source of such spiritual experiences in recovery is participation in a 12-step program such as AA. The 12-step approach to spiritual experience is one that specialists in addiction psychiatry should understand, clinically support, and communicate to their colleagues who care for patients addicted to alcohol and other drugs.

Definitions and Theory

Spirituality can be defined as the relationship between an individual and a transcendent or Higher Being or force or mind of the universe.[11] This relationship is personal to the individual and does not require affiliation with any religion. In fact, religion is not necessary for a person to have a spiritual experience or to develop his or her own spirituality. Religion does, however, provide the most common path to spiritual experience in growth and development. Weil comments that "restoring that which is broken is the function of religion; the word means 'to bind again.' Religion is the medicine of the soul."[12] Although spirituality does not require religion, it does require theology—that is, a theory of this Higher Being, mind, or power.

Why should a person make any effort to develop spirituality or work on his or her spiritual health? The main reason for making the effort has to do with the benefits that can result, as discussed in the paragraphs that follow.

HUMILITY

Khantzian and Mack, both academic psychoanalysts, state that "the power and awe engendered by an outside universe and our humble place in it instill a sense of a force or power greater than ourselves."[13] They believe that this experience "may be a step in the direction of taming and transforming infantile omnipotence and serving in early childhood to establish a capacity for object love. In this context God serves as a 'self-object love' in transition from self love to object love and provides much needed authority and structure within the self."

Humility can be a powerful stimulus for healing. It probably does this by engendering honesty and a willingness to accept help. In humility, we know ourselves as fallible individuals who make mistakes. It then is unnecessary to make excuses, blame others, or tell lies when a problem arises. It has been said that humility is not thinking less of myself, but thinking of myself less. A relevant 12-step saying is that "humility is our acceptance of ourselves."[2] When this acceptance occurs, defensiveness subsides. With this acceptance comes a willingness to ask for and receive help. "The smartest thing an AA member can say is 'Help me.' "[2]

INNER STRENGTH

The experience of a Higher Power within oneself leads to a sense of being able to deal with adversity. This makes it possible for the individual to face painful situations and to continue the struggles that so often are necessary in life. This inner strength is closely related to the AA saying, "Serenity is not freedom from the storm, but peace amid the storm."[2] The challenge for addiction psychiatry is to help stressed and troubled individuals work toward attaining this experience. Kurtz and Ketcham recount some poignant stories that reflect this characteristic.[14]

A SENSE OF MEANING AND PURPOSE

Spiritual experience often leads to a greater interest and intention in living. This may be as specific as promoting healing in medical practice or as general as working to improve or sustain the quality of life on earth. This experience is a major reason for associating service with spiritual health.

Coles, a child analyst, spent years studying children from different cultures and various religious backgrounds.[15] He concluded that most if not all children struggle with the concept of God and attempt to find meaning and purpose in their lives. His concluding comment is, "So it is that we connect with one another, move in and out of one another's lives, teach and heal and affirm one another, across space and time—yet how young we are when we start wondering about it all, the nature of the journey and of the final destination!"

ACCEPTANCE AND TOLERANCE

The internal experience of being accepted and cared for by a power greater than oneself leads to acceptance of oneself. This is the first step toward accepting others as they are. Acceptance and tolerance are facilitated by humility, recognizing the fact that it is difficult enough to live our own lives without trying to direct, control, or destroy the lives of others. Acceptance and tolerance develop into affection, caring, and love. These qualities greatly enhance human relationships. The willingness of AA and Narcotics Anonymous (NA) to accept and tolerate any alcoholic or addict who wants to stop drinking or using drugs, no matter how disreputable or repugnant their appearance and smell, provides an excellent model for these characteristics. These 12-step programs also pay serious attention to minority opinion, no matter how much it differs from the majority.

The antithesis of spirituality is hatred, prejudice, and resentment directed toward oneself and others. It is a sad fact that many religions, including Christianity, have been unable to help their adherents develop spiritual health and overcome the behaviors associated with these negative emotions. These problems were noted by both Bill W. and Dr. Bob S., the cofounders of AA, and given as their reasons for separating AA from any religion.[16]

HARMONY

Closely related to acceptance is the experience of being in harmony with the universe. This leads to an interest in preserving and protecting our environment. It also leads to a sense of connectedness to all other human beings and living things.

Other qualities could be described, including the sobriety that is so important in addiction medicine. More benefit is to be derived, however, from focusing on a few key issues rather than dwelling on complex theoretical issues that atheist and agnostic healthcare professionals can more justifiably ignore.

Booth described spirituality as "an inner attitude that emphasizes energy, creative choice, and a powerful force for living. . . . There are four qualities that increasingly reflect healthy spirituality the more we develop them in our lives. They are truth (honesty), energy (vitality), love, and acceptance."[17]

How Is Spiritual Health Attained?

Attainment of physical and mental health requires more than the belief that they can be experienced. Both require active effort and practice on the part of each individual. The roles of exercise, nutrition, and physiological monitoring have been well established in developing and maintaining physical health. Less is known about the ways in which mental health can be maintained, but most of us practice thinking, problem solving, management and expression of feelings, and the maintenance of long-term relationships in a social support system.

What areas of practice and exercise are needed if we are to attain and maintain a relationship with a Higher Power? Five activities could be postulated as useful for developing spiritual experiences and spiritual health. Examples from working a 12-step program of recovery are used where applicable.

PRAYER

Attempts to communicate with a Higher Power have been effective for many people. Books have been written on how to pray. One simple fact to remember is that communication with another includes listening as well as talking. Anyone can pray. At issue are the results. As one recovering alcoholic said, "I came into this program as a drunken atheist. Today I pray. . . . As an atheist, I faked prayer in the beginning. The results have altered my view of the cosmos. . . . This change in a drunken, hardcore, cynical atheist is a miracle beyond human comprehension."[18] Step 2, in which belief in the existence of a Power greater than oneself, sets the stage for this activity. Step 3 involves turning over one's life and will to this Higher Power. I have come to appreciate the therapeutic benefit of this step so much that I sometimes try teaching psychiatric patients the third step to help them let go of tenaciously held beliefs and ideas that are causing pain to both them and others. Step 5 consists in part of an honest opening of oneself to a loving and accepting Higher Power. This type of prayer is an antidote to both shame and guilt. It is built on by step 7, when an individual asks for help in changing character defects, a task that we psychiatrists and other mental health professionals have found to be very difficult. Step 11 continues to build on the contact already made with one's Higher Power. It gives a very useful direction, advising the person to ask for only knowledge and power to carry out life's tasks. This direction provides a continuing antidote for the selfishness and self-centeredness that interfere so powerfully with intimacy and caring relationships.

MAINTAIN AN OPEN MIND

Clearing the mind through meditation may be a way of opening one's self to the experience of a Higher Power. Many people experience new ideas and energy, in addition to mental and physical benefits, when they practice meditation. The best results appear to be obtained through disciplined practice.

There are many barriers to developing an open mind, including our reluctance to give up beliefs that were developed in childhood. The "Big Book" of AA quotes Herbert Spencer's admonition that one sure way of maintaining a closed mind is to have contempt before investigation.[16] Open-mindedness is encouraged in the 12-step programs by encouraging individuals to look for things to identify with in the experience of others. This attitude, combined with the focus on welcoming and accepting newcomers, no matter how unpleasant they may appear, has helped AA and NA become true democracies.

DISCUSSION

We can learn much from the experience of others. Unfortunately, social prohibitions make discussion about spiritual issues difficult; for example, servicemen are cautioned not to talk about religion because of the arguments and fights that so often ensue. Anxiety at the prospect of ridicule and rejection poses another barrier to discussion of spiritual issues. The 12-step programs, by valuing personal experience and refusing to evaluate or judge anyone's experience, have created a forum where people can be comfortable discussing their spiritual beliefs and experiences or lack of them. Psychiatrists are now expected to be able to facilitate discussion about spiritual and religious issues. The new residency training requirements and addition to DSM-IV-R indicate that knowledge and skill in this area are expected of us. Addiction psychiatrists are fortunate in having easy and close access to the 12-step programs. In my experience, it is easier to discuss spiritual issues with people working a 12-step program of recovery than it is with church members.

READING

The recorded thoughts and experiences of others can be useful in developing one's own ideas and experiences. The classical literature of each of the world's great religions provides examples that often are stimulating and inspiring. Kurtz and Ketcham have gathered stories from both religious and secular sources to illustrate the spirituality of imperfection.[14] The "Big Book" of AA provides useful reading in the spiritual area.[16] Chapter 4, entitled "To the Agnostic," makes as much sense today as when it was written in 1939. Many medical students have found this chapter helpful in distinguishing spirituality from religion. An addiction psychiatrist who is an atheist or agnostic would do well to become familiar with the various spiritual experiences that have helped people recover from addiction. It does not require belief in a Higher Power to acknowledge that there are many mysteries about health and illness that medicine and science cannot explain. We can help our addicted patients remain open to the experience described by Bill W. in a talk to physicians.[19] He described what AA members mean when they talk about a spiritual experience: "They mean a certain quality of personality change which, in their belief, could not have occurred without the help and presence of the creative spirit of the universe."

RELIGIOUS ACTIVITY

Worship services in all religions are designed to help participants strengthen their contact with a Higher Power and improve their spiritual health. That this activity alone is insufficient to attain spiritual health is evidenced by the unspiritual behavior of many religious people when they are not in a place of worship.

No empirical data support the relationship of these activities to healing. The amount of time and energy that should be devoted to the attainment of spiritual health is unknown. In this regard, it is useful to recall the example of aerobic exercise. Although the aspects of such exercise are easily measurable, it took years for scientists to demonstrate its beneficial effect on physical health and longevity. Those of us who had experienced the benefits of aerobic exercise in our own lives did not wait for the controlled studies. We made the effort, noted how much better we felt, and modified our lifestyles.

The same is true of activities that contribute to mental and spiritual health. As potentially beneficial activities, such as step 11, are identified and practiced on a regular basis, it will be possible to measure their effects on different areas of health.

Suggestions for Clinical Practice

Specialists in addiction medicine or addiction psychiatry must have a working knowledge of the potential role of spirituality in enhancing recovery from alcoholism and other drug addictions. Knowledge and skill in supporting a patients' spiritual experience, as well as the work necessary to develop and maintain spiritual health, do not require spiritual beliefs on the part of the healthcare professional. An atheist or agnostic physician is at no greater disadvantage than is a physician who smokes or is overweight in helping patients deal with those problems. In any case, it is important that physicians refrain from any attempt to persuade patients to adopt or discard a particular set of religious beliefs. In this context, addiction psychiatrists are offered the following guidelines, which have been adapted from principles articulated by the American Psychiatric Association[6]:

- Maintain respect for each patient's beliefs.
- Obtain information about the religious or ideological orientation and beliefs of patients so that they can be attended to in the course of treatment.
- If conflict arises in relation to such beliefs, handle it with a concern for the patient's vulnerability to the physician's attitudes.
- Develop empathy for the patient's sensibilities and particular beliefs.
- Do not impose your own religious, antireligious, or ideological concepts in the course of therapeutic practice.

Some patients may wish to enter a religiously based treatment program. There is no reason to discourage this. After studying several programs in New York and surveying the literature, Muffler and colleagues concluded that "religious programs have demonstrated successful outcomes comparable to those of secular treatment regimens. Religious commitment and treatment by religious practitioners are playing a vital role for many in addictive treatment care."[20]

KNOW ALCOHOLICS ANONYMOUS

AA is recommended because it provides the best practical example of a spiritual program that is not a religion. This fact is not always recognized in the professional literature. For example, Galanter, although he recommends the clinical use of AA, refers to it as a zealous self-help group and compares it with cults.[21] After describing Bill W.'s initial spiritual experience, he states, "Bill went on from this experience to preach to other alcoholics and, as with the cultic groups described above, the forces of shared belief and group cohesiveness have become central in the engagement process of

AA." The key fact missed in this description is that after a few months of preaching, which failed to sober up a single alcoholic, Bill W. stopped preaching and began sharing his experience. It took less than 3 years for AA to discover that a religious approach did not work for many alcoholics. AA then separated from the Oxford Group and emphasized only a uniquely personal spiritual experience with a Higher Power as each individual alcoholic understood this.

INQUIRE ABOUT THE BENEFITS ASSOCIATED WITH SPIRITUAL HEALTH

The benefits of spiritual health include the humility, inner strength, sense of meaning and purpose, evidence of acceptance and tolerance, and sense of harmony with others and the world already described. Kurtz and Ketcham add gratitude and forgiveness as benefits of spiritual health; indeed, their research in this area found that "the experience of being able to forgive was preceded by some experience of being forgiven."[14] This observation illustrates the close association of social support and intimacy with spiritual experience and health.

Conclusion

Although powerful arguments can be made against including spiritual issues in addiction medicine, an even stronger case can be made for their inclusion. The experiences of so many recovering alcoholics and other drug addicts cannot be ignored. As physicians, we find it useful to practice acceptance of the varied spiritual experiences of our patients and to support them as helping their recovery.

As practitioners of addiction psychiatry and addiction medicine, we have an obligation to demonstrate knowledge and skill in supporting spiritual issues in the treatment of addictive disorders.

ACKNOWLEDGMENTS

This chapter is based on an earlier chapter, Spiritual Components of the Recovery Process, which appeared in *Principles of Addiction Medicine*, Section XIV, published by ASAM in 1994.

REFERENCES

1. Ornstein R, Swencionis C (eds): The Healing Brain: A Scientific Reader. New York, Guilford Press, 1990.

2. Pittman B: Stepping Stones to Recovery. Seattle, WA, Glen Abbey Books, 1988.
3. Veach TL, Chappel NN: Measuring spiritual health: A preliminary study. Substance Abuse 13(3):139–147, 1992.
4. Lukodd S, Lu F, Ruenwe E: Towards a more culturally sensitive DSM-IV. J Nerv Ment Dis 180(11):673–682, 1992.
5. Sansone RA, Khatain K, Rodenhauser P: The role of religion in psychiatric education: A national survey. Academic Psychiatry 14:34–38, 1990.
6. American Psychiatric Association (APA), Committee on Religion and Psychiatry: Guidelines regarding possible conflict between psychiatrists' religious commitments and psychiatric practice. Am J Psychiatry 47:542, 1990.
7. APA: Diagnostic and Statistical Manual of Mental Disorders, 4th ed. Washington, DC, APA, 1994.
8. Engel GL: The need for a new medical model: A challenge for biomedicine. Science, 196:129, 1977.
9. Hiatt JF: Spirituality, medicine and healing. South Med J 79:736–743.
10. Kuhn C: A spiritual inventory of the medically ill patient. Psychiatric Medicine 6:87–89, 1988.
11. Peterson EA, Nelson K: How to meet your client's spiritual needs. Journal of Psychological Nursing 25:34–39, 1987.
12. Weil A: Health and Healing: Understanding Conventional and Alternative Medicine. Boston, Houghton Mifflin, 1983.
13. Khantzian EJ, Mack JE: Alcoholics Anonymous and contemporary psychodynamic theory. Recent Dev Alcohol 7:67–89, 1989.
14. Kurtz E, Ketcham K: The Spirituality of Imperfection: Modern Wisdom From Classic Stories. New York, Bantam Books, 1992.
15. Coles R: The Spiritual Life of Children. Boston, Houghton Mifflin, 1990.
16. Alcoholics Anonymous. AA: Alcoholics Anonymous: The Story of How Many Thousands of Men and Women Have Recovered from Alcoholism, 3rd ed. New York, AA Grapevine, 1976.
17. Booth L: When God Becomes a Drug: Breaking the Chains of Religious Addiction and Abuse. New York, Tarcher/Perigree Books, 1991.
18. Alcoholics Anonymous: AA: Best of the Grapevine. New York, AA Grapevine, 1985.
19. William W: Basic Concepts of Alcoholics Anonymous. N Y State Med J 44:1805–1810, 1944.
20. Muffler J, Langrod JG, Larson D: "There is a balm in Gilead": Religion and substance abuse treatment. In Lowinson J (ed): Substance Abuse: A Comprehensive Textbook. Baltimore, Williams & Wilkins, 1992, pp 584–595.
21. Galanter M: Cults and zealous self-help movements: A psychiatric perspective. Am J Psychiatry 147(5):543–551, 1990.

46

Pathological Gambling

Sheila B. Blume, MD

There is nothing new about gambling or gambling problems in human history. Archaeologists have identified gambling-related artifacts and records dating back as far as the ancient Babylonians in 3000 B.C.[1] Both the Old and New Testaments make mention of the casting of lots. For example, Moses is instructed by God to divide the land west of the Jordan among the tribes of Israel by this means (Numbers 25:55). Gambling is also mentioned prominently in the literature and tradition of the Eastern cultures. In Europe, organized lotteries date back to the middle ages. The first government-sponsored lottery was chartered by Queen Elizabeth I in 1566.[2]

European settlers brought their tradition to North America, and each of the 13 original colonies authorized lotteries to raise money, as did the young nation's major universities (Harvard, Yale, Princeton, Columbia).[2]

Gambling, like the use of psychoactive substances, has been looked on as a source of pleasure and recreation by most cultures. However, as with alcohol and other drug use, societies have recognized the potential for harm related to gambling and have found it necessary to regulate and control the activity. Such controls are aimed at preventing fraudulent games, preventing minors from gambling, placing controls on the amounts of money wagered, limiting the amount of credit that can be extended by the sponsors of games, and regulating the numbers, types, and sponsors of gambling establishments. Such laws have been enacted in all parts of the world during many historical periods. Only recently, however, have a small number of gambling control laws included the provision of resources to prevent and treat gambling-related problems.

Gambling in the United States

Despite its early history of helping establish the country, gambling has not always been welcome in the United States. Public opinion and public policy have vacillated between extremes of prohibition and acceptance. The 1980s and 1990s have witnessed an overwhelming trend toward the establishment of state lotteries, legalization of many additional forms of wagering (e.g., off-site sports betting, gambling machines, cards, bingo), and the establishment of casino gambling on Native American reservations and riverboats in a growing number of states.

Gambling in the United States today is big business. In 1992, Americans wagered approximately $330 billion (the so-called handle, or gross amount bet), representing more than $1300 for every man, woman, and child in the country. Profit from this volume of wagering amounted to nearly $30 billion.[3] Most Americans (between 80% and 90% of adults) report having some experience with gambling,[4] and about a third report gambling at least once a week. The spread and popularity of gambling have raised concerns about the relationship between increasing the availability of gambling and possibly producing a corresponding increase in the prevalence of gambling problems. Present epidemiological evidence indicates that such a relationship exists.[5]

Pathological Gambling

DEFINITIONS

There is sometimes confusion, particularly in evaluating individual behavior, between gambling and other behaviors involving risk. Can a person who defuses bombs or skydives be considered gambling with his or her life, or is crossing the street, marrying, or life itself a gamble? The act of gambling or wagering is defined as either (1) playing a game for money or (2) staking money (or any other thing of value) on an uncertain event, one influenced by chance.[6] In practical terms, gambling includes risking money (or valuables) on the possibility (influenced to a greater or lesser degree by chance) of attaining more money within a relatively short period of time. Thus, a long-term investment in government bonds would not usually be considered gambling, whereas short-term stock market transactions such as options, or "puts" and "calls," do fall into the category. Thus, skydiving (risk taking without the short-term wagering of something valuable) is not gambling for the purpose of defining gambling problems.

The term *problem gambling* is used as an overall umbrella term for gambling problems including but not limited to pathological gambling.[7] The term *pathological gambling* was coined when diagnostic criteria for the disorder were first published in the American Psychiatric Association's *Diagnostic and Statistical Manual of Mental Disorders* (DSM-III) in 1980.[8] The disorder is commonly referred to as *compulsive gambling* by the public and by Gamblers Anonymous (GA), but this term was thought likely to cause confusion with obsessive-compulsive disorder and obsessive-compulsive personality disorder in the diagnostic nomenclature.

DSM-IV-R[9] describes pathological gambling as "persistent and recurrent maladaptive gambling behavior" and requires at least five of the ten diagnostic criteria listed in Table 46–1 for a diagnosis.

Inclusion as a mental disorder in the standard nomenclature lends credence to the conceptualization of pathological gambling as a

Table 46–1. DIAGNOSTIC CRITERIA FOR PATHOLOGICAL GAMBLING

A. A persistent and recurrent maladaptive gambling behavior as indicated by at least five of the following:
  (1) Preoccupation with gambling (e.g., preoccupied with reliving past gambling experiences, handicapping or planning the next venture, or thinking of ways to get money with which to gamble)
  (2) The need to gamble with increasing amounts of money in order to achieve the desired excitement
  (3) Repeated unsuccessful efforts to control, cut back, or stop gambling
  (4) Restlessness or irritability when attempting to cut down or stop gambling
  (5) Gambles as a way of escaping from problems or of relieving dysphoric mood (e.g., feelings of helplessness, guilt, anxiety, depression)
  (6) After losing money gambling, often returns another day in order to get even ("chasing" one's losses)
  (7) Lies to family members, therapists, or others to conceal the extent of involvement with gambling
  (8) Has committed illegal acts such as forgery, fraud, theft, or embezzlement, in order to finance gambling
  (9) Has jeopardized or lost a significant relationship, job, or educational or career opportunity because of gambling
  (10) Reliance on others to provide money to relieve a desperate financial situation caused by gambling
B. Is not better accounted for by a manic episode.

From the American Psychiatric Association: Diagnostic and Statistical Manual of Mental Disorders, 4th ed. Washington, DC, American Psychiatric Association, 1994, p 618.

disease,[10] although this model is not universally accepted.[11] Although both behavioral psychology and psychodynamic theory add to the understanding of pathological gambling,[7] an addiction model of the disorder and its treatment have become popular, especially in the United States.[10, 12] The addiction model is discussed in this chapter.

EPIDEMIOLOGY

Two articles by Volberg[4, 5] review epidemiological studies of gambling problems in the United States during the past two decades. These epidemiological surveys have used two different methods to study random populations of adults reached by telephone.[4, 13] The six studies performed in the 1980s, using the South Oaks Gambling Screen, involved eastern and western states (New York, New Jersey, Maryland, Massachusetts, and California). These surveys found a lifetime prevalence of problem gambling among adults of 3.9% to 4.2%. Probable pathological gambling was identified in 1.2% to 2.3% of the adult population (about a third of problem gamblers). In Iowa, in contrast, a similar survey during the 1980s found 1.6% problem gamblers and 0.1% pathological gamblers. Later surveys conducted during the 1990s in seven states (Michigan, Connecticut, Missouri, North Dakota, South Dakota, Texas, and Washington) found a lifetime prevalence of pathological gambling of 3.5% to 6.3% and a current (6 months or 1 year) prevalence of 1.4% to 2.8%.[4] Although further study is warranted, these differences in findings may be interpreted as reflecting both an absolute increase in the prevalence of the disorder and regional differences, all related to the spread of legalized gambling, especially lotteries. In addition, a 1990 Iowa study found that lottery participation correlated with other forms of gambling behavior, including loss of control and gambling-related problems.[14]

RISK FACTORS

Risk factors for pathological gambling include having a family history of gambling problems,[15] being male, being younger than 30 years, being unmarried, gambling frequently, beginning gambling at a young age, having a low household income,[4, 5] and having a family history of alcoholism.[16] Higher rates of pathological gambling are also found among adults[15, 16] and adolescents[17] in chemical dependence treatment and among adult inpatients on a psychiatric admission service.[18]

PATHOPHYSIOLOGY

It is somewhat curious that despite the significant prevalence and social cost of pathological gambling, little research attention has been paid to biological components in the etiology and psychopathology of the disorder. Electroencephalographic studies have shown patterns of decreased hemispheric differentiation between the left and right sides of the brain in response to a task. This pattern is similar to that seen in children with attention deficit/hyperactivity disorder.[19, 20] A study of neurotransmitters and their metabolites in bodily fluids compared newly abstinent male pathological gamblers with normal male subjects.[21] Elevated levels of the norepinephrine metabolite 3-methoxy-4-hydroxyphenylglycol (MHPG) were found in the cerebrospinal fluid (CSF), and elevated levels of norepinephrine were found in the urine of gamblers. Further study of this population found a correlation between the extraversion scale of the Eysenck Personality Questionnaire and both CSF and plasma MHPG and with urinary norepinephrine metabolites.[22] A single study of beta-endorphins found lower baseline levels in racetrack compulsive gamblers than in gambling machine addicts and normal subjects.[23] Elevated central and peripheral norepinephrine may explain the highly aroused "high" described by pathological gamblers. Endorphin abnormalities may link pathological gambling with other addictive disorders. However, far more study is needed before conclusions can be drawn.

PERSONALITY FACTORS

Lesieur and Rosenthal, in their review of the literature on problem gambling, briefly summarize personality trait research in pathological gamblers.[7] Minnesota Multiphasic Personality Inventory studies have shown increased scores on the psychopathic deviate scale and on the depression scale (similar to the findings in alcoholics). Other studies have indicated several personality constructs relevant to pathological gamblers: mood, obsessive-compulsive symptoms, life stressors, socialization, and substance addiction.[24]

SYMPTOMS AND COURSE

Pathological gambling has been conceptualized as an addiction to being "in action," an aroused euphoric state described by pathological gamblers as comparable to the high produced by cocaine. A gambler is in action when risking a significant amount on an outcome that is not yet decided. The term describes the gambler's experience while watching a horse race or a sports competition, playing cards, or reading the daily market reports. Another experience postulated to be part of gambling addiction is a feeling of dissociation, called by Jacobs a "state of altered identity."[25] This trancelike state experienced while gambling permits an escape from worries and dysphoria, lowers self-critical consciousness, and permits wish-fulfillment fantasies.

Pathological gambling is usually described as developing in the three phases delineated by Custer and Milt[26] (the winning, losing, and desperation phases). To this, Rosenthal has added a *giving up* phase.[7] In reviewing these phases, it is important to note that there is no uniformity in the course followed and that women often do not experience a winning phase.

Most pathological gamblers begin to gamble in adolescence, although females may begin later. A preoccupation with gambling sometimes begins with a "big win." Such a progression is described in Dostoyevsky's novel *The Gambler*, which the author wrote in the desperation phase of his own pathological gambling to relieve his gambling debts.[27] For most pathological gamblers, however, a winning phase depends on the skilled playing of cards, handicapping of horses, or playing the market, as more and more time, energy, and concentration are devoted to gambling-related activities. Although a gambler both wins and loses during the winning phase, wins tend to be acknowledged and losses denied, leading to an occasional or repeated inability to account for money claimed to be won. A gambler's self-esteem becomes increasingly dependent on being both smarter than the average person and favored by luck, therefore able to achieve wealth, power, and social status without hard labor. During this early phase, the size and frequency of betting increase, but indebtedness is not a major problem because the gambler continues to work and wins frequently enough to support the growing need to stay in action. During this period, there is also an increasing psychological dependence on gambling as a remedy for dysphoric states such as depression, boredom, resentment, and anxiety as well as a source of pleasure and self-esteem. Preoccupation with gambling is evident.

The losing phase characteristically begins with the kind of chance loss common in all gambling experiences. To early-stage pathological gamblers, however, losses are experienced as injuries to the self-esteem and begin to lead to "chasing" (i.e., gambling increasing amounts to try to win back money lost).[28] The pattern of chasing accelerates losses, although there are ups and downs with accompanying euphoria and depression that sometimes mimic bipolar disorder. During this period, pathological gamblers gamble away all available resources and go into debt. Time and energy spent on gambling displace social and vocational pursuits. Interpersonal relationships suffer, and somatic symptoms are often experienced, including headaches, palpitations, insomnia, and gastrointestinal upsets. Comorbid psychiatric disorders, including major depression, anxiety disorders, hypomanic episodes, and bipolar disorder, have been described. However, pathological gambling is not diagnosed if the gambling-related symptoms are present only during a manic episode. Suicide attempts are common.[7] Personality disorders often diagnosed include narcissistic and antisocial types. Substance-related disorders are frequent (discussed later).

Pathological gamblers describe various withdrawal symptoms when they become abstinent from gambling. Symptoms include craving, restlessness, insomnia, and sometimes headaches and gastrointestinal or respiratory symptoms.[7]

The desperation phase of pathological gambling includes massive lying and behaviors (e.g., stealing from family members and white collar crime) inconsistent with the individual's customary moral standards. This phase is often ushered in by one or more "bailouts" (gifts or loans by significant others meant to relieve a desperate financial situation but often, at least in part, gambled away). Wagering becomes more reckless, and the fantasy that a big win is about to occur and solve all problems dominates the gambler's thinking. The irrational belief in such a win may be striking. The gambler may become isolated from family and friends. Arrests and convictions characterize this phase. Depression and suicide are common.

The giving-up phase is characterized by the loss of the fantasy of winning and by gambling for its own sake.

Families of pathological gamblers are often destroyed by this disease. Spouses are subjected to financial insecurity and theft of their savings and property and are often abused (verbally and sometimes physically). They are also harassed by bill collectors and coerced into cosigning for loans. They suffer from physical (headache, gastrointestinal problems, respiratory symptoms) and psychiatric (anxiety, depression, suicide) symptoms and disorders. Their ability to function as parents also suffers.[7] The few studies of children of compulsive gamblers in the literature have found increased health-threatening behaviors (e.g., smoking, overeating, substance use, gambling), psychological risk factors, dysphoria, and deficits in functioning.[29] Children from multiproblem families (e.g., substance dependence in addition to pathological gambling) fared worse than those whose parents suffered from pathological gambling alone.[30]

SPECIAL POPULATIONS

Female compulsive gamblers differ from males in that they more often state that they gambled to escape from a difficult situation from the beginning and never gambled for pleasure or excitement. They are also more likely to miss the winning phase.[31] Women are clearly underrepresented in specific treatment for gambling problems,[5] although many have histories of psychiatric or psychological treatment aimed at associated problems (e.g., depression, substance dependence) without confronting the gambling.[31] They are also underrepresented in GA.[5]

Minorities, including black, Hispanic, Asian, and Native American populations, are also underrepresented in treatment and GA. The recent spread of legalized gambling among Native American tribes has led to special concern about this group. Volberg reports that preliminary data from North Dakota show a higher rate of probable pathological gambling among Native Americans than in the population at large.[5]

Because young people are thought to be at special risk for problem gambling, state laws restrict their access to legal wagering. Epidemiological evidence confirms the clinical observation that gambling at a young age and gambling during adolescence predict pathological gambling in adulthood.[5] Relatively little research attention has been focused on adolescent gamblers, and very little in the way of prevention or treatment programming has been developed. Young people's GA groups are not widely available. One researcher has proposed developing a special scale for measuring pathological gambling in young people.[32] She found that 9% of 284 schoolchildren (11 to 16 years of age) in a seaside English town where gambling machines were available scored in the probable pathological gambling range on her DSM-IV-J (for juvenile) scale.

Relationship Between Pathological Gambling and Substance-Related Disorders

Several studies have demonstrated a markedly increased prevalence of gambling problems among alcoholics and other drug-dependent persons.[16, 17] Among 458 adult alcohol/drug-dependent inpatients (average age 37 years), 9% satisfied a lifetime diagnosis of pathological gambling and an additional 10% had a history of some gambling problems but did not meet criteria for the disorder. Thus, a total of 19% qualified as problem gamblers.[16] Drinking and drug use often accompanied gambling in these subjects. A further study of 100 alcohol/drug-dependent adolescent inpatients (average age 17 years) found that 14% met diagnostic criteria for pathological gambling and an additional 14% had gambling-related problems, for a total of 28%.[17]

Conversely, studies of populations in treatment for pathological gambling have shown a higher prevalence of alcohol and drug problems than are characteristic of the general public. For example, 47% of 51 male compulsive gamblers met alcohol/drug abuse or dependence criteria.[33]

The relationships between psychoactive substance use disorders and gambling problems are complex but important for the treatment of both disorders.[34] It is common for gambling and substance use to occur together. Alcoholic beverages are served at casinos and card games and are sold at racetracks and sports arenas. Both gambling activities such as bookmaking and illicit drug sales are often conducted in neighborhood bars. Dependence on alcohol or other drugs may develop concurrently with dependence on gambling. In other cases, when dependence on a substance develops, gambling activities decrease. However, the excitement caused by gambling or the feelings of disappointment on losing money may trigger a relapse in addicts who are working at abstinence. In chemically dependent patients with a history of pathological gambling in remission, alcohol/drug abstinence may lead to a return to gambling, which then causes a chemical relapse.

An additional pattern observed in the natural history of chemically dependent patients is a switch of addictions to pathological gambling.[35] This pattern is seen in abstinent addicts who may or may not have had an intense interest in gambling or overt gambling problems in the past. Recovering addicts discover that the high or the feeling of altered consciousness attained through gambling is easily substituted for the altered feelings previously sought through substance use. The addictive behavior pattern now centers around gambling instead of alcohol or other drugs. In such cases, the progression of pathological gambling is accelerated, and the individual may reach the desperation state in a period of a year or two.

For this reason, pathological gambling screening of all patients entering treatment for chemical dependence is recommended[35] (discussed later). This screening is able to identify patients in need of intervention and concurrent treatment for gambling problems as well as those at special risk for switching addictions (because of family history of gambling problems, a strong interest in gambling, or a history of gambling problems in the past).

In addition, recreational activities in residential or outpatient addiction treatment programs should not include games usually associated

Table 46–2. SOUTH OAKS GAMBLING SCREEN (SOGS)

Name _____ Date _____

1. Please indicate which of the following types of gambling you have done in your lifetime. For each type, mark one answer: "not at all," "less than once a week," or "once a week or more."

	not at all	less than once a week	once a week or more	
a.	_____	_____	_____	Play cards for money
b.	_____	_____	_____	Bet on horses, dogs, or other animals (at OTB, the track, or with a bookie)
c.	_____	_____	_____	Bet on sports (parlay cards, with a bookie, or at jai alai)
d.	_____	_____	_____	Played dice games (including craps, over and under, or other dice games) for money
e.	_____	_____	_____	Gambled in a casino (legal or otherwise)
f.	_____	_____	_____	Played the numbers or bet on lotteries
g.	_____	_____	_____	Played bingo for money
h.	_____	_____	_____	Played the stock, options, and/or commodities market
i.	_____	_____	_____	Played slot machines, poker machines, or other gambling machines
j.	_____	_____	_____	Bowled, shot pool, played golf or some other game of skill for money
k.	_____	_____	_____	Pull tabs or "paper" games other than lotteries
l.	_____	_____	_____	Some form of gambling not listed above (please specify) _____

2. What is the largest amount of money you have ever gambled with on any one day?

_____ Never have gambled ⠀⠀⠀⠀ _____ More than $100 up to $1,000

_____ $1 or less ⠀⠀⠀⠀ _____ More than $1,000 up to $10,000

_____ More than $1 up to $10 ⠀⠀⠀⠀ _____ More than $10,000

_____ More than $10 up to $100

3. Check which of the following people in your life has (or had) a gambling problem.

_____ Father ⠀⠀⠀ _____ Mother ⠀⠀⠀ _____ A brother or sister ⠀⠀⠀ _____ A grandparent

_____ My spouse or partner ⠀⠀⠀ _____ My child(ren) ⠀⠀⠀ _____ Another relative

_____ A friend or someone else important in my life

4. When you gamble, how often do you go back another day to win back money you lost?

_____ Never

_____ Some of the time (less than half the time I lost)

_____ Most of the time I lost

_____ Every time I lost

5. Have you ever claimed to be winning money gambling but weren't really? In fact, you lost?

_____ Never (or never gamble)

_____ Yes, less than half the time I lost

_____ Yes, most of the time

6. Do you feel you have ever had a problem with betting money or gambling?

_____ No

_____ Yes, in the past but not now

_____ Yes

7. Did you ever gamble more than you intend to? .... _____ Yes _____ No

Table continued on following page

Table 46–2. SOUTH OAKS GAMBLING SCREEN (SOGS) *Continued*

8. Have people criticized your betting or told you that you had a gambling problem, regardless of whether or not you thought it was true? .... _____ Yes _____ No

9. Have you ever felt guilty about the way you gamble or what happens when you gamble? .... _____ Yes _____ No

10. Have you ever felt like you would like to stop betting money or gambling but didn't think you could? .... _____ Yes _____ No

11. Have you ever hidden betting slips, lottery tickets, gambling money, I.O.U.s, or other signs of betting or gambling from your spouse, children, or other important people in your life? .... _____ Yes _____ No

12. Have you ever argued with people you live with over how you handle money? .... _____ Yes _____ No

13. (If you answered yes to question 12): Have money arguments ever centered on your gambling? .... _____ Yes _____ No

14. Have you ever borrowed from someone and not paid them back as a result of your gambling? .... _____ Yes _____ No

15. Have you ever lost time from work (or school) due to betting money or gambling? .... _____ Yes _____ No

16. If you borrowed money to gamble or to pay gambling debts, who or where did you borrow from? (check "yes" or "no" for each)

	No	Yes
a. from household money _____	( )	( )
b. from your spouse _____	( )	( )
c. from other relatives or in-laws _____	( )	( )
d. from banks, loan companies, or credit unions _____	( )	( )
e. from credit cards _____	( )	( )
f. from loan sharks _____	( )	( )
g. you cashed in stocks, bonds, or other securities _____	( )	( )
h. you sold personal or family property _____	( )	( )
i. you borrowed on your checking account (passed bad checks) _____	( )	( )
j. you have (had) a credit line with a bookie _____	( )	( )
k. you have (had) a credit line with a casino _____	( )	( )

From South Oaks Foundation, 400 Sunrise Highway, Amityville, NY 11701.

with gambling, such as cards, dice games, or bingo. Although in most cases house rules prohibit gambling, side bets are often made, and gambling on sports or numbers is conducted within the program. Patients attempting to give up drinking and drug use should not be encouraged to fill their leisure time with gambling-related recreational pursuits. Programs of physical exercise and constructive hobbies are preferable recreational activities for addiction facilities. In addition, all patients in chemical dependence treatment should be educated about their risk for pathological gambling and the process of switching addictions. Such prevention and intervention activities improve program effectiveness. Pathological gambling can be effectively treated concurrently with other addictive disorders.[36]

Screening for Pathological Gambling

The South Oaks Gambling Screen (SOGS) a valid and reliable screening tool for the identification of pathological gamblers, was introduced in 1987.[37] A total of 1616 subjects were involved in its development (867 patients in addiction treatment, 213 members of GA, 384 university students, and 152 hospital employees). The screen yields information about family history, lifetime involvement in gambling, and gambling-related problems (Table 46–2). The score sheet should be used (Table 46–3), because not all positive responses are counted toward the total score. The maximum SOGS score is 20. A score of 5 or more is indicative

Table 46–3. SOUTH OAKS GAMBLING
SCREEN (SOGS) SCORE SHEET

Scores on the SOGS itself are determined by adding up
the number of questions that show an at-risk response:

Questions 1, 2, and 3 not counted:

_____ Question 4—most of the time I lose
or
every time I lose

_____ Question 5—yes, less than half the time I
lose
or
yes, most of the time

_____ Question 6—yes, in the past but not now
yes

_____ Question 7—yes

_____ 8—yes

_____ 9—yes

_____ 10—yes

_____ 11—yes

12 not counted

_____ 13—yes

_____ 14—yes

_____ 15—yes

_____ 16a—yes

_____ b—yes

_____ c—yes

_____ d—yes

_____ e—yes

_____ f—yes

_____ g—yes

_____ h—yes

_____ i—yes

_____ Questions 16 j and k not counted

Total = ___ (there are 20 questions which are counted)

0 = no problem

1–4 = some problem

5 or more = probable pathological gambler

From South Oaks Foundation, 1992, 400 Sunrise Highway, Amityville, NY 11701.

of probable pathological gambling. It should be
noted that the SOGS is written in terms of lifetime experience (e.g., "Have you ever. . . ."").
Persons with high SOGS scores should be evaluated for a past or active DSM-IV-R diagnosis
of pathological gambling. The SOGS may be
adapted to local conditions.[38]

At South Oaks, the SOGS is given to all
addiction inpatients and outpatients at the time
of admission. Those who indicate a positive
family history or an intense interest in gambling are given special education about gam-

bling risk in addition to the general education
about gambling problems given to all patients.
With patients scoring 1 to 4, staff explore gambling behavior and recommend gambling
abstinence. Patients scoring 5 or more and diagnosed as pathological gamblers receive gam-
bling-specific treatment and are introduced to
meetings of GA. All significant others atending
the South Oaks family program are asked to fill
out the South Oaks Leisure Activities Screen
(SOLAS) about the patient's gambling (Table
46–4). When compared with the patient's
SOGS responses, the SOLAS may reveal denial
or misrepresentation by a patient covering up
his or her gambling history.

Treatment of Pathological Gambling

Addiction-model treatment for pathological
gambling uses both outpatient[39] and inpatient[40]
settings. Inpatient care is usually reserved for
patients unable to cooperate with outpatient
treatment, those with serious comorbid psychopathology, or those for whom other help
is unavailable. Compulsive gamblers may be
treated separately or in a special track within
a general addictions program. Alcoholics or
other drug addicts found to have a gambling
problem through SOGS screening are best
treated for both problems at the same time.

Pathological gamblers are motivated to seek
treatment by various means. Structured intervention by a group of significant others may
be used to break down denial in a compulsive
gambler, as it is used in alcoholism treatment.
Many pathological gamblers reach treatment
after a crisis such as a suicide attempt or an
arrest. Employee assistance programs sometimes identify and refer problem gamblers.
Routine screening of patients in treatment for
addictive disorders identifies additional pathological gamblers in need of help.

Initial treatment aims at establishing abstinence, breaking down denial and omnipotent
defenses, and establishing stable motivation
for treatment.[41] Techniques are similar to those
used in other addiction treatment: individual,
group, and family counseling; psychoeducation; and self-help (GA for the patient and
Gam-Anon for family members). Group therapy,[42] including psychodrama,[40] is often particularly helpful.

Continuing treatment concentrates on relapse prevention and rehabilitation, with measures to improve family and interpersonal relationships, work, and social functioning.

Table 46–4. SOUTH OAKS LEISURE ACTIVITIES SCREEN (SOLAS)

Please indicate the level of interest and involvement of the patient in the following activities. Circle a number or question mark for each activity.

	No interest at all	Moderate interest	Heavy interest	Obsessive interest	I don't know
Watching television _____	0	1	2	3	?
Playing cards _____	0	1	2	3	?
Playing cards for money _____	0	1	2	3	?
Betting on sports _____	0	1	2	3	?
Betting on horses, dogs, or jai alai _____	0	1	2	3	?
Playing the lottery or numbers _____	0	1	2	3	?
Playing dominoes or dice for money _____	0	1	2	3	?
Playing video games _____	0	1	2	3	?
Playing slot or video machines for money _____	0	1	2	3	?
Playing bingo for money _____	0	1	2	3	?
Gambling in casinos _____	0	1	2	3	?
Stocks, commodities, or options _____	0	1	2	3	?
Other gambling or betting activities _____	0	1	2	3	?

If the patient's interest in the above is causing family problems due to the amount of time devoted to it or financial problems due to the amount of money involved, please describe:

_____

_____

_____

_____

_____

_____

Patient's name: _____ Date: _____

Your signature: _____ Relation to patient: _____

From South Oaks Foundation, 1992, 400 Sunrise Highway, Amityville, NY 11701.

Financial problems require special attention. Recovering pathological gamblers often turn control of their finances over to a significant other, and checking accounts, credit cards, and all ready sources of cash or credit are discontinued. Gradual planned repayment of debts is preferred to a declaration of bankruptcy or a family bailout. The gradual attainment of self-esteem through repaying debts and otherwise making amends to those injured as a result of the patient's illness is as effective in pathological gambling as it is in other addictions.

Long-term follow-up involves individual, group, or family counseling and continuing GA attendance. Psychodynamic psychotherapy may be indicated in some patients. Psychopharmacological therapy is reserved for comorbid conditions such as major depression or bipolar disorder.

Treatment of family members is important,

whether or not the identified pathological gambler remains in treatment and recovers. Children of pathological gamblers are a special population in need of help.[29, 30]

GA is an important part of recovery for many pathological gamblers. Although based on the 12 steps of Alcoholics Anonymous (AA), GA is different in many respects from AA. Language used in the program puts less emphasis on God. For example, the third GA step uses the term "this Power of our own understanding" rather than the AA "God, as we understand Him."[43]

Although the literature on treatment outcome is not extensive, several studies have found inpatient rehabilitation programs effective, both for treating pathological gambling separately[44] and in a special track of an addiction program.[36] In the latter study, in which 72 patients at South Oaks Hospital were monitored for 6 to 14 months, a modification of the addiction severity index was used to measure clinical status. Marked improvement in all areas except employment and medical condition was found. Treatment for multiple addictions yielded abstinence from gambling in 64%, from alcohol in 65%, and from drugs in 80%.

Prevention

Little is known about prevention of gambling problems in the general public. Some attempts at public education have been made, but most efforts have been directed at setting up toll-free telephone numbers that can be called for help. These, in turn, refer to GA, Gam-Anon, and the few existing gambling treatment programs within the public and private sectors. There is a great unmet need for more treatment resources and for more research into the epidemiology, etiology, pathology, treatment, and prevention of this disease. Until public and professional interest in pathological gambling begins to approach the interest of governments and business interests in the promotion of legalized gambling, the vast majority of individuals and families suffering from this serious illness will continue to go without services.

REFERENCES

1. Fleming AM: Something for Nothing: A history of Gambling. New York, Delacorte Press, 1978. Cited by McGurrin MC (ed): Pathological Gambling: Conceptual, Diagnostic, and Treatment Issues. Sarasota, Professional Resource Press, 1992.
2. Clotfelter CT, Cook PJ: Selling Hope: State Lotteries in America. Cambridge, MA, Harvard University Press, 1989.
3. Christiansen EM: The 1992 gross annual wagering of the United States: Parts I and II. International Gaming and Wagering Business, Part I 14(7):12–33, Part II 14(8):12–30, 1993.
4. Volberg RA: Prevalence studies of problem gambling in the United States. J Gambl Stud (in press).
5. Volberg RA: The prevalence and demographics of pathological gamblers: Implications for public health. Am J Public Health 84(2):237–241, 1994.
6. Webster's New International Dictionary, 2nd ed. Springfield, IL, G&C Meriam, 1946.
7. Lesieur HR, Rosenthal RJ: Pathological gambling: A review of the literature (prepared for the American Psychiatric Association Task Force on DSM-IV Committee on Disorders of Impulse Control Not Elsewhere Classified). J Gambl Stud 7(1):5–39, 1991.
8. American Psychiatric Association (APA): Diagnostic and Statistical Manual of Mental Disorders, 3rd ed. Washington, DC, Author, 1980.
9. APA: Diagnostic and Statistical Manual of Mental Disorders, 4th ed. Washington, DC, APA, 1994.
10. Blume SB: Compulsive gambling and the medical model. J Gambl Behav 3:237–247, 1988.
11. Blaszczynski AP, McConaghy N: The medical model of pathological gambling: Current shortcomings. J Gambl Behav 5(1):42–52, 1989.
12. Walker MB: Some problems with the concept of "gambling addiction": Should theories of addiction be generalized to include excessive gambling? J Gambl Behav 5(3):179–200, 1989.
13. Volberg RA, Banks SM: A review of two measures of pathological gambling in the United States. J Gambl Stud 6(2):153–163, 1990.
14. Hraba J, Mok W, Huff D: Lottery play and problem gambling. J Gambl Stud 6(4):355–377, 1990.
15. Gambino B, Fitzgerald R, Shaffer H, et al: Perceived family history of problem gambling and scores on South Oaks Gambling Screen. J Gambl Stud 9(2):169–184, 1993.
16. Lesieur HR, Blume SB, Zoppa RM: Alcoholism, drug abuse and gambling. Alcohol Clin Exp Res 10(1):33–38, 1986.
17. Lesieur HR, Heineman M: Pathological gambling among youthful multiple substance abusers in a therapeutic community. Br J Addict 83:765–771, 1988.
18. Lesieur HR, Blume SB: Characteristics of pathological gamblers identified among patients on a psychiatric admissions service. Hosp Community Psychiatry 41(9):1009–1012, 1990.
19. Carlton P, Goldstein L: Physiological determinants of pathological gambling. In Galski T (ed): The Handbook of Pathological Gambling. Springfield, IL, Charles C Thomas, 1987, pp 111–122.
20. Goldstein L, Manowitz P, Nora R, et al: Differential EEG activation and pathological gambling. Biol Psychiatry 20:1232–1234, 1985.
21. Roy A, Adinoff B, Roehrick L, et al: Pathological gambling: A psychobiological study. Arch Gen Psychiatry 45:369–373, 1988.
22. Roy A, DeJong J, Linnoila M: Extraversion in pathological gamblers, correlates with indices of noradrenergic function. Arch Gen Psychiatry 46:679–681, 1989.
23. Blaszczynski AP, Winter SW, McConaghy N: Plasma endorphin levels in pathological gambling. J Gambl Behav 2:3–14, 1986.
24. McCormick RA, Taber JI: The pathological gambler: Salient personality variables. In Galski T (ed): The Handbook of Pathological Gambling. Springfield, IL, Charles C Thomas, 1987, pp 9–39.
25. Jacobs DF: Evidence for a common dissociative-like reaction among addicts. J Gambl Behav 4(1):27–37, 1988.
26. Custer R, Milt H: When Luck Runs Out: Help for Compulsive Gamblers and Their Families. New York, Facts On File Publications, 1985.
27. Dostoyevsky F: The Gambler/Bobok/A Nasty Story (translated by J Coulson). New York, Penguin Books, 1966, pp 7–16.
28. Lesieur HR: The Chase: Career of the Compulsive Gambler. Cambridge, MA, Schenkman, 1984.
29. Jacobs DF, Marston AR, Singer RD, et al: Children of problem gamblers. J Gambl Behav 5(4):261–268, 1989.
30. Lesieur HR, Rothschild J: Children of Gamblers Anonymous members. J Gambl Behav 5(4):269–281, 1989.
31. Lesieur HR, Blume SB: When lady luck loses: Women and compulsive gambling. In Van Den Bergh N (ed): Feminist Perspectives on Addictions. New York, Springer, 1991, pp 181–197.
32. Fisher S: Measuring pathological gambling in children: The case of fruit machines in the U.K. J Gambl Stud 8(3):263–285, 1992.
33. Ramirez LF, McCormick RA, Russo AM, et al: Patterns of substance abuse in pathological gamblers undergoing treatment. Addict Behav 8:425–428, 1984.

34. Blume SB: Gambling problems in alcoholics and drug addicts. In Miller NS (ed): Comprehensive Handbook of Drug and Alcohol Addiction. New York, Marcel Dekker, 1991, pp 967–980.

35. Blume SB: Pathological gambling and switching addictions: Report of a case. J Gambl Studies 10(1):87–96, 1994.

36. Lesieur HR, Blume SB: Evaluation of patients treated for pathological gambling in a combined alcohol, substance abuse and pathological gambling treatment unit using the addiction severity index. Br J Addict 86:1017–1028, 1991.

37. Lesieur HR, Blume SB: The South Oaks Gambling Screen (SOGS): A new instrument for the identification of pathological gamblers. Am J Psychiatry 144(9):1184–1188, 1987.

38. Lesieur HR, Blume SB: Revising the South Oaks gambling screen in different settings. J Gambl Behav 9(3):213–219, 1992.

39. Maurer CD: Practical issues and the assessment of pathological gamblers in a private practice setting. J Gambl Studies 10(1):5–20, 1994.

40. Blume SB: Treatment for the addictions in a psychiatric setting. Br J Addict 84:727–729, 1989.

41. Rosenthal RJ, Rugle LJ: A psychodynamic approach to the treatment of pathological gambling: Part I. Achieving abstinence. J Gambl Behav 10(1):21–42, 1994.

42. Taber JI, Chaplin MP: Group psychotherapy with pathological gamblers. J Gambl Behav 4(3):183–196, 1988.

43. Browne BR: The selective adaptation of the Alcoholics Anonymous program by Gamblers Anonymous. J Gambl Behav 7(3):187–206, 1991.

44. Russo AM, Taber JI, McCormick RA, et al: An outcome study of an inpatient treatment program for pathological gamblers. Hosp Community Psychiatry 35:823–827, 1984.

Eating Disorders and Addictions: Behavioral and Neurobiological Similarities

Karen A. Stennie, M.D. • Mark S. Gold, M.D.

Eating Disorders as Addictions

As the twentieth century concludes, DSM-IV may have defined, established, and operationalized addiction, but America through the media has expanded its own definition of addictions. Our pop culture appears to have broadened its concept of addictions to encompass most other self-destructive yet seemingly compulsive behaviors such as workaholism, gambling, compulsive spending, excessive sex, endless talking on the phone, and food addiction, with numerous self-confessed foodaholics. This chapter addresses the compelling issue of whether evidence exists to consider eating disorders as forms of addiction. It appears that this tendency to consider addictions as including every compulsive or repetitive behavior that is potentially harmful is one of the major reasons for *not* considering some eating disorders as addictive, autoaddictive disorders. Experts worry whether such a discussion might lead to a proposal to include gambling or compulsive sexual behaviors as addictions. However, on the basis of the well-known adage "if it looks like a duck, acts like a duck, and quacks . . . it must be a duck," eating disorders look like addictions. Patients with

anorexia and bulimia have a chronic disorder characterized by loss of control, compulsivity, reprioritization, and continuation despite severe and adverse consequences, loss of job and social performance, and so on. The DSM-IV eating disorder category naturally encompasses a diverse patient group. Some patients have a history of anorexia nervosa without obesity, others are restrictors, some purge, and still others have amenorrhea. Arguments have been made to consider eating disorders as personality disorders, obsessive-compulsive disease (OCD), depression, and addictive disorders. Addiction treatment programs have alerted us to the high comorbidity of eating disorders in patients with addiction, the commonness of eating disorders in several members of a family, the predominance of eating binges or starvation as relapse triggers in newly abstinent patients, and patients' reports of enhancing a drug's euphoric properties through starvation or purging. These observations support the hypothesis that eating disorders are related to tobacco and alcohol addiction and other addictive disorders.

Behavioral Similarities

Addiction has been defined as a disease characterized by the repetitive and destructive use of one or more mood-altering drugs that stems from a biological vulnerability manifested or induced by environmental factors.[1] It is a maladaptive pattern of substance use leading to clinically significant impairment or distress, with three or more of the following occurring in the same 12 months: (1) tolerance; (2) withdrawal; (3) taking the substance in larger amounts or for a longer period than was intended; (4) persistent desire or unsuccessful efforts to cut down or control; (5) spending a great deal of time in activities necessary to obtain the substance, use the substance, or recover from its effects; (6) neglect or reduction of important social, occupational, or recreational activities because of substance use; and (7) continued substance use despite knowledge of having a persistent or recurrent physical or psychological problem that was likely to have been caused or exacerbated by the substance.

If DSM-IV did not define addiction in terms of a psychoactive substance, would eating disorders qualify? With the change away from considering tolerance and withdrawal as essential aspects of dependence, eating disorders share many of the most salient features of addictions. In the eating disorders currently classified in DSM-IV—anorexia nervosa, bulimia nervosa, and binge eating disorder—food is a substance used both repetitively and destructively by either its prolonged restriction or episodic overconsumption.[2] Many young men and women experiment with severe diets, starvation, fasting, and self-induced vomiting, yet few apparently lose control and become anorectic or bulimic. These behaviors occur and continue independently of harm, loss, and risk caused by the activity. Despite the significant negative consequences, including a mortality rate of 5% to 17% for anorexia nervosa,[3] these behaviors are engaged in by approximately 0.5% of women between the ages of 15 and 40 years in the case of anorexia nervosa[4] and 1% to 1.5% of women in the case of bulimia.[5] The majority of patients are females, with males constituting only approximately 5% of the total.[6] As with classical addictions, eating disorders are chronic and relapsing, interfering with normal life patterns. Preoccupation with the food or the substance in question, such as supermarket browsing and cooking for others, is common.[7] Just as with other addictive substances, the overconsumption of food or bingeing is frequently conducted at night or in secret, historically as well as in present-day binge eating practice.[8] The chronic compromised nutritional state induced by both of these eating disorders[9] produces cognitive changes, mood lability, apathy, irritability, decreased libido, and sleep disturbances commonly observed in other addictions. Eating disorders, like classical addictions, can have quite tragic outcomes with a high degree of mortality. Mortality due to anorexia nervosa, as estimated from 42 published studies in a meta-analysis, is substantially greater than that among female psychiatric inpatients, 200 times greater than the suicide rate in the general population, at approximately 5.6% per decade.[10] Cocaine is self-administered to the point of death in rodents, nonhuman primates, and humans. Untreated alcoholism, nicotine dependence, and other addictive disorders are accompanied by increased death and disability. Bulimics, like other addicts, appear to have a favorite drug of abuse, consuming proportionally more sweet, high-fat foods in larger meals.[11] It is quite common to hear of a bulimic trigger in the same way an addict describes a drug cue that precipitates intense cravings and use. Bulimics describe external and internal cues such as seeing a pizza delivery truck or feeling depressed as triggering thoughts that they are fat or in need or a binge-purge episode. They describe rituals similar to drug-using rituals, with similar foods and environments.

Vandereycken suggests that the true addiction underlying both anorexia and bulimia is the craving to control body weight and appearance.[12] Additionally, he considers the bingeing addictive, inasmuch as the only identifiable peak experience occurs with self-induced vomiting. However, he notes pitfalls in attempting to overgeneralize the partial similarities between eating disorders and the addiction model. For example, the neuroadaptation phenomenon, which results in tolerance and withdrawal, includes events that are not readily translatable in terms of the eating disorders. Although weight loss is progressive in severe anorectics and it is unknown if the magnitude of bulimic episodes increases during the course of the disease process, the reduction in diagnostic emphasis on neuroadaptation diminishes the importance of this reservation. Eating disorders are addiction disorders in which food is the addicting substance.

We should keep in mind that the importance placed on a patient's obsession with body weight and appearance in our current concept of eating disorders may be a misleading bias of Western culture.[13] Despite the popular thesis that anorexia nervosa is the pathological expression of a need for control in twentieth century women overwhelmed by conflicting societal pressures, anorexia was described as early as 1694 by Morton and in the reports of Marce (1980), Gull (1873), and Laseque (1873). In a review of 360 cases of self-inflicted fasting from 1900 to 1939, the major subgroup in each century was categorized by having an abnormal attitude to food, eating, or weight. Similar to their contemporary counterparts, 85% of the group were female and more than half were younger than 20 years. Unlike their modern counterparts, however, historical female anorectics, although concerned about their shape and appearance, only sporadically expressed a fear of becoming fat. Furthermore, it has been noted that in present-day cases of anorexia reported from non-Western cultures, such as Hong Kong and India, patients express little concern about body weight.

As for the mostly male bulimics who have been described since the sixth century, they also have expressed no concern about body weight. Vomiting occurred frequently (bulimia emetica) but was never reported as self-induced, and there was no evidence of the use of either purgatives or laxatives. Weight concern and subsequent dieting may serve as the typical entry route into the disease process in our present culture. In all probability, the frequency of eating disorders and other addictions continues to rise because of the increasing prevalence of dieters and drug experimenters in our society. Nonetheless, the phenomena of self-induced food restriction and episodic overconsumption have transcended the cultures of many centuries, and the psychobiological vulnerabilities that led to the pious self-starvation of medieval saints continues to be expressed in the eating disorders of teenage American girls.[14]

Neurobiology

What is the nature of the psychobiological vulnerabilities that are expressed in the symptom cluster of the eating disorders? Many data suggest that the eating disorders represent dysregulations in the neurotransmitter pathways involving the dopamine, serotonin, and endogenous opioids. The involvement of the dopaminergic systems in the eating disorders links them with the pathway of brain reward on which all classical addictions appear to converge. The reality of this convergence seems obvious when one reflects on the common desire for a cigarette or coffee after a good meal and the stereotypical use of alcohol before sex, with a cigarette afterward.

DOPAMINE

Dopamine neurons discharge under conditions consistent with an attribution of incentive salience, suggesting that dopamine functions to give survival meaning to a particular occurrence.[15, 16] Wise suggested on the basis of this evidence that dopamine systems in the mesotelencephalon mediate the subjective pleasure produced by food, drugs, electrical brain stimulation, sex, and so forth.[17] The so-called dopamine hypothesis of the reinforcing properties of cocaine and resultant effects of chronic self-administration have been reviewed.[18–20] This work has led to the proposal of a common mesocorticolimbic dopamine system in drug and survival behavior reward. Drugs that are abused by humans have been shown to preferentially increase synaptic dopamine concentrations in the mesolimbic system of freely moving rats in microdialysis studies.[21, 22] This theory has been supported by these animal studies and the reports of dopamine increase produced during ethanol self-administration or the anticipation of ethanol availability for self-administration. Both are reversed or prevented by the opioid antagonist naloxone or naltrexone. Naltrexone itself, through opioid receptor blockade, appears to have an antiethanol reward effect in humans or increases the aversive effects as a working mechanism for its efficacy in alcohol dependence. The brain's perception of important events is integrally related to these chemical changes.

Pleasure is normally activated by an encounter with a natural incentive, such as when a hungry person eats food. However, neither the experience of pleasure nor the expectation of impending pleasure by itself causes wanting.[23] Stimuli that are attributed to incentive salience become attractive and demand attention. Drugs can acquire such a significance, and so can food. For example, the sight of cocaine to a cocaine user on a binge or the site of food to a starving bulimic person demands attention and cannot be easily ignored. Such notions are described as brain rewarding or reinforcing, yet they are not always pleasurable. They are acquired drives or pathological attachments. Dopamine neurons are common to the experience of eating and drug taking, yet they do not discharge when an animal actually eats food or when an animal would experience sensory pleasure. They change firing as the stimulus becomes more salient or attention grabbing.[24] The ability of drugs to elevate dopamine neurotransmission beyond that which normally occurs may be the feature of drugs that makes them such potent incentives, making stimuli perceived as brighter and more attractive and more able to dominate other competing interests.

SEROTONIN

In animal studies, serotonin produces satiety and inhibition of feeding. It has been proposed that anorexia nervosa reflects a state of serotonergic hyperactivity, and cerebrospinal fluid (CSF) levels of 5-hydroxyindoleacetic acid (5-HIAA) were found to be elevated in long-term weight-restored anorectic subjects.[25] The hypophagic effect of serotonergic agonists is greater in female than male rats and has been shown to vary with the stage of the menstrual cycle in humans.[26, 27] Hormone-related differences in serotonergic effects may help explain the overwhelming female prevalence and peripubertal onset of anorexia nervosa. The biologically rewarding aspects of eating may be exaggerated in females as well. In several species, female sexual behavior is inhibited by serotonin activity,[28] which may explain the fear or repression of sexuality commonly found in anorectics. Arousal and stress increase central serotonin release,[29, 30] allowing for a role of environmental influences in the development of anorexia nervosa in biologically vulnerable individuals.

Serotonin administration in the rat hypothalamus produces a decrease in total food intake, meal size, rate of eating, and percentage of carbohydrates eaten, and it has been hypothesized that binge behavior reflects a deficiency in serotonergic function. Bulimic anorectics had lower CSF levels of 5-HIAA than nonbulimic anorectics,[31] as did bulimic patients with high binge frequency, compared with other bulimics and controls. As for other addictions, bingeing may be an attempt by dysphoric bulimics to self-medicate—that is, to improve their mood by elevating their central nervous system (CNS) serotonin activity.[32] Patients with bulimia have reported relatively more negative moods before they binge.[33] The mechanism is as follows: During a binge, the preferential consumption of sweet, high-fat foods causes an insulin-mediated decrease in levels of large neutral amino acids in plasma. There amino acids compete with L-tryptophan for transport into the CNS, and thus the transport of L-tryptophan into the CNS is favored. This increased substrate availability results in increased 5-HT synthesis by the CNS.

ENDOGENOUS OPIOIDS

Biological models based on dysregulation of opiate reward systems have been proposed for anorexia and bulimia nervosa. Such a model has also been proposed for alcoholism and has resulted in the successful trials of naltrexone in alcoholism. In the autoaddiction opioid model, a potential anorectic develops a phobic fear of eating because of psychological maturation fears, which induces obsession dieting.[34] In biologically vulnerable individuals, the ensuing weight loss stimulates the release of endogenous opioids and the positive reward of the opioids then perpetuates the weight loss behavior despite its other negative consequences. The hyperphagic effect of opioids could be responsible for the food preoccupation exhibited by anorectics. Although opiates typically produce sedation, the vigorous exercising engaged in by many anorectics could be related to its ability to stimulate endorphin release. The ability of opiates to inhibit reproductive function through their luteinizing hormone, follicle-stimulating hormone, and gonadal hormone release suggests a possible mechanism for the prepubertal hormone patterns and amenorrhea sometimes observed even before weight loss below a critical body weight defined as healthy for that individual has occurred.[35] Sexual maturation and conflicts, rather than causing anorexia, may be secondary to opioid peptide dysfunction. The opioid model is supported by the presence of increased CSF opioid activity in severely underweight anorectics but not in those with maintained or restored body weight.[36] Also, the facilitation of perifornical lateral hypothalamic stimulation (a form of brain reward) that occurs with weight loss is blocked by naltrexone.[37, 38] Although case reports using naltrexone in the treatment of anorexia nervosa were promising, no successful controlled clinical trials have yet been conducted.

Evidence for involvement of endogenous opioids in bulimic behavior is suggested by successful clinical treatment with the opioid antagonist naltrexone.[39-43] A low dose of naltrexone was ineffective,[44] but in a double-blind placebo-controlled trial, naltrexone significantly decreased binge duration but not binge frequency.[44] Naltrexone was also shown to be effective, in conjunction with psychotherapy, in reducing bingeing behavior in a case study of binge eating disorder.[45] It is interesting to note that while on naltrexone, patients showed transient improvement in dysfunctional personality traits such as interpersonal distrust maturity fears and drive for thinness, suggesting that these traits are part of a behavioral cluster rather than a cause of the disease process. CSF beta-endorphin levels in bulimic patients have been found to be lower than in controls, but an effect for coexisting depression could not be precluded.[46]

Comorbidity

Several reports have described comorbidity of eating disorders and substance abuse,[47, 48] and the relationship was noted in the first current-day description of bulimia.[49] Eating disorders are common in families with addiction, and vice versa.[50] A review of 51 comorbidity studies conducted since 1977 found greater comorbidity with substance abuse among bulimics than anorectics and among bulimic anorectics than restrictor anorectics.[51] In a comorbidity study of 105 female inpatients with eating disorders, 37% met DSM-III-R criteria for either alcohol or drug dependence.[52] Restrictor anorectics were significantly less likely to be alcohol or drug dependent than the group as a whole. Substance abuse was more common in patients with comorbid personality disorders, and the most common among bulimics was borderline personality disorder. In a retrospective review of female psychiatric inpatient records from 1978 to 1990, the high incidence of alcohol abuse in the patients with eating disorders was accounted for by the subset of patients with borderline personality disorders.[53] A review of 12 studies found the prevalence of borderline personality disorder in bulimics to range from 25% to 48%.[54] Like substance abusers and patients with borderline personality disorders, bulimics also display mood lability and a tendency toward impulsive self-destructive behaviors such as stealing[55] and suicide attempts.[56] Obese bingers appear to be a subgroup of obese patients who are similar to normal-weight bulimics with increased frequency of depression and personal and family history of substance abuse. The comorbidity of bulimia with substance abuse and borderline personality disorder as well as their shared symptoms suggests a common, underlying serotonin dysregulation.[57] Alcoholics have been reported to have low 5-HIAA levels, as do nonhuman primates with notable alcohol preference. Anorexia nervosa and possibly bulimia nervosa are also highly comorbid with OCD.[58, 59] Selective serotonin reuptake inhibitors (SSRIs) and other serotonergic agents are currently being used to treat all of these disorders.

Family Studies

The apparent aggregation of anorexia nervosa and bulimia nervosa found in families would support a genetically acquired biological basis. Unfortunately, the twin studies to date have been deemed too small or subject to selection bias to allow valid conclusions to be drawn.[60]

Conclusion

If addictive disorders are defined by the presence of a pathological attachment to a substance, preoccupation with that substance, inability to modulate use of that substance, pathological attachment that results in consequences that are life threatening, loss of quality of life, relapse, and an overall change in priority given to activities, then eating and addictive disorders are quite similar. Both, however, have obsessional and compulsivity features that suggest the possibility that some patients may share features with OCD and others share features with alcoholism.

The overlap between addictive and eating disorders and OCDs underlines problems in the descriptive approach to psychiatric nosology. Naturally it is important to have diagnostic criteria that are operational. Uniformity in diagnostic classification has allowed pharmacological research studies to be conducted in various sites and settings with comparable results. Certainly, the high placebo response rate in OCD before the addition of distress thresholds speaks to the limitations of existing criteria. The success of fluoxetine (Prozac) in treating major depression, dysphoria, OCD, and bulimia suggests a critical need to redefine our nosology. Medications work at the level of pathophysiology and not according to a DSM committee. The idea of subdividing syndromes by agreeing to new operational criteria has had an important role in the past but has not allowed us to look at the disease or the disease process. Patients with eating disorders are prone to a number of other comorbid psychiatric and addictive disorders, but a disease could mimic multiple DSM-defined syndromes. The goal of SSRI development research was to develop medications that specifically and selectively inhibited the serotonin uptake pump without involving other systems. Although designed to retain antidepressant efficacy and reduce side effects, SSRIs have revitalized the treatment of eating disorders, alcoholism, dysphoria, and other DSM-defined groups.

In answer to the initial question about whether eating disorders should be classified as addictions, we would propose that both disorders involve similar brain systems and result in similar behaviors and feeling states. Both are important diseases in which loss of control and compulsive use are preeminent. Both involve acquired pathological attachment with the agent(s) of their ultimate compromise and possible destruction. Both involve patients' denial and reluctance to accept that they are in fact ill and in need of treatment. Both can be relapse triggers for each other. The similarities are numerous and striking, but as long as the diagnostic scheme is descriptive and not neurobiological, it will be difficult to identify which patients have one disorder and which have two. Food is a mood-altering substance that is repetitively and destructively used (or restricted) in eating disorders, and considerable experimental evidence shows biological vulnerability.

As our understanding of neurochemistry expands in the next century, the various dysfunctional personality traits that were thought to predispose a young female to acquire an eating disorder may be shown to be part of the phenotypical expression of the underlying chemical abnormality. The treatment implications in regarding eating disorders as addictions with a biochemical basis are that future treatments should be designed to address the underlying neurotransmitter abnormalities. In support of this, in a prospective naturalistic study of 98 bulimic patients, it was observed that sustained recovery in the first year was associated with receipt of pharmacotherapy within the first 13 weeks.[61] In earlier times, anorexia was believed to result from divine or supernatural intervention. Perhaps someday our own psychosocial theories about the etiology of the eating disorders will be seen as equally unenlightened.

REFERENCES

1. Gold MS: The Good News About Drugs and Alcohol. New York, Villard Books, 1991.
2. American Psychiatric Association: Diagnostic and Statistical Manual of Mental Disorders, 4th ed. Washington, DC, American Psychiatric Press, 1994.
3. Ratnasuriya RH, Eisler I, Szmukler GI, et al: Anorexia nervosa: Outcome and prognostic factors after 20 years. Br J Psychiatry 158:495–502, 1991.
4. Willi J, Giacometti G, Limacher B: Update on the epidemiology of anorexia nervosa in a defined region of Switzerland. Am J Psychiatry 147:1514–1517, 1990.
5. Fairburn CG, Beglin SJ: Studies of the epidemiology of bulimia nervosa. Am J Psychiatry 147:401–408, 1990.
6. Kaplan AS, Garfinkel PR: General Principles of Outpatient Treatment—Eating Disorders. In Gabbard GO (ed): Treatments of Psychiatric Disorders, vol 2. Washington, DC, American Psychiatric Press, 1995.
7. Treasure J, Campbell I: A biological hypothesis for anorexia nervosa (editorial). Psychol Med 24:3–8, 1994.
8. Parry-Jones WL, Parry-Jones B: Implications of historical evidence for the classification of eating disorders. Br J Psychiatry 165:287–292, 1994.
9. Pirke KM, Pahy S, Schweiger V, Warnoff M: Metabolic and endocrine indices of starvation in bulimia: A comparison with anorexia nervosa. Psychiatry Res 15:33–39, 1985.
10. Sullivan PF: Mortality in anorexia nervosa. Am J Psychiatry 152:1073–1074, 1995
11. Kaye WH, Weltzin T: Neurochemistry of bulimia nervosa. J Clin Psychiatry 52:21–28, 1991.
12. Vandereycken W: The addiction model in eating disorders: Some critical remarks and a selected bibliography. Int J Eating Dis 9:95–101, 1990.
13. Palmer R: Weight concern should not be a necessary criteria for the eating disorders: A polemic. Int J Eating Dis 14:459–465, 1993.
14. Halmi K: Images in psychiatry: Princess Margaret of Hungary. Am J Psychiatry 151:1242–1271, 1994.
15. Berridge KC, Valenstein ES: What psychological process mediated feeding evoked by electrical stimulation of the lateral hypothalmus? Behav Neurosci 105:3–15, 1991.
16. Robinson TE, Berridge KC: The neural basis of drug craving: An incentive-sensitization theory of addiction. Brain Res 18:247–291, 1993.
17. Wise RA: The anhedonia hypothesis: Mark III. Behav Brain Sci 8:178–186, 1985
18. Kuhar MJ, Ritz MC, Boja JW: The dopamine hypothesis of the reinforcing properties of cocaine. Trends Neurosci 14:299–302, 1991.
19. Wise RA, Bozarth MAA: A psychomotor stimulant theory of addiction. Pharmacol Rev 94:469–492, 1987.
20. Wise RA: Catecholamine theory of reward: A critical review. Brain Res 152:215–247, 1978.
21. Bradbury CW, Roth RH: Cocaine increases extracellular dopamine in rat nucleus accumbens and ventral tegmental area as shown by in vivo microdialysis. Neurosci Lett 103:97–102, 1989.
22. Kalivas PW, Duffy P: Effect of acute and daily cocaine treatment on extracellular dopamine in the nucleus accumbens. Synapse 5:48–58, 1990.
23. Robinson TE, Berridge KC: The neural basis of drug craving: An incentive-sensitization theory of addiction. Brain Res Rev 18:247–291, 1993.
24. Schultz W: Activity of dopamine neurons in the behaving primate. Soc Neurosci 4:129–138, 1992.
25. Kaye WH, Ebert MH, Gwirtsman HE, et al: Differences in brain serotonergic metabolism between nonbulemic and bulemic patients with anorexia nervosa. Am J Psychiatry 141:1598–1601, 1984.
26. Leiter LA, Huboticky N, Anderson GH: Effects of L-trytophan on food intake and selection in lean men and women. Ann N Y Acad Sci 499:327–328, 1987.
27. Hill AJ, Blundell JE: Food selection, body weight and the premenstrual syndrome. (PMS effect of D-fenfluramine.) Int J Obesity 15:215, 1991.
28. Carter A, Davis ST: Biologenic animes, reproductive hormones and female sexual behavior. Behav Res 1:213–225, 1977.
29. Lalan P, Rosegren E, Lindvall O, Bjorklund A: Hippo-

campal noradrenaline and serotonin release over 24 hours as measured by the dialysis techniques in freely moving rats: Correlation to behavioral activity state, effect of handling and tail pinch. Eur J Neurosci 1:181–188, 1989.

30. Dunn AJ, Welsh J: Stress and endotoxin-induced increases in brain tryptophan and serotonin metabolism depend on sympathetic nervous system activation. J Neurochem 57:1615–1622, 1991.
31. Kaye WH, Ebert MH, Gwirtsman HE, et al: Differences in brain serotonergic metabolism between nonbulemic and bulemic patients with anorexia nervosa. Am J Psychiatry 141:1598–1601, 1984.
32. Weltzin TE, Fernstrom MH, Kaye WH: Serotonin and bulimia nervosa. Nutr Rev 52:399–408, 1994.
33. Davis R, Freeman RJ, Garner DM: A naturalistic investigation of eating behaviors in bulimia nervosa. J Consult Clin Psychol 2:273–279, 1988.
34. Marazzi MA, Luby ED: Anorexia nervosa as an autoaddiction. Ann N Y Acad Sci 575:545–547, 1989.
35. Marrazzi MA, Luby ED: An auto-addiction model of chronic anorexia nervosa. Int J Eating Dis 5:191–208, 1986.
36. Kaye WH, Pickar DM, Naber D, Ebert MH: Cerebrospinal fluid opioid activity in anorexia nervosa. Am J Psychiatry 139:643–645.
37. Carr KD, Wolinsky TD: Chronic food restriction and weight loss produce opioid facilitation of periforniical hypothalamic self-stimulation. Brain Res 607:141–148, 1993.
38. Carr KD, Papadouka V: The role of multiple opioid receptors in the potentiation of reward by food restriction. Brain Res 639:253–260, 1994.
39. Jonas JM, Gold MS: Opiate antagonists a clinical probes in bulimia. In Hudson JL, Pope HF Jr (eds): The Psychobiology of Bulimia. Washington, DC, American Psychiatric Association Press, 1987, pp 115, 127.
40. Jonas JM, Gold MS: Naltrexone reverses bulimic symptoms. Lancet 1(8444):390, 1986.
41. Jonas JM, Gold MS: Naltrexone treatment of bulimia: Clinical and theoretical findings linking eating disorders and substance abuse. Adv Alcohol Subst Abuse 7(1):29, 37, 1988.
42. Jonas JM, Gold MS: The use of opiate antagonists in treating bulimia: A study of low dose versus high dose naltrexone. Psychiatry Res 24:195, 199, 1988.
43. Gold MS: Are eating disorders addictions? Adv Biosci 90:455–463, 1993.
44. Alger SA, Schwalberg MD, Bigaouette JM, et al: Effect of trycyclic antidepressant and opiate antagonist on binge eating subjects. Am J Clin Nutr 53:865–871, 1991.

45. Marazzi MA, Markham KN, Kinzie J, Luby E: Binge eating disorder response to naltrexone. Int J Obesity 19:143–145, 1995.
46. Brewerton TD, Lydiard RB, Laraia MT, et al: CSF beta-endorphin and dynorphin in bulimia nervosa. Am J Psychiatry 149:1086–1090, 1992.
47. Gold MS: Cocaine. New York, Plenum, 1993.
48. Jonas JM, Gold MS: Cocaine abuse and eating disorders. Lancet 1(8477):390, 1986.
49. Russell G: Bulimia nervosa: Ominous variant of anorexia nervosa. Psychol Med 9:429–448, 1979.
50. Halmi K, Eckert E, Marchi P, et al: Comorbidity of psychiatric diagnoses in anorexia nervosa. Arch Gen Psychiatry 48:712–718, 1991.
51. Holderness CC, Brooks-Gunn J, Warren MP: Co-morbidity of eating disorders and substance abuse. Review of the literature. Int J Eating Dis 16:1–34, 1994.
52. Braun DL, Sunday SR, Halmi KA: Psychiatric comorbidity in patients with eating disorders. Psychol Med 24:859–867, 1994.
53. Koepp W, Schildbach S, Schmager C, Rohner R: Borderline diagnosis and substance abuse in female patients with eating disorders. Int J Eating Dis 14:107–110, 1993.
54. Rossiter EM, Agras WS, Telch CF, Schneider JA: Cluster B personality characteristics predict outcome in the treatment of bulimia nervosa. Int J Eating Dis 13:349–357, 1993.
55. Pyle RL, Mitchell JE, Eckert ED, et al: Maintenance treatment and 6-month outcome for bulimic patients who respond to initial treatment. Am J Psychiatry 9:291–293, 1990.
56. Hatsukami D, Eckert E, Mitchell JR, Pyle R: Affective disorder and substance abuse in women with bulimia. Psychol Med 14:701–704, 1984.
57. Apter A, van Praag M, Plutchik R, et al: Interrelationships among anxiety, aggression, impulsivity, and mood: A serotonergically linked cluster? Psychiatry Res 32:191–199, 1990.
58. Pigott TA, L'Heureax F, et al: Obsessive compulsive disorder: comorbid conditions. J Clin Psychiatry 55:15–27, 1994.
59. Rubenstein C, Pigott TA, Altemeis MA, et al: High rates of co-morbid OCD in patients with bulemia nervosa. Eating Disorders 1(2):147–155, 1994.
60. Strober M: Family-genetic studies of eating disorders. J Clinical Psychiatry 52:9–12, 1991.
61. Herzog DB, Sacks NR: Bulimia nervosa: Comparison of treatment responders vs. non-responders. Psychopharmacol Bull 29:121–125, 1993.

Addictive Sexual Disorders

Richard R. Irons, MD •
Jennifer P. Schneider, MD, PhD

Indulgence in the gratification of sexual desires and appetites to excess has been a major subject in literature, myths, and the creative arts from the beginning of recorded history. One example of the hypersexual predatory male is Don Juan, the legendary lover of many women, who suffered a multitude of adverse consequences, including death, as a result of his behavior. He is immortalized as the sexual athlete who worshipped the female body as the ideal object of desire, created for him to be consumed and ravished, and who had to make his escape from each one before potential engulfment by intimacy in a relationship. His story was immortalized in the plays of Corneille, Molière, Shaw, and Rostand, in Byron's unfinished poem, and in Mozart's *Don Giovanni*. He has become an infamous symbol for a hedonistic, narcissistic male who engages in recurrent sexual affairs. Women with culturally defined excessive sexual appetite were given the diagnosis of nymphomania, a term no longer in clinical use.

We have evolved into a society obsessed with the pursuit of pleasure and materialism—and for some, sexual materialism. In our sensually driven society, sexual excesses and deviances are regularly reported by the media and served up as entertainment in books, movies, and television. Corporations have learned through advertising campaigns that sex sells. The majority of adolescents, adult men, and women in our society can engage in fantasy and seductive behavior without significant consequences to their personal or professional life. However, for some, it is not possible to limit the intensity of their desire or expression of sexual behavior. For them, sexual excesses can become addictive in nature and represent a serious mental disorder.

A distinction must be made between a situational and a pervasive use of sex. Two surveys[1, 2] confirm that unmarried persons have more sexual partners than married people. For most, sexual variety is situational. Others, dealing with a life crisis such as the breakup of a relationship, may find themselves using sex compulsively for a brief period. For those with addictive sexual disorders, on the other hand, sex is the pervasive organizing principle of their lives.

Current Nosology According to the Diagnostic and Statistical Manual of Mental Disorders

The DSM-IV[3] classification of sexual disorders includes sexual dysfunctions and paraphilias. The sexual dysfunctions are characterized by disturbance in sexual desire and in the psychophysiological changes that constitute the sexual response cycle and cause marked distress and interpersonal difficulty. The sexual dysfunctions include sexual desire disorders, sexual arousal disorders, orgasmic disorders, sexual pain disorders, sexual dysfunction due to a general medical condition, substance-induced sexual dysfunction, and sexual dysfunction not otherwise specified (NOS).

The paraphilias are characterized by recurrent intense sexual urges, fantasies, or behaviors that involve unusual objects, activities, or situations and cause clinically significant distress or impairment in social, occupational, or other important areas of functioning. The paraphilias include exhibitionism, fetishism, frotteurism, pedophilia, sexual masochism, sexual sadism, transvestic fetishism, voyeurism, and paraphilia NOS.

Gender identity disorders are characterized by strong and persistent cross-gender identification accompanied by persistent discomfort with one's assigned sex.

Sexual disorder NOS is included for coding disorders of sexual functioning that are not classifiable in any of the specific categories. It is important to note that notions of deviance, standards of sexual performance, and concepts of appropriate gender role can vary from culture to culture.[3]

The essential feature of impulse control disorders is the failure to resist an impulse, drive, or temptation to perform an act that is harmful to oneself or to others. For most of the disorders in this section, the individual feels an increasing sense of tension or arousal before committing the act and then experiences pleasure, gratification, or relief at the time of committing the act. After the act, the person may or may not feel regret, self-reproach, or guilt.[3]

The types of sexual improprieties and excesses that are considered addictive sexual disorders can usually be classified into one of three major categories: paraphilia, impulse control disorder NOS, or sexual disorder NOS. When the behavior does not fit easily into one of these categories and is not considered a manifestation of some other DSM-IV axis I diagnosis, then it is reasonable to use the work-related problem (V 62.2) or relationship problem (V 6.) descriptors. Frequent and infrequent DSM axis I diagnoses associated with sexual excesses are presented in Table 48–1. It is helpful to complete the differential diagnosis on axis I before considering axis II and axis III. Sexual disorders, impulse control disorders, and paraphilias, when identified, should be described as precisely as possible. If the NOS category is used, it is important to apply appropriate descriptors that define the features observed. In our experience, the most frequent

Table 48–1. AXIS I DIFFERENTIAL DIAGNOSIS OF EXCESSIVE SEXUAL BEHAVIORS

Common	Infrequent
Paraphilias	Substance-induced anxiety disorder (obsessive-compulsive symptoms)
Sexual disorder NOS	
Impulse control disorder NOS	
	Substance-induced mood disorder (manic features)
Bipolar affective disorder (type I or II)	
	Dissociative disorder
Cyclothymic disorder	Delusional disorder (erotomania)
Posttraumatic stress disorder	Obsessive-compulsive disorder
Adjustment disorder [disturbance of conduct]	Gender identity disorder
	Delirium, dementia, or other cognitive disorder

NOS, not otherwise specified.

features noted in addition to specific paraphilic behaviors are those of addiction, exploitation, predation, romance, coercion, professional misconduct, sexual offense, and sexual assault. The severity of the disorder, the duration, the current level of activity, and amenability to treatment should also be presented. In the differential diagnosis of sexual improprieties and excesses, axis II characterological disorders and traits are often contributory or may be considered the primary cause of paraphilic sexual behavior.

A discussion of these disorders is included in this text on addiction psychiatry because they often have distinct parallels with other addictive disorders, commonly coexist with substance-related disorders, may themselves have features associated with addiction, and may respond to an addiction model of treatment and therapy. Unrecognized and untreated symptoms of these sexual disorders currently are frequently being recognized as significant factors leading to return to substance use in substance-related disorders. Compulsive sexual behavior has significantly contributed to the growth of the current epidemic of acquired immunodeficiency syndrome.

Evolution of the Addiction Model

Bill Wilson, in his classic Big Book,[4] describes an alcoholic's difficulties with sexual behavior:

"Now about sex. Many of us needed an overhauling there. But above all, we tried to be sensible on this question. It's so easy to get way off the track. Here we find human opinions running to extremes—absurd extremes perhaps.... We do not want to be the arbiter of anyone's sex conduct. We all have sex problems. We'd hardly be human if we didn't. What can we do about them?

We reviewed our conduct over years past. ... We got this all down on paper and looked at it. In this way we tried to shape a sane and sound ideal for our future sex life. We subjected each relation to this test—was it selfish or not? We asked God to mould our ideals and help us to live up to them....Whatever our ideal turns out to be, we must be willing to grow toward it.... Suppose we fall short of our ideal and stumble? Does this mean we are going to get drunk? It depends on us and on our motives.... If we are not sorry, and our conduct continues to harm others, we are quite sure to drink. We are not theorizing. These are facts out of our experience.

To sum up about sex: We earnestly pray for the right ideal, for guidance in each questionable situation, for sanity, and for the strength to do the right thing. If sex is troublesome, we throw ourselves the harder into helping others. We think of their needs and work for them. This takes us out of ourselves. It quiets the imperious urge, when to yield would mean heartache.''

Clearly, even in the early development of Alcoholics Anonymous (AA), it was difficult for many to work the 12-step program of AA without coming to terms with their sexual behavior and applying the principles of the program to this as well as to their drinking.

In proposing an addiction framework, Orford[5] reviewed some examples of excessive sexual behavior and concluded that "a theory of dependence must take into account forms of excessive appetitive behavior which do not have psychoactive drugs as their object." His analogy, in a 1985 book,[6] is still relevant today:

"Debate over definitions in this area is intriguingly reminiscent of debates on the same subject when drug-taking, drinking, or gambling are under discussion. In none of these areas is there agreement about the precise points on the continuum at which normal behavior, heavy use, problem behavior, excessive behavior, 'mania' or 'ism' are to be distinguished from one another. When reading of the supposed characteristics of the 'real nymphomaniac,' one is haunted by memories of attempts to define the 'real alcoholic' or the 'real compulsive gambler.'"

Carnes[7] posited that out-of-control sexual behaviors represent an addiction and defined sexual addiction as a "pathological relationship with a mood-altering behavior." The emphasis on the *behavior* or the *experience* as causa-

tion rather than on a particular chemical was earlier supported by Peele, who in a popular book[8] described addiction as having as much to do with love as with drugs. After critically reviewing research on addiction, he concluded,[9] "Drug addiction is based on the experience a drug gives a person and the place this experience has in the person's life. Anything that produces a comparable experience can likewise be addictive." Ironically, Peele has become an outspoken critic of the epidemic of addiction in America. Persons who are dually addicted to drugs and to sexual experiences describe a euphoria during their sexual acting out similar to that experienced when using mood-altering chemicals.

Quadland[10] characterized the disorder as sexual compulsivity, whereas Barth and Kinder[11] suggested the term *sexual impulsivity* and reserved the term *addiction* only for substance dependence. Schwartz,[12] noting the high frequency of sexual victimization of children who later become sexually compulsive, views sexual compulsivity as an aspect of posttraumatic stress disorder. According to Coleman,[13, 14] sexual excesses represent a variant of obsessive-compulsive disorder (OCD). Countering this view, Shaffer[15] identifies psychodynamic distinctions between addiction and OCD:

"The loss of insight among addicts and the maintenance of discrimination among OCD sufferers distinguishes these populations. While the excessive behavior patterns of OCD are disconnected from the dysphoric affect that energizes their activity, addictive behavior remains attached to these noxious emotions. Consequently, addicts *escape* their discomfort by acting out through excess behavior patterns, while OCD patients *avoid* the conscious experience of psychic pain through repetitive intemperate activity."

Renshaw[16] presented a primarily negative critique of the concept of sexual addiction, and Levine and Troiden[17] believed that sexual compulsivity was altogether a myth. DSM-III-R[18] identified sexual addiction under the psychosexual disorders, NOS descriptor, but this reference was dropped in DSM-IV, a reflection of the continuing controversy about the addiction model. In addiction medicine, the existence of sexual addiction (and of all so-called process addictions) remains theoretical[19] and continues to be questioned by many. Further research is required to establish this entity as an accepted disease.

Although sexual addiction is not classified in DSM-IVr as a mental disorder, a diagnostic

Table 48–2. DIAGNOSTIC CRITERIA FOR SUBSTANCE DEPENDENCE

A maladaptive pattern of substance use, leading to clinically significant impairment or distress, as manifested by three (or more) of the following, occurring at any time in the same 12-month period:

(1) Tolerance, as defined by either of the following:
  a. A need for markedly increased amounts of the substance to achieve intoxication or desired effect
  b. Markedly diminished effect with continued use of the same amount of the substance
(2) Withdrawal, as manifested by either of the following:
  a. The characteristic withdrawal syndrome for the substance
  b. The same (or a closely related) substance is taken to relieve or avoid withdrawal symptoms
(3) The substance is often taken in larger amounts or over a longer period than was intended.
(4) There is a persistent desire or unsuccessful efforts to cut down or control substance use.
(5) A great deal of time is spent in activities necessary to obtain the substance, use the substance, or recover from its effects.
(6) Important social, occupational, or recreational activities are given up or reduced because of substance use.
(7) The substance use is continued despite knowledge of having a persistent or recurrent physical or psychological problem that is likely to have been caused or exacerbated by the substance.

From the American Psychiatric Association: Diagnostic and Statistical Manual of Mental Disorders, 4th ed. Washington, DC, American Psychiatric Association, 1994, p 181.

framework for the use of the term can be extrapolated from the DSM-IV diagnostic criteria for substance dependence. These criteria are listed in Table 48–2. According to the manual, three of seven criteria must be met for a diagnosis of substance dependence. If the term *sexual fantasy, desire,* or *behavior* is substituted for *substance use,* these diagnostic criteria can be used to define what we are considering addictive features of sexual disorders.

Goodman[20, 21] proposed a set of diagnostic criteria for addictive disorders that could be applied to either behavior or substance use (Table 48–3). By his definition of addiction, any behavior that is used to produce gratification and to escape internal discomfort can be engaged in compulsively and can constitute an addictive disorder. The similarities between his proposed criteria and DSM-IV are self-evident. Both define the essential elements of addiction as loss of control, continuation despite adverse consequences, and obsession.

Multiple Addictions, Switching Addictions

Sexual fantasy or behavior and substance use are often combined through the repetition of ritualized behavior. When one wishes to engage in sexual activity, mood-altering substances can be used ritualistically to (1) reenact scenarios from movies, books, fantasy, or past experience; (2) create mood and intensify sexual pleasure; (3) decrease inhibitions and fears; (4) treat sexual dysfunction or performance anxiety; (5) permit the expression of sexual aggression or paraphilia; or (6) provide a later rationalization or excuse for shameful or objectionable behavior. Mood-altering substances can be used ritualistically alone or with a potential sexual partner to (1) reenact scenarios from movies, books, or past experience; (2) increase the partner's vulnerability; (3) decrease inhibitions; (4) attempt to overcome a

Table 48–3. CRITERIA FOR ADDICTIVE DISORDER

Recurrent failure to resist impulses to engage in a specified behavior
Increasing sense of tension immediately before initiating the behavior
Pleasure or relief at the time of engaging in the behavior
At least five of the following:
  1. Frequent preoccupation with the behavior or with activity that is preparatory to the behavior
  2. Frequent engaging in the behavior to a greater extent or for a longer period than intended
  3. Repeated efforts to reduce, control, or stop the behavior
  4. A great deal of time spent in activities necessary for the behavior, engaging in the behavior, or recovering from its effects
  5. Frequent engaging in the behavior when expected to fulfill occupational, academic, domestic, or social obligations
  6. Important social, occupational, or recreational activities given up or reduced because of the behavior
  7. Continuation of the behavior despite knowledge of having a persistent or recurrent social, financial, psychological, or physical problem that is caused or exacerbated by the behavior
  8. Tolerance: need to increase the intensity or frequency of the behavior in order to achieve the desired effect, or diminished effect with continued behavior of the same intensity
  9. Restlessness or irritability if unable to engage in the behavior
Some symptoms of the disturbance have persisted for at least 1 month or have occurred repeatedly for a longer period.

From Goodman A: Diagnosis and treatment of sex addiction. J Sex Marital Ther, 19(3):225–242, 1993.

partner's resistance, objections, or sexual dysfunction; (5) manipulate and control events; (6) promote emotional numbness; (7) distort reality and memory; or (8) provide compensation for sexual services.

When a person develops a pathological relationship with mood-altering substances and behaviors, he or she typically goes through multiple cycles of "acting in" and "acting out," moving from satisfying cravings in excess to abstinence or avoidance. When acting out, boundaries collapse, one is physically present but emotionally absent, anger is expressed either actively or passively, and life becomes chaotic. When one moves to the opposite extreme and acts in, boundaries become rigid, one becomes physically or emotionally isolated from others, experiences fear and anxiety, and finds life dull and empty. One then moves from acting in to acting out, from being in control to being out of control. Increasingly polarized extremes intensify pain and suffering. Among sexual disorders, acting in can present as a sexual desire disorder, sexual arousal disorder, or orgasmic disorder; acting out is expressed through paraphilic and non-paraphilic sexual behavior.

Addictive disorders tend to coexist. Nicotine dependence, for example, is highly correlated with alcohol dependence. The same is true of sex addiction and chemical dependence. In an anonymous survey of 75 recovering sex addicts,[22] 39% were also recovering from chemical dependence, 32% had an eating disorder, 13% characterized themselves as compulsive spenders, and 5% were compulsive gamblers. Only 17% believed they had no other addiction. Similar percentages have been reported by Carnes.[23] In another study,[24] 70% of cocaine addicts entering an outpatient treatment program were found also to be engaging in compulsive sex.

In Irons and Schneider's population of health professionals assessed for sexual impropriety,[25] those with addictive sexual disorders were almost twice as likely to have concurrent chemical dependence (38% prevalence) than were those who were not sexually addicted (21%). Thus, the presence of sexual compulsivity was a comorbid marker for chemical dependence.

Addictive sexual disorders are frequently found during assessment for chemical dependence. For example, during a 4-year period in one treatment facility, approximately 33% of the chemically dependent patients were also found to be sexually compulsive, as were approximately 25% of the chemically dependent physician patients.[26] Many of the patients at this facility had been previously treated for drug dependence, but the dually addicted patients had more relapses before the present admission. In the presence of concurrent drug and sexual dependence, relapse or failure to treat one of the addictions is likely to lead to relapse in the other. This conclusion is supported by the earlier finding by Washton[24] that many of his cocaine-dependent patients had become trapped in a reciprocal relapse pattern, in which compulsive sexual behavior precipitated relapse to cocaine use and vice versa.

A related phenomenon in early recovery is the tendency to switch addictions or to intensify a concurrent addiction. A well-known example is the increased use of cigarettes, caffeine, and sugar by new AA members. "Thirteenth stepping," the seeking of sexual partners at 12-step meetings, may in some cases represent a flight into addictive sexual activity. Substituting one addiction for another may temporarily help an addict refrain from drinking, but this approach is unlikely to lead to sustained sobriety.

Milkman and Sunderwirth, in their book *Craving for Ecstasy,*[27] described three basic types of neurobiochemical responses we may experience when we pursue any given desire to gratification—arousal, satiation, or an increase in fantasy or preoccupation with the object. Mood-altering behaviors can create the same central nervous system responses as mood-altering substances. In the pursuit of satisfaction, one may often combine behaviors with the use of drugs. We are just beginning to understand brain neurobiochemistry. We currently associate arousal with the neurotransmitters norepinephrine and dopamine, satiation with gamma-aminobutyric acid and endorphins, and fantasy with serotonin. It is important to observe that sex can easily fit into any or all of the foregoing categories, making it an extremely powerful mood-altering activity. Some individuals may have a propensity for behavior that provides a sense of excitement, such as gambling, using stimulants, or participating in high-risk stunts. Others may prefer sedation through self-medication with alcohol or satiation through sexually exploitive relations or compulsive overeating. Still others escape via fantasy, use of psychedelic drugs, preoccupation with work, or compulsive religious practice pursued to excess. When kept in balance, these activities may provide comfort and status, assuaging the sense of unworthiness. When carried to extremes, however, they often represent a personal variation on the theme of addiction.

Disease Expression and Progression

Carnes[28] described the progression of untreated sexual addiction. The *initiation phase* is characterized by an exceptionally intense impact of observed or experienced sexual activities during development as an adolescent and young adult. At some point, sex becomes the drug of choice, used to escape or cope. Catalytic environments and catalytic experiences lead to the *establishment phase*, in which there is repetition of an addictive cycle of preoccupation, ritualization, sexual acting out, then despair, shame, and guilt, which are alleviated by renewed preoccupation. With time, the addiction may *escalate*, with greater intensity, more frequency, more risk, and greater loss of control. The behavior may intermittently *deescalate*, at times through the means of substituting another addictive behavior (such as a period of heavy drug use), or it may progress to the *acute phase*, when the individual becomes alienated from significant others and is constantly preoccupied with the addiction cycle. In some, the addiction becomes immutable and behavior is limited only by opportunity, physical consequences, or incarceration.

Physical Manifestations

Sexual addicts may present with various physical health problems such as genital injury as a direct result of sexual activity; sexually transmitted diseases (STDs) including hepatitis, human immunodeficiency virus (HIV) infection, herpes simplex, gonorrhea, syphilis, and *Chlamydia*; physical injuries associated with engagement in high-risk sexual behaviors or sadomasochistic activity; unnecessary operations (such as breast implants, hair transplants, plastic surgery, liposuction) used to enhance sexual appeal; binge-purge cycles in an attempt to regulate weight; abuse of agents reputed to be sexual performance enhancers ("poppers," other inhalants, yohimbine, papaverine); and unwanted pregnancies or the complications of abortions. Associated secondary (reactive) mental disorders include depressive disorders, posttraumatic stress, dissociative disorders, and anxiety disorders. Self-destructive and self-defeating behavior is not unusual, including suicidal ideation or suicide attempts.

The use of alcohol and other drugs in conjunction with sexual activity is associated with an increased risk of HIV infection, even when drugs are not injected. Among heterosexuals entering alcohol treatment in San Francisco, unsafe sexual practices were common: 54% had multiple sexual partners in the previous year and 97% of nonmonogamous respondents did not use condoms during all sexual encounters.[29] In a review of 16 epidemiological studies relating crack cocaine use, sexual behavior, and STDs[30] 15 of the studies reported a connection, often related to an exchange of drugs for sex and lack of self-care while high on the drug. An additional reason, not mentioned in this review, was the likelihood that the sexual behavior was compulsive in many of the cocaine users. Given the high concordance between cocaine addiction and sex addiction,[24] it is clear that both addictions must be addressed in order to decrease a cocaine addict's risk of HIV disease.

Compulsive sexual behavior, even in the absence of drug use, is often unsafe. Addicts report that once they find themselves in the ritual phase of the addictive cycle, they are on automatic pilot and do not even think about safe versus unsafe sex. It is only after the sexual contact is completed that remorse, guilt, and fear of infection set in.

Disease Expression in the Family

Addictive sexual disorders, like substance addictions, affect an entire family directly or indirectly. Substance addiction correlates directly with an increase in domestic violence and family conflict and in accidents around the home and in automobiles. Families in which a member has a sex addiction but not chemical dependence tend to appear less chaotic and fragmented early in the course of the disease. However, as the stress and consequences of addiction accumulate, family members of both types of addicts often react with common behaviors.

A number of self-help books describe how various family members may respond to addiction—for example, the phenomenon of codependence and the "adult child" from an alcoholic family. These stereotypes represent the adaptation of an individual's personality to the experience of living with addiction. The evolution of compulsive and maladaptive behaviors in family members is recognized less often. Profound shame, unconscious denial, and minimization of the consequences, for example, may lead the spouse to try to bolster self-esteem through excessive involvement in vocational, religious, or parenting activities or through episodes of compulsive shopping or eating.

Addiction and coaddiction often have their roots in a dysfunctional family system in which the child is either abused or neglected. In Carnes' survey[23] of recovering sexual addicts, 83% reported they had been sexually abused as children. For such children, a confusion of sex with nurturing becomes a lifelong problem. When the survey respondents were asked to categorize their family of origin along the two axes of Olson and colleagues' circumplex model of marital and family systems,[31] a clear majority (68%) fell into just one of the 16 cells, the rigid disengaged family. The rigidly religious family is a prototype and had inflexible rules and insufficient nurturing. Sex addicts' families of origin typically have a multigenerational history of addictions, with various combinations of addictions to chemicals, sex, food, work, and gambling.

Partners of sex addicts most commonly come from a family background remarkably similar to that of sex addicts[23, 32]—a dysfunctional family often riddled with addiction problems, where their emotional needs as children were not met. Many were sexually abused and grew up believing that sex is the most important sign of love or that love must be earned with sex; alternatively, they may fear sex and have disorders of sexual desire, arousal, or orgasm. They have a great need for approval from others and have difficulty setting appropriate boundaries. They often have a history of relationships with addicts or other emotionally unavailable people. Choosing a sex addict for a relationship is generally no accident.[32] An example of a couple whose dysfunctions complement each other is an addict who prefers prostitutes to marital sex, and his wife, who was sexually abused in childhood, has no interest in sex and is grateful for her husband's lack of sexual interest in her. This wife represents the other extreme from disorders of sexual excess and struggles with a sexual disorder that inhibits desire or sexual function.

The sexual coaddict (partner of an addict) is often intensely fearful of abandonment and is overinvested in the relationship. Coaddicts may be aware of serious family problems but often believe that they are responsible for the problems and that if they try hard enough they can solve them. With the addict's top priority being the addiction and the coaddict focusing on the addict, the children may receive inadequate or inconsistent nurturing.

One child may become the family hero and eventually a compulsive worker who speculates on commodities and periodically flies off to Las Vegas—with disastrous financial consequences. Another child may develop an eating disorder, and a third may indulge in a series of devastating sexual affairs. Of course, all the children vow that "it will never happen to me," and family shame and consternation are reinforced when yet another family member succumbs to addictive disease.

When addiction is evident, developing appreciation of how these patterns are expressed within the family may promote better self-understanding for all. Addiction treatment, family therapy, and the experience, strength, and hope found in 12-step programs often provide comfort and needed support for addicts and their families. As people at risk for addiction come to understand the creative and destructive forces that have shaped their family, they may gain greater freedom to make conscious, informed choices that promote personal and family health.

Dynamic Formulation

Stoller[33] described how a personal, specific vulnerability may develop during male separation and individuation. Disruptions or failures in integration result in a psychological wounding, unique to the individual. Once this wound is formed, it has an autonomous existence that may be expressed years later as personal insensitivity toward others, ambivalence in complex, demanding relationships, or misogyny.

We experience certain critical events, which Maslow called *peak experiences,* that have a profound effect on us for the rest of our lives. Some of these are not peaks, however; they are canyons. Each of us can recall them, and each brings up specific emotions and images. Some of them may be sexual and may have profound effects on our future sexuality and intimacy, such as the time when, as children, we explored and compared anatomy with an age mate; the first time we masturbated; the first time we looked at pornography; our first sexual feelings; our first experience of love; the pleasure of touching another's genitalia; the time we were uncomfortable with the embrace of our mother or father; the night when we were unable to perform sexually; the sexual partner we used and then discarded; and the person who used or rejected us. Some of these experiences are suffused with shame and guilt. Others we recall with warmth, joy, and perhaps a wish to return to that moment once again. Hudson and Jacot[34] believe that such experiences are a central feature in mental architecture and exert a formative influence on imaginative needs. Some may be carried forward in life as wounds that remain with us as an inner source of unresolved tension, expressed in characteristic biases or patterns, unique to the individual. Such wounds are evidenced by a loose-knit group of telltale signs. Needs and desires related to these wounds tend to reassert themselves over time, although their influence can be temporarily overridden. They have protean forms of expression, both creative and destructive.

Years later, wounds may be reopened, perhaps derepressed when our interaction with another creates associations with images or feelings we experienced long ago. We may not recall the wound directly, but unresolved feelings from the past affect our current emotions and actions. We are often experiencing the effects of a wound when we feel paradoxical feelings toward our sexual partner. On one hand, we might revere and adore the partner, and on the other, fear the power he or she has over us. We may find ourselves in a conflict about what we believe is healthy sexuality and that which is unhealthy and potentially addictive. When our sexual interactions with another leave us with a Jekyll-and-Hyde feeling about ourselves and sex brings a sense of unreality, isolation, and grief, further exploration of the old wound is avoided or thoughts and emotions are repressed.

Young boys who are sexually abused often find the experience confusing. Films such as *The Summer of '42*, in which a teenage boy is seduced by an attractive, newly widowed woman, promote the view that such a boy "got lucky." Yet the boy may find the experience frightening. He may respond by developing chronic anger at women and may detach emotionally from sexual experiences, considering them nothing more than another "score." He may find himself making a clear distinction between the idealized "good" woman and the deprecated "bad" woman, developing a "madonna-whore complex," which may make it difficult for him in later years to enjoy a sexual relationship with a woman he loves.

Emotional abuse in childhood was experienced by 97% of sex addicts in a large survey.[23] In many homes, the abuse took the form of criticism and humiliation by a parent, of never being able to measure up. A boy who grows up feeling inadequate may seek to compensate by having many female partners. The goal of his behavior is not to have many orgasms but rather to receive validation of his sexual attractiveness from many women.

These early injuries may be sexual, but they are by no means invariably so. Whatever their source, these wounds need to be honored and nurtured; some have to be recalled and brought to consciousness so that we can better understand ourselves and others. To develop insight into the nature of addictive sexual disorders, appreciation of these wounds is crucial. As portrayed in the Arthurian legend of the Fisher King and effectively interpreted dynamically by Johnson,[35]

> "As in the story of the Fisher King coming upon the roasting salmon, a boy in his early adolescence touches something [of spiritual/sexual nature] too soon. He is unexpectedly wounded by it and drops it immediately as being too hot. His first contact with what will be redemption for him in later life is a wounding. This is what turns him into a wounded Fisher King. The first touch of consciousness in a youth appears as a wound or suffering. Most western men are Fisher Kings. Every boy has naively blundered into something that was too big for him. He proceeds halfway through his masculine development and then drops it as being too hot. Often a certain bitterness arises, because like the King, he can neither live with the new consciousness he has touched or entirely drop it. Every adolescent receives his Fisher King wound. He would never proceed into consciousness if it were not so."

The roots of sexual addiction often lie in the absence of adequate parenting, coupled with sexual abuse or a sexualized atmosphere in the home. Each young child must developmentally evolve through a narcissistic stage. When a child is sexually, physically, or emotionally abused or, by contrast, when abandoned or neglected, the child may become convinced that his or her misbehavior or inherent "badness" must be the cause of the adult actions; the alternative, that one's caregivers are unloving or unreliable, is intolerable to the child. Low self-esteem and shame are predictable consequences.

Sexual abuse affects sexuality in three areas[36]: (1) Sexual emergence in early adulthood—Survivors seem either to become socially and sexually withdrawn or to plunge into a phase of hypersexual and sometimes self-destructive sexual activity. In adulthood, they may continue this behavior, developing a full-blown sex addiction. Males may view their female partners merely as objects to be used and discarded; females may use sex to gain power over men. (2) Sexual orientation and influence—Males who have been abused by other males tend as adults to relate homosexually more often than do nonabused males.[36] In adulthood, some men may compulsively reenact the abuse with other males, even if they believe themselves to be primarily heterosexual.[37] Others may need to repeatedly prove their masculinity at the expense of a large number of female partners. (3) Sexual arousal, response, and satisfaction—Survivors of sexual abuse frequently lack sexual desire. Women in particular may develop sexual dysfunctions and may avoid sex throughout their adulthood. Some may remain celibate, marry a man who has low sexual desire or finds other sexual outlets, or turn to female partners. Some find they are comfortable sexually only when intoxicated; a majority of female alcoholics were sexually abused in childhood.

Victims of childhood abuse may themselves become victimizers. An important aspect of treatment of sexually addicted sex offenders involves resolution of their childhood trauma experience.[12, 38, 39]

Patterns of Sexual Addiction, Sexual Offense, and Sexual Exploitation

Based on a survey of nearly 1000 patients (81% male, 19% female) admitted for treatment of addictive sexual disorders, Carnes[23] found that out of 104 behavioral items, 10 behavior types emerged; each type had a specific sexual focus with common characteristics. The ten patterns and examples of each are listed in Table 48–4.

Carnes and colleagues[40] observed significant gender differences in the incidence of these behavior types. Under the influence of addiction, men tended to engage in behavioral excesses that objectify their partners and require little emotional involvement (voyeuristic sex, paying for sex, anonymous sex, and exploitive sex). A trend toward emotional isolation was clear. Women, in contrast, tended to be excessive in behaviors that distort power—either in gaining control over others or being a victim (fantasy sex, seductive role sex, trading sex, and pain exchange). Carnes and associates found that women sex addicts use sex for power, for control, and for attention. Similar conclusions were reached by Kasl,[41] who treated many women with addictive sexual disorders. Sex addiction, according to Carnes, seems to "intensify the wounds already present in each gender." In women,[42] these wounds involve power and victimization issues, whereas men have difficulty with bonding, intimacy, and the tendency to objectify others.

Carnes' typology of addictive sexual behaviors includes both paraphilic (exhibitionism, voyeurism, frotteurism [indecent liberties], pedophilia, sadism, masochism, sex with animals) and nonparaphilic behaviors (seductive role sex, anonymous sex). In other words, both paraphilia NOS and sexual disorder NOS can have addictive features. In his early writings, Carnes[7] separated addictive behaviors according to another criterion—the extent to which the behavior victimizes others. The

Table 48–4. PATTERNS AND THEMES OF SEXUAL ADDICTION

Fantasy sex: Items focused on sexual fantasy life and consequences due to obsession. Themes include denial, delusion, and problems due to preoccupation.

Seductive role sex: Items focused on seductive behavior for conquest. Multiple relationships, affairs, and unsuccessful serial relationships.

Anonymous sex: Engaging in sex with anonymous partners; having one-night stands.

Paying for sex: Paying prostitutes for sex; paying for sexually explicit phone calls.

Trading sex: Receiving money or drugs for sex or using sex as a business. Highly correlated were swapping partners and using nudist clubs to find sex partners.

Voyeuristic sex: Items focused on forms of visual sex, including pornography, window peeping, and secret observation. Highly correlated with excessive masturbation, even to the point of injury.

Exhibitionist sex: Exposing oneself in public places or from the home or car; wearing clothes designed to expose.

Intrusive sex: Touching others without permission; using position or power (e.g., professional, religious) to sexually exploit another person; rape.

Pain exchange: Causing or receiving pain to enhance sexual pleasure. Use of dramatic roles, sexual aids, and animals were common themes.

Exploitive sex: Use of force or partner vulnerability to gain sexual access.

From Carnes P: Don't Call It Love: Recovery from Sexual Addiction. New York, Bantam Books, 1991, pp 42–44.

greater the victimization or the risk involved, the greater the addict's lack of control and unmanageability. Level one comprises behaviors regarded as normal, acceptable, or tolerable, such as masturbation, visits to pornographic bookstores and theaters, anonymous sex in parks and bathrooms, and prostitution. Level two includes nuisance crimes such as exhibitionism, voyeurism, obscene telephone calls, and frotteurism. Level three behaviors are serious crimes such as incest, child molestation, or rape. Addicts who are compulsive at level three are usually also compulsive at levels two and one; level two addiction is generally accompanied by addictive behaviors at level one as well. Although one specific behavior type may precipitate the crisis that brings a sexual addict to intervention, experience has shown that when a thorough sexual history is taken, an average of three compulsive sexual behaviors is found.

Sexual offense is a legal rather than a clinical term and refers to behaviors that directly traumatize and harm another individual. Sex offenders exploit available power, influence, opportunity, or vulnerability to gain control over their victim and advance their sexual agenda. Although sex offenses such as rape by physical force and pedophilia *may* result from sexual addiction, many sex offenders are not sexually addicted. Blanchard[43] examined the prevalence of sexual addiction among 109 imprisoned male sex offenders at the Wyoming State Penitentiary. Based on written instruments, personal interviews, and review of arrest records and presentence reports, he found that 55% of the sex offenders were sexually addicted. Of 63 child molesters, 71% were sexually addicted, compared with 39% of the rapists. Sex offenders who do not meet the diagnostic criteria for an addictive sexual disorder often have significant characterological pathology, such as antisocial, paranoid, schizotypal, or narcissistic personality disorders. Such individuals are sometimes eager to flee into illness and claim to be sexual addicts to excuse and justify their sexual assaults. In such situations, the self-proclaimed diagnosis should be viewed with skepticism unless strongly supported by clinical experience. Blanchard[43] also reported that sexually addicted offenders had different antecedent emotions than nonaddicts. The former felt sad, alienated, unworthy, and socially inadequate and needed constant signals of acceptance and approval; in contrast, the nonaddicted offenders were outwardly angry and had a hostile attitude toward society, especially toward women. The nonaddicted offenders had a greater incidence of violent assault against age mates. Many in both groups had suffered abuse during childhood, but the sexually addicted offenders had suffered less violent forms of maltreatment.

Compared with nonaddicted sex offenders, sexually addicted offenders have a higher number of prior offenses and fewer intrusive offenses, engage in rituals around offense behaviors rather than impulsive actions, have a higher level of shame about the offense behavior, make greater use of pornography, have a higher incidence of concomitant substance addictions, feel unworthy and out of control (whereas nonaddicted offenders feel anger, frustration, and hatred), are more in touch with their own past victimization, and are likely to have a history of child sexual abuse or sexualized home environment (whereas nonaddicted offenders are more likely to have a history of childhood physical abuse).[44]

That there are at least two different subsets of sex offenders with differing dynamics may explain why traditional one-size-fits-all models for treatment of sex offenders have been so notoriously unsuccessful. New models that selectively and individually incorporate behavioral, cognitive, and addiction approaches for treating these different groups are being developed[45, 46] and should lead to improved outcomes.

Professional Sexual Exploitation

One category of sexual offending that is receiving increasing attention is sexual exploitation by professionals, in which violation of a fiduciary relationship is used to advance a personal sexual agenda. Examples of such professionals include physicians, psychotherapists, counselors, teachers, lawyers, dentists, and ministers. There are two primary categories of sexual exploitation of power. *Professional sexual misconduct* is the overt or covert expression of erotic or romantic thoughts, feelings, or gestures by a professional toward a patient or client that are sexual or may reasonably be construed by the patient or client as sexual. *Sexual offense* is a nontherapeutic, nondiagnostic attempt by a professional to touch, or any actual contact with, any of the anatomical areas of a patient's or client's body commonly considered reproductive or sexual. Offending may also involve forcing or manipulating a client to touch the professional in these anatomical areas.

Professional sexual exploitation can occur within a diverse array of scenarios, examples of which are listed in Table 48–5. Gonsiorek[47] edited a text that provides a comprehensive review of current knowledge in this area, and Schoener[48] reviewed current experience with rehabilitation.

Professional sexual exploitation is surprisingly common, although often not reported by victims. Anonymous surveys of physicians and other helping professionals have consistently yielded a lifetime prevalence of 6% to 9% of those surveyed admitting to sexual contact with at least one patient or client[49–51]; 30% to 40% of respondents who had sexual contact with one patient or client admitted to such contact with more than one, suggesting a pattern of recurrent sexual exploitation. In addition to professionals who have had sexual contact with active patients or clients, many others have engaged in sexual contact with *former* clients, an activity that is also considered exploitive[52] and unethical.

Irons and Schneider[25] reported the results of an intensive inpatient assessment of 137 healthcare professionals (85% of them physicians, 98% male) referred because of allegations of personal or professional sexual impropriety. After assessment, half (54%) of the total group were found to have sexual disorder NOS with addictive features (i.e., to be sexually addicted). Two thirds (66%) of the entire group were found to have engaged in professional sexual exploitation, and of this subpopulation, two thirds (66%) were sexually addicted. Thus, addictive sexual disorders are a common feature of sex offending by professionals. In addition, one third (31%) of the entire group was incidentally found to be chemically dependent, a condition for which many had not been previously treated.

Although the incidence of antisocial personality disorder in incarcerated sex offenders is high, this characterological disorder is uncommon in sexually exploitive professionals. Among a group of 157 helping professionals assessed by Irons, only one had this disorder and another had antisocial personality traits (total 1.2%). The most common axis II disorder in this group of professionals was narcissistic personality disorder (9.5%), followed by dependent personality disorder (3.8%). In addition, 18.5% had a mixed personality disorder. Overall, 62 of the 157 consecutive professionals evaluated (39.5%), met the DSM diagnostic criteria for a personality disorder. Many more had axis II traits, in particular narcissistic (21.7%) and dependent (21.7%) personality features.

Contribution of Characterological Pathology

As we have shown, many cases involving sexual impropriety are associated with and at least partially attributable to characterological pathology, particularly when exploitation, assault, or sexual offense is involved. It is appropriate if not essential to diagnose a personality disorder during assessment or treatment. This characterological diagnosis can be the primary diagnosis, or the patient can be viewed as having comorbid conditions involving an axis I

Table 48–5. SEXUAL EXPLOITATION SCENARIOS

Therapeutic touch becomes erotic or is experienced by patient as sexual
Caretaking or emotional support extends beyond professional boundaries
Romantic enmeshment with patient
Use of power and position to advance sexual agendas
"Fatal Attraction" or enactment of a rescue fantasy
Paternal or maternal nurturance of a younger patient
Involvement with family member of patient
Frotteurism, voyeurism, or exhibitionism in a professional role
Unnecessary or overextensive genital examination
Rude/abusive/verbally inappropriate solicitation
Professional offers of sexually enhancing procedures
Personal sexual therapy for a patient's sexual or relationship problems
Cultural dissonance between professional and patient becomes sexualized
Molestation of patient who is physically, mentally, or emotionally unable to offer resistance or is under the influence of mood-altering substances or anesthesia
Attempt by professional to resolve conflicts involving sexual preference by sexual involvement with patient or client
Reenactment of patient or professional's incestuous desires or past sexual abuse

From Irons RR, Schneider JP: Sexual addiction: Significant factor in sexual exploitation by health care professionals. Sexual Addiction and Compulsivity 1:198–214, 1994.

diagnosis and an axis II diagnosis of characterological pathology. Many mental health professionals are reluctant to make a diagnosis of personality disorder, and such a diagnosis is viewed by some as a characterological curse—immutable, untreatable or poorly treatable, and auguring a poor prognosis. In our clinical experience, defects of character and other types of self-destructive or self-defeating behavior are often noted as part of addictive disease. If a patient is capable of honesty and at least partial insight, is able to identify characterological defects, and can work with them in steps 4 through 9 of a 12-step program, such defects are treatable using addiction model treatment and therapy. Dramatic characterological change is not infrequently observed as part of personal transformation achieved through dedicated participation in 12-step programs, insight-oriented or analytical therapy, and other avenues that promote spiritual awakening.

Evaluation for Sexual Addiction

All chemically dependent patients and all persons whose sexual behavior has been problematical should be screened for the presence of addictive sexual disorders. An appropriate starting place is the 25-item sexual addiction screening test developed by Carnes.[28] If 13 of the 25 questions are answered in the affirmative, the likelihood that an addictive sexual disorder is present is 96%. This tool must be used with caution in homosexual men, whose behavior and lifestyle are often characterized by secrecy and shame even though most are not sexual addicts. Also, the test has not been validated for women or adolescents. An additional adjunct to assessment is the checklist of collateral indicators that is reproduced in Table 48–6. Carnes compiled these indicators from research and therapy and believes that the presence of six or more collateral indicators is strongly suggestive of sexual addiction.

Because a multigenerational family history of addictive disorders is common among sex addicts, obtaining a genogram and a detailed biopsychosocial history can also assist diagnosis.

If the screening test suggests addiction, a more detailed sexual history should be obtained. One helpful tool is the Sexual Dependency Inventory, Revised,[53] a detailed, self-administered inventory that asks 184 questions about specific sexual behaviors and the frequency and power of each for the person. When given in the first 3 days after the initial intervention or admission, this inventory makes patients aware of the many areas in which their sexual behavior is out of control and helps break patients' denial about the seriousness of their life situation (Carnes P: Personal communication).

A thorough physical and neurological examination should be part of assessment. Persons who have had several sexual partners must be checked for HIV infection and other STDs. Female patients should have pregnancy testing. Rarely, endocrine disorders or central nervous system diseases such as a brain tumor or infection can cause a change in behavior.

The axis I differential diagnosis of sexual addiction was presented in Table 48–1. The clinical interview, along with standard psychological tests such as the Minnesota Multiphasic Personality Inventory and Millon and projective tests such as the Rorschach and Thematic Apperception Tests can help work through the differential diagnoses as well as define characterological pathology that can either exacerbate or simulate addictive disease.

Primary Treatment

Because a large percentage of persons with addictive sexual disorders are also chemically dependent, the initial decision often facing a treatment professional is which addiction to treat first. By the time many sex addicts seek help for this disorder, they are already in recovery from their substance dependence. If not, then regardless of which addiction is primary, the drug dependence must be treated first, or else sex addiction treatment is unlikely to be successful.

Decisions about inpatient versus outpatient primary care for addictive sexual disorders can be based on criteria analogous to the American Society of Addiction Medicine's *Patient Placement Criteria for the Treatment of Psychoactive Substance Use Disorders.*[54] Inpatient admission is appropriate for those who are unlikely to be able to engage in treatment as outpatients, are a danger to themselves or others, or have significant concurrent medical or psychiatric conditions requiring close observation.

Early treatment is similar to that for chemical dependence, comprising education about addiction in general and sex addiction in particular, a combination of group and individual therapy, introduction to 12-step programs and to mutual-help meetings, and, if possible,

Table 48–6. CHECKLIST OF COLLATERAL INDICATORS

1. Patient has severe consequences because of sexual behavior
2. Patient meets the criteria for depression and it appears related to sexual acting out
3. Patient reports history of sexual abuse
4. Patient reports history of physical and emotional abuse
5. Patient describes sexual life in self-medicating terms (intoxicating, tension relief, pain reliever, sleeping pills)
6. Patient reports persistent pursuit of high-risk or self-destructive behavior
7. Patient reports much greater sexual arousal with high-risk or self-destructive behavior than with safe sexual behavior
8. Patient describes pleasure or relief at time of sexual acting out but experiences despair afterward
9. Patient meets diagnostic criteria for other addictive disorders
10. Patient simultaneously uses sexual behavior in concert with other addictions (gambling, eating disorders, substance addiction, alcoholism, compulsive spending) to the extent that desired effect is not achieved without both sexual activity and other addiction present
11. Patient has history of deception around sexual behavior
12. Patient reports other members of the family are addicts
13. Patient expresses extreme self-loathing because of sexual behavior
14. Patient describes periods of time when all sexual interest and behavior cease
15. Patient has a pattern of bingeing followed by periods of being compulsively nonsexual
16. Patient is sexually excessive in some areas and compulsively nonsexual in others
17. Patient has few intimate relationships that are not sexual
18. Patient has attempted self-mutilation as an attempt to disrupt cycle
19. Patient is in crisis because of sexual matters
20. Patient has a history of crisis around sexual matters
21. Patient experiences anhedonia in the form of diminished pleasure for same experiences
22. Patient has mood lability around sexual behavior

From Carnes PJ: Personal communication, Minneapolis, 1995.

involvement of family members in family week, a program of education and confrontation. Shame, a major issue for sex addicts, is best addressed in group, where other recovering persons can provide support, confrontation, and shame reduction. Goodman[20] provides a review of the different aspects of treatment of sex addiction.

Recovery from sexual addiction is better viewed as analogous to recovery from eating disorders than to recovery from chemical dependence. Unlike the goal in treatment of chemical dependence, which most often is abstinence from use of all psychoactive substances, the initial therapeutic goal in addictive sexual disorders is abstinence only from compulsive sexual behavior. Development of healthy sexuality is a primary goal that is usually achieved only through continued commitment to a program of continued recovery and therapy. Early in the treatment period, it is suggested that patients refrain from all sexual activities, including masturbation, for 30 to 90 days. This enables them to learn that they can indeed survive without sex and allows them to get in touch with feelings that have been avoided and covered up with sexual activity. When they stop all sexual activity, some addicts report withdrawal symptoms similar to those experienced by cocaine addicts.

Pharmacotherapy has a definite place in the treatment of addictive sexual disorders. Some addicts report that the selective serotonin reuptake inhibitors (SSRIs) such as fluoxetine, sertraline, and paroxetine modulate the intensity of their sexual preoccupation and allow them to participate fully in treatment and self-help groups.[55, 56] For others, the tendency of the SSRIs to inhibit orgasm is a benefit. SSRIs are also useful, of course, in alleviating the depression that so often accompanies addiction. Progestational agents are occasionally used in the treatment of sex offenders.

Recovery Contracting with Sexual Addicts

PERSONAL

In the process of developing awareness of ritualized behavior and appreciation of powerlessness over compulsive sexual thoughts and actions, patients become ready and able to define certain bottom-line behaviors that they are willing to avoid as part of a continuing care contract. Engagement in one of these behaviors is considered either a slip or a relapse, depending on the behavior involved and the circumstances. Behavioral modification, by applying the 3-second rule to limit the length of time one focuses on an object or thought associated with sexual desire, and arousal reconditioning are also useful for some recovering addicts.

PROFESSIONAL

Some subgroups of sexually exploitive professionals have a better prognosis than others for return to professional practice. In contrast to professionals who have exploited primarily as an expression of an axis II characterological disorder, sexually addicted professionals who have successfully completed comprehensive assessment and primary treatment can often return to work without compromising public health and safety. Irons[57] devised a set of proposed contractual provisions for reentry. Such a contract can be part of a binding legal stipulation between the professional and a state professional licensing board or other regulatory agency and can define a standard care for potentially impaired healthcare professionals.

Course of Recovery Over Time

Compared with recovery from drug dependence, improvement in the quality of life of a recovering sex addict takes longer.[28] The first year is characterized by great turmoil. Most relapses, if they occur, take place in the second 6 months. Health, legal, occupational, and relationship consequences of the addiction take their greatest toll during the first year.

Because sex addicts were often sexually abused as children and because they have distorted ideas about sex, they generally lack experience that facilitates development of healthy sexuality. In the early recovery period, sex addicts and their partners frequently have sexual difficulties, often to a greater degree than they had during the active addiction phase.[22] Therapists can provide reassurance during this phase. If the compulsive sexual behavior was with same-sex partners, as is quite common even among men who identify themselves as heterosexual,[37] therapists can help patients work through conflicts about sexual preference.

In the second and third years, significant rebuilding starts. Patients experience improvement in career status, finances, friendships, and self-esteem. It is possible finally to define and work for healthy sexuality and intimacy in a relationship. In the fourth and fifth years, relationships with the significant other, parents, children, and life in general continue to improve.

Partners of sex addicts follow a similar path,[28] except that they experience their worst health problems and relapses to other addictions during the first 6 months. By the second 6 months, they begin experiencing improvement in self-image, career status, and communication with a partner. This means that for a couple working for recovery in the first year, each may be at a different phase, contributing to relationship stress. Couples need to be counseled to avoid making relationship decisions during this period; the couple relationship typically finds significant improvement only after this time.

Continuing Care

Like other addicts, sex addicts need ongoing support for establishing and maintaining a healthy lifestyle and avoiding relapse. Regular attendance at 12-step meetings (discussed later), coupled with ongoing therapy for dealing with shame, childhood trauma, false beliefs, and the consequences of past actions, all can facilitate recovery.

Lapses and relapses in the addictive sexual disorders often have more severe consequences than in substance dependence: A single incident of exhibitionism may lead to arrest or imprisonment; another sexual encounter may precipitate the end of the marriage. Accordingly, relapse prevention is a key component of treatment of sex addiction. Marlatt and Gordon's cognitive-behavioral approach to relapse prevention in drug dependence[58] has been adapted for the treatment of sex offenders. The volume edited by Laws[59] on relapse prevention for sex offenders is a very useful guide to treatment for all sex addicts.

Sex therapy is generally most effective at a later stage of treatment, in the second year and beyond. When treating patients with addictive sexual disorders, sex therapists may need to modify some of their beliefs (e.g., views on masturbation) and to honor recovery boundaries of clients.[60] Some traditional sex therapy techniques may also require modification. Irons[61] described healthy sexuality in recovery from substance dependence.

By the time sex addicts seek help, their marriage or relationship is often in great distress. Communication is lacking, and distrust, anger, and resentment are chronic. Couples counseling by a therapist who is knowledgeable about sex addiction can facilitate forgiveness and rebuilding of trust.[62] Such counseling is unlikely to be effective, however, as long as the significant other persists in viewing himself or herself as the victim. The significant other should be encouraged to obtain individual therapy to deal with his or her probable dependence issues, fear of abandonment, external locus of control, and low self-esteem. Attendance at 12-step programs for partners of sex addicts can facilitate recovery.

Community and National Resources

TWELVE-STEP PROGRAMS

The 12 steps of AA have been adapted for use in programs for sexual disorders. Programs modeled after Al-Anon (the mutual-help program for families and friends of alcoholics) are also available in many cities. Group support can be a powerful tool for overcoming the shame that most sex addicts and their family members feel. Table 48–7 provides addresses of the national offices of the 12-step programs. These offices can provide information about meeting locations as well as literature about the addiction.

Because the goal in recovery from addictive sexual disorders is abstinence only from the addictive behaviors, the definition of *sexual sobriety* has room for interpretation. The various 12-step programs listed in Table 48–7 differ primarily in their definition of sexual sobriety. For Sexaholics Anonymous, it is limited to sex within marriage. In the other programs, members define their own recovery plans and determine which behaviors to avoid. The members of Sexual Compulsives Anonymous are primarily gay men and lesbians. The two recovery programs for family members have no significant differences. Recovering Couples Anonymous is a program for couples recovering from all addictions; approximately 50% of the members are recovering from addictive sexual disorders.

OTHER RESOURCES

Professionals seeking additional information on addictive sexual disorders can contact the National Council on Sexual Addiction and Compulsivity, located at P.O. Box 16104, Atlanta, GA 30321-9998. Their help-line telephone number is (770) 968-5002. This organization has an annual educational conference, sponsors a refereed journal, *Sexual Addiction and Compulsivity*, and publishes a quarterly newsletter.

Patients seeking information for themselves and family members can be referred to the books for laypeople by Carnes,[7] Earle and Crow,[63] Kasl,[41] Schneider,[32] and Schneider and Schneider.[22]

The Interfaith Sexual Trauma Institute (ISTI), located at Saint John's University, Collegeville, MN 56321 ([612] 363-3931), affirms the goodness of human sexuality and advocates respectful relationships through appropriate use of power within communities of all religious traditions. ISTI promotes prevention of sexual abuse, exploitation, and harassment through research, education, and publication. In areas of sexuality, ISTI offers leadership, gives voice, and facilitates healing of victims, communities of faith, and offenders, as well as those who care for them.

The Walk-In Counseling Center, 2421 Chi-

Table 48–7. TWELVE-STEP PROGRAMS FOR SEX ADDICTION

For the Addict	For the Partner
Sexaholics Anonymous P.O. Box 111910 Nashville, TN 37222-1910 (615) 331-6901	S-Anon P.O. Box 111242 Nashville, TN 37222-1242 (615) 833-3152
Sex Addicts Anonymous P.O. Box 70949 Houston, TX 77270 (713) 869-4902	Codependents of Sex Addicts P.O. Box 14537 Minneapolis, MN 55414 (612) 537-6904
Sex and Love Addicts Anonymous P.O. Box 119, New Town Branch Boston, MA 02258 (617) 332-1845	Co-SLAA P.O. Box 1449 Brookline, MA 02146
Sexual Compulsives Anonymous Old Chelsea Station P.O. Box 1585 New York, NY 10013-0935 (800) 977-HEAL	**For Couples** Recovering Couples Anonymous P.O. Box 11872 St. Louis, MO 63105 (314) 830-2600

cago Avenue South, Minneapolis, MN 55404 ([612] 870-0565), is nationally recognized as a leader in providing resources and counseling to those who have been victims of professional sexual exploitation. The center is also known for its expertise in approaching, intervening in, and recommending evaluation for sexually exploitive professionals.

REFERENCES

1. Billy JOG, Tanfer K, Grady WR, et al: The sexual behavior of men in the United States. Fam Plann Perspect 25(2):52–60, 1993.
2. Michael RT, Gagnon JH, Lauman EO, et al: Sex in America: A Definitive Survey. Boston, Little-Brown & Co, 1994.
3. American Psychiatric Association: Diagnostic and Statistical Manual of Mental Disorders, 4th ed. Washington, DC, American Psychiatric Association, 1994, pp 493–538.
4. Alcoholics Anonymous, 3rd ed. New York, Alcoholics Anonymous World Services, 1976, pp 68–70.
5. Orford J: Hypersexuality: Implications for a theory of dependence. Br J Addict 73:299–310, 1978.
6. Orford J: Excessive Appetites: a Psychologist's View of Addictions. New York, John Wiley & Sons, 1985.
7. Carnes P: Out of the Shadows: Understanding Sexual Addiction. Minneapolis, CompCare Publications, 1983, p 40.
8. Peele S: Love and Addiction. New York, Signet Books, 1975, p 1.
9. Peele S: How Much Is Too Much? New York, Prentice-Hall, 1981.
10. Quadland MC: Compulsive sexual behavior: Definition of a problem and approach to treatment. J Sex Marital Ther 11:121–132, 1985.
11. Barth RJ, Kinder BN: The mislabeling of sexual impulsivity. J Sex Marital Ther 13(1):15–23, 1987.
12. Schwartz MF: Sexual compulsivity as post-traumatic stress disorder: Treatment perspectives. Psychiatr Ann 22(6):333–338, 1992.
13. Coleman E: The obsessive-compulsive model for describing compulsive sexual behavior. Am J Prev Psychiatr Neurol 2:9–14, 1990.
14. Coleman E: Sexual compulsion versus addiction: The debate continues. SIECUS Report 14(6):7–11, 1986.
15. Shaffer HJ: Considering two models of excessive sexual behaviors: Addiction and obsessive-compulsive disorder. Sexual Addiction and Compulsivity 1:6–18, 1994.
16. Renshaw DC: What is sexual addiction? Proceedings of the Institute of Medicine, Chicago 39:67–68, 1986.
17. Levine MP, Troiden RR: The myth of sexual compulsivity. Journal of Sex Research 37:347–363, 1988.
18. American Psychiatric Association: Diagnostic and Statistical Manual of Mental Disorders, 3rd ed, revised. Washington, DC, American Psychiatric Association, 1987, p 284.
19. Schneider JP: Sexual addiction: controversy in mainstream addiction medicine, DSM-III-R diagnosis, and physician case histories. Sexual Addiction and Compulsivity 1:19–46, 1994.
20. Goodman A: Diagnosis and treatment of sex addiction. J Sex Marital Ther 19(3):225–242, 1993.
21. Goodman A: Addiction: Definition and implications. Br J Psychiatry 85:1403–1408, 1990.
22. Schneider JP, Schneider BH: Sex, Lies, and Forgiveness: Couples Speak on Healing from Sex Addiction. Center City, MN, Hazelden Educational Materials, 1991, p 17.
23. Carnes P: Don't Call It Love: Recovery from Sexual Addiction. New York, Bantam Books, 1991, p 35.
24. Washton A: Cocaine may trigger sexual compulsivity. USJ Drug Alcohol Dependency 13(6):8, 1989.
25. Irons RR, Schneider JP: Sexual addiction: Significant factor in sexual exploitation by health care professionals. Sexual Addiction and Compulsivity 1:198–214, 1994.
26. Gordon LJ, Fargason PJ, Kramer JJ: Sexual behaviors of chemically dependent physicians and nonphysicians in comparison to sexually compulsive chemically dependent physicians and nonphysicians. Sexual Addiction and Compulsivity 2:233–255, 1995.
27. Milkman H, Sunderwirth S: Craving for Ecstasy. Lexington, MA, Lexington Books, 1987.
28. Carnes P: Contrary to Love: Helping the Sexual Addict. Minneapolis, CompCare Publishers, 1989, pp 77–79.
29. Avins AA, Woods WJ, Lindan CP, et al: HIV infection and risk behaviors among heterosexuals in alcohol treatment programs. JAMA 271(7):515–518, 1994.
30. Marx R, Aral SO, Roles RT, et al: Crack, sex, and STD. Sex Transm Dis 18:92–101, 1991.
31. Olson DH, Sprenkle D, Russell C: Circumplex model of marital and family systems. I. Cohesion and adaptability dimensions, family types and clinical application. Fam Process 18:3–28, 1979.
32. Schneider JP: Back From Betrayal: Recovering From His Affairs. Center City, MN, Hazelden Educational Materials, 1988, p 55.
33. Stoller R: Symbiosis anxiety and the development of masculinity. Arch General Psychiatry 30:164, 1974.
34. Hudson L, Jacot B: The Way Men Think: Intellect, Intimacy and the Erotic Imagination. New Haven, Yale University Press, 1991, pp 42–45.
35. Johnson R: He: Understanding Masculine Psychology. New York, Harper Perennial, 1989, p 9.
36. Maltz W, Holman B: Incest and Sexuality. Lexington, MA, Lexington Books, 1987, pp 69–77.
37. Schneider JP, Schneider BH: Marital satisfaction during recovery from self-identified sexual addiction among bisexual men and their wives. J Sex Marital Ther 16(4):230–250, 1990.
38. Schwartz MF: The Masters and Johnson treatment program for sex offenders: Intimacy, empathy, and trauma resolution. Sexual Addiction and Compulsivity 1:261–277, 1994.
39. Schwartz MF, Masters WM: Integration of trauma-based, cognitive, behavioral, systemic, and addiction approaches for treatment of hypersexual pair-bonding disorder. Sexual Addiction and Compulsivity 1:57–76, 1994.
40. Carnes P, Nonemaker D, Skilling N: Gender differences in normal and sexually addicted populations. Am J Prev Psychiatr Neurol 3(1):16–23, 1991.
41. Kasl CD: Women, Sex, and Addiction. New York, Ticknor & Fields, 1989.
42. Lewis HB: Psychic War in Men and Women. New York, New York University Press, 1976.
43. Blanchard G: Differential diagnosis of sex offenders: Distinguishing characteristics of the sex addict. Am J Prev Psychiatr Neurol 2:45–47, 1990.
44. Delmonico D, Griffin E: Yes, Virginia, there are sexually addicted offenders. Presented at the Annual Conference of the National Council on Sexual Addiction and Compulsivity, Atlanta, GA, March 24, 1995.
45. Herman JL: Considering sex offenders: A model of addiction. Signs: J Women Culture Soc 13(4):695–724, 1988.

46. Blanchard G: The Difficult Connection: The Therapeutic Relationship in Sex Offender Treatment. Brandon, VT, The Safer Society Press, 1995.

47. Gonsiorek J (ed): Breach of Trust: Sexual Exploitation by Health Care Professionals and Clergy. Thousand Oaks, CA, Sage Publications, 1995.

48. Schoener G: Rehabilitation of professionals who have sexually touched patients. In Schwebel M, Skorina J, Schoener G (eds): Assisting Impaired Psychologists. Washington, DC, American Psychological Association, 1994.

49. Gartrell N, Herman J, Olarte S, et al: Psychiatrist-patient sexual contact: Results of a national survey. I. Prevalence. Am J Psychiatry 143:1126–1130, 1986.

50. Gartrell N, Milliken N, Goodson, W III, et al: Physician-patient sexual contact: Prevalence and problems. West J Med 157:139–143, 1992.

51. Wilbers D, Veenstra G, van de Will HBM, et al: Sexual contact in the doctor-patient relationship in the Netherlands. Br Med J 304:1531–1534, 1992.

52. Gabbard GO, Pope KS: Sexual intimacies after termination: Clinical, ethical, and legal aspects. In Gabbard GO (ed): Sexual Exploitation in Professional Relations. Washington, DC, American Psychiatric Association, 1989, pp 115–128.

53. Carnes P, Delmonico D: Sexual Dependency Inventory, revised (in press). Available through Workshop Design Associates, (612) 925-0134.

54. American Society of Addiction Medicine: Patient Placement Criteria for the Treatment of Psychoactive Substance Use Disorders. Washington, DC, American Society of Addiction Medicine, 1991.

55. Kafka MP: Successful antidepressant treatment of nonparaphilic sexual addictions and paraphilias in men. J Clin Psychiatry 52(2):60–64, 1991.

56. Stein DJ, Hollander E, Anthony DT, et al: Serotonergic medications for sexual obsessions, sexual addictions, and paraphilias. J Clin Psychiatry 53(8):267–271, 1992.

57. Irons RR: Sexually addicted professionals: Contractual provisions for re-entry. Am J Prev Psychiatr Neurol 3:57–59, 1991.

58. Marlatt GA, Gordon JR (eds): Relapse Prevention. New York, Guilford Press, 1985.

59. Laws DR: Relapse Prevention with Sex Offenders. New York, Guilford Press, 1989.

60. Manley G: Sexual health recovery in sex addiction: Implications for sex therapists. Am J Prev Psychiatr Neurol 3(1):33–39, 1991.

61. Irons RR: Healthy sexuality in recovery. Sexual Addiction and Compulsivity 1(4):322–336, 1994.

62. Schneider JP: Rebuilding the marriage during recovery from compulsive sexual behavior. Family Relations 38:288–294, 1989.

63. Earle R, Crow G: Lonely All the Time. New York, Pocket Books, 1989.

Forensic and Ethical Issues in Addiction Psychiatry

Amin N. Daghestani, MD

As the impact of addictive illnesses permeates the various societal matrices, forensic and ethical questions are increasingly raised. Practicing psychiatrists are now faced with issues that were in the experimental realm only a few years ago, such as decisions on liver transplantation in alcoholics. Other issues that have been discussed in psychiatry for many years, such as countertransference, are assuming new importance as more comorbidities of alcohol and drug addiction are recognized. Positions that were addressed by the Hippocratic oath, such as patient confidentiality and physician-patient relationships, continue to be refined and often debated.

The close association between ethics and addiction traces its roots to the way our attitudes are shaped. The behavioral consequences of alcohol and substance addiction are first manifested by addicted patients. The social symptoms often present even before the psychological or physiological complications take place. An arrest for driving while intoxicated often precedes the discovery of liver pathology in an alcoholic. It is no wonder that personal attitudes toward addictive disorders far exceed any negative attitudes society might have toward other physical or psychological disorders.

Two possible reasons for the recent interest in ethics and addiction are the enhanced role of the media and the increased rate of diagno-sis of addiction with comorbid psychiatric conditions.

A distinction needs to be made between ethical and forensic issues. One could ascertain situations that pertain solely to ethics, to law, or to both. Breach of patient confidentiality by a physician is illegal, but performing a urine screen on every job applicant certainly raises some genuine ethical questions. On the other hand, a sexual relationship between a doctor and patient clearly has both ethical and legal implications. It is also of interest to note that some ethical questions will spontaneously resolve by changes in economics (i.e., better coverage by managed care or by improved medical technology) and by having organs more easily available for transplantation, when the issues associated with the waiting list will become less significant.

This chapter outlines the main forensic and ethical issues involved in working with addicted and dually-diagnosed patients.

Confidentiality

Maintaining a confidential relationship between the physician and patient has been a hallmark of the practice of medicine throughout recorded history. With advanced communication technology, the need to ensure confidentiality between physician and patient becomes more acute. It is believed that by ensuring strict confidentiality, addicted patients are encouraged to seek treatment actively. It is the responsibility of physicians to protect their patients' confidentiality regardless of the nature of the complaint or illness. However, such protection becomes paramount in dually diagnosed patients, who exhibit such a wide range of vulnerabilities. Personal sensitivities, inner conflicts, shame, guilt, rage, betrayal, hurt, and abandonment are but examples of a long list of emotions usually uncovered in the course of treatment with addicted patients.

The first law to protect patients with alcohol and drug addiction was introduced by Congress in 1975 and later amended in 1987 under Confidentiality of Alcohol and Drug Abuse Patients Records. The law specifies that the disclosure of information about any patient in a federally assisted alcohol or drug addiction program is prohibited. This prohibition supersedes any state provision in this regard. If confidentiality is not maintained, it is considered an invasion of privacy. When information is authorized to be released, an accompanying statement should emphasize the confidential nature of the information and prohibit redisclosure.

Consent given by patients should be written, informed, intentional, and voluntary. Contents of the written consent should specifically include the name of the patient, the names of the disclosing program and receiving agency, the purpose of the disclosure, what information is to be revealed, and a statement that the patient may revoke the consent in writing at any time.

The amount of information to be released is usually specified on the consent form. The disclosing party should reveal only the minimum information required and should reveal only what is pertinent to the request. Examples of this would be disclosures made to third-party payors, to employers, and to collection agencies. Newer technologies have the potential of disseminating information indiscriminately, and additional caution should be taken when using fax machines, voice mail, or E-mail.

Exceptions to confidentiality rules are made by federal and individual state laws. These involve disclosure with patient consent, disclosure to other staff within the treatment program, disclosure in response to medical emergencies or a court order, reporting of child abuse or neglect, or as part of an audit or examination of the program. In circumstances involving patients' criminal activities or arrest warrants against registered patients, a legal opinion should be obtained. Furthermore, subpoenas should be distinguished from the type of court order exempted by federal law. The subpoena compels the psychiatrist only to appear and should not be ignored.

Commitment

Commitment refers to the involuntary hospitalization of psychiatric patients to a closed inpatient psychiatric unit. This usually follows the filing of certificates by a witness, citizen, or a family member, plus a certificate by a psychiatrist stating that the patient is imminently in danger of hurting himself or herself or others or that the patient is unable to take care of his or her basic needs. The initial petition is usually made for a limited period and varies from state to state, generally between 3 and 14 days. To prepare for a certificate of need for involuntary hospitalization, an examination of the patient, including an adequate mental status examination, should be conducted and the findings recorded. This examination should describe the specific reasons, events, acts, behaviors, or threats made by the patient or witnessed by a reliable individual to justify the need for this form of admission.

Most substance addiction treatment programs do not admit patients involuntarily. Those substance addicts who are suicidal or homicidal are admitted to closed psychiatric inpatient units on a certificate. Once they no longer become actively suicidal or homicidal, they are usually discharged to a different level of care such as an inpatient substance addiction program, a day program, or an outpatient treatment facility.

Documentation

Medical records serve the important function of sharing needed patient information among various treatment personnel. They serve as a basis for therapeutic interventions or aftercare planning. In addition to this, they are considered a legal document that could be used at a later point for litigation, prosecution, or defense. Therefore, it is important to have medical records that are detailed, accurate, legible, and timely.

Medical records should have meaningful and pertinent information about a patient. This should include findings of a patient's history and physical examination, psychiatric assessment, laboratory workup including Breathalyzer readings, and urine and blood toxicology screens; medication names, doses, and instructions for use; progress notes; consent forms; and all correspondence. Medical records should be kept for not less than 6 years for adult patients and longer for children. Records should not be altered.

Under most state laws, patients have the right to see their records. In malpractice cases, the plaintiff's attorney is also permitted to review the records.

Physicians with Substance Addiction Problems

Being a physician does not preclude an individual from becoming addicted to alcohol or other drugs. Despite the practice-related stresses and the availability of abusable drugs to physicians, research suggests that the incidence of substance addiction among physicians is no less and no more than that in the general population. Older physicians tend to become addicted to alcohol, and younger physicians tend to become addicted to multiple drugs. *Physician's impairment* refers to the inability to practice medicine with reasonable skills and safety for patients by reasons of physical or mental illness, including alcohol or drug dependence. The concept of impairment is more of a legal term than a medical one.

Any physician who suspects a colleague of having an impairment that negatively affects the practice of medicine has an ethical obligation to report the suspicion. The physician assistance committee in the hospital or the medical society can be contacted. Those members of the committee will be able to conduct a careful, confidential, and proper assessment to ascertain the presence or absence of an impairment and to map out an empathic intervention plan. Impaired physicians are the group with the best treatment outcome among substance-addicted patients in general.

Suicidal Patients

Suicide by a patient is a tragic event for the patient, family, and friends. It is a risk inherent in treating patients with psychiatric disorders, especially depression. Research findings have proved that alcohol and drug addiction adds significantly to patients' suicide risk. The pharmacological effects of alcohol lead to an impairment of judgment. Alcohol is often taken before a suicide attempt to give patients "the courage" to kill themselves. The combination of alcohol and other sedative-hypnotic tranquilizers is a well-known lethal mix in serious suicide attempts. The comorbid association of drugs and depression in patients raises concern about their suicide potential.

Despite the fact that the prediction of dangerousness to oneself is difficult to establish, a psychiatrist has two obligations to suicidal patients: a duty to assess and a duty to protect. Assessment of suicide risk is a part of every psychiatric evaluation. All suicide risk factors such as age, social support availability, stressors and losses, gender, and history of suicide attempts by the patient or the patient's family are to be considered. Records should document that such an assessment has been carried out.

If a patient is judged to be suicidal, adequate measures should be taken to protect him or her from self-harm. Appropriate communication with family members and other treatment team members should not be overlooked, and adequate follow-up discharge plans should be put in place.

Homicidal Patients

Substance addicts typically have a major problem in dealing with their impulse control. The disinhibiting effects of abusable drugs and the impairment of judgment that result from psychoactive drug use precipitate in vulnerable individuals fits of anger and rage, as well as assaultive and violent tendencies. Antisocial personality or traits are considered predisposing factors. Social factors of urban congestion, unemployment, poverty, and family dissolutions all increase the predisposition to violence. The availability of weapons such as handguns presents the opportunity for violent acts to be more lethal.

As with suicidal patients, a psychiatrist has two obligations when dealing with homicidal patients: a duty to assess and a duty to protect.

Every dually diagnosed patient should receive a comprehensive evaluation including a history of violence, imprisonments, and arrest. Gathering data of a legal history should be a regular part of every social history. Assessment of both suicidal and homicidal potential, ideations, tendencies, and plans becomes more important as more patients with comorbid psychiatric and addictive disorders are seen in emergency rooms or in clinical practice.

The duty to warn intended victims was initially established by the landmark case of *Tara-*

soff v. *Regents of the University of California*. It becomes a delicate balancing act for therapists to follow the Tarasoff responsibility on one hand and protect a patient's right to confidentiality on the other hand.

The duty to protect gives a psychiatrist the ability to initiate a certificate for involuntary hospitalization of a patient who is suspected of having homicidal ideations or plans. Before such patients are discharged from inpatient care, a clearly documented evaluation should establish the changes in the patient's mental status and behavior, as well as the kind of follow-up plans needed to maintain the absence of homicidality.

Toxicology Testing

Urine toxicology testing is used as a screening method for suspicion of drug use. A number of variables are involved in this testing, such as the type of drugs, dose, frequency of use, type of body fluid tested, individual metabolism, and sample collection time. Toxicological testing of urine or blood has been a subject of increasing public debate. Both ethical and legal questions have been raised in connection with this screening method. The two issues involved are individual privacy on one hand and ensuring public safety on the other hand. Some have felt that preemployment urine screening might stereotype certain individuals because of their age or their ethnic, social, or racial backgrounds.

The legal profession has questioned the validity of certain test results. Forensic experts want to protect the due process rights. Under forensic circumstances or in special monitoring situations (e.g., recovering physicians), a special procedure of chain of custody is followed to ensure the accuracy of the collection, handling, and delivery of specimens. Screening tests are usually followed up by a more sensitive test for confirmation purposes by using gas chromatography–mass spectrometry methods.

Child Abuse and Reporting Duties

It is not unusual for mental health and substance addiction professionals to encounter numerous cases of child abuse and neglect among parents who are substance addicts. A history of physical, sexual, and emotional abuse during childhood is also reported by substance addicts. To protect minors, most states have enacted laws requiring health professionals to report any suspected cases of child abuse to special state agencies such as the Department of Children and Family Services. Reporting of incidents of suspected abuse has been extended by some states to include the reporting of disorders that impair the ability to drive a motor vehicle and the reporting of elder abuse in homes or at nursing home facilities.

Patient Intervention

Intervention in addiction psychiatry refers to an organized, prearranged confrontation or meeting with a substance addict who is in denial. Employers, family members, or friends of the patient present to the addict concrete evidence of the adverse effects of substance use on the individual's behavior and functioning. This includes problems in performing work responsibilities and family, physical, legal, or social problems associated with alcohol or drug addiction.

Some patients have perceived the experience of intervention as an intrusion on their privacy, coercion, or unnecessary pressure. It is important that intervention meetings be diligently prepared. Supporting data have to be well documented and not based on guessing. Patients should be approached with empathy, care, and understanding yet must be led to realize that their denial of their illness is perpetuating the destructive results of their substance addiction.

Physician's Prescribing Practices

Physician's prescribing practices refers to a physician's patterns of working with patients, their families, and the public and the way he or she runs the office and handles records, documentation, and paperwork.

With every drug-seeking patient, a physician should take a comprehensive history focusing on the possibility of substance addiction and referring potential substance addicts to chemical dependence programs for further assessment and treatment. Some drug addicts are known for "doctor shopping"—attempting to get prescription tranquilizers and pain killer drugs from various doctors or clinics at the same time. Physicians should keep their prescription pads locked and not scattered or within easy reach of patients.

Human Immunodeficiency Virus

Drug addicts are at high risk for contracting human immunodeficiency virus (HIV) infections. Some women have used sex in exchange for drugs such as cocaine, thereby exposing themselves to increased risk for contracting HIV by having multiple partners and indiscriminate patterns of sexual behavior. Courts in many states have held that healthcare providers have a duty to warn their parties that they may have been exposed to HIV or may be at risk for infection.

Issues of Countertransference

Working with addicted patients often evokes feelings and emotional reactions that could have detrimental effects on the therapeutic relationship itself. These situations may sometimes lead to serious ethical or legal questions. Following are examples of these situations:

1. Identification with patients. This leads to difficulty in establishing limit setting with patients, which is often needed to treat the behavioral correlates of drug addiction.
2. Denial of drug addiction. Some therapists tend to minimize the impact of drug addiction on the lives of patients or their families. Such denial may constitute a misdiagnosis, which only prolongs identification of the problem at an early stage.
3. Rationalization of drug addiction. This is an attempt by the therapist to explain or excuse a patient's act of using drugs based on a poorly supported theory of self-medication by drug addicts.
4. Undertreatment or overtreatment. In either case, a therapist is not responding appropriately to the treatment needs of a patient or, on the other hand, is showing signs of enabling behavior, thus perpetuating the cycle of drug addiction.
5. Withholding or rejection of a patient. Therapists may have cold, distant, and aloof attitudes toward their patients or may experience empathic failure. They may have these same feelings because of treatment noncompliance or dropout.

6. Sexualization. Sexualization of physician-patient relationships leads to destruction of this relationship and of the element of trust, which is essential in this professional relationship.

Addiction, Pregnancy, and Breast-Feeding

To protect fetuses or infants who are born to addicted mothers, some states have tried to prosecute addicted mothers for exposing fetuses or newborns to the impacts of psychoactive substances on physical and emotional development. More specialized drug addiction treatment for women is needed to educate addicts about this major public health problem and to offer active treatment interventions and support.

Managed Care

With reductions in healthcare benefits, substance addiction treatment programs have been forced to downsize, leaving large numbers of patients without available treatment. When dealing with health maintenance organizations and other groups, physicians should obtain patient consent to provide information about the patient to the managed care company. Only pertinent information is to be released. When no insurance benefits are provided, a physician must avoid abandonment of patients. Instead, an orderly transfer to other treatment facilities in the public sector such as county hospitals, veterans affairs hospitals, state-run hospitals, or local community mental health centers should be arranged.

Liver Transplantation

As the techniques for performing liver transplantation improve, the ethics of establishing a priority list for potential transplant recipients becomes the center of debates. Alcoholics who need liver transplants should not be discriminated against in terms of transplant decisions simply because they carry the diagnosis of alcoholism. The decision to prioritize liver recipients should be based on many factors, such as the acuteness of the condition, the prognosis, and a patient's motivation for recovery.

Ethics in Substance Addiction Research

Investigators must pay attention to the well-being of the participants in research studies. All research proposals should meet the approval of institutional review boards. The protection of human subjects was dictated by a federal policy known as 45CFR46. Researchers must obtain the subjects' informed consent to participate in the study. Informed consent has three components: information, voluntariness, and competence. Obviously, every research proposal must make a clear assessment of potential risks and benefits involved in the study.

SELECTED READINGS

American Medical Association: Council on Ethical and Judicial Affairs, American Medical Association Code of Medical Ethics: Current Opinions with Annotations. Chicago, American Medical Association, 1992.

American Psychiatric Association: The Principles of Medical Ethics with Annotations Especially Applicable to Psychiatry. Washington, DC, American Psychiatric Association, 1989.

Bissel L, Royce J: Ethics for Addiction Professionals. Center City, MN, Hazelden, 1987.

Brooks MK: Ethical and legal aspects of confidentiality. In Lowinson JH, Ruiz P, Millman RB, Langrad JG (eds): Substance Abuse: A Comprehensive Textbook, 2nd ed. Baltimore, Williams & Wilkins, 1992.

Brown-Miller A: Ethical dilemmas in the drug free workplace. Addiction and Recovery 12(4):12–14, 1992.

Chankin W, Walker NA, Paone D: Drug using families and child protection: Results of a study and implications for change. University of Pittsburgh Law Review 54(1):295–324, 1993.

Cohen C, Benjamin M: Alcoholics and liver transplantation: The ethics and social impact committee of the transplant and health policy center. JAMA 265(10):1299–1301, 1991.

Cohen S: Drugs for pleasure: Ethical issues. Drug Abuse and Alcoholism Newsletter: Vista Hill Foundation. 8(7): 1979.

Council on Ethical and Judicial Affairs, American Medical Association: Sexual misconduct in the practice of medicine. JAMA 226:2741–2745, 1991.

Fingarette H: Alcoholism: Can honest mistakes about one's capacity for self-control be an excuse? Int J Law Psychiatry 13(102):77–93, 1990.

Imhof JE: Countertransference issues in alcoholism and drug addiction. Psychiatr Ann 21(5):292–306, 1991.

Landwirth J: Fetal abuse and neglect: An emerging controversy. Pediatrics 79:508–514, 1987.

Loewy EH: Drunks, livers, and values. Should social value judgements enter into liver transplant decisions? J Clin Gastroenterol 9(4):436–441, 1987.

Lundberg GD: Mandatory unindicated urine drug screening: Still chemical McCarthyism. JAMA 256(21):3003–3005, 1986.

Macbeth JE, Wheeler AM, Sitber JW, Onek JN: Legal and Risk Management Issues in the Practice of Psychiatry. Washington, DC, Psychiatrists Group, 1994.

Nadelson CC: Ethics, empathy, and gender in health care. Am J Psychiatry 150:1309–1314, 1993.

Oberman M: Sex, drugs and pregnant addicts: Ethical and legal critiques of societal responses to pregnant addicts. J Clin Ethics 1(2):145–152, 1990.

Popivits RM: Confidentiality vs. the courts: Your legal obligations. Addiction and Recovery. 12(7):9–10, 1992.

Wilms J, Schneiderman H: The ethics of impaired physicians. In Brock DH, Ratzan RM (eds): Literature and Bioethics. Baltimore, Johns Hopkins University Press, 1988, pp 123–131.

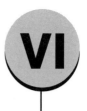

PHARMACOLOGICAL TREATMENTS

Pharmacological Treatment of Alcoholism: Clinical Management

Robert M. Swift, MD, PhD

Although ethanol is a drug that does not act through a specific neurotransmitter receptor, certain neurotransmitter systems are important for the modulation of behaviors produced by ethanol. Ethanol appears to have effects on several brain neurotransmitter systems, including dopamine, serotonin, gamma-aminobutyric acid (GABA), N-methyl-D-aspartate (NMDA), norepinephrine, and opioids. Because of these effects of alcohol on selective neurotransmitters, psychotropic medications that selectively modify neurotransmitters have efficacy as potential treatments for alcohol use disorders.[1] This chapter discusses the use of pharmacological agents in the treatment of alcohol dependence and withdrawal.

General Considerations in Alcoholism Treatment

The word *alcoholism* has many definitions and encompasses a number of alcohol-related behaviors. Generally defined, it is a condition in which a patient has "repetitive, but inconsistent and sometimes unpredictable loss of control of drinking which produces symptoms of serious dysfunction or disability."[2] Alcohol withdrawal, alcohol dependence, and alcohol abuse are medical diagnoses developed by the

Diagnostic and Statistical Manual of Mental Disorders (DSM) of the American Psychiatric Association, currently in its 4th edition.[3] Although it is estimated that as many as 7% to 10% of adult Americans have alcohol addiction or dependence, alcoholism is often underrecognized and left untreated by physicians. The reasons for these deficiencies include poor education about alcoholism, negative biases about the etiology of the condition, and a lack of knowledge of treatment resources.[4] In an American Medical Association–sponsored poll, 71% of physicians believed they were either not competent enough or were too ambivalent to treat alcoholic patients correctly.[5]

Pharmacological treatment of alcohol withdrawal and dependence must occur in the context of a comprehensive treatment program that addresses the multiple psychological, social, and medical needs of patients. The treatment of alcoholic patients comprises several components. First, the primary task of the clinician is to establish an effective therapeutic relationship. Second, a treatment plan should be developed that is practical, cost-effective, and based on well-established principles. Optimal treatment of substance use and dependence requires knowledge about therapies for the acute management of intoxicated or withdrawing patients, as well as knowledge about long-term treatment and rehabilitation. Figure 50–1 shows some of the treatment modalities available.

Several factors determine the type and intensity of treatment to be received. The severity of alcohol dependence, the occurrence of previous treatment and its success or failure, the presence of comorbid psychiatric or medical problems, and the amount of psychosocial support all are factors that can influence the intensity of the treatment required.

Cost of treatment and who pays for it have become major factors in determining patient placement. Treatment plans often need to be approved by third-party payors such as insurance companies or managed care programs, for whom cost is a major consideration. It is important, therefore, to act as a patient's advocate and to negotiate for the most effective, optimal treatment, consistent with the patient's coverage. Treatment standards, such as those developed by the American Society of Addiction Medicine,[6] can assist clinicians in matching the intensity of treatment to the severity of the substance use disorder and the medical and psychiatric condition. The so-called ASAM criteria for determination of treatment placement have been widely adopted and accepted by many third-party payors.

The treatment process should address both the physical and psychological consequences of alcohol use and the physical and psychological factors that contribute to use. Treatment is often described as occurring in two phases: detoxification and rehabilitation. Medications can play an important part in the treatment process. The objectives of detoxification treatment include (1) establishment of a drug- or alcohol-free state, (2) relief of distress and discomfort due to intoxication or withdrawal, (3) treatment of comorbid medical or psychiatric conditions, and (4) preparation and referral for longer-term treatment or rehabilitation. The objectives for longer-term treatment or rehabilitation include (1) long-term maintenance of the alcohol- or drug-free state and (2) psychological, family, and vocational interventions to ensure its persistence. Changes in living situation, work situation, or friendships may be necessary to decrease availability of drugs and alcohol and to reduce peer pressure to use drugs and alcohol. For patients with severe dependence and few social supports, halfway houses, therapeutic communities, and other residential treatment situations may be useful. Individual and group counseling can be useful for understanding the role of drugs in an individual's life, improving self-esteem, and

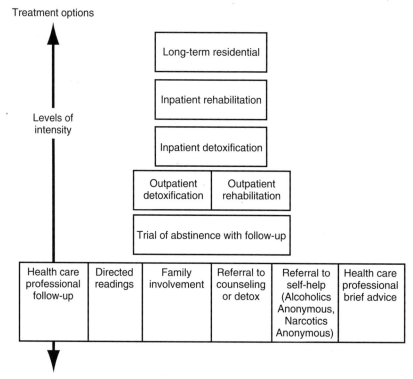

Figure 50–1. Levels of alcoholism treatment. (From Project ADEPT, vol 1. Providence, RI, Brown University Center for Alcohol and Addiction Studies, 1987.)

providing alternative coping skills for relieving psychological distress and for avoiding drugs and alcohol. The identification and treatment of underlying psychiatric or medical illness may reduce the impetus for self-medication. Twelve-step programs such as those of Alcoholics Anonymous (AA) and Narcotics Anonymous (NA) and Al-Anon and other self-help groups such as Rational Recovery can provide effective treatment, education, emotional support, and hope.[7]

Most patients presenting for treatment do so in a family structure, which is usually also experiencing dysfunction. It is important for clinicians to be aware of dysfunctional family dynamics and the denial, defensiveness, and hostility often present in family members. Family members need education and emotional and social support. Self-help organizations such as Al-Anon and Alateen also may provide meaningful education and support for spouses and family members. It is important to involve family members in a patient's treatment as much as possible and to recommend treatment for other family members when appropriate.

Treatment of Alcohol Intoxication

Although alcohol is generally considered to be a sedative drug, it also possesses stimulant effects and may produce behavioral disinhibition and confusion, resulting in agitation or even violent behavior. Also, alcoholics may have significant medical or psychiatric problems that complicate their presentation. A complete medical evaluation, including laboratory studies, should be conducted to rule out complicating problems. Illnesses such as liver disease, pancreatitis, gastrointestinal bleeding, head trauma, seizures, renal and electrolyte abnormalities, heart disease, and pulmonary disease should be assessed and appropriately treated. Patients presenting with extremely high blood alcohol levels (>400 mg/dl) are particularly at risk for complications and need careful assessment.

The treatment of uncomplicated alcohol intoxication is essentially supportive: support vital functions, maintain physiological homeostasis, and manage behavioral problems. Minimally intoxicated patients need a safe environment, behavioral and emotional support, and observation if they have a history of behavioral or medical problems due to alcohol. Severely intoxicated individuals may need life support measures because of the respiratory suppressant effects of alcohol. Unruly or agitated individuals may respond to reassurance, a structured setting, and low sensory input. However, patients who are potentially violent, dangerous to themselves or others, or actively suicidal require restraint, isolation, and a safe setting. If chemical restraint with sedatives or neuroleptics is required, these medications must be carefully titrated in an already intoxicated individual to prevent oversedation.

Patients using alcohol should be hydrated and should *always* be medicated with thiamine and other vitamin B supplements to prevent the development of Wernicke-Korsakoff syndrome. This condition is characterized by ocular disturbances (nystagmus and sixth-nerve ophthalmoplegia), ataxia, and mental status changes, although most patients do not have the full triad of signs. The cause is primarily thiamine deficiency. Its presence should be considered a medical emergency, because delay in treatment diminishes its reversibility. Although low doses of oral thiamine probably are effective, most patients are administered 25 to 100 mg of thiamine intramuscularly daily for 3 days to ensure proper dosing.

Treatment of Alcohol Withdrawal

Detoxification may be defined as removal of a drug in a manner that minimizes signs and symptoms of withdrawal. Detoxification can occur in both inpatient and outpatient treatment settings. The determination of the level of treatment to be used in detoxification should depend on the expected severity of withdrawal and the presence of past and present medical and psychiatric complications.

The alcohol withdrawal syndrome is defined as a state of increased neuronal activity in the central and peripheral nervous systems that follows the cessation of chronic alcohol use or a reduction in use. The range of signs and symptoms constitutes a continuum from mild (tremor and insomnia) to severe (autonomic hyperactivity, seizures, delirium, and general physiological dysregulation).[8] Most alcohol-dependent individuals can taper or stop alcohol use and develop only minor withdrawal signs and symptoms. Studies suggest that approximately 5% of alcohol-dependent individuals undergoing detoxification develop severe withdrawal delirium (delirium tremens). Studies conducted before the 1930s suggested that the mortality of severe alcohol withdrawal was as high as 50%, although current sources quote much lower mortality figures of 5%.[9] For those patients who do not develop delirium tremens, alcohol withdrawal still may be associated with various serious medical complications, including seizures, pneumonia and other infections, myocardial infarction, cardiac arrhythmias, electrolyte disturbances, and serious physiological derangements, including hypertension, tachycardia, tremors, agitation, insomnia, and so forth.[10]

Physical dependence on alcohol and the alcohol withdrawal syndrome are due to compensatory central nervous system (CNS) changes in response to a chronically administered depressant substance (ethanol). Studies of the physiology of alcohol dependence and withdrawal suggest that the CNS effects of alcohol may be mediated through modification of neurotransmitter signal-transduction mechanisms involving inhibitory GABA receptors and excitatory NMDA receptors.[11] Alcohol modifies the binding of GABA to its receptors and augments the electrophysiological and behavioral effects of GABA.[12] Alcohol also appears to have effects on the binding of other sedative drugs to the GABA receptor–chloride channel complex, presumably by dissolving in the membrane and altering its fluidity.[13, 14] In the case of NMDA receptors, acute low doses of ethanol cause NMDA receptor inhibition, and chronic ethanol use results in an increase in the number of these excitatory receptors. Alcohol also affects other neurotransmitters, including norepinephrine, serotonin, opioids, dopamine, and adenosine.

Treatment of the alcohol withdrawal syndrome includes correction of physiological abnormalities, hydration, nutritional support, and pharmacological therapy for the increased activity of the nervous system.[15] Patients who present with high blood alcohol levels need careful observation. Clinicians should be aware that signs and symptoms of withdrawal may obscure an underlying illness. For example, fever and change in mental status associated with withdrawal may coexist with an infection or head trauma. All patients who are experiencing significant withdrawal should have a complete physical examination and laboratory work, including pregnancy testing in women of childbearing age. Because many alcoholics also use other psychoactive substances in addition to alcohol, toxicological screening should be performed to identify other substance addiction and dependence, because these may complicate treatment. It is important to obtain as detailed a past history of alcohol withdrawal

complications as possible. The previous occurrence of withdrawal seizures or delirium tremens is predictive of an increased chance of recurrence of these complications. Elderly alcoholics appear to experience more cognitive impairment, weakness, and hypertension than younger patients.[16]

Table 50–1 lists several general methods that can be used in treating drug and alcohol withdrawal. These are described next.

TREATMENT OF ALCOHOL WITHDRAWAL WITH ETHANOL

Many alcoholics detoxify themselves using a gradual reduction in the amount of alcohol that they drink. Tapering oral or intravenous ethanol has occasionally been used in medical settings. Intravenous ethanol as a 5% solution and beer or brandy persist as medications on hospital formularies. However, given the short half-life of ethanol, the difficulty in titrating ethanol blood levels, and the therapeutic contradiction between administering alcohol and promoting abstinence, this method should not be used in treatment settings.

TREATMENT OF ALCOHOL WITHDRAWAL WITH CROSS-TOLERANT SEDATIVE AGENTS

Many pharmacological agents have historically been observed to reduce the signs and symptoms of the withdrawal syndrome. In particular, it has long been observed that administration of depressant medications during alcohol withdrawal markedly attenuates the signs and symptoms of withdrawal and greatly reduces the medical morbidity and mortality. Medications used to treat withdrawal have included alcohol, chloral derivatives, paraldehyde, barbiturates, antihistamines, neuroleptics, antidepressants, lithium, adrenergic blocking agents, and benzodiazepines.[17–19] Indeed, almost any CNS depressant substance may have efficacy in reducing alcohol withdrawal. Readers are referred to two excellent

Table 50–1. GENERAL METHODS OF DETOXIFICATION FROM ALCOHOL

Controlled administration of ethanol, with a slow decrease in ethanol level

Administration of a cross-tolerant sedative agent such as a benzodiazepine (chlordiazepoxide or diazepam) or a barbiturate

Administration of an alternate agent to suppress signs and symptoms of withdrawal (clonidine or atenolol)

Nonpharmacological detoxification, with supportive care

articles that review the pharmacological treatment of alcohol withdrawal and alcoholism.[1, 20]

Today, benzodiazepine derivatives are the treatment of choice for the alcohol withdrawal syndrome, and their efficacy is well established by double-blind controlled studies.[21] Benzodiazepines are superior to other agents because of their high degree of effectiveness, low toxicity, and anticonvulsant effects. Studies suggest that benzodiazepines are optimally used when the dose is titrated according to a withdrawal severity scale such as the Clinical Institute Withdrawal Assessment for Alcohol (CIWA-A) scale.[22, 23] Several methods have been described for titrating medication dosage to symptoms. The benzodiazepine loading method appears to have utility in many patients.[21] The advantages of this method include matching dose of medication to an individual patient's tolerance and avoiding cumulative pharmacokinetics. During this procedure, patients receive an initial oral or intravenous dose of a long-half-life benzodiazepine (10 to 20 mg of diazepam or 50 to 100 mg chlordiazepoxide), repeated every hour until the patient is sedated, develops nystagmus, or has a significant decrease in withdrawal signs and symptoms as shown by a reduced withdrawal scale score.

The vast majority of patients treated in this way respond within several hours with a marked reduction in withdrawal signs and symptoms. Many patients require no additional medication for the duration of their detoxification, presumably because of the long half-life of the drugs. Patients may occasionally require additional doses of medication after several days, to suppress emergent symptoms. During the period of benzodiazepine loading, patients must be closely observed to avoid undermedication or overmedication. In particular, close attention must be paid to patients with respiratory, cardiovascular, or hepatic disease. In patients receiving adrenergic blocking drugs, some signs of withdrawal such as hypertension, tachycardia, and tremor may be obscured.

Some clinicians prefer using shorter-half-life benzodiazepines, such as oxazepam or lorazepam, for detoxification. Because these medications have a shorter duration of action, they pose less chance of overmedication, particularly in the elderly or in patients with compromised hepatic function.

Gamma-hydroxybutyrate (GHB) is a sedative, GABA analogue that has been used successfully in Europe for the treatment of alcohol withdrawal and dependence.[24]

Alcoholics are frequently hypomagnesemic and require magnesium replacement. Magnesium levels should always be determined as part of the laboratory screening, and plasma magnesium levels found to be less than 2.0 mEq/L should be treated with oral or parenteral replacement. Magnesium at high doses has sedative and anticonvulsant effects and has been used to treat alcohol withdrawal. Magnesium is also effective for the CNS hyperactivity occurring in preecclampsia/ecclampsia. The sedative effects of magnesium may be due to an inhibitory action at the excitatory NMDA receptor ion channel.[11]

THE USE OF ALTERNATE AGENTS FOR WITHDRAWAL

Other pharmacological agents such as beta-adrenergic blocking drugs, anticonvulsants, and antipsychotics often are administered to control alcohol withdrawal symptoms. Carbamazepine appears effective in reducing most signs and symptoms of alcohol and other sedative withdrawal.[25] Patients receive 200 to 400 mg of carbamazepine in divided doses the first day and 400 to 600 mg thereafter, with the dose adjusted to achieve therapeutic (anticonvulsant) blood levels. Therapeutic carbamazepine blood levels are maintained for 10 days to 2 weeks, and then the medication is tapered and discontinued.

The major side effects of carbamazepine include sedation, ataxia, and hematological abnormalities. Using a lower dose on the first day of treatment and then increasing the dose subsequently appears to reduce the initial sedative side effects. Blood levels of carbamazepine can be accurately measured 2 to 3 days after a dose adjustment. The hematological side effects include a dose-dependent lowering of white blood cell count and idiosyncratic agranulocytosis. A complete blood count should be performed before starting carbamazepine and at weekly intervals thereafter. The medication should be discontinued in patients with a white blood cell count less than 3000/ mm^3.

During alcohol withdrawal, adrenergic activity increases as a result of increased autonomic nervous system activity and increased sensitivity of beta-adrenergic receptors.[26] Beta-adrenergic blocker drugs such as propranolol and atenolol, which reduce this activity, have been used successfully as primary agents in the treatment of alcohol withdrawal.[15] However, beta blockers are most effective in reduction of peripheral autonomic signs of withdrawal and less so for CNS signs such as delirium or seizures. The drugs are particularly useful for controlling tachycardia and hypertension, especially in patients with coronary disease. The dose of the beta blocker is titrated to symptoms, with an effective dose reducing autonomic signs without producing significant side effects. Major side effects of beta blockers include hypotension, sleep disturbance, and fatigue. Beta blockers may be safely combined with benzodiazepines.

Several studies have reported that the alpha-2-adrenergic agonist clonidine hydrochloride suppresses many of the autonomic signs and symptoms of alcohol and opioid withdrawal. However, because clonidine does not have anticonvulsant activity, patients may still be at risk for withdrawal seizures. Clonidine is thought to act at presynaptic noradrenergic nerve endings in the locus caeruleus of the brain and blocks the adrenergic discharge that occurs during drug and alcohol withdrawal.[27, 28] Clonidine has been reported as effective for suppressing opioid withdrawal after discontinuation of opioids in dependent patients.[29-31] In the treatment of alcohol withdrawal, clonidine is probably best used to control autonomic hyperactivity, as an adjunct to other medications, such as benzodiazepines. An effective dose is usually 0.3 to 0.6 mg daily, in three divided doses, titrated to symptoms and to blood pressure. The major side effects of clonidine are hypotension and sedation.

Neuroleptic medications such as haloperidol are useful for the treatment of hallucinosis and paranoid symptoms that can occur during withdrawal. Although neuroleptic medications by themselves have been shown to be effective in reducing withdrawal signs and symptoms, they can reduce the seizure threshold and are usually used in combination with other medications, such as benzodiazepines. Usually 1 to 5 mg of haloperidol twice daily for several days controls psychotic symptoms. If psychotic symptoms persist past this time, a psychiatric evaluation should be conducted to determine whether a patient has a comorbid psychiatric illness.

Controversy surrounds the use of anticonvulsant medications to control withdrawal seizures. Single seizures do not require anticonvulsant treatment; for patients who have multiple seizures during withdrawal or who have a chronic seizure disorder, anticonvulsants such as phenytoin may be useful. Because many alcoholics are noncompliant with treatment, the erratic use of anticonvulsants on an outpatient basis may actually worsen a seizure problem.[32]

NONPHARMACOLOGICAL METHODS FOR ALCOHOL DETOXIFICATION

The widespread use of pharmacological agents in the detoxification from alcohol has been called into question. Alcohol treatment facilities have been experimenting with social setting detoxification, a nondrug method. This procedure relies on the extensive use of peer and group support and usually occurs in nonmedical settings. This method seems effective in reducing withdrawal signs and symptoms, without an increased incidence of medical complications. Some questions have been raised about the possible bias in selection of healthier patients for detoxification in these nonmedical settings. Shaw and colleagues[33] have shown that even within a medical setting, most patients respond to supportive care and do not require pharmacological intervention. In a double-blind study comparing parenteral diazepam treatment with placebo, more than half the patients receiving a placebo injection responded with marked attenuation of withdrawal symptoms within 5 hours.[21] British practitioners routinely detoxify most alcohol-dependent patients as outpatients, with minimal use of psychotropic drugs.[34]

Thus, the available evidence suggests that many alcohol-dependent individuals may be detoxified with minimal use of sedatives or other psychotropic drugs. However, some researchers have expressed concerns that repeated episodes of even mild alcohol withdrawal may sensitize patients to experiencing more severe withdrawal in the future through kindling effect.[35] Judicious use of sedative medications to minimize symptoms could protect against this process. This hypothesis needs to be more carefully studied. Nevertheless, a subgroup of patients apparently do require careful monitoring and pharmacological treatment during the withdrawal process. A history of delirium tremens or seizures or the presence of medical or psychiatric comorbidities increases the need for closer medical supervision. However, few data are available for clinicians to use to predict which alcohol-dependent patients have an absolute requirement for pharmacological treatment. The existence of predictive data would optimize clinical care for patients and reduce the cost of care, because patients who do not require drug administration within a hospital setting may be detoxified out of hospital at lower cost.

During and after detoxification, many alcoholic patients appear to suffer from major or minor depression. Some mood disturbances are directly related to alcohol or resolve within several weeks of detoxification. Major depressive symptoms persisting beyond this time should be considered for treatment with antidepressants. Patients previously known to have recurrent mood disorders or family histories of mood disorders may be treated immediately after detoxification if mood symptoms are severe.

Rehabilitation and Long-Term Treatment

The goals of long-term treatment include maintaining a state of abstinence from alcohol. Psychological, family, and social interventions help to maintain this recovery. Continued abstinence is best achieved through patients' participation in a comprehensive treatment program, beginning during the initial detoxification phase. The task of patients in recovery is to develop skills to avoid alcohol, better methods of coping with stress, and improved self-esteem and self-efficacy. A wide range of treatment options and treatment intensities are available, although today, the specific treatment modalities to be used may be dictated by a patient's insurance coverage. The spectrum of treatment ranges from outpatient psychotherapy and counseling to more intensive residential treatment. Attending self-help groups such as AA and Rational Recovery should be suggested for all patients.

Pharmacological treatment can be used to assist rehabilitation. Pharmacotherapies may reduce drug craving, lessen protracted withdrawal symptoms, or decrease positive reinforcing effects of the drugs. Pharmacotherapies can also treat comorbid psychiatric disorders that provide part of the impetus for drinking. However, it should be emphasized that the use of pharmacotherapies should be part of a comprehensive treatment plan and integrated into that plan. Types of pharmacotherapies used in long-term treatment and rehabilitation are listed in Table 50-2.

MAINTENANCE SEDATIVE MEDICATIONS IN ALCOHOLISM

The use of maintenance pharmacological agents to reduce drinking and to prevent relapse has a long history and is controversial. In the past, some alcoholics were maintained on daily doses of benzodiazepines, barbiturates, or other sedatives in a poorly monitored

Table 50-2. PHARMACOTHERAPIES USED IN LONG-TERM TREATMENT

Sedative maintenance treatment with a cross-tolerant sedative agent such as a benzodiazepine; used historically, not currently used
Aversive therapy—disulfiram
Administration of an alternate agent, such as naltrexone, to suppress craving and effects of alcohol
Pharmacotherapy of comorbid psychiatric disorders, such as schizophrenia

and uncontrolled manner. This uncontrolled use frequently led to deleterious consequences, including the development of benzodiazepine dependence or combined alcohol and benzodiazepine dependence. At present, the use of benzodiazepines or other sedatives for maintenance treatment is strongly discouraged by most addiction professionals.

AVERSIVE THERAPY—DISULFIRAM

Disulfiram (Antabuse) is an irreversible inhibitor of the enzyme acetaldehyde dehydrogenase and is used as an adjunctive treatment in selected alcoholics. Figure 50-2 shows the site of action of disulfiram. Disulfiram was originally used as a chemical in the rubber industry, and its effect on alcohol intoxication was discovered serendipitously by workers who were exposed to the chemical and then consumed alcohol. If alcohol is consumed in the presence of this drug, the toxic metabolite acetaldehyde accumulates in the body, producing tachycardia, flushing of skin, intense diaphoresis, dyspnea, nausea, and vomiting. Hypotension, cardiac problems, and death may occur if large amounts of alcohol are consumed after ingesting of disulfiram. The presence of this unpleasant reaction provides a strong deterrent to the consumption of alcohol for some alcoholic patients.[36] A double-blind treatment study comparing the effectiveness of disulfiram with placebo found the medication most effective for those who believed in its efficacy and who remained compliant with treatment.[37] Direct supervision of disulfiram consumption has been shown to increase its effectiveness.[38] A few professional groups have questioned whether the toxicity of disulfiram justifies its therapeutic use under any circumstances.

Disulfiram is available in 250-mg tablets, and the usual dose is 250 mg once daily. Daily doses of 125 to 500 mg are sometimes used, depending on side effects and patient's response. Disulfiram is best used in conjunction with ongoing psychosocial treatment for alco-

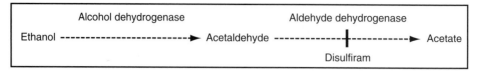

Figure 50–2. Effect of disulfiram on alcohol metabolism.

holism. The optimal duration of treatment is unknown. Most patients use the medication for brief periods of high risk of relapse; however, some patients use the medication continuously for years. Some clinicians administer an alcohol challenge—a small dose of alcohol—to all their patients receiving disulfiram. The disulfiram-alcohol reaction that develops is thought to provide an excellent deterrent to future alcohol drinking.

Because the disulfiram-alcohol reaction can be severe, patients started on disulfiram must be informed about the dangers of even small amounts of alcohol. Alcohol present in foods, shaving lotion, mouthwashes, or over-the-counter medications may produce a disulfiram reaction. Disulfiram may have interactions with other medications, notably anticoagulants and phenytoin. It is contraindicated in patients with severe liver disease. A complete blood count and liver function tests should be performed before starting disulfiram therapy and periodically during treatment.

BLOCKADE OF CRAVING—NALTREXONE AND OTHER OPIOID ANTAGONISTS

The opioid neurotransmitter system has been strongly implicated in mediating certain aspects of ethanol consumption. Animals administered μ-opioid agonists, such as morphine, typically increase alcohol consumption.[39] Humans receiving chronic opioids as methadone maintenance also appear to increase their alcohol drinking. Furthermore, although opioid agonists seem to increase ethanol consumption, opioid antagonists have the opposite effect. Animal studies reported by Froelich and colleagues,[40] George and associates,[41] and Volpicelli and coworkers[42] indicated that μ-opioid receptor antagonists reduce alcohol consumption.

Two laboratories have conducted controlled clinical trials with the opioid antagonist naltrexone in recently abstinent alcoholics. O'Malley and colleagues[43] compared double-blind naltrexone with placebo in 97 alcoholics receiving supportive therapy or coping skills therapy for a 12-week period. They found that the naltrexone-treated subjects had lower rates

of relapse to heavy drinking, consumed fewer drinks per drinking day, and had lower dropout than did the placebo group. Volpicelli and associates[44] conducted a 12-week double-blind placebo-controlled outpatient naltrexone trial with 70 male alcohol-dependent patients. They found that the group treated with naltrexone had a lower relapse rate, fewer drinking days, longer time to relapse, and greater success in coping with a drinking relapse. Subjects in the naltrexone group also reported decreased craving during the medication trial. In both studies, naltrexone-treated subjects consumed fewer drinks per drinking day. These findings suggest that subjects in both the placebo and naltrexone groups sampled alcohol, but the naltrexone-treated patients were less likely to continue to drink.

O'Malley's and Volpicelli's initial clinical studies have now been supported by other researchers. Bohn and coworkers[45] conducted a single-blind study with two doses of naltrexone in abstinent alcoholics and found reduced drinking. Mason and colleagues[46] at the University of Miami conducted a pilot study with a related opioid antagonist, nalmefene, and also found increased abstinence in the medication group. Swift and associates[47] conducted a double-blind placebo-controlled study of the effects of naltrexone on alcohol intoxication in nonalcoholic social drinkers and found less positive reinforcement and more intense sedative effects when the subjects received naltrexone and alcohol than placebo and alcohol.

On the basis of these positive treatment results, the Food and Drug Administration (FDA) approved naltrexone (ReVia) as an adjunct in the treatment of alcoholism. The usual dose of naltrexone is 50 mg/day, although doses of 25 to 100 mg/day have been reported to be effective. Naltrexone should be used only in the context of a comprehensive alcoholism treatment program, which includes counseling and other psychosocial therapies. The most common side effects include anxiety, sedation, and nausea in approximately 10% of patients. Hepatic toxicity with use of the drug is also a potential issue. High doses of naltrexone (300 mg/day) have been associated with hepatotoxicity. No deleterious hepatic effects were observed in the clinical studies performed using a 50-mg/day dose of naltrexone. However, naltrexone should probably be avoided by patients with hepatitis or severe liver disease. It is recommended that liver functions be monitored before naltrexone treatment and periodically thereafter.

The mechanism of action of naltrexone in reducing alcohol consumption is unknown. Wise and Bozarth[48] hypothesize that the reinforcement and dependence-producing properties of several drugs, including ethanol, are mediated through dopamine in the nucleus accumbens of the brain. Ethanol increases dopamine turnover in the nucleus accumbens. Benjamin and colleagues[49] report that naltrexone and other opioid antagonists block the ethanol-induced release of dopamine. The reduced dopamine release due to naltrexone would be associated with less psychomotor stimulation and positive reinforcement due to ethanol and may thus result in decreased ethanol intake.

Lukas and Mendelson[50] hypothesize that certain euphoric mood effects of ethanol are increased and that general stress is decreased through these endocrine hormones. Ethanol consumption is associated with activation of the hypothalamic-pituitary-adrenal axis and release of adrenocorticotropic hormone (ACTH), beta-endorphin, and glucocorticoids. Acute administration of opioid antagonists such as naltrexone also activates the hypothalamic-pituitary-adrenal axis and produces increases in ACTH, cortisol, and beta-endorphin.

SEROTONERGIC MEDICATIONS

Manipulations that augment central serotonergic function appear to reduce ethanol consumption in animals and humans. Serotonergic agonists, such as D-fenfluramine, which release serotonin (5HT) from neurons, have also been reported to decrease ethanol consumption in rats.[51]

Buspirone (Buspar) is a nonbenzodiazepine anxiolytic medication that has partial agonist activity at the 5HT-1a receptor and 5HT-2 receptor, as well as having dopamine-2 receptor antagonist activity. Buspirone reduces alcohol consumption in alcohol-drinking rats and may reduce drinking in alcoholic patients, particularly those with anxiety disorders.[52-54] In a study of 50 alcoholic subjects in treatment, Bruno[53] found reduced drinking, less craving, and improved social and psychological status in the patients receiving buspirone, in comparison with those receiving placebo. A double-

blind placebo-controlled trial of study of buspirone versus placebo in 61 anxious alcoholics also receiving behavioral therapy found that buspirone treatment was associated with less drinking and less anxiety in those completing the study.[54] However, a double-blind placebo-controlled study of buspirone in 67 anxious alcoholics found little effect of the medication, compared with placebo.[55] In this study, the patients were more ill and the response rate to placebo was higher, and thus the effects of the medication may have been obscured.

Selective serotonin reuptake inhibitors (SSRIs), such as fluoxetine (Prozac) and sertraline (Zoloft), zimeldine, and citalopram, which augment serotonergic function, also appear to reduce alcohol consumption in animals[56] and humans.[57, 58] In several different animal models of alcohol consumption, pretreatment with various SSRIs reduces alcohol intake.[59] Several human studies of heavy drinkers found SSRIs to reduce overall alcohol consumption by small but significant amounts (approximately 15% to 20%).[57, 58] Other studies have yielded less impressive results. A 3-week prospective study by Gorelick[60] on the effects of fluoxetine on drinking found reductions in alcohol intake during the first week only. A recent double-blind fluoxetine-placebo study on relapse to drinking, in which both groups received cognitive-behavioral psychotherapy, found no difference between groups.[61] In placebo-controlled outpatient trials with alcohol-dependent patients, SSRIs decreased desire and liking for alcohol.[62] At least in the case of fluoxetine, the drug does not appear to alter ethanol pharmacokinetics.[63]

Two serotonin antagonist medications have been reported as efficacious in reducing alcohol consumption in animals and humans. Ritanserin, a 5HT-2 receptor antagonist, has been reported to reduce alcohol consumption in animals and humans.[51, 64, 65] 5HT-3 receptor antagonists are marketed as antiemetics, for the treatment of chemotherapy-induced nausea in cancer patients. These antiemetic drugs, including ondansetron, zacopride, and ICS 250-930, also reduce ethanol consumption in ethanol-drinking rats.[51, 64, 65] Johnson and colleagues[66] reported that ondansetron reduced the euphoric effects of alcohol in nonalcoholic human subjects tested in a laboratory setting. An outpatient trial with male alcohol abusers treated with ondansetron found low oral doses of ondansetron to reduce alcohol consumption.[67] These medications are currently being tested in clinical trials with alcoholic patients.

In several studies, lithium carbonate has been found to reduce alcohol consumption in animal models and in some patients.[51, 68] In laboratory studies, lithium blocks the intoxicating effects of alcohol in human social drinkers.[69] However, a double-blind placebo-controlled study of 457 alcoholics stratified for depression found no significant improvement in drinking due to lithium.[70] A review of the published controlled and uncontrolled clinical studies of lithium in the treatment of alcoholism concluded that lithium was not an effective treatment of affective disorders in alcoholics and does not reduce alcohol intake or decrease craving in nondepressed patients.[71]

Thus, although considerable neurochemical evidence points to involvement of the 5HT system of the brain in the subjective and behavioral effects of ethanol, including discrimination, reinforcement, and consumption, the effects of serotonergic medications appear to be only modest in reducing alcohol consumption in alcoholics. Data on agents such as lithium and buspirone are equivocal. In patients with comorbid major depression and alcohol dependence, in whom SSRI antidepressants would be expected to have the greatest effect, no well-controlled double-blind studies have been conducted.

OTHER AGENTS

Acamprosate (calcium acetylhomotaurine) is a structural analogue of GABA that appears to have agonist activity at GABA receptors[72, 73] and inhibitory activity at NMDA receptors.[74] Acamprosate reduces alcohol consumption in several animal models of alcoholism.[75] In two European clinical trials involving alcoholic human subjects, acamprosate reduced relapse drinking and craving for alcohol and had minimal side effects.[76, 77] Acamprosate is not yet available for clinical treatment, but the initial results with this agent appear quite promising.

Affective disorders, especially major depression, are frequently associated with alcohol dependence. Several investigators have studied antidepressant agents in depressed alcoholics. Mason and Kocsis[78] conducted a double-blind placebo-controlled trial of the tricyclic antidepressant desipramine in 42 recently abstinent alcoholics. The patients were stratified according to the presence of current depression. Depressed subjects receiving desipramine had improved depression, compared with placebo. There were no significant differences in sobriety between the groups, although there was a trend for desipramine-treated subjects to re-

main sober for a longer period. In an open antidepressant trial with imipramine in alcoholics with major depression or dysthymia, Nunes and colleagues[79] reported improved mood and decreased drinking in those who completed the trial. An open trial of fluoxetine in 12 depressed suicidal alcoholics showed decreased depression and alcohol consumption, compared with pretreatment.[80]

Summary

Pharmacological agents are important adjuncts in the treatment of alcohol withdrawal; they reduce withdrawal signs and symptoms and medical morbidity. Several pharmacological agents have shown efficacy as adjuncts in the treatment of alcohol dependence by decreasing drinking and reducing relapse in patients in rehabilitation treatment. Pharmacological agents should always be used as adjuncts in treatment, as part of a comprehensive treatment program that addresses the psychological, social, and spiritual needs of patients.

REFERENCES

1. Litten RZ, Allen JP: Pharmacotherapies for alcoholism: Promising agents and clinical issues. Alcohol Clin Exp Res 15(4):620–633, 1991.
2. Clark WD: Alcoholism: Blocks to diagnosis and treatment. Am J Med 71:275–285, 1981.
3. American Psychiatric Association: Diagnostic and Statistical Manual of Mental Disorders, 4th ed. Washington, DC, American Psychiatric Association, 1994.
4. Holden C: The neglected disease in medical education. Science 229:741–742, 1985.
5. Kennedy W: Chemical dependency: A treatable disease. Ohio State Med J 71:77–79, 1985.
6. American Society of Addiction Medicine (ASAM): Patient Placement Criteria, Psychoactive Substance Use Disorders. Chicago, ASAM, 1993.
7. Emrick CD: Alcoholics Anonymous: Affiliation processes and effectiveness as treatment. Alcoholism 11:416–423, 1987.
8. Gross M, Lewis E, Hastey J: Acute alcohol withdrawal syndrome. In Kissin B, Begleiter H (eds): The Biology of Alcoholism, vol 3. New York, Plenum, 1974.
9. Lewis DC, Gomolin IH: Emergency treatment of drug and alcohol intoxication and withdrawal. Brown University Program in Alcoholism and Drug Abuse Medical Monograph II. Providence, RI, Brown University.
10. McIntosh I: Alcohol-related disabilities in general hospital patients: A critical assessment of the evidence. Int J Addict 17:609–639, 1982.
11. Hoffman PL, Rabe CS, Grant KA, et al: Ethanol and the NMDA receptor. Alcohol 7:229–231, 1990.
12. Hunt WA: The effect of ethanol on GABAergic transmission. Neurosci Biobehav Rev 7:87–95, 1983.
13. Seeman P: Membrane effects of anesthetics and tranquilizers. Pharmacol Rev 24:583–655, 1972.
14. Skolnick P, Moncada V, Barker J, Paul SM: Pentobarbi-

tal: Dual action to increase brain benzodiazepine receptor affinity. Science 211:1448–1450, 1981.

15. Sellers EM, Kalant H: Drug therapy: Alcohol intoxication and withdrawal. N Engl J Med 294:757–752, 1976.

16. Brower KJ, Mudd S, Blow FC, et al: Severity and treatment of alcohol withdrawal in elderly versus younger patients. Alcohol Clin Exp Res 18:196–201, 1994.

17. Golbert TM, Sanz CJ, Rose HD, Leitschuh TH: Comparative evaluation of treatments of alcohol withdrawal syndromes. JAMA 201:113–116, 1967.

18. Palestine ML, Alatorre E: Control of acute alcoholic withdrawal symptoms: A comparative study of haloperidol and chlordiazepoxide. Curr Ther Res 20:289–299, 1976.

19. Sellers EM, Kalant H: Drug therapy: Alcohol intoxication and withdrawal. N Engl J Med 294:757–762, 1976.

20. Liskow BI, Goodwin DW: Pharmacological treatment of alcohol intoxication, withdrawal and dependence: A critical review. J Stud Alcohol 48:356–370, 1987.

21. Sellers EM, Narango CA, Harrison M, et al: Diazepam loading: Simplified treatment for alcohol withdrawal. Clin Pharmacol Ther 6:822–827, 1983.

22. Foy A, March S, Drinkwater V: Use of an objective clinical scale in the assessment and management of alcohol withdrawal in a large general hospital. Alcohol Clin Exp Res 12:360–364, 1988.

23. Saitz R, Mayo-Smith MF, Roberts MS, et al: Individualized treatment for alcohol withdrawal: A randomized double-blind clinical trial. JAMA 272:519–523, 1994.

24. Gallimberti L, Ferri M, Ferrara SD, et al: Gamma-hydroxybutyric acid in the treatment of alcohol dependence. Alcohol Clin Exp Res 16(4):673–676, 1992.

25. Malcolm R, Ballenger JC, Sturgis ET, Anton R: Double blind controlled trial comparing carbamazepine to oxazepam treatment of alcohol withdrawal. Am J Psychiatry 146(5):617–621, 1989.

26. Swift RM, DePetrillo P: Human leukocyte beta-adrenergic stimulated cyclic AMP in ethanol intoxication and withdrawal. Alcohol Clin Exp Res 14(1):58–62, 1990.

27. Aghajanian GK: Tolerance of locus ceruleus neurons to morphine and inhibition of withdrawal response by clonidine. Nature 276:186–188, 1976.

28. Gold MS, Redmond DE Jr, Kleber HD: Noradrenergic hyperactivity in opiate withdrawal supressed by clonidine. Am J Psychiatry 136:100–102, 1979.

29. Gold MS, Pottash AC, Sweeney DR, Kleber HD: Opiate withdrawal using clonidine: A safe effective and rapid non-opiate treatment. JAMA 243(4):343–346, 1979.

30. Charney DS, Sternberg DE, Kleber HD, et al: Clinical use of clonidine in abrupt withdrawal from methadone. Arch Gen Psychiatry 38:1273–1278, 1981.

31. Washton AM, Resnick RB: Clonidine for opiate detoxification: Outpatient clinical trials. J Clin Psychiatry 43:39–41, 1981.

32. Hillbom ME, Hjelm-Jager M: Should alcohol withdrawal seizures be treated with anti-epileptic drugs? Acta Neurol Scand 69:39–42, 1984.

33. Shaw JM, Kolesar GS, Sellers EM, et al: Development of optimal treatment tactics for alcohol withdrawal: Assessment and effectiveness of supportive care. J Clin Psychopharmacol 1:382–387, 1981.

34. Whitfield CL, Thompson G, Lamb A, et al: Detoxification of 1024 alcoholic patients without psychoactive drugs. JAMA 239:1409–1410, 1978.

35. Fuller RK, Gordis E: Editorial on pharmacologic treatment of alcohol withdrawal. JAMA 272:557–558, 1994.

36. Keventus J, Major LF: Disulfiram in the treatment of alcoholism. Q J Stud Alcohol 40:428–446, 1979.

37. Fuller RK, Branchley L, Brightwell DR, et al: Disul-

38. Brewer C: Recent developments in disulfiram treatment. Alcohol Alcohol 28(4):383–395, 1993.

39. Reid LD, Hubbell CL: Excess of drinking related to excess activity of opioid systems. Alcohol 4:149–168, 1987.

40. Froelich JC, Harts J, Lumeng L, Li TK: Naloxone attenuates voluntary ethanol intake in rats selectively bred for high ethanol preference. Pharmacol Biochem Behav 35(2):385–390, 1990.

41. George SR, Roldan L, Lui A, Naranjo CA: Endogenous opioids are involved in genetically determined high preference for alcohol consumption. Alcohol Clin Exp Res 15:668–672, 1991.

42. Volpicelli J, Davis M, Olgin J: Naltrexone blocks the post-shock increase of ethanol consumption. Life Sci 38:841–847, 1986.

43. O'Malley SS, Jaffee AJ, Chang G, et al: Naltrexone and coping skills therapy for alcohol dependence. Arch Gen Psychiatry 49:881–887, 1992.

44. Volpicelli JR, Alterman AI, Hayashida M, O'Brien CP: Naltrexone in the treatment of alcohol dependence. Arch Gen Psychiatry 49:876–880, 1992.

45. Bohn MJ, Kranzler HR, Beazoglou D, Stachler BA: Naltrexone and brief counseling to reduce heavy drinking. Am J Addict 3:91–99, 1994.

46. Mason BJ, Ritvo EC, Morgan RO, et al: A double-blind, placebo-controlled trial of nalmefene in the treatment of alcoholism. Alcohol Clin Exp Res 18(5):1162–1167, 1994.

47. Swift RM, Whelihan W, Kuznetsov O, et al: Naltrexone-induced alterations in human ethanol intoxication. Am J Psychiatry 151:1463–1467, 1994.

48. Wise R, Bozarth M: A psychomotor stimulant theory of addiction. Psychol Rev 94:469–492, 1987.

49. Benjamin D, Grant ER, Pohorecky LA: Naltrexone reverses ethanol-induced dopamine release in the nucleus accumbens in awake, freely moving rats. Brain Res 621:137–140, 1993.

50. Lukas SE, Mendelson JH: Electroencephalographic activity and plasma ACTH during ethanol-induced euphoria. Biol Psychiatry 23:141–148, 1988.

51. Sellers EM, Higgins GA, Tomkins DM: Serotonin receptor subtypes and alcohol consumption. Proceedings of American College of Neuropsychopharmacology, Annual Meeting, San Juan, Puerto Rico, December, 1991, p 84.

52. Collins DM, Myers RD: Buspirone attenuates volitional alcohol intake in the chronically drinking monkey. Alcohol 4:49–56, 1987.

53. Bruno F: Buspirone in the treatment of alcoholic patients. Psychopathology 22 (Suppl 1):49–59, 1989.

54. Kranzler H, Meyer R: An open trial of buspirone in alcoholics. J Psychopharmacol 9:379–380, 1989.

55. Malcolm R, Anton R, Randall CF, et al: A placebo-controlled trial of buspirone in anxious inpatient alcoholics. Alcohol Clin Exp Res 16:1007–1013, 1992.

56. Lawrin MO, Naranjo CA, Sellers EM: Identification and testing of new drugs for modulation of alcohol consumption. Psychopharmacol Bull 22:1020–1025, 1986.

57. Naranjo CA, Sellers EM, Roach CA, et al: Zimelidine-induced variations in alcohol intake by non-depressed heavy drinkers. Clin Pharmacol Ther 35:374–381, 1984.

58. Naranjo CA, Sellers EO, Sullivan JT, et al: The serotonin uptake inhibitor citalopram attenuates ethanol intake. Clin Pharmacol Ther 41:266–274, 1987.

59. Linnoila M, Eckardt M, Durcan M, et al: Interactions of serotonin with ethanol: Clinical and animal studies. Psychopharmacol Bull 23:452–457, 1987.

60. Gorelick DA: Serotonin uptake blockers and the treatment of alcoholism. Recent Dev Alcohol 6:267–279, 1989.
61. Kranzler HR, Burleson JA, Korner P, Del Boca, et al: Placebo-controlled trail of fluoxetine as an adjunct to relapse prevention in alcoholics. Am J Psychiatry 152(3):391–397, 1995.
62. Naranjo CA, Bremner KE: Serotonin uptake inhibitors decrease desirability, liking and consumption of alcohol. Proceedings of American College of Neuropsychopharmacology, Annual Meeting, San Juan, Puerto Rico, December, 1991, p 84.
63. Lemberger L, Rowe H, Bergstrom RF, et al: The effect of fluoxetine on psychomotor performance, physiologic response and kinetics of ethanol. Clin Pharmacol Ther 37:658–664, 1985.
64. Knapp DJ, Pohorecky LA: Zacopride, a 5HT3 receptor antagonist reduces voluntary ethanol consumption in rats. Pharmacol Biochem Behav 41:847–850, 1992.
65. Hodge CW, Samson HH, Lewis RS, Erickson HL: Specific decreases in ethanol but not water-reinforced responding produced by the 5-HT antagonist ICS 205-930. Alcohol 10(3):191–196, 1993.
66. Johnson BA, Campling GM, Griffiths P, Cowen PJ: Attenuation of some alcohol-induced mood changes and the desire to drink by 5HT$_3$ receptor blockade: A preliminary study in healthy male volunteers. Psychopharmacology 112:142–144, 1993.
67. Toneatto T, Romach MK, Sobell MK, et al: Ondansetron, a 5HT$_3$ antagonist reduces alcohol consumption in alcohol abusers. Alcohol Clin Exp Res 15:382, 1991.
68. Fawcett J, Clark DC, Aagesen CA, et al: A double-blind, placebo controlled trial of lithium carbonate therapy for alcoholism. Arch Gen Psychiatry 44:248–256, 1987.
69. Judd L, Hubbard R, Huey L, et al: Lithium carbonate and ethanol induced "highs" in normal subjects. Arch Gen Psychiatry 34:463–467, 1977.
70. Dorus W, Ostrow DG, Anton R, et al: Lithium treatment of depressed and nondepressed alcoholics. JAMA 262:1646–1652, 1989.
71. LeJoyeux M, Ades J: Evaluation of lithium treatment in alcoholism. Alcohol Alcohol 28(3):273–279, 1993.
72. Daoust M, Legrand E, Gewiss M, et al: Acomprosate modulates synaptosomal GABA transmission in chronically alcoholised rats. Pharmacol Biochem Behav 41(4):669–674, 1992.
73. Gewiss M, Heidbreder C, Opsomer L, et al: Acamprosate and diazepam differentially modulate alcohol-induced behavioral and cortical alterations in rats following chronic inhalation of ethanol vapor. Alcohol Alcohol 26(2):129–137, 1991.
74. Zeise ML, Kasparov S, Capogna M, Zieglgansberger W: Acamprosate (calciumacetylhomotaurine) decreases postsynaptic potentials in rat neocortex: Possible involvement of excitatory amino acid receptors. Eur J Pharmacol 231(1):47–52, 1993.
75. Nalpas B, Dabadie H, Parot P, Paccalin J: Acamprosate: From pharmacology to therapeutics. Encephale 16(3):175–179, 1990.
76. Lhuintre JP, Moore N, Tran G, et al: Acamprosate appears to decrease alcohol intaake in weaned alcoholics. Alcohol Alcohol 25(6):613–622, 1990.
77. Ladewig D, Knecht T, Leher P, Fendl A: Acamprosate—a stabilizing factor in long-term withdrawal of alcoholic patients. Ther Umsch 50(3):182–188, 1993.
78. Mason BJ, Kocsis JH: Desipramine treatment of alcoholism. Psychopharmacol Bull 27(2):155–161, 1991.
79. Nunes EV, McGrath PJ, Quitkin FM, et al: Imipramine treatment of alcoholism with co-morbid depression. Am J Psychiatry 150:963–965, 1993.
80. Cornelius JR, Salloum IM, Cornelius MD, et al: Fluoxetine trial in suicidal, depressed alcoholics. Psychopharmacol Bull 29:195–199, 1993.

Pharmacological Interventions for Withdrawal Syndromes Other Than Alcohol and Nicotine

William W. Weddington, MD

Clinicians in various settings (i.e., medical, obstetrical, surgical, psychiatric, or emergency room) are confronted with diagnosing and treating patients experiencing withdrawal from many addicting substances. Developments have been made in diagnosing substance withdrawal as well as delineating specific pharmacological interventions for withdrawal.

The purpose of this chapter is to describe substance-specific withdrawal syndromes and offer clinical pharmacological interventions for substance-dependent individuals who meet criteria for withdrawal from substances other than alcohol and nicotine. Specifically, pharmacological management strategies for withdrawal from opioids, sedative-hypnotics, and stimulants are described. Medications used for sedative-hypnotic withdrawal syndrome are usually cross-tolerant (i.e., benzodiazepines or barbiturates) with alcohol or are efficacious (i.e., carbamazepine) for alcohol withdrawal syndrome and thus intervene with concurrent alcohol withdrawal if administered in appropriate doses and frequencies.

It should be noted that withdrawal syndromes are not associated with the addicting substances cannabis, hallucinogens (LSD, mescaline, MDMA, and other compounds), inhalants, or phencyclidine.[1]

Criteria for Withdrawal Syndromes

Changes have been made in the *Diagnostic and Statistical Manual of Mental Disorders*, fourth edition (DSM-IV)[1] in terms of criteria for diagnosing substance withdrawal. Three criteria for diagnosing substance withdrawal are now required rather than two in the previous manual, DSM-III-R.[2] These criteria offer the diagnosis of substance withdrawal and more specificity and rigor.

Criterion A remains the development of a substance-specific syndrome due to the cessation of or reduction in substance use but is revised to require substance use to be heavy and prolonged[1] rather than just regular use[2] before substance-specific withdrawal. A new criterion, now criterion B,[1] has been added. This specifies that withdrawal syndromes cause clinically significant distress or impairment in social, occupational, or other important areas of functioning. Criterion C in DSM-IV[1] is essentially the same as criterion B in DSM-III-R[2] and requires that the symptoms in question not be attributable to a general medical condition or another mental condition. In addition, DSM-IV[1] points out that most if not all individuals experiencing substance withdrawal meet criteria for substance dependence and have cravings to use the substance.

In contrast to substance intoxication syndrome, withdrawal is considered a de novo syndrome with acute emergence of specific signs and symptoms after reduction or cessation of a substance. Signs and symptoms attributable to substance intoxication improve, albeit gradually, after substance use ceases. However, there is often overlap between intoxication and withdrawal symptoms and signs. Substance withdrawal symptoms usually improve after administration of the substance, whereas substance intoxication symptoms are made more severe on readministration of the substance.

General Medical Care Issues

For patients who are being detoxified from substances, medical and laboratory examinations are essential. Patients addicted to opioids or cocaine, especially those who administer these substances intravenously, are at high risk for concurrent medical disorders such as human immunodeficiency virus infection, syphilis, hepatitis, abscesses, endocarditis, pneumonia, tuberculosis, arrhythmias, malnutrition with weight loss, and anemias.[3] Moreover, patients may present with cognitive clouding or confusion as well as severe depressive symptoms and suicidal or homicidal ideation during early withdrawal. These phenomena usually dissipate as withdrawal symptoms are relieved.

It is important that the attending physician inform a patient about detoxification measures to be used, the expected course of symptoms during withdrawal, and that he or she will sustain some discomfort during medically supervised withdrawal.[3] Patients undergoing withdrawal are particularly reactive to perceived staff support and rapport.[3] They benefit from a sense of confidence in the medical staff by having a less stressful clinical course.

Finally, it is most important that patients be encouraged to participate in treatment planning and to pursue substance abuse treatment and rehabilitation after withdrawal. It is useful to emphasize to patients that withdrawal is but an early yet important step in recovery from addiction to substances.

Opioid Withdrawal

By DSM-IV criteria,[1] opioid withdrawal typically follows cessation or reduction in heavy and prolonged use of opioids, typically illicit heroin but also prescribed opioid drugs. Opioid withdrawal can also be precipitated by administration of an opioid antagonist, such as naloxone or naltrexone, after a period of opioid use. In addition to craving, three or more of the following symptoms/signs develop acutely or within days after substance cessation and are severe enough to impair a patient's functioning: dysphoric mood, nausea or vomiting, muscle aches, lacrimation or rhinorrhea, pupillary dilation, piloerection, diaphoresis, diarrhea, yawning, fever, or insomnia. Heroin withdrawal peaks 36 to 72 hours after the last use, and symptoms of insomnia, weakness, gastrointestinal problems, chills, abdominal pain, and muscle spasm are predominant.[3, 4]

Because of increased risk to the fetus, opioid withdrawal is contraindicated in pregnant women; methadone maintenance is the only accepted treatment for pregnant opioid addicts.[5] In addition, other acutely medically impaired patients with concurrent opioid dependence, such as those with acute myocardial infarction or heart failure, may be untowardly distressed physiologically and psychologically by opioid withdrawal. For such patients, temporary opioid agonist therapy with methadone is recommended, followed by gradual methadone taper, as described later.

Although methadone and clonidine are commonly used pharmacological interventions for opioid withdrawal, as described later, other opioids such as morphine, meperidine, or propoxyphene may be used in a tapering dose to help ameliorate acute psychological and physiological distress associated with opioid withdrawal. In addition, buprenorphine, a mixed opioid agonist-antagonist, is being evaluated as an agent to detoxify heroin-dependent patients. However, only methadone is approved by the Food and Drug Administration (FDA) as a pharmacological treatment of opioid dependence.

L-Alpha-acetyl-methadol (LAAM), a long-acting opioid agonist, has been approved by the FDA for treatment of opioid dependence, but there is limited experience with detoxification, either with LAAM-dependent patients or with using LAAM to treat opioid withdrawal. Thus, methadone is the preferred agent for opioid withdrawal.

Detoxification from Opioids Using Methadone

Opioid withdrawal typically occurs in an inpatient setting, although outpatients can also be withdrawn using a slow taper of methadone for up to 6 months.[6] Outpatient treatment with methadone is restricted to outpatient clinics that are licensed to dispense methadone.

Persons addicted to heroin typically administer the drug three or four times a day by either nasal insufflation or intravenous injection. Drug use can be elicited by asking a patient about the number of days on which he or she used heroin during the prior 30 days, as well as an estimated average dollar amount per day of use. Amounts of heroin use may range from $10 to $20 per day to more than $100 per day. Regardless of the amounts of opioids used, patients in inpatient settings can usually be stabilized with 20 to 40 mg of methadone per day orally, given once or twice a day.[7] Once a patient is stabilized in 1 to 3 days, methadone is tapered by 5 mg/day until a dose of 10 mg/day is reached. Methadone is then reduced by 5 mg every other day.[7] Patients addicted to methadone or medical professionals who have access to pure opioid drugs usually have more severe physical dependence. They need higher stabilizing doses of methadone and require more gradual withdrawal.[7] For patients who cannot ingest methadone orally, methadone can be administered intramuscularly using doses similar or slightly lower than orally administered doses.[8]

Prominent symptoms during opioid withdrawal are drug craving, insomnia, and various physical symptoms. Patients respond to limit setting and support as well as to being engaged in activities on the unit with other patients. Insomnia can be treated with short-term oral administration at bedtime of 25 to 50 mg of diphenhydramine or hydroxyzine pamoate or 500 mg of chloral hydrate.

Encouraging patients to participate in developing their treatment plans and detoxification schedules helps withdrawing patients feel more in control and mitigates against power struggles and suspiciousness about medication.[7]

Outpatient opioid withdrawal using methadone is less successful than inpatient withdrawal.[7] Once outpatients are stabilized on a fixed dose, which may range from 20 to 80 mg or more of methadone for patients who are no longer using illicit substances, methadone can be gradually reduced by 10% of the starting dose per week until 20 mg/day is reached. After this, the dose is reduced by 3% per week.[6] FDA regulations permit extended opioid detoxification for up to 6 months. However, many patients are not able to free themselves of illicit drug use even when on an appropriate dose of methadone. They may resume illicit drug administration during detoxification if psychosocial aspects of their addiction disorder have not changed. Such phenomena point out that withdrawal symptoms often have only a limited role in continued substance use among patients with substance use disorder.

Clonidine Hydrochloride

The alpha-2 agonist antihypertensive medication clonidine hydrochloride has been used to assist opioid withdrawal for both inpatients and outpatients.[7] Clonidine in doses of 0.6 to 2.0 mg/day reduces autonomic hyperactivity.[7] However, psychological symptoms such as craving, insomnia, depression, and myalgias are less relieved.[9] Because clonidine has side effects of sedation and hypotension and is not approved by the FDA for opioid withdrawal, its use is usually limited to inpatient detoxification because of patient safety issues.[7] However, carefully selected methadone-maintained patients who have reached stability in treatment have been withdrawn from methadone as outpatients using clonidine.[7, 10]

Clonidine is used with caution for patients who have hypertension or who are taking antihypertensive medications.[7] Other exclusions for clonidine administration are recent use of tricyclic antidepressants, severe insomnia, pregnancy, psychosis, and cardiac arrhythmias.[7]

Doses of clonidine are gradually increased for inpatients withdrawing from longer-acting opioids such as methadone and more quickly increased for patients withdrawing from the shorter-acting heroin.[7] A starting dose of clonidine for methadone withdrawal is 0.1–0.2 mg three times a day, increasing to 0.2–0.4 mg three times a day by day 3.[7] Blood pressure is monitored and confirmed to be 85/55 mm Hg or higher before clonidine is administered.[7] The dose is maintained until the patient's symptoms stabilize for several days and then is reduced by 0.2 to 0.4 mg/day.[7]

Sedative-Hypnotic Withdrawal

Sedative-hypnotics are essentially barbiturates and benzodiazepines. Other sedative-hypnotic drugs are meprobamate, glutethimide (Doriden), and methaqualone.[5] Sedative-hypnotic withdrawal is characterized by two or more symptoms that are similar to alcohol withdrawal. These include autonomic hyperactivity, hand tremor, insomnia, anxiety, nausea sometimes accompanied by vomiting, and psychomotor agitation after cessation or reduced use of the drug.[1] A grand mal seizure may occur in perhaps as many as 20% to 30% of patients undergoing detoxification from sedative-hypnotics.[1] The time course of onset and intensity of withdrawal syndromes are generally predicted by the half-life of the substance.

Medications with short- to intermediate-enduring actions typically last about 10 hours or less (e.g., lorazepam, oxazepam, and temazepam) and produce withdrawal symptoms within 6 to 8 hours of decreasing blood levels.[1] Symptoms peak in intensity on the second day and improve markedly by the fourth or fifth day. For substances with longer half-lives (e.g., diazepam), withdrawal symptoms may not develop for more than a week after the last use, peak in intensity during the second week, and decrease markedly during the third or fourth week.[1] Low-intensity symptoms such as anxiety, moodiness, and sleep disturbances constitute a protracted withdrawal syndrome and may persist for several months after acute withdrawal symptoms subside.

BARBITURATE WITHDRAWAL

Barbiturates that are associated with withdrawal syndromes have a short to intermediate half-life.[11] These include pentobarbital, secobarbital, amobarbital, and butalbital. Combinations products, such as Fiorinal, contain butalbital and may be abused by patients.[11] Barbiturate withdrawal occurs later than alcohol withdrawal and has a more variable course.[11] Severe withdrawal is characterized by seizures and delirium.[11] Convulsions, likely to be multiple, occur between 24 and 115 hours after last use.[11] Mortality may be associated with barbiturate withdrawal.[11]

BENZODIAZEPINE WITHDRAWAL

Growing data suggest that continuous treatment with benzodiazepines for months to years within a low-dose or therapeutic dose range is associated with mild to moderate withdrawal symptoms.[12] Even after gradual tapering of therapeutic doses of benzodiazepines, symptoms of anxiety, agitation, tachycardia, anorexia, muscle cramps, delirium, insomnia, and hypersensitivity to sounds and light may emerge 1 to 7 days after cessation or dose reduction of benzodiazepines.[12]

High-dose (greater than the therapeutic dose range) benzodiazepine withdrawal consists of symptoms of anxiety, insomnia, nightmares, seizures, delirium, hyperpyrexia, and even death.[12] Signs and symptoms of withdrawal occur 1 to 2 days after discontinuation of a short-acting benzodiazepine, such as oxazepam, alprazolam, and triazolam. Withdrawal symptoms occur 3 to 8 days after discontinuing a long-acting benzodiazepine, such as diazepam.[12]

MANAGEMENT OF SEDATIVE-HYPNOTIC WITHDRAWAL

Abrupt withdrawal of sedative-hypnotics is contraindicated because of morbidity and mortality risks to patients who are physiologically dependent. Several pharmacological approaches to detoxification from sedative-hypnotic drugs have evolved. One method is gradually reducing the drug on which a patient is dependent.[5] This method is marked by problems of continued reinforcement by use of the substance and variable blood levels at lower doses when tapering shorter-acting drugs. The preferred method is substitution of a longer-acting, cross-tolerant medication such as a benzodiazepine or phenobarbital or use of the anticonvulsant carbamazepine[5] and instituting a gradual stepwise reduction in dose.

Phenobarbital substitution techniques allow use of a longer-acting drug, which permits a more stable blood level at smaller doses.[13] Phenobarbital has a greater safety factor than shorter-acting barbiturates and is less likely to produce disinhibition euphoria associated with shorter-acting barbiturates.[13] Moreover, phenobarbital is rarely abused.[5] Thus, phenobarbital serves as the preferable agent in treating withdrawal from sedative-hypnotic substances.[13]

Smith and Wesson[14] developed the phenobarbital substitution technique.[5] A patient's daily barbiturate, benzodiazepine, other sedative-hypnotic drug, and alcohol use is estimated during the prior 30 days. Daily amounts of each substance are converted to their equivalent phenobarbital dose.[5] The sum of doses is the daily dose of phenobarbital, not to exceed 500 mg/day. Phenobarbital is administered two to four times per day. If the daily dose is calculated to be greater than 180 mg, a challenge dose of one third the estimated daily dose is administered. After 90 minutes, if a patient's vital signs are stable and the patient is not oversedated, the remainder of the dose is given. If a patient becomes oversedated, the dose is recalculated.[5]

The pentobarbital challenge test may also be used to calculate a starting dose of phenobarbital. Exclusion criteria for this drug challenge test include pregnancy, severe hypertension, or severe medical illness.[12] Two hundred milligrams of pentobarbital is administered orally, and the patient is observed for the next 60 to 90 minutes. If the patient is sedated, medical detoxification may not be necessary.[5] If the patient has slurred speech and ataxia but is not sedated, then 400 to 600 mg/day of phenobarbital could be required.[5] If lateral nystagmus is the only sign after 200 mg pentobarbital is administered, then 600 to 1000 mg of phenobarbital per day may be necessary.[5] If 200 mg of pentobarbital has no effects, as much as 1000 to 1200 mg/day of phenobarbital may be initially needed for detoxification.[5]

Signs of barbiturate toxicity (e.g., nystagmus, sedation, or dysarthria) are noted during stabilization and stepwise dose reduction. Patients are stabilized on phenobarbital during 3 to 5 days for alcohol and barbiturate dependence, 7 days for a short-acting benzodiazepine, and 14 days for a longer-acting benzodiazepine.[5] After stabilization occurs, the phenobarbital dose is tapered by 30 mg/day or 30 mg every other day until 90 mg/day is reached, after which the taper is slowed.[5]

Another use of phenobarbital for detoxification from combined alcohol-sedative-hypnotic dependence is to administer a loading dose of phenobarbital. Phenobarbital is given orally, 120 mg/hour until a patient develops three of the following five symptoms: dysarthria, ataxia, nystagmus, confusion, or drowsiness. The patient's urine is maintained at a pH of less than 6.5 in order to slow phenobarbital excretion, thus allowing a smoother withdrawal course.[15, 16]

Another modality for sedative-hypnotic detoxification is use of carbamazepine,[5, 17] which is initiated at 200 mg/day on day 1 of withdrawal and increased to 600 to 800 mg/day as tolerated. Once the daily dose of carbamazepine has reached at least 400 mg/day, the abused sedative-hypnotic substance is then discontinued or tapered over 3 to 6 days.[5] After the sedative-hypnotic drug is discontinued, carbamazepine is reduced over 5 to 14 days.[5]

Carbamazepine is not approved by the FDA for sedative-hypnotic withdrawal. Because of a potential for carbamazepine to cause aplastic anemia, determination of baseline complete blood counts with differential and platelet count, liver functions tests, and electrolyte measurements are needed.[5]

Stimulants

AMPHETAMINE WITHDRAWAL

According to DSM-IV,[1] an amphetamine withdrawal syndrome develops within a few hours to several days after cessation of or reduction in heavy or prolonged amphetamine use. The syndrome is characterized by dysphoric mood and two or more of the following: fatigue, vivid and unpleasant dreams, insomnia or hypersomnia, increased appetite, and psychomotor retardation or agitation.[1] Anhedonia and drug craving may also be present. The diagnosis requires that these symptoms cause distress or impairment in functioning, and they cannot be due to a medical or another mental disorder. Marked withdrawal symptoms ("crashing") often follows an episode of intense amphetamine use.[1] This crashing is marked by dysphoria and is comparable to an acute alcohol hangover.[18]

There are no controlled, systematic studies of humans undergoing acute cessation of amphetamines in order to examine psychological and physiological changes during early amphetamine cessation. Thus, concepts of amphetamine withdrawal have been formed from clinical impressions and inferences from pharmacological phenomena in animal studies.

COCAINE WITHDRAWAL

The existence of a cocaine withdrawal syndrome is controversial. Because of a perceived lack of physiological withdrawal signs and symptoms from cocaine, cocaine dependence was not a category in DSM-III.[19] However, given the serious cocaine epidemic of the 1980s and considerable clinical evidence of addicting properties of cocaine, cocaine dependence, abuse, and withdrawal were diagnostic categories in DSM-III-R.[2]

The definition of cocaine withdrawal in DSM-IV[1] has been revised. Cocaine withdrawal is defined as a characteristic withdrawal syndrome that develops within hours to days after cessation or reduction in cocaine use that has been prolonged and heavy. Like amphetamine withdrawal, the syndrome is characterized by the development of dysphoria and is accompanied by two or more of the following physiological changes: fatigue, vivid and unpleasant dreams, insomnia or hypersomnia, increased appetite, and psychomotor retardation or agitation.[1] Anhedonia and drug craving may also be present. Withdrawal symptoms must cause significant clinical distress or impairment in functioning. Finally, the symptoms cannot be due to a medical condition or accounted for by another mental disorder.

Unlike the dearth of studies of amphetamine, several studies have investigated the phenomenology of short-term abstinence from cocaine in persons addicted to cocaine. A study of therapists' clinical impressions of patients addicted to cocaine undergoing outpatient treatment proposed a triphasic cocaine withdrawal syndrome: crash, withdrawal, and indefinite extinction.[20] This proposed model has received considerable clinical acceptance. However, two residential studies[21, 22] of cocaine-dependent subjects demonstrated that mood distress and craving for cocaine were highest immediately after recent cocaine use. These phenomena decreased steadily in a linear pattern for several weeks, with no phases.[23]

Differences between these outpatient and residentially based studies may be secondary to important environmental differences. Conditioned cues as well as cocaine use (although lesser than at intake) occurred among the outpatient subjects, thus probably affecting patient reports.[21]

DSM-IV[1] points out that substantial numbers of persons with cocaine dependence have few or no clinically evident withdrawal symptoms after cessation of heavy, prolonged cocaine use. This observation suggests that cocaine withdrawal probably is associated with considerable heterogeneity and that further study is required.

TREATMENT OF STIMULANT WITHDRAWAL

Unfortunately, there are few and mostly inconsistently controlled studies of medications used to treat stimulant addiction.[24, 25] Almost all of these studies were for treatment of cocaine dependence. Results of these studies offer no support for using pharmacological agents to treat stimulant withdrawal per se.[22, 24, 25]

Medication trials with cocaine-dependent outpatients have been carried out using desipramine, bromocriptine, amantadine, carbamazepine, and flupenthixol decanoate.[23] Desipramine has been the most promising pharmacological intervention for decreasing symptoms and cocaine use during early cocaine abstinence, but results are mixed.[23, 26] Moreover, desipramine appears to have only a modest, time-limited effect in increasing periods of abstinence and decreasing cocaine use. Desipramine does not affect treatment attrition during early cocaine abstinence.[23, 27]

Although no specific pharmacological intervention may be available for early stimulant cessation in outpatients, medication interventions are possible for certain symptoms that may occur during early stimulant abstinence. Patients with comorbid mood disorders are reported to benefit from administration of antidepressant medication.[28, 29] Patients with insomnia may benefit from time-limited use of 25 to 50 mg of diphenhydramine or hydroxyzine pamoate or 500 mg of chloral hydrate at bedtime. Dysphoric states during early cocaine cessation are reported to be ameliorated by use of several nutritional supplements, along with vitamins and minerals.[5] However, whether these products have a specific pharmacological effect beyond a placebo effect has not been determined.[5]

Summary

Withdrawal syndromes occurring with cessation of or reduction in use of opioids, sedative-hypnotics, and stimulants (amphetamine and cocaine) have been described. Systematic studies of psychological and physiological phenomena on cessation of substance use have clearly demonstrated a withdrawal syndrome of a de novo emergence of dysphoric mood and hyperexcitable physiological phenomena after discontinuing use of opioids and sedative-hypnotics but not stimulants. Moreover, specific pharmacological interventions for opioid and sedative-hypnotic withdrawal have been demonstrated, whereas no definitive pharmacological intervention has been found for stimulant withdrawal.

Further research is needed to facilitate development of better methods to predict severe withdrawal syndromes among subgroups of patients who are at risk for undergoing withdrawal syndromes. Such research may help to delineate more precisely the phenomenology of withdrawal, clarify specificity of interventions, and add to our understanding of the course of addictive disorders.

REFERENCES

1. American Psychiatric Association (APA): Diagnostic and Statistical Manual of Mental Disorders, 4th ed. Washington, DC, APA, 1994.
2. APA: Diagnostic and Statistical Manual of Mental Disorders, 3rd ed, revised. Washington, DC, APA, 1987.

3. Schuckit MA: Drug and Alcohol Abuse, 3rd ed. New York, Plenum, 1989.
4. Himmelsbach CK: The morphine abstinence syndrome, its nature and treatment. Ann Intern Med 15:829–839, 1941.
5. Sees KL: Pharmacological adjuncts for the treatment of withdrawal syndromes. J Psychoactive Drugs 23:179–193, 1991.
6. Senay ED, Dorus W, Goldberg G, et al: Withdrawal from methadone maintenance. Arch Gen Psychiatry 34:361–367, 1977.
7. Jaffe JH, Kleber HD: Opioids: General issues and detoxification. In APA Task Force on Treatment of Psychiatric Disorders (eds): Treatment of Psychiatric Disorders. Washington DC, APA, 1989, pp 1309–1341.
8. Novick DM: The medically ill substance abuser. In Lowinson JH, Ruiz P, Millman RB (eds): Substance Abuse: A Comprehensive Textbook, 2nd ed. Baltimore, Williams & Wilkins, 1992, pp 657–674.
9. Jasinski DR, Johnson RE, Kocher TR: Clonidine in morphine withdrawal: Differential effects on signs and symptoms. Arch Gen Psychiatry 42:1063–1066, 1985.
10. Kleber HD, Riordan CE, Rounsaville B, et al: Clonidine in outpatient detoxification from methadone maintenance. Arch Gen Psychiatry 42:391–394, 1985.
11. Sellers EM: Alcohol, barbiturate and benzodiazepine withdrawal syndromes: Clinical management. Can Med Assoc J 139:113–120, 1988.
12. Wesson DR, Smith DE, Seymour RB: Sedative-hypnotics and tricyclics. In Lowinson JH, Ruiz P, Millman RB (eds): Substance Abuse—A Comprehensive Textbook, 2nd ed. Baltimore, Williams & Wilkins, 1992, pp 271–279.
13. Smith ED, Landry MJ, Wesson DR: Barbiturate, sedative, hypnotic agents. In APA Task Force on Treatments of Psychiatric Disorders (eds): Treatment of Psychiatric Disorders. Washington, DC, APA, 1989, pp 1294–1308.
14. Smith DE, Wesson DR: Benzodiazepine dependency syndromes. In: Smith DE, Wesson DR (eds): The Benzodiazepines: Current Standards for Medical Practice. Lancaster, UK, MTP Press, 1985, pp 235–248.
15. Robinson GA, Sellers EM, Janacek E: Barbiturate and hypnosedative withdrawal by multiple oral phenobarbital loading dose techniques. Clin Pharm Ther 28:71–76, 1981.
16. Gallant DM: Treatment of organic mental disorders. In APA Task Force on Treatment of Psychiatric Disorders (eds): Treatment of Psychiatric Disorders. Washington, DC, APA, 1989, pp 1076–1092.
17. Reis RK, Roy-Byrne PP, Ward NG, et al: Carbamazepine treatment for benzodiazepine withdrawal. Am J Psychiatry 146:536–537, 1989.
18. Gawin FH, Ellinwood EH: Cocaine and other stimulants. N Engl J Med 318:1173–1182, 1988.
19. APA: Diagnostic and Statistical Manual of Mental Disorders, 3rd ed. Washington, DC, APA, 1980.
20. Gawin FH, Kleber HD: Abstinence symptomatology and psychiatric diagnoses in cocaine abusers: Clinical observations. Arch Gen Psychiatry 43:107–113, 1986.
21. Weddington WW, Brown BS, Haertzen CA, et al: Changes in mood, craving and sleep during short-term abstinence reported by male cocaine addicts: A controlled, residential study. Arch Gen Psychiatry 47:861–868, 1990.
22. Satel SL, Price LH, Palumbo JM, et al: Clinical phenomenology and neurobiology of cocaine abstinence: A prospective inpatient study. Am J Psychiatry 148:1712–1716, 1991.
23. Weddington WW: Cocaine: Diagnosis and treatment. Psychiatr Clin North Am 16:87–95, 1993.
24. Weddington WW: Use of unproven and non-approved drugs to treat cocaine addiction (letter). Am J Psychiatry 147:1576, 1990.
25. Meyer RE: New pharmacotherapies for cocaine dependence . . . revisited. Arch Gen Psychiatry 49:900–904, 1992.
26. Weiss RD, Mirin SM: Psychological and pharmacological treatment strategies in cocaine dependence. Ann Clin Psychiatry 2:239–243, 1991.
27. Gawin FH, Ellinwood EH: Stimulants. In APA Task Force on Treatments of Psychiatric Disorders (eds): Treatment of Psychiatric Disorders. Washington, DC, APA, 1989, pp 1218–1241.
28. Kosten TR, Morgan CM, Falcione J, et al: Pharmacotherapy for cocaine abusing methadone maintained patients using amantadine or desipramine. Arch Gen Psychiatry 49:904–908, 1992.
29. Gastfriend DR: Pharmacotherapy of psychiatric syndromes with comorbid chemical dependence. J Addict Dis 12:155–170, 1992.

Pharmacological Treatments for Psychiatric Symptoms in Addiction Populations

David R. Gastfriend, MD

Given the range of psychiatric symptoms that are a direct result of substance use and the lack of research on efficacy, prescribing restraint is usually the better part of psychiatric valor. However, when deteriorating function occurs despite motivated recovery efforts or recovery itself is jeopardized by objective symptoms, nonreinforcing pharmacotherapy can offer benefits. Psychiatrists must be aware of the temporal range of psychoactive substance effects, must identify target symptoms, and must determine an expected time frame for their effects. Many therapeutic agents have potential interactions with alcohol or drug use. Patients are at risk for protracted dysfunction, relapse, or medical morbidity and mortality from either nonspecific prescribing or failure to treat. The pharmacotherapeutic approach may make the difference between mere abstinence or stable recovery from addictive disease. Finally, by emphasizing nonpharmacological treatments and using a formal treatment contract, the highest likelihood of successful pharmacotherapy outcome is possible.

Alcohol and drug dependence syndromes mimic the symptoms of all major psychiatric illnesses.[1-6] Adding to this complexity is the fact that psychiatric severity is one of the most important predictors of failure of addictions treatment. Several temporal relationships are possible: Psychiatric symptoms may either precede, *co-occur* with, or follow cessation of the substance use. The context of psychiatric symptoms may also vary, because symptoms may be isolated problems or may be part of a constellation of symptoms that meet criteria for a syndrome. Because the latter have been discussed elsewhere, this chapter focuses on discrete psychiatric symptoms and options for approaching these with pharmacotherapy.

Psychiatric symptoms that co-occur with ongoing substance use may be difficult if not impossible to treat with pharmacotherapy. As a rule, a patient who is actively using alcohol or drugs represents an unstable platform on which to build pharmacotherapeutic homeostasis. For example, a patient who has depressed mood, insomnia, and weight loss and who is actively dependent on heroin is unlikely to benefit from the addition of antidepressant therapy. These pharmacotherapies require predictable pharmacokinetic (e.g., steady-state levels of medication) and pharmacodynamic (e.g., unperturbed neurotransmitter and receptor interaction) states in order to be effective.

Many psychiatric symptoms are known to *follow* cessation of chronic alcohol or drug dependence. These symptoms may result from withdrawal, receptor system dysregulation, reward system disruption, neurotoxicity, and neuronal degeneration. Different drug classes have unique effects and time courses. Research on the underlying mechanisms for these effects is revealing important neurobiological relationships that clarify these parameters.[7, 8] A summary of DSM-IV categories is presented in Table 52–1.

The following examples illustrate the complex range of symptoms that occur and the time courses in which they may be expected to resolve. The earliest neurobehavioral process that can be observed to produce serious symptoms is withdrawal. Withdrawal from chronic alcohol, sedative, and opiate dependence produces anxiety via the abrupt loss of modulation of noradrenergic neurotransmission. These symptoms usually remit in hours to days. In the next phase after discontinuing use of a substance such as cocaine, anhedonia and depressed mood emerge, presumably via catecholamine receptor up-regulation. This early effect may not remit for days to weeks as receptor down-regulation proceeds. Further along the temporal course, cessation of most drugs of addiction after chronic dependence is associated with poor frustration tolerance, dependence on quick gratification, and existential malaise. These symptoms may be ascribed to disruption of the brain's reward system and may require weeks to months to resolve. Prolonged amnestic or interictal symptoms may also occur after alcohol-induced neurotoxicity, and these symptoms may require months to resolve. Finally, dementia subsequent to alcohol-induced neuronal degeneration may be irreversible.

The key question that psychiatrists must weigh before considering pharmacotherapy for psychiatric symptoms in an addicted patient

Table 52–1. PSYCHIATRIC SYMPTOMS OF SUBSTANCE ABUSE AND DEPENDENCE

Symptom	Substance	Temporal State
Delirium	Alcohol and sedatives	Intoxication and withdrawal
	Amphetamines and cocaine	Intoxication
	Hallucinogens and phencyclidine	Intoxication
	Inhalants	Intoxication
	Opioids	Intoxication
Psychosis	Alcohol and sedatives	Intoxication and withdrawal
	Amphetamines and cocaine	Intoxication
	Cannabis	Intoxication
	Hallucinogens and phencyclidine	Intoxication and flashbacks
	Inhalants	Intoxication
	Opioids	Intoxication
Amnestic disorder/dementia	Alcohol and sedatives	Persisting
	Inhalants	Persisting
Mood disorder	Alcohol	Intoxication and withdrawal
	Sedatives	Withdrawal
	Amphetamines and cocaine	Intoxication and withdrawal
	Hallucinogens and phencyclidine	Intoxication
	Inhalants	Intoxication
	Opioids	Intoxication
Anxiety disorder	Alcohol and sedatives	Intoxication and withdrawal
	Amphetamines and cocaine	Intoxication
	Caffeine	Intoxication
	Cannabis	Intoxication
	Hallucinogens	Intoxication
	Inhalants	Intoxication
Sexual disorder	Alcohol and sedatives	Intoxication
	Amphetamines and cocaine	Intoxication
	Opioids	Intoxication
Sleep disorder	Alcohol and sedatives	Intoxication and withdrawal
	Amphetamines and cocaine	Intoxication and withdrawal
	Caffeine	Intoxication
	Opioids	Intoxication and withdrawal

Adapted from the American Psychiatric Association: Diagnostic and Statistical Manual of Mental Disorders, 4th ed. Washington, DC, American Psychiatric Association, 1994; reprinted from Gastfriend DR: When substance abuse is the cause of treatment resistance. In Pollack M, Otto M, Rosenbaum J (eds): Clinical Challenges in Medical Psychiatry. New York, Guilford Press, in press.

is, *Do the symptoms seriously disturb the patient's function or recovery effort?* This operationalizes the issue via treatment goals and objective behavioral outcomes. It avoids the moral and theoretical extremes of both pharmacological Calvinism ("the only good drug is a dead drug") or pharmacological hedonism ("better living through chemistry"). In practice, these polar ideologies place patients at unnecessary risk, either influencing patients to reject psychotropics altogether or promoting iatrogenic substitute dependencies. Another ill-considered strategy is the use of the pill transference, in which reinforcing agents are prescribed in an attempt to attach a handle to a hard-to-hold patient. The functional criterion for pharmacotherapy is the best approach because its basis of decision making is careful assessment of prior function, the severity of target symptoms, the recovery effort of the patient, and the risk versus benefit of pharmacological agents.

Pharmacotherapy for Anxiety Symptoms

Central nervous system depressant withdrawal may produce symptoms of generalized anxiety and agoraphobia for 3 to 6 months, but these remit over time. For this reason, pharmacotherapy may be unnecessary.[9] Other causes of anxiety symptoms should be considered, such as use of caffeine, over-the-counter diet pills, and androgenic steroids. It is true, however, that alcohol, stimulants, marijuana, and hallucinogens may provoke the onset of an anxiety disorder, presumably in someone with a biological vulnerability to the anxiety disorder. Patients often stop using marijuana and hallucinogens when these become associated with increased anxiety, whereas alcohol dependence may persist or become substituted with anxiolytic dependence. Many alcoholic and drug-dependent patients believe they initiated substance use in an effort to self-medicate. This is not necessarily an indication for treatment, because there is a notable lack of objective data to support the self-medication hypothesis.

An anxiety disorder can be extremely difficult to stabilize without initial detoxification and the benefit of a period of drug-free observation. If a patient with severe anxiety rejects hospitalization because of fear of confinement, it may be helpful to contract with the patient for intensive outpatient treatment or an extended outpatient evaluation for several weeks, after which the patient will agree to reconsider hospitalization if still not abstinent.

These measures are usually safer than immediately proceeding to pharmacotherapy without a contract.

After detoxification, substance-dependent patients with anxiety require exceptional efforts to engage in behavior therapy because of their conditioning for immediate (i.e., pharmacological) gratification. This effort is essential, because behavior therapy can address both anxiety and substance addiction with relaxation, meditation, self-hypnosis, in vivo exposure, and addiction relapse prevention training.

Serotonin uptake inhibitor (SUI) antidepressants are the first-line agents for symptoms of panic attacks, compulsions, and possibly generalized anxiety in addicted patients. In addition to the proven efficacy of SUIs for depression and the foregoing symptoms at standard doses, numerous studies have demonstrated that SUIs exert a modest antiappetitive effect on reducing drug consumption, at least in alcoholics. Data exist to support the use of fluoxetine,[10] citalopram,[11] sertraline,[12] and others. Therefore, it is possible that SUIs may be a parsimonious class of agents for these symptoms even in patients who may continue episodic alcohol consumption. Important caveats remain, however, given that long-term studies are not yet available. It is unclear to what extent antiappetitive pharmacotherapies are effective in patients with severe substance dependence. Further, it is doubtful whether SUI benefits for these other psychiatric symptoms are effective in patients who continue to drink heavily. Trazodone may be useful for anxiety symptoms in benzodiazepine withdrawal and has been reported to reduce relapse risk, in comparison with placebo.[13]

Tricyclic antidepressants may also relieve anxiety and pose low risk for substance addiction relapse. Both imipramine and trazodone have been reported in one controlled trial to relieve generalized anxiety symptoms as well as diazepam, without substantial risk of inducing dependence.[14] An open trial in patients with substance dependence and anxiety (many with posttraumatic stress symptoms) found that trazodone, 50 to 150 mg/day, relieved anxiety and was associated with decreased use of benzodiazepines.[15] Monitoring plasma levels of tricyclics (e.g., nortriptyline, desipramine) is important because of altered rates of elimination in drug-dependent individuals and for determining compliance. Patients may be noncompliant with antidepressants because of a covert preference for benzodiazepines. Also, these agents, being less specific than the SUIs, may themselves contribute to addiction. For example, in my practice, imipramine, with catecholamine, cholinergic, and histaminergic effects, was abused by a cocaine-dependent patient who took the drug only intermittently for its sedative effect. Important interactions between agents of addiction and treatment are listed in Table 52–2.

Buspirone offers many clinical benefits without dependence risk. Buspirone has a high safety profile and may be combined with antidepressants at doses of up to 60 to 80 mg/day. The price of this long-term safety is the burden of vigorous patient education and support to help patients tolerate the slow onset (up to 6 weeks) and the imperceptibility of its unique response.[16] Buspirone may offer parsimonious relief of combined anxiety and depression[17] and may augment incomplete antidepressant response. In substance dependence with anxiety symptoms, most reports indicate benefit.[18–21] Despite early caveats reserving its use for "benzodiazepine virgins," buspirone has been an effective anxiolytic in cases with benzodiazepine dependence, when adequate patient education was provided.[16, 22]

Benzodiazepines, despite their safety in the general population, put addicted patients at risk via pharmacological tolerance and physiological dependence.[23] Pharmacological tolerance is not a pharmacokinetic process (i.e., there is no induction of metabolism) but is rather pharmacodynamic in nature (decreased receptor binding).[24] Single doses of benzodiaz-

Table 52–2. INTERACTIONS BETWEEN DRUGS OF ABUSE AND COMMON THERAPEUTIC AGENTS

Drug of Abuse	Therapeutic Agent	Interaction and Mechanism (If Known)
Ethanol	• Disulfiram	Acetaldehyde dehydrogenase inhibition produces flushing, hypotension, nausea, tachycardia. Fatal reactions possible.
	• MAO inhibitors	Impaired hepatic metabolism of tyramine in some beverages produces a dangerous, possibly fatal pressor response.
	• Tricyclic antidepressants	Acute ethanol may inhibit first-pass TCA metabolism, yielding additive CNS impairment. Chronic ethanol use induces hepatic TCA metabolism up to three-fold.
	• Neuroleptics	Cumulative CNS impairment of psychomotor skills, judgment, and behavior. Possible increased risk of akathisia and dystonia.
	• Anticonvulsants	Chronic ethanol use produces prolonged hepatic microsomal enzyme induction, reducing phenytoin levels. Possible seizure risk.
Barbiturates	• Tricyclic antidepressants	Increased TCA metabolism may reduce efficacy. Acutely, combination may potentiate respiratory depression.
	• MAO inhibitors	MAO inhibitors may also inhibit barbiturate metabolism, prolonging intoxication.
	• Neuroleptics	Induced hepatic microsomal enzymes may reduce chlorpromazine levels.
	• Anticonvulsants	Valproic acid increases phenobarbital levels and toxicity. Induced hepatic microsomal enzymes may lower carbamazepine levels. Combined induction and competitive inhibition yield unpredictable phenytoin levels.
Benzodiazepines	• Disulfiram	Inhibited hepatic oxidation may enhance benzodiazepine effects. Oxazepam and lorazepam (inactivated by glucuronidation) are not thus affected.
	• MAO inhibitors	Two reports describe edema with chlordiazepoxide.
Opiates	• MAO inhibitors	Meperidine has produced severe excitation, diaphoresis, rigidity, hypertension or hypotension, coma, and death.
	• Neuroleptics	Chlorpromazine and meperidine may produce hypotension and excessive CNS depression.
	• Anticonvulsants	Propoxyphene inhibits oxidation of carbamazepine, yielding toxic levels. Methadone metabolism may be increased by carbamazepine or phenytoin via hepatic enzyme induction, causing withdrawal.
Stimulants	• MAO inhibitors	MAO inhibitors increase neuronal catecholamine storage; amphetamines and cocaine provoke abrupt release, hyperpyrexia, severe hypertension, and death.
	• Neuroleptics	Amphetamines and cocaine exacerbate positive symptoms of chronic psychosis. Conversely, neuroleptics may effectively treat stimulant-induced psychosis.

MAO, monoamine oxidase; TCA, tricyclic antidepressant; CNS, central nervous system.
From Gastfriend DR: Pharmacotherapy of psychiatric syndromes with comorbid chemical dependency. J Addict Dis 12(3):155–170, 1993.

epines produce pharmacological tolerance,[25] and chronic therapeutic doses produce symptoms of physiological dependence in as many as 100% of patients.[23, 26]

Benzodiazepine agents with the most rapid absorption are the most addicting. Patients have learned this for themselves, sometimes chewing alprazolam and lorazepam to achieve more rapid sublingual absorption. The rate of transfer across the blood-brain barrier may vary by as much as 50-fold. For this reason, diazepam is particularly dangerous because of the "rush" it produces, in contrast to an agent such as clonazepam. In any case, the classical problem is iatrogenically induced substitute addiction from alcohol to benzodiazepines, or relapse as a result of the reinforcing psychological and physical dependence on benzodiazepines. Further, the goal of treatment is not just abstinence but *recovery*. Recovery is the process of restoring intrapsychic growth and maturation. Benzodiazepines offer a degree of immediate gratification that appears to impede initiation of recovery.

In severe conditions that prove refractory to behavioral and antidepressant approaches, a slow-onset and long-acting agent such as clonazepam may be the safest of this class,[27] yet even clonazepam has addictive potential in severe drug dependence. Thus, the use of benzodiazepines should be reserved for patients who have a well-documented failure to respond to antidepressants or other agents and who have demonstrated continued distress and a commitment to treatment.

Finally, it is important to teach patients that the goal of treatment is not elimination of anxiety. Anxiety is a normal adaptive stimulus in recovering addicts who are in the process of acquiring new coping behaviors. This process may require months or years of stressful effort.

Pharmacotherapy for Depressive Symptoms

Most depressed addicted patients do not benefit from pharmacotherapy but rather require detoxification and abstinence. Antidepressant efficacy in anhedonic, depressed early remission is not proved, and overdose is a serious risk in the event of relapse. A high rate of spontaneous remission of these symptoms follows withdrawal. Premature introduction of an agent also makes it difficult to determine whether treatment will be needed over the longer term. These patients need vigorous edu-

cation and reinforcement to accept that these symptoms are expectable and transient and therefore should simply be endured. In patients who meet the functional criterion of a depressed mood that threatens employment or poses a suicide risk, standard pharmacotherapy serves several purposes, including restoration of the euthymic state, treatment retention, and relapse prevention.

SUI antidepressants may be useful in addicted patients who remain dysfunctionally depressed despite abstinence. SUIs show great promise for reducing alcohol consumption as well as reducing affective symptoms, even in alcoholics who resist psychosocial treatments.[10–12, 28, 29] Despite the improved side effect profile compared with tricyclic antidepressants, some cautions do apply. Fluvoxamine has been reported to potentiate alcohol's psychomotor effects. SUIs may displace protein-bound compounds. A moderate adverse interaction has been reported in which fluvoxamine increases alprazolam plasma concentrations, causing increased psychomotor impairment.[30] SUIs may also inhibit rapid-eye-motion (REM) sleep, increasing nocturnal wakefulness and stage I (light) sleep. Nefazodone, a $5HT_2$ antagonist and 5HT reuptake inhibitor with little or no effect at cholinergic, histamine, and alpha-1-adrenergic receptors, does not have this limitation at doses to 300 mg twice a day.

Tricyclic antidepressants and dopamine agonists (e.g., bromocriptine, amantadine) have been reported to benefit cocaine withdrawal depressive symptoms such as anhedonia in open trials.[31] Unfortunately, other trials have been contradictory.[32] Effects of these agents for patients who do not meet full criteria for major depression are probably modest, at best, for normalizing mood, enhancing treatment activity, retaining patients in treatment, and preventing early relapse.[33] Desipramine should be initiated gradually to avoid provoking relapse. Newer agents with specificity for both serotonin and norepinephrine uptake blockade (e.g., venlafaxine) may achieve more consistent benefits.

Nicotine dependence produces numerous interactions with psychotropic agents. Also, the incidence of alcoholism among smokers may be tenfold greater than among non-smokers.[34] Women may be particularly at risk for nicotine dependence and comorbid depression.[35] The implications for pharmacotherapy are that smoking increases the hepatic metabolism of tricyclic antidepressants sufficiently to reduce clinical efficacy and warrants plasma level monitoring. Fortunately, smoking cessation may safely coexist with substance dependence inpatient treatment and with outpatient recovery as well.[36]

In opiate addicts with comorbid psychiatric symptoms, it is common to find continued illicit drug use and increased high-risk behavior for human immunodeficiency virus (HIV) transmission. Depressive symptoms are frequent, but antidepressants may yield no better response than placebo.[37] Depression in opiate-dependent patients, even those on methadone treatment, is usually transient and may be situational or related to withdrawal.[38] Therefore, antidepressants should be reserved for patients who are receiving methadone maintenance and who have a discrete major depressive disorder.

Buprenorphine, a mixed opiate agonist, may benefit opiate addicts who have concurrent cocaine dependence and who also manifest depressive symptoms.[39, 40] Buprenorphine is a long-acting sublingually administered agent, recently submitted for Food and Drug Administration review, that has been shown to reduce opiate use in a manner that is similar to methadone. It may also reduce craving for cocaine and use of cocaine by individuals with combined opiate and cocaine dependence. An antidepressant effect has also been proposed for this agent.[62]

Monoamine oxidase (MAO) inhibitors have demonstrated efficacy for depression and may be useful in related mood symptoms associated with cluster B personality disorders; such symptoms may be noted in some addicted patients in postwithdrawal states. Their usefulness is limited, however, by the dangers of relapse to tyramine-rich beverages such as beer and wine. Cocaine relapse is another serious risk, as is impulsive noncompliance with food restrictions. For depressed patients who are addicted to opiates, a severe and fatal serotonin syndrome can occur between MAO inhibitors and meperidine (Demerol).[30] A similar interaction with propoxyphene (Darvocet-N, Darvon) is also possible.[30]

Pharmacotherapy for Insomnia

A leading, preventable cause of insomnia following alcohol or drug withdrawal is ongoing nicotine dependence. Alternatively, patients may suffer a prolonged sleep disorder in the absence of nicotine. In the past, patients with protracted or severe insomnia following alcohol or hypnosedative withdrawal often faced a high risk for relapse or pressured psychiatrists to prescribe benzodiazepines, at considerable risk of producing iatrogenic dependence. The only alternative would be to prescribe anticholinergics. Patients seeking abstinence usually rejected these because of complaints of feeling drugged. Opiate addicts have long sought anticholinergic agents to enhance the euphoric state of opiate intoxication and to diminish opiate withdrawal side effects rather than for treatment of insomnia. Insomnia over this situation has been shared by patients and physicians alike.

Trazodone appears to be an effective, safe solution to this need. Trazodone increases total sleep time in normal adults.[41] In depressed insomniacs, it increases stage IV sleep and increases REM latency.[42] Too sedating for first-line use as an antidepressant, particularly in recovering persons who are sensitized to feeling drugged, at lower doses of 50 to 200 mg, trazodone is nonreinforcing even in methadone-maintained heroin addicts, in the author's experience. An important consideration, however, is that trazodone does not provide cross-tolerance for seizure threshold reduction. Therefore, benzodiazepines must be slowly tapered when trazodone is used concurrently for anxiety reduction. Patients who complain of feeling lethargic on awakening in the morning should be advised to decrease the dose or administer the agent earlier in the evening (e.g., after the evening meal).

Pharmacotherapy for Mood Lability

Lithium is effective in the treatment of mania in addicted patients who are abstinent, at standard plasma levels. In early studies, lithium also appeared to promote cocaine abstinence in patients with bipolar and cyclothymic disorder, but this finding has not been replicated.[43, 44] In patients without comorbid bipolar disorder, lithium does not appear to be useful in treating alcohol, cocaine, or other drug dependence.

Anticonvulsants are another class of agents that may be useful for controlling elevated mood in addicted patients. Carbamazepine has antimanic and antikindling effects that may be helpful for patients with recurrent cyclothymia/mania at standard therapeutic levels.[45, 46] Whether carbamazepine has benefits for cocaine dependence itself remains a topic of study, but double-blind studies are needed.[47] Valproic acid is another option for manic patients, although studies on the efficacy of these agents are few. In a multicenter comparison trial using valproic acid, the two offer similar control of generalized tonic-clonic seizures, but carbamazepine is superior for complex partial seizures with fewer long-term adverse effects.[48] How these findings reflect on their relative control of elevated mood is unclear.

Pharmacotherapy for Psychotic Symptoms

Dopamine (D2) receptor antagonists are effective for short-term control of transient hallucinations during alcohol or drug intoxication and withdrawal. High-potency agents such as haloperidol (5 to 10 mg intramuscularly) have been effective for control of severe, even violent agitation during alcohol intoxication with minimal risk of seizure potentiation or extrapyramidal symptoms.[49] Psychosis may be the most difficult comorbid psychiatric symptom to treat when it occurs in addicted patients. Psychotic symptoms during abstinence may have many causes and represent a serious public health problem, because nearly half of individuals with schizophreniform illness have comorbid alcohol or drug problems.[50] These patients tend to be young males, suffer from poor living skills, and have increased likelihood of multiple substance use, violent behavior, and suicide.[51]

Clozapine, with dopamine D1, cholinergic, muscarinic, and serotonergic antagonist activity, is not practical as an agent for acute transient symptoms because of the monitoring that is required to protect against agranulocytosis, which occurs in 1% to 2% of patients. In patients with chronic symptoms of psychosis, particularly those who are treatment resistant or who have substantial negative symptoms of schizophrenia, clozapine has been reported to diminish psychosis, improve inertia, and decrease substance addiction.[52] Benzodiazepines may have an adverse interaction with clozapine, with loss of consciousness and respiratory depression, according to one report.[53]

Benzodiazepines may be useful both therapeutically and diagnostically when alcohol or hypnosedative withdrawal is a suspected cause of acute psychosis. Alcoholic hallucinosis may occur in 5% of alcoholics, and stimulant- or hallucinogen-induced psychosis, which is not uncommon, resolves in hours to days. Prolonged antipsychotic administration may not be needed, and side effects may alienate patients from providers. High-dose benzodiazepines may be required, depending on tolerance

or the presence of alcohol withdrawal delirium. Benzodiazepine dependence may be a covert problem in the chronic schizophrenic population, given that in one sample, 41% of schizophrenic patients were receiving both neuroleptics and long-term benzodiazepines.[54] Inpatient hospitalization is usually essential because the first priority is to achieve abstinence and then initiate antipsychotic pharmacotherapy. Dopamine-blocking agents do not block cocaine or amphetamine craving or euphoria in humans. Therefore, antipsychotics should be reserved for psychotic symptoms. In most cases, standard antipsychotic doses are indicated. Occasional drug-drug interactions may warrant higher than usual doses. Barbiturates may reduce chlorpromazine levels through hepatic microsomal enzyme induction. Some agents may aggravate psychosis and counteract effects of antipsychotics, such as disulfiram, which inhibits dopamine beta-hydroxylase, and bromocriptine and amantadine, via dopamine agonism. Patients with vulnerabilities to psychosis should first be stabilized on an antipsychotic dose before initiation of other pharmacotherapy.

Patients with opiate dependence and chronic psychosis generally fare best with methadone maintenance for initial treatment as opposed to detoxification and abstinence. Aside from the benefit of the stabilizing routine of daily outpatient methadone administration, methadone treatment staff tend to be more supportive and reinforcing of pharmacotherapy compliance than do staff at abstinence-oriented treatment programs.[55]

Carbamazepine may be useful for cocaine-induced paranoia,[45] although the mechanism for this effect is unknown. The anticonvulsant properties of carbamazepine may be mediated through calcium channel effects via a subtype of benzodiazepine receptors. These properties may have an antikindling effect that may benefit the paranoia that accompanies compulsive cocaine use. Standard levels are the goal (i.e., 8 to 12 μg/ml).

Nicotine dependence has been associated with decreased phenothiazine effects in several studies.[30] Meta-analysis of smoking cessation treatment indicates the usefulness of both nicotine replacement[56] and clonidine,[57] particularly when combined with psychosocial approaches.[58] However, these studies did not examine the population with psychosis, who may experience unique interactions between nicotine and antipsychotic pharmacotherapy and between nicotine and psychosis.

Pharmacotherapy for Symptoms of Late Luteal Phase Dysphoric Disorder

Symptoms of late luteal phase dysphoric disorder, also known as premenstrual syndrome (PMS), may include a bloated feeling, irritability, tension, and depression. These symptoms may be cyclical triggers for relapse. There are few data on this relationship, however. Standard pharmacotherapies for these symptoms may be helpful in recovering patients, as well, with the caveats against benzodiazepine use. Low-dose antidiuretics such as hydrochlorothiazide, 25 to 50 mg/day for the week before the anticipated menses, may reduce bloating and its related headache. Nonsteroidal anti-inflammatory agents are also palliative for headache. Treatments for insomnia may also help during this phase, as described earlier.

Nefazodone may also benefit PMS symptoms, as suggested in one comparison with placebo and progesterone, and it may cause fewer side effects than the SUIs (Rickels K: Personal communication Philadelphia, PA, 1994).

Pharmacotherapy for Inattention and Distractibility

Although many patients in early recovery may report some difficulty maintaining concentration, attention deficit hyperactivity disorder (ADHD) is thought to occur with the highest prevalence among patients with cocaine dependence and, even in this group, has been diagnosed in only 2% to 5% of patients.[59] Inattention and distractibility alone without childhood stigmata usually respond in time to abstinence, recovery counseling, psychosocial stabilization, and restoration of healthy sleep patterns. Alcohol- and drug-dependent adults without ADHD have not been found to benefit from stimulants and may develop rapid tolerance and dependence.[60]

Interactions of Drugs of Abuse with Psychopharmacotherapies

Drug-drug interactions may be serious in patients who require psychotropics for psychiatric symptoms and who use alcohol or drugs concurrently. Table 52–2 presents the major classes of agents that are used in the treatment of psychiatric symptoms, listed according to their degree of interaction with some drugs of abuse, from most to least severe.[30] It is valuable to remember several general principles of management. MAO inhibitors are contraindicated in patients who are still at risk for using ethanol, stimulants, or meperidine. Plasma level determinations are needed when prescribing tricyclic antidepressants, carbamazepine, or valproic acid for patients who have consumed ethanol or barbiturates heavily or chronically.

Other interactions may result from combinations of two therapeutic agents in the context of substance addiction. Clonidine in combination with chlorpromazine, haloperidol, or fluphenazine has produced isolated cases of severe hypotension or delirium. Antipsychotics with bromocriptine (e.g., in a psychotic patient with severe cocaine withdrawal) would theoretically be expected to counteract each other. This may not be a problem if a patient is first stabilized on the antipsychotic. Trazodone may produce hypotension when added to a neuroleptic.

More important than the choice of agent is painstaking psychoeducation and a formal treatment contract.[61] An example of such a contract is presented in Table 52–3. The essential

Table 52–3. KEY COMPONENTS OF A PHARMACOTHERAPY CONTRACT WITH RECOVERING PATIENTS

1. Medication is part of a rational psychosocial treatment package and is discontinued if key psychosocial components are neglected.
2. Urine or blood testing may be required at any time to provide an independent source of data about the course of the chemical dependence or to determine if a prescribed medication is reaching adequate levels in blood.
3. Medication is to be used only as prescribed. Any need for changes must first be discussed with the physician. A unilateral change in medication by the patient often is an early sign of relapse.
4. Changes in medication are prescribed one at a time (i.e., two agents are not initiated simultaneously).
5. The purpose of medication, when used, is to treat predetermined target symptoms. If medication proves ineffective for these, it is discontinued.
6. Once target symptoms remit, a process of dose tapering may be initiated to determine the minimum dose necessary to maintain healthy function. The medication strategy periodically includes a period of discontinuation, or drug holiday. Medication may not be necessary on a long-term basis.

From Gastfriend DR: Pharmacotherapy of psychiatric syndromes with comorbid chemical dependency. J Addict Dis 12(3):155–170, 1993.

principles are that pharmacotherapy should target specific symptoms, in time-limited objectives, modifying only one change at a time while monitoring compliance and proceeding only in the context of a comprehensive psychosocial treatment plan. Underlying all aspects of the contract is the need for continual reevaluation of a patient's condition in terms of medication response and active treatment participation. The latter involves initiating lifestyle changes such as participating in a self-help group, using sober supports such as a sponsor(s), and engaging in longitudinal (i.e., aftercare) treatment for both addiction and the comorbid illness. Patients with addiction and psychiatric symptoms who invest in these modalities often have gratifying responses to pharmacotherapy when indicated.

ACKNOWLEDGMENTS

Supported by NIDA Grants DA08781 and DA07693.

REFERENCES

1. American Psychiatric Association: Diagnostic and Statistical Manual of Mental Disorders, 4th ed. Washington, DC, American Psychiatric Association, 1994.
2. Hall RC, Stickney SK, Gardner ER, et al: Relationship of psychiatric illness to drug abuse. J Psychedelic Drugs 11:337–342, 1979.
3. O'Farrell TJ, Connors GJ, Upper D: Addictive behaviors among hospitalized psychiatric patients. Addict Behav 8:329–333, 1983.
4. Hasin DS, Grant BF: Psychiatric diagnosis of patients with substance abuse problems: A comparison of two procedures, DIS and the SADS-L. J Psychiatr Res 21(1):7–22, 1987.
5. Lehman AF, Meyers CP, Corty E: Assessment and classification of patients with psychiatric and substance abuse syndromes. Hosp Community Psychiatry 40(10):1019–1025, 1989.
6. Galanter M, Egelko S, De Leon G, et al: Crack/cocaine abusers in the general hospital: Assessment and initiation of care. Am J Psychiatry 149(6):810–815, 1992.
7. Gold MS: Neurobiology of addiction and recovery: The brain, the drive for the drug, and the 12-step fellowship. J Subst Abuse Treat 11(2):93–97, 1994.
8. Tsai G, Gastfriend DR, Coyle JT: The glutamatergic basis of human alcoholism. Am J Psychiatry 152:332–340, 1995.
9. Schuckit MA, Irwin M, Brown SA: The history of anxiety symptoms among 171 primary alcoholics. J Stud Alcohol 51(1):34–41, 1990.
10. Cornelius JR, Salloum IM, Cornelius MD, et al: Fluoxetine trial in suicidal depressed alcoholics. Psychopharmacol Bull 29(2):195–199, 1993.
11. Naranjo CA, Poulos CX, Bremner KE, et al: Citalopram decreases desirability, liking, and consumption of alcohol in alcohol-dependent drinkers. Clin Pharmacol Ther 51(6):729–739, 1992.
12. Brands B, Sellers EM, Kaplan HL: The effects of the 5-HT uptake inhibitor, sertraline, on ethanol, water and food consumption. Alcohol Clin Exp Res 14(2):273, 1990.
13. Ansseau M, De Roeck J: Trazodone in benzodiazepine dependence. J Clin Psychiatry 54(5):189–191, 1993.
14. Rickels K, Downing R, Hassman H: Antidepressants for the treatment of generalized anxiety disorder: A placebo-controlled comparison of imipramine, trazodone, and diazepam. Arch Gen Psychiatry 50:884–895, 1993.
15. Liebowitz NR, el Mallakh RS: Trazodone for the treatment of anxiety symptoms in substance abusers (letter). J Clin Psychopharmacol 9(6):449–451, 1989.
16. Gastfriend DR, Rosenbaum JF: Adjunctive buspirone in benzodiazepine treatment of four patients with panic disorder. Am J Psychiatry 146:914–916, 1989.
17. Gammans RE, Stringfellow JC, Hvizdos AJ, et al: Use of buspirone in patients with generalized anxiety disorder and coexisting depressive symptoms—a meta-analysis of eight randomized, controlled studies. Pharmacopsychiatry 25:1–9, 1992.
18. Bruno F: Buspirone in the treatment of alcoholic patients. Psychopathology 1:49–59, 1989.
19. Giannini AJ, Loiselle RH, Graham BH, et al: Behavioral response to buspirone in cocaine and phencyclidine withdrawal. J Subst Abuse Treat 10:523–527, 1993.
20. Udelman HD, Udelman DL: Concurrent use of buspirone in anxious patients during withdrawal from alprazolam therapy. J Clin Psychiatry 51(Suppl 9):46–50, 1990.
21. Kranzler HR, Burleson JA, Del Boca FK, et al: Buspirone treatment of anxious alcoholics. A placebo-controlled trial. Arch Gen Psychiatry 51(9):720–731, 1994.
22. Kranzler HR: Buspirone treatment of anxiety in a patient dependent on alprazolam. J Clin Psychopharmacol 9(2):153, 1989.
23. Busto U, Sellers EM, Naranjo CA, et al: Withdrawal reaction after long-term therapeutic use of benzodiazepines. N Engl J Med 315:854–859, 1986.
24. Ciraulo DA: Clinical Manual of Chemical Dependence. Washington, DC, American Psychiatric Association, 1991.
25. Greenblatt DJ, Shader RI: Dependence, tolerance, and addiction to benzodiazepines: Clinical and pharmacokinetic considerations. Drug Metab Rev 8:13–28, 1978.
26. Rickels K, Schweizer E, Case WG, et al: Long-term therapeutic use of benzodiazepines. I. Effects of abrupt discontinuation. Arch Gen Psychiatry 47:99–107, 1990.
27. Herman JB, Rosenbaum JF, Brotman AW: The aprazolam to clonazepam switch for the treatment of panic disorder. J Clin Psychopharmacol 7:175–178, 1987.
28. Naranjo CA, Sellers EM: Serotonin uptake inhibitors attenuate ethanol intake in problem drinkers. Recent Dev Alcohol 7:255–266, 1989.
29. Naranjo CA, Sellers EM, Sullivan JT, et al: The serotonin uptake inhibitor citalopram attenuates ethanol intake. Clin Pharmacol Ther 41(3):266–274, 1987.
30. Hansten PD, Horn JR: Drug Interactions and Updates: A Clinical Perspective and Analysis of Current Developments. Malvern, PA, Lea & Febiger, 1990.
31. Kosten TR, Gawin FH, Kosten TA, et al: Six-month follow-up of short-term pharmacotherapy for cocaine dependence. Am J Addict 1(1):40–49, 1992.
32. Kosten TR, Morgan CM, Falcione J, et al: Pharmacotherapy for cocaine-abusing methadone-maintained patients using amantadine or desipramine. Arch Gen Psychiatry 49(11):894–899, 1992.
33. Vaughan DA: Frontiers in pharmacologic treatment of alcohol, cocaine, and nicotine dependence. Psychiatr Ann 20:695–708, 1990.
34. DiFranza JR, Guerrera MP: Alcoholism and smoking. J Stud Alcohol 51(2):130–135, 1990.

35. Kendler KS, Neale MC, MacLean CJ, et al: Smoking and major depression. A causal analysis. Arch Gen Psychiatry 50(1):36–43, 1993.
36. Covey LS, Glassman AH, Stetner F, et al: Effect of history of alcoholism or major depression on smoking cessation. Am J Psychiatry 150(10):1546–1547, 1993.
37. Kleber HD, Weissman MM, Rounsaville BJ: Imipramine as treatment for depression in addicts. Arch Gen Psychiatry 40:649–653, 1983.
38. Rounsaville BJ, Kosten TR, Kleber HD: Long term changes in current psychiatric diagnoses of treated opiate addicts. Compr Psychiatr 27:480–498, 1986.
39. Gastfriend DR, Mendelson JH, Mello NK, et al: Buprenorphine pharmacotherapy for concurrent heroin and cocaine dependence. Am J Addict 2(4):269–278, 1993.
40. Schottenfeld RS, Pakes J, Ziedonis D, et al: Buprenorphine: Dose related effects on cocaine and opioid use in cocaine abusing opioid dependent humans. Biol Psychiatry 3:66–74, 1993.
41. Ware JC, Pittard JT: Increased deep sleep after trazodone use: A double-blind palcebo-controlled study in healthy young adults. J Clin Psychiatry 51(Suppl 9):18–22, 1990.
42. Scharf MB, Sachais BA: Sleep laboratory evaluation of the effects and efficacy of trazodone in depressed insomniac patients. J Clin Psychiatry 51(Suppl 9):13–17, 1990.
43. Nunes EV, McGrath PJ, Wager S, et al: Lithium treatment for cocaine abusers with bipolar spectrum disorders. Am J Psychiatry 147(5):655–657, 1990.
44. Lemere F: Lithium treatment of cocaine addiction. Am J Psychiatry 148(2):276, 1991.
45. Halikas JA, Crosby RD, Carlson GA, et al: Cocaine reduction in unmotivated crack users using carbamazepine versus placebo in a short-term, double-blind crossover design. Clin Pharmacol Ther 50:81–95, 1991.
46. Halikas JA, Kuhn K, Carlson GA, et al: The effect of carbamazepine on cocaine use. Am J Addict 1(1):30–39, 1992.
47. Campbell JL, Thomas HM, Gabrielli W, et al: Impact of desipramine or carbamazepine on patient retention in outpatient cocaine treatment: preliminary findings. J Addict Dis 13(4):191–199, 1994.
48. Mattson RH, Cramer JA, Collins JF: A comparison of valproate with carbamazepine for the treatment of complex partial seizures and secondarily generalized tonic-clonic seizures in adults. The Department of Veterans Affairs Epilepsy Cooperative Study No. 264 Group. N Engl J Med 327(11):765–771, 1992.
49. Lenehan GP, Gastfriend DR, Stetler C: Use of haloperidol in the management of agitated or violent, alcohol-intoxicated patients in the emergency department: A pilot study. J Emerg Nursing 11(2):72–79, 1985.
50. Regier DA, Farmer ME, Rae DS, et al: Comorbidity of mental disorders with alcohol and other drug abuse. Results from the Epidemiologic Catchment Area (ECA) Study. JAMA 264(19):2511–2518, 1990.
51. Caton CLM, Gralnick A, Bender S, et al: Young chronic patients and substance abuse. Hosp Community Psychiatry 40(10):1037–1040, 1989.
52. Buckley P, Thompson P, Way L, et al: Substance abuse among patients with treatment resistant schizophrenia: Characteristics and implications for clozapine therapy. Am J Psychiatry 151(3):385–389, 1994.
53. Albanese MJ, Khantzian EJ, Murphy SL, et al: Decreased substance use in chronically psychotic patients treated with clozapine (letter). Am J Psychiatry 151(5):780–781, 1994.
54. Pecknold JC: Survey of the adjuvant use of benzodiazepines for treating outpatients with schizophrenia. J Psychiatry Neurosci 18(2):82–84, 1993.
55. McLellan AT, Luborsky L, Woody GE, et al: Predicting response to alcohol and drug abuse treatments. Arch Gen Psychiatry 40:620–625, 1983.
56. Lam W, Sze PC, Sacks HS, et al: Meta-analysis of randomized controlled trials of nicotine chewing-gum. Lancet 2(8549):27–30, 1987.
57. Covey LS, Glassman AH: A meta-analysis of double-blind placebo-controlled trials of clonidine for smoking cessation. Br J Addict 86(8):991–998, 1991.
58. Imperial Cancer Research Fund General Practice Research Group: Effectiveness of a nicotine patch in helping people stop smoking: Results of a randomised trial in general practice. Br Med J 306:1304–1308, 1993.
59. Weiss RD, Mirin SM, Michael JL, et al: Psychopathology in chronic cocaine abusers. Am J Drug Alcohol Abuse 12:17–29, 1986.
60. Gawin FH, Riordan C, Kleber H: Methylphenidate treatment of cocaine abusers without attention deficit disorder: A negative report. Am J Drug Alcohol Abuse 11:193–197, 1985.
61. Gastfriend DR: Pharmacotherapy of psychiatric syndromes with comorbid chemical dependency. J Addict Dis 12(3):155–170, 1993.
62. Bodkin JA, Zornberg GL, Lukas SE, Cole JO: Buprenorphine treatment of refractory depression. J Clin Psychopharmacol 15:49–57, 1994.

Pharmacological Treatments for Addiction in Pregnant Populations

Laura J. Miller, MD

Most infants in the United States are born having been exposed to an addictive drug in utero. Although exact figures are difficult to determine, the best available recent estimates are that about 73% of neonates have been exposed to alcohol, about 20% to 25% to nicotine, about 4.5% to cocaine, and about 2% to 3% to opiates.[1, 2] Because approximately 50% of pregnancies in the United States are unplanned,[3] much of this exposure occurs before a woman realizes she is pregnant. Even if she then stops or cuts down on drug use, significant adverse effects can arise from first-trimester exposure.

For women with severe addictive disorders, complete cessation of drug use during pregnancy is not always possible, even with optimal nonpharmacological intervention. Further, abrupt cessation of drug use may adversely affect a fetus or a pregnant woman. In these cases, pharmacological treatment may be the safest alternative.

This chapter summarizes what is known about the effects during pregnancy of pharmacological agents used to treat addiction to alcohol, cocaine, opiates, and nicotine. This information should be taken into account when weighing the risks and benefits of pharmacological treatment, not only for patients known to be pregnant but for any potentially pregnant woman of reproductive age.

Addiction to Alcohol

Untreated alcohol addiction during pregnancy poses major risks to pregnant women and their offspring. The most notable result of in utero exposure is fetal alcohol syndrome, characterized by growth retardation, facial dysmorphism, and enduring central nervous system dysfunction.[1] The full syndrome affects about 1 in 300 to 1 in 1000 births. Partial expressions of the syndrome, known as *fetal alcohol effects*, occur in about 1 in 100 babies.[1]

Pharmacotherapy for alcohol addiction may be used for two main purposes: during detoxification, to treat complications of withdrawal, and later to decrease the likelihood of return to drinking. Each of these is addressed next.

DETOXIFICATION

Optimal management of alcohol withdrawal during pregnancy begins with recognition of its occurrence. Some signs of early withdrawal may be missed because they resemble normal pregnancy-related changes. These include tachypnea, respiratory alkalosis, tachycardia, nausea, vomiting, restlessness, and, in cases of preeclampsia or eclampsia, hypertension and seizures. However, symptoms such as pronounced tremor, diaphoresis, fever, agitation, distractibility, impaired memory, and hallucinosis are not characteristic of pregnancy and are more likely to be recognized as symptoms of alcohol withdrawal. A careful history and laboratory screening remain the most reliable ways to make the diagnosis.

Untreated alcohol withdrawal can result in risks to both a woman and her fetus if accompanied by agitation, hypertension, tachycardia, or seizures. If these remain severe despite supportive measures, pharmacotherapy is indicated. The agents most often used are carbamazepine, benzodiazepines (primarily for agitation and seizures), and beta-adrenergic–blocking agents (primarily for hypertension and tachycardia). Antipsychotic agents may also be needed for severe or prolonged alcohol hallucinosis.

Benzodiazepines During Pregnancy

The use of benzodiazepines during pregnancy is controversial owing to conflicting results from studies of teratogenicity. Some studies found an increased incidence of oral clefts after first-trimester diazepam exposure,[4–6] but others did not.[7] A widespread increase in diazepam use among women did not result in a population-wide increase in the incidence of oral clefts. A weak association, if any, is found between diazepam and oral clefts. Lorazepam has not been linked to oral clefts or other congenital anomalies[8] and has a theoretical advantage in that it does not accumulate in a fetus.[9]

Data on behavioral teratogenicity are also contradictory. One group of researchers reported impaired motor and cognitive development after in utero benzodiazepine exposure.[10, 11] However, major methodological shortcomings have been found in the studies on which these conclusions are based. Other studies have found no link between in utero benzodiazepine exposure and lower IQ[12] or mental retardation,[13] although it was difficult to separate out the effects of benzodiazepines from the effects of alcohol.

It is not uncommon for alcohol withdrawal to occur during labor, because a mother may then be hospitalized and not have access to alcoholic beverages. If high doses of benzodiazepines are needed right before birth (the equivalent of 30 mg of diazepam or more), neonatal toxicity is likely.[14] This is manifested as the floppy baby syndrome: hypotonia, hyporeflexia, lethargy, difficulty sucking, poor respiratory efforts, and difficulty maintaining body temperature. These effects are temporary and can be reversed with flumazenil.[15] Because

flumazenil has a short half-life, the baby must be carefully monitored to assess whether repeat doses are needed. Overall, using benzodiazepines when needed is less risky than allowing delirium tremens or severe agitation to remain untreated.

One advantage of benzodiazepines during alcohol withdrawal is that they can be administered intravenously. However, during pregnancy, this presents a unique complication. Intravenous benzodiazepines are usually stored in a solution with a sodium benzoate/benzoic acid buffer. This buffer tends to displace bilirubin from albumin, raising free bilirubin levels and increasing the risk of kernicterus.[16] During pregnancy, oral preparations of benzodiazepines should be used whenever possible.

If benzodiazepines are used for prolonged periods during pregnancy, neonatal withdrawal may result.[17–19] Symptoms include hypertonia, hyperreflexia, and tremor. These symptoms resolve spontaneously.

Carbamazepine During Pregnancy

Carbamazepine is a weak human teratogen. First-trimester use increases the risk of spina bifida and minor congenital anomalies.[20–22] One study suggested an association with mental retardation,[20] but others found no decrease in IQ after in utero carbamazepine exposure.[23, 24]

Third-trimester carbamazepine use can lower vitamin K–dependent clotting factors,[25] thus rendering a newborn more vulnerable to hemorrhage. This risk can be prevented by administering 20 mg of vitamin K orally to a woman during her last 1 to 2 months of pregnancy and 1 mg intramuscularly to the baby at birth. Another potential but rare complication is transient hepatic dysfunction.[26]

In most cases, benzodiazepines are preferred during pregnancy for the treatment of alcohol withdrawal. In some instances, a concomitant illness, such as epilepsy or bipolar mood disorder, warrants the use of carbamazepine. If carbamazepine is necessary, folate should be given daily to decrease the risk of neural tube defects.[27] Alpha-fetoprotein screening for neural tube defects is indicated if a woman has had first-trimester exposure. Vitamin K should be given as described earlier. Serum levels of carbamazepine can be misleading during pregnancy because protein binding is decreased; thus, clinical condition or levels of free carbamazepine should guide dosing.[28]

Beta-Adrenergic Blocking Agents During Pregnancy

Hypertension during pregnancy, whether or not it is caused or exacerbated by alcohol withdrawal, can worsen fetal outcome. Propranolol and atenolol have been widely used to treat hypertension during pregnancy, with no adverse effects reported in systematic studies.[29] By blocking the beta-2 receptors in the uterine wall, propranolol can increase myometrial tone.[30] Although this has not been demonstrated to result in premature labor, it has swayed some clinicians to prefer a selective beta-1–blocking agent such as atenolol.

Antipsychotic Agents During Pregnancy

For severe or persistent alcohol hallucinosis, antipsychotic agents may be required. Most studies of in utero exposure to antipsychotic agents have not shown any link with teratogenicity.[31–36] However, two studies demonstrated an increase in nonspecific congenital anomalies with phenothiazines.[37, 38]

For that and other reasons, phenothiazines are best avoided during pregnancy. Women with alcoholism are especially prone to hypotension and liver damage, both of which can be side effects of phenothiazines. Higher-potency neuroleptics, such as haloperidol and trifluoperazine, are less likely to contribute to hypotension or hepatotoxicity and have not been associated with teratogenicity. They are also better tolerated during pregnancy because they are less sedating and have fewer anticholinergic side effects.

Although antipsychotic use during pregnancy does not seem to affect IQ, children exposed to dopamine blockade in utero may be taller or heavier than other children.[39] This may be related to dopamine's influence on growth hormone.

If neuroleptic use is prolonged during pregnancy, a mild neonatal withdrawal syndrome can result.[40] This includes hypertonia, tremor, and poor motor maturity. In rare cases, withdrawal dyskinesia occurs in the baby.[41] In addition to tremor and hypertonia, this can include hyperreflexia, irritability, abnormal posturing, tongue thrusting, irregular respiration, and a shrill cry. These symptoms resolve over several months and are sometimes alleviated by diphenhydramine elixir.

PROPHYLAXIS AGAINST FUTURE DRINKING

The pharmacological agent most commonly used to prevent future drinking is disulfiram. In some patients, especially those with a concomitant mood disorder or mood disturbance that persists after several weeks of abstinence,

lithium is tried. Considerations for using these agents during pregnancy are discussed next.

Disulfiram During Pregnancy

Disulfiram poses a number of risks to a fetus. If a pregnant woman drinks alcohol while using disulfiram, the resultant hypotension may decrease placental perfusion. Further, the combination of disulfiram and even small amounts of ethanol may be teratogenic.[42] This is thought to be because disulfiram inhibits aldehyde dehydrogenase, allowing an accumulation of acetaldehyde as ethanol is metabolized. Acetaldehyde may be a potent teratogen.

An additional risk arises if a pregnant woman taking disulfiram is exposed to lead. A metabolite of disulfiram functions as a chelating agent for lead, allowing it to cross the blood-brain barrier easily. This means that even small amounts of lead may enter the fetal brain in sufficient amounts to cause damage.[43] Women may be exposed to lead via homemade alcoholic beverages, lead-based paint chips, occupational sources, or soldering.

Before embarking on a course of disulfiram therapy for a woman of reproductive age, it is useful to obtain a urine pregnancy test. Potential risks during pregnancy should be explained, and family planning should be discussed when appropriate.

Lithium During Pregnancy

Early data on in utero lithium exposure suggested that lithium increased the risk of cardiovascular anomalies. More recent studies, including the first prospective study, have shown that the risk is less than it previously seemed.[44] Lithium may be a weak teratogen, with some predilection for the cardiovascular system.

In some animal species, the combination of lithium and ethanol is especially teratogenic, significantly more so than either agent alone.[45] This may be because of a disulfiram-like effect of lithium, which inhibits aldehyde dehydrogenase so that acetaldehyde accumulates as ethanol is metabolized.[46] Although this has not been directly studied in humans, it suggests the possibility that lithium is more teratogenic in women who drink.

In addition to its teratogenicity, lithium has been associated with a number of other adverse effects during pregnancy. It may produce side effects in a fetus or neonate that are similar to those it causes in adults. Fetal diabetes insipidus can result in polyhydramnios. In rare instances, this may become so extreme that the volume of fetal urine does not allow enough room for the woman's lungs to expand, and some amniotic fluid thus must be withdrawn.[47] Thyroid function can be inhibited in a fetus, although this is reversible and has not been reported to lead to permanent sequelae.[48] Lithium may be associated with an increased rate of prematurity and in some reports has been linked with macrosomia.[49] Even when a pregnant woman has a therapeutic serum lithium level, neonatal lithium toxicity can occur.[50] Symptoms include poor sucking, abnormal respiratory patterns, cyanosis, hypotonia, decreased Moro reflex, cardiac arrhythmias, poor myocardial contractility, and hypoglycemia.

Lithium's efficacy for the treatment of primary alcoholism is not well established. Given its potential risks, it is not recommended for this purpose during pregnancy. However, its use may be necessary for patients with concomitant lithium-responsive bipolar mood disorder. The combination of untreated mania and active drinking probably presents a much greater risk to a pregnant woman and her fetus than does lithium.

In patients for whom lithium is necessary during pregnancy, certain practices can minimize the risks. Days 18 to 55 after conception, the period of cardiac formation, should be kept lithium free if possible.[51] Electroconvulsive therapy is a reasonable alternative if manic symptoms arise during that time.[52] If lithium must be given during that period or was given before pregnancy was diagnosed, an ultrasonogram at about 16 weeks of pregnancy may be useful to assess cardiac formation.[53] Fluid volume increases as pregnancy progresses, and higher doses may be needed to maintain therapeutic serum levels. Toward the end of pregnancy, lithium can be given in small divided doses to avoid toxic peaks in the neonate. At the time of labor, the patient and her obstetrician should be instructed to cut the lithium dose in half. Because labor results in substantial fluid loss, lithium toxicity may result if this is not done. However, because women with bipolar disorder are at high risk for postpartum psychosis,[54] discontinuing lithium totally is not advisable. Serum level should be checked about 2 days after delivery, and the dose adjusted accordingly.

Addiction to Cocaine

Certain sociocultural aspects of cocaine use contribute to its association with unplanned pregnancies.[55] Although it actually suppresses sexual desire, it is thought of as an aphrodisiac in some circles and therefore is often associated with sexual intercourse. Further, a number of women pay for cocaine habits through prostitution. Pregnancies in women addicted to cocaine have a far greater likelihood of poor outcomes, including prematurity, growth retardation, placental abruption, miscarriage, stillbirth, fetal distress, and neurobehavioral abnormalities. However, it is not yet clear how much of that can be attributed to the direct effects of cocaine and how much to associated conditions such as inadequate prenatal care, poor nutrition, other drugs, infections, and so forth.[56]

The pharmacological agents most often used to provide acute relief of "crash" symptoms are benzodiazepines and neuroleptics, which were discussed earlier. Agents sometimes used to prevent relapse by reducing cocaine craving are amantadine, bromocriptine, and tricyclic antidepressants. Their use during pregnancy is summarized next.

AMANTADINE DURING PREGNANCY

No large-scale systematic studies have investigated outcome after in utero amantadine exposure. In a study of 18 pregnant women with Parkinson's disease, all 4 who took amantadine had complications, including miscarriage, hydatidiform mole, preeclampsia, and first-trimester bleeding.[57] Another infant was born with a single cardiac ventricle and pulmonary atresia after first-trimester amantadine exposure.[58] Although some reports describe safe use of amantadine during pregnancy,[59] it is best avoided until further data are available.

BROMOCRIPTINE DURING PREGNANCY

Bromocriptine is often used to treat certain forms of infertility. When a woman becomes pregnant, bromocriptine is discontinued. For this reason, there are several studies of brief first-trimester exposure to bromocriptine[60] but no data about second- or third-trimester exposure. Available studies have demonstrated no adverse effects. Because of insufficient data, it is best to avoid prescribing bromocriptine as an anticraving agent during pregnancy. However, if its therapeutic efficacy is clear in an individual case, it is probably far worse to risk ongoing cocaine use. Brief, inadvertent exposure to bromocriptine before a pregnancy is discovered is no cause for alarm.

TRICYCLIC ANTIDEPRESSANTS DURING PREGNANCY

A number of studies have uncovered no increased incidence of congenital anomalies after in utero exposure to tricyclic antidepressants.[61–63] Although some of these studies are small and methodologically flawed, the overall pattern of similar results over several decades in several countries suggests that tricyclic antidepressants do not cause morphological teratogenicity in humans. No data are yet available to determine whether there are enduring behavioral effects on exposed offspring. However, adverse behavioral outcomes are probably far more likely with ongoing cocaine use than with addiction successfully treated with an antidepressant.

The anticholinergic activity of tricyclic antidepressants may account for side effects occasionally observed in a fetus or neonate, such as urinary retention[61] and tachycardia.[64] In addition, some infants may experience mild withdrawal phenomena after prolonged tricyclic use during pregnancy.[40] Relatively common symptoms include irritability, tachycardia, and tachypnea. More rarely, these may progress to tremor, clonus, or seizures. In these rare instances, the infant may be treated with a low dose of the antidepressant agent, which is gradually withdrawn.

Some common side effects of tricyclics, such as constipation, sedation, tachycardia, and orthostatic hypotension, may be more difficult to tolerate during pregnancy. This is because pregnancy itself may cause those symptoms, which are then intensified by the medication. Further, as pregnancy progresses, serum levels of tricyclics usually decline owing to increased fluid volume.[65] If a tricyclic that appeared to be working seems to lose its effectiveness during pregnancy, the serum level should be checked to see whether a previously therapeutic dose has become subtherapeutic.

GUIDELINES FOR PHARMACOLOGY OF COCAINE ADDICTION DURING PREGNANCY

Whenever possible, nonpharmacological measures should be attempted first. Severe, lingering psychotic symptoms during detoxification can be safely treated with haloperidol or trifluoperazine. Severe agitation can be managed with short-term use of lorazepam or clonazepam.

When a coexisting major depression persists after postintoxication dysphoria, treatment with desipramine or nortryptiline is indicated if psychotherapeutic measures are insufficient. Levels should be monitored carefully, at least once per trimester or whenever symptoms recur. If a patient is symptom free and has supportive surroundings, the dose can be gradually tapered beginning about 3 weeks before her due date in order to minimize withdrawal symptoms in her newborn.

In the absence of major depression, tricyclics or bromocriptine may be used during pregnancy in cases in which they clearly decrease the risk of resuming cocaine use. The use of amantadine for this purpose may pose greater risk to a fetus.

Addiction to Opiates

Untreated opiate addiction poses major hazards to pregnant women and their offspring.[1] This is probably not because opiates are teratogenic but because of numerous associated complications. Women addicted to opiates have a high incidence of associated social problems such as poverty, homelessness, physical and sexual abuse, poor nutrition, inadequate prenatal care, and prostitution or other criminal activity. The addiction and associated behavior severely compromise a woman's ability to plan for and meet the needs of a newborn baby. These women have a high rate of concomitant psychiatric and medical illness, including human immunodeficiency virus infection. All of these factors contribute to a high rate of obstetrical complications, custody loss, and enduring physical and psychological problems in offspring.

Many of these risks can be greatly alleviated by methadone maintenance during pregnancy. As compared with pregnant women using "street" heroin, methadone-maintained women have babies with higher birth weights,[66] suffer fewer obstetrical complications,[67] are less likely to engage in criminal activity, have less concomitant drug use, and are more aware of their children's needs.[68] These gains seem to result partly from accompanying supportive treatment. They may also be due to receiving a steady dose of a pure agent instead of chaotic dose changes, unknown additives, and repeated cycles of intoxication and withdrawal. The one adverse effect that is worse with methadone than with street heroin is neonatal withdrawal.[69] Because of methadone's longer half-life, withdrawal in a newborn is more frequent, more severe, and more likely to have a delayed onset.

Given these data, three approaches to pharmacological treatment of opiate addiction can reasonably be considered during pregnancy, as discussed next.

METHADONE MAINTENANCE AT DOSES NEEDED TO MAINTAIN A PATIENT FREE OF WITHDRAWAL SYMPTOMS

This choice is the least likely to result in recurrence of street use and therefore is the most likely to be accompanied by improvements in prenatal care, nutrition, lifestyle, and planning for the baby, as well as diminished risk of medical and obstetrical complications. It is the most likely to result in neonatal withdrawal. However, neonatal withdrawal is a self-limited condition, unlike the far more serious complications resulting from street heroin use. For this reason, this choice is appropriate for most pregnant women addicted to opiates.

Methadone maintenance during pregnancy is, for the most part, conducted according to the same guidelines as methadone maintenance in general. However, a few pregnancy-related modifications must be kept in mind. As pregnancy progresses, a given dose of methadone often results in a lower serum level, primarily because of increased fluid volume. Dosage requirements may increase accordingly. Further, methadone may produce a false impression of fetal distress on a nonstress test, an obstetrical procedure commonly used to assess fetal well-being.[70] Methadone should be administered after scheduled nonstress tests, not beforehand. Finally, provisions should be made for close observation of a newborn baby for the first 4 weeks of life. Although neonatal withdrawal symptoms usually appear within the first 48 hours, delayed onset between 2 and 4 weeks after birth has been noted in 10% of methadone-addicted babies.[69]

LOW-DOSE METHADONE MAINTENANCE

Although studies have come to contradictory conclusions, most available evidence suggests that the severity of neonatal withdrawal depends on the maternal methadone dose.[71] This has prompted some attempts to maintain pregnant women on low-dose methadone (e.g., 20 mg/day instead of the 60 mg/day or more typically needed to avoid craving). Two major risks are involved in this choice. One is that the mother will resume illicit drug use; the other is fetal morbidity, including fetal distress,

preterm delivery, or impaired fetal growth resulting from too rapid a decline in dose.[71, 72] It is hypothesized that a rapid, rather than gradual, dose reduction causes rapid replenishment of neurotransmitters. In the presence of increased brain receptors due to addiction, this could produce central nervous system excitability, manifested as intrauterine seizures or other signs of fetal distress.[71]

Reducing the dose slowly while carefully monitoring a fetus may be a reasonable option for a few highly motivated women in intensive psychosocial treatment programs.

METHADONE DETOXIFICATION

The primary motivation for methadone detoxification is to avoid neonatal withdrawal. If detoxification is attempted too rapidly, marked fetal distress and even fetal death can result.[73] Detoxification during pregnancy has been safely accomplished slowly and with frequent fetal monitoring. Such a program begins with substituting the best estimate of the equivalent dose of methadone for the prior heroin intake. The dose is reduced by about 0.2 to 1 mg/day; thus, detoxification may take as long as 8 weeks.[72] If any sign of fetal distress is noted, detoxification is stopped and methadone is maintained. Even when carried out safely, detoxification poses the risk of resumption of illicit drug use. For this reason, it is best begun in an inpatient setting and followed by a highly structured residential facility for pregnant addicted women.

Addiction to Nicotine

The harmful effects of cigarette smoking during pregnancy have been well publicized. After evidence accumulated that cigarette smoking substantially increases infant mortality, miscarriage, prematurity, and low birth weight, a massive public education campaign was mounted. As a result, pregnancy is a time when many women are highly motivated to quit smoking. Behavioral methods of smoking cessation have a high rate of success.

Unfortunately, about 20% to 25% of pregnant women in the United States continue to smoke during pregnancy.[2] Heavy smokers (those who smoke one pack or more per day) are especially likely to continue smoking throughout a pregnancy. When nonpharmacological attempts at smoking cessation fail, clinicians must assess whether nicotine replacement systems will improve maternal and fetal outcome.

A key difference between nicotine replacement systems and cigarette smoking is that the latter delivers thousands of substances in addition to nicotine.[2] It is not known which adverse fetal effects of smoking can be attributed to nicotine alone and which to other cigarette toxins such as carbon monoxide. Existing evidence supports the idea that nicotine adversely affects placental circulation. As a result, fetal heart rate may initially be increased via sympathetic nervous system activation. Later (usually in the third trimester), nicotine may decrease fetal heart rate owing to hypoxia. This in turn may contribute to behavioral problems later in life. Other cigarette toxins probably amplify poor outcomes. For example, carbon monoxide contributes to fetal hypoxia by binding to fetal hemoglobin.

Another important difference between cigarette smoking and nicotine delivery systems is the dose of nicotine.[2] A pack-per-day smoker consumes about 20 mg of nicotine per day. A person chewing 12 pieces of nicotine polacrilex gum per day (more than most smokers use) takes in about 12 mg of nicotine per day. A person wearing a transdermal nicotine patch absorbs about 15 to 20 mg of nicotine per day (depending on the strength), but less if it is removed at night.

In conclusion, smoking cessation should be a top priority during pregnancy. In cases in which nonpharmacological attempts at quitting are unsuccessful, nicotine delivery systems are likely to be substantially less harmful than heavy cigarette smoking. Because nicotine gum delivers a lower total dose and is more easily titrated, it is preferred when possible during pregnancy.

Conclusion

Treating women with addictive disorders during their pregnancies can be a complex challenge and a golden opportunity. For many women, the desire to protect their babies may kindle new hope and motivation to enter treatment. In some cases, this may allow success with supportive nonpharmacological treatment, especially in the context of programs geared specifically to pregnant addicted women. In other cases, pharmacological intervention is needed. When properly chosen and administered, pharmacotherapy poses fewer risks to both a woman and her fetus than does uncontrolled use of addictive substances.

REFERENCES

1. Finnegan LP, Kandall SR: Maternal and neonatal effects of alcohol and drugs. In Lowinson JH, Ruiz P, Millman RB (eds): Substance Abuse: A Comprehensive Textbook, 2nd ed. Baltimore, Williams & Wilkins, 1992, p 628.
2. Benowitz NL: Nicotine replacement therapy during pregnancy. JAMA 266(22):3174–3177, 1991.
3. Jones EF, Forrest JD, Henshaw SK, et al: Pregnancy, Contraception and Family Planning Services in Industrialized Countries. New Haven, Yale University Press, 1989, p 12.
4. Saxen I: Associations between oral clefts and drugs taken during pregnancy. Int J Epidemiol 4(1):37–44, 1975.
5. Aarskog D: Association between maternal intake of diazepam and oral clefts. Lancet 2:921, 1975.
6. Safra MJ, Oakley GP: Association between cleft lip with or without cleft palate and prenatal exposure to diazepam. Lancet 2:478–480, 1975.
7. Rosenberg L, Mitchell AA, Parsells JL, et al: Lack of relation of oral clefts to diazepam use during pregnancy. N Engl J Med 309(21):1282–1285, 1983.
8. St. Clair SM, Schirmer RG: First-trimester exposure to alprazolam. Obstet Gynecol 80(5):843–846, 1992.
9. Whitelaw AGL, Cummings J, McFadyen IR: Effect of maternal lorazepam on the neonate. Br Med J 282:1106–1108, 1981.
10. Laegreid L, Hagberg G, Lundberg A: Neurodevelopment in late infancy after prenatal exposure to benzodiazepines—a prospective study. Neuropediatrics 23:60–67, 1992.
11. Viggedal G, Hagberg BS, Laegreid L, et al: Mental development in late infancy after prenatal exposure to benzodiazepines—a prospective study. J Child Psychol Psychiatry 34(3):295–305, 1993.
12. Hartz SC, Heinonen OP, Shapiro S, et al: Antenatal exposure to meprobamate and chlordiazepoxide in relation to malformations, mental development, and childhood mortality. N Engl J Med 292(14):726–728, 1975.
13. Bergman U, Rosa FW, Baum C, et al: Effects of exposure to benzodiazepine during fetal life. Lancet 340:694–696, 1992.
14. Cree JE, Meyer J, Hailey DM: Diazepam in labour: Its metabolism and effect on the clinical condition and thermogenesis of the newborn. Br Med J 4:251–255, 1973.
15. Stahl MM, Saldeen P, Vinge E: Reversal of fetal benzodiazepine intoxication using flumazenil. Br J Obstet Gynaecol 100:185–188, 1993.
16. Schiff D, Chan G, Stern L: Fixed drug combinations and the displacement of bilirubin from albumin. Pediatrics 48:139–141, 1971.
17. Athinarayanan P, Peirog SH, Nigam SK, et al: Chlordiazepoxide withdrawal in the neonate. Am J Obstet Gynecol 124(2):212–213, 1976.
18. Mazzi E: Possible neonatal diazepam withdrawal: A case report. Am J Obstet Gynecol 129(5):586–587, 1977.
19. Anderson PO, McGuire GG: Neonatal alprazolam withdrawal—possible effects of breast feeding. Drug Intell Clin Pharm 23:614, 1989.
20. Jones KL, Lacro RV, Johnson KA, et al: Pattern of malformations in the children of women treated with carbamazepine during pregnancy. N Engl J Med 320(25):1661–1666, 1989.
21. Rosa FW: Spina bifida in infants of women treated with carbamazepine during pregnancy. N Engl J Med 324(10):674–676, 1991.
22. Little BB, Santos-Ramos R, Newell JF, et al: Megadose

carbamazepine during the period of neural tube closure. Obstet Gynecol 82(4):705–708, 1993.

23. Van der Pol MC, Hadders-Algra M, Huisjes HJ, et al: Antiepileptic medication in pregnancy: Late effects on the children's central nervous system development. Am J Obstet Gynecol 164(1):121–128, 1991.

24. Scolnik D, Nulman I, Rovet J, et al: Neurodevelopment of children exposed in utero to phenytoin and carbamazepine monotherapy. JAMA 271(10):767–770, 1994.

25. Moslet U, Hansen ES: A review of vitamin K, epilepsy and pregnancy. Acta Neurol Scand 85:39–43, 1992.

26. Merlob P, Mor N, Litwin A: Transient hepatic dysfunction in an infant of an epileptic mother treated with carbamazepine during pregnancy and breastfeeding. Ann Pharmacother 26:1563–1565, 1992.

27. Dansky LV, Rosenblatt DS, Andermann E: Mechanisms of teratogenesis: Folic acid and antiepileptic therapy. Neurology 42(Suppl 5):32–42, 1992.

28. Yerby MS, Friel PN, McCormick K: Antiepileptic drug disposition during pregnancy. Neurology 42(Suppl 5):12–16, 1992.

29. Rubin PC: Beta-blockers in pregnancy. N Engl J Med 305(22):1323–1326, 1981.

30. Ryan CL, Pappas BA: Prenatal exposure to antiadrenergic antihypertensive drugs: Effects on neurobehavioral development and the behavioral consequences of enriched rearing. Neurotoxicol Teratol 12:359–366, 1990.

31. Sobel DE: Fetal damage due to ECT, insulin coma, chlorpromazine, or reserpine. Arch Gen Psychiatry 2:606–611, 1960.

32. Rawlings WJ, Ferguson R, Maddison TG: Phenmetrazine and trifluoperazine. Med J Aust 1:370, 1963.

33. Van Waes AV, Van de Velde E: Safety evaluation of haloperidol in the treatment of hyperemesis gravidarum. J Clin Pharmacol 224–227, 1969.

34. Scanlan FJ: The use of thioridazine (Melleril) [sic] during the first trimester. Med J Aust 1:1271–1272, 1972.

35. Rieder RO, Rosenthal D, Wender P, et al: The offspring of schizophrenics; fetal and neonatal deaths. Arch Gen Psychiatry 32:200–211, 1975.

36. Slone D, Siskind V, Heinonen O, et al: Antenatal exposure to the phenothiazines in relation to congenital malformations, perinatal mortality rate, birth weight, and intelligence quotient score. Am J Obstet Gynecol 128(5):486–488, 1977.

37. Rumeau-Rouquette C, Goujard J, Huel G: Possible teratogenic effect of phenothiazines in human beings. Teratology 15:57–64, 1977.

38. Edlund MJ, Craig TJ: Antipsychotic drug use and birth defects: An epidemiologic reassessment. Compr Psychiatry 25(1):244–248, 1976.

39. Platt JE, Friedhoff AJ, Broman SH, et al: Effects of prenatal exposure to neuroleptic drugs on children's growth. Neuropsychopharmacology 1(3):205–212, 1988.

40. Auerbach JF, Hans SL, Marcus J, et al: Maternal psychotropic medication and neonatal behavior. Neurotoxicol Teratol 14:399–406, 1992.

41. Sexson WR, Barak Y: Withdrawal emergent syndrome in an infant associated with maternal haloperidol therapy. J Perinatol 9:170–172, 1989.

42. Gardner RJM, Clarkson JE: A malformed child whose previously alcoholic mother had taken disulfiram. NZ Med J 93:184–186, 1981.

43. Oskarsson A, Ljungberg T, Stahle L, et al: Behavioral and neurochemical effects after combined perinatal treatment of rats with lead and disulfiram. Neurobehav Toxicol Teratol 8:591–599, 1986.

44. Cohen LS, Friedman JM, Jefferson J, et al: A reevalua-

tion of risk of in utero exposure to lithium. JAMA 271(2):146–150, 1994.

45. Sharma A, Rawat AK: Teratogenic effects of lithium and ethanol in the developing fetus. Alcohol 3:101–106, 1986.

46. Messiha FS: Lithium and the neonate: Developmental and metabolic aspects. Alcohol 3:107–112, 1986.

47. Krause S, Ebbesen F, Lange AP: Polyhydramnios with maternal lithium treatment. Obstet Gynecol 75(3):504–506, 1990.

48. Karlsson K, Lindstedt G, Lundberg PA, et al: Transplacental lithium poisoning: Reversible inhibition of fetal thyroid. Lancet 1:1295, 1975.

49. Troyer WA, Pereira GR, Lannon RA, et al: Association of maternal lithium exposure and premature delivery. J Perinatol 13(2):123–127, 1993.

50. Simard M, Gumbiner B, Lee A, et al: Lithium carbonate intoxication: A case report and review of the literature. Arch Intern Med 149:36–46, 1989.

51. Wisner KL, Perel JM: Psychopharmacologic agents and electroconvulsive therapy during pregnancy and the puerperium. In Cohen RL (ed): Psychiatric Consultation in Childbirth Settings: Parent- and Child-Oriented Approaches. New York, Plenum, 1988, p 184.

52. Miller LJ: Use of electroconvulsive therapy during pregnancy. Hosp Community Psychiatry 45(5):444–450, 1994.

53. Long WA, Willis PW: Maternal lithium and neonatal Ebstein's anomaly: Evaluation with cross-sectional echocardiography. Am J Perinatol 1(2):182–184, 1984.

54. Kendell RE, Chalmers JC, Platz C: Epidemiology of puerperal psychoses. Br J Psychiatry 150:662–673, 1987.

55. Winick C: Substances of use and abuse and sexual behavior. In Lowinson JH, Ruiz P, Millman RB (eds): Substance Abuse: A Comprehensive Textbook, 2nd ed. Baltimore, Williams & Wilkins, 1992, p 727.

56. Mayes LC, Granger RH, Bornstein MH, et al: The problem of prenatal cocaine exposure: A rush to judgment. JAMA 267(3):406–408, 1992.

57. Golbe LI: Parkinson's disease and pregnancy. Neurology 37:1245–1249, 1987.

58. Nora JJ, Nora AH, Way GL: Cardiovascular maldevelopment associated with maternal exposure to amantadine. Lancet 2:607, 1975.

59. Levy M, Pastuszak A, Koren G: Fetal outcome following intrauterine amantadine exposure. Reprod Toxicol 5:79–81, 1991.

60. Turkalj I, Braun P, Krupp P: Surveillance of bromocriptine in pregnancy. JAMA 247(11):1589–1591, 1982.

61. Elia J, Katz IR, Simpson GM: Teratogenicity of psychotherapeutic medications. Psychopharmacol Bull 23(4):531–586, 1987.

62. Misri S, Sivertz K: Tricyclic drugs in pregnancy and lactation: A preliminary report. Int J Psychiatry Med 21:157–171, 1991.

63. Pastuszak A, Schick-Boschetto B, Zuber C, et al: Pregnancy outcome following first-trimester exposure to fluoxetine (Prozac). JAMA 269(17):2246–2248, 1993.

64. Prentice A, Brown R: Fetal tachyarrhythmia and maternal antidepressant treatment. Br Med J 298(6667):190, 1989.

65. Wisner KL, Perel JM, Wheeler SB: Tricyclic dose requirements across pregnancy. Am J Psychiatry 150(10):1541–1542, 1993.

66. Kandall SR, Albin S, Lowinson J, et al: Differential effects of maternal heroin and methadone use on birthweight. Pediatrics 58(5):681–685, 1976.

67. Harper RG, Solish GI, Purow HM, et al: The effect of a methadone treatment program upon pregnant heroin addicts and their newborn infants. Pediatrics 54(3):300–305, 1974.

68. Keenan E, Dorman A, O'Connor J: Six year follow up of forty five pregnant opiate addicts. Irish J Med Sci 162(7):252–255, 1993.
69. Levy M, Spino M: Neonatal withdrawal syndrome: Associated drugs and pharmacologic management. Pharmacotherapy 13(3):202–211, 1993.
70. Archie CL, Lee MI, Sokol RJ, et al: The effects of methadone treatment on the reactivity of the nonstress test. Obstet Gynecol 74(2):254–255, 1989.
71. Doberczak TM, Kandall SR, Friedmann P: Relation-ships between maternal methadone dosage, maternal-neonatal methadone levels, and neonatal withdrawal. Obstet Gynecol 81(6):936–940, 1993.
72. Maas U, Kattner E, Weingart-Jesse B, et al: Infrequent neonatal opiate withdrawal following maternal metha-done detoxification during pregnancy. J Perinat Med 18:111–118, 1990.
73. Zuspan FP, Gumpel JA, Mejia-Zelaya A, et al: Fetal stress from methadone withdrawal. Am J Obstet Gyne-col 122(1):43–46, 1975.

Pharmacotherapy for Adolescents with Psychoactive Substance Use Disorders

Yifrah Kaminer, MD

Adolescence is a crucial developmental phase for the onset and diagnosis of psychiatric disorders, including psychoactive substance use disorders (PSUD).[1] The co-occurrence of PSUD with other psychiatric disorders has been termed *dual diagnosis.*

Psychiatric comorbidity is highly prevalent among children and adolescents in the general population.[2] Adolescents with a dual diagnosis constitute the largest subgroup of adolescents with PSUD in clinical settings.[3, 4]

The literature on treatments of adolescents diagnosed with PSUD is replete with descriptive publications on treatment philosophies, modalities, and programs. Very little empirical research on treatment outcome has been reported, and virtually no studies have yet documented the differential efficacy of various therapies or packages of treatment components.[5] Pharmacotherapy for PSUD in this age group appears to be the most neglected therapeutic modality.

In this chapter, relevant adult-oriented literature on psychopharmacotherapy is described and relied on whenever necessary. These publications also serve as a basis for generalization; however, these generalizations are made cautiously, and their limitations are noted whenever possible. Also, although this chapter deals exclusively with pharmacological treatment, a comprehensive treatment plan using various individualized therapeutic interventions must be designed to meet the needs of adolescents (i.e., behavioral-cognitive therapy, self-help groups) in order to achieve a beyond-threshold treatment dosage effect.[6]

The objectives of this chapter are fourfold: to improve our understanding of the scarcity of publications and research on pharmacological interventions of PSUD in adolescents, to review the present knowledge about treatment outcome and its relationship with pharmacotherapy of adolescents with PSUD, to provide an update on the pharmacotherapy of PSUD and of dual diagnosis in adolescents, and to outline suggestions for future directions for the development of pharmacotherapies for this age group.

Difficulties in the Development of Pharmacotherapy for Adolescents with Psychoactive Substance Use Disorders

In contrast to the increased acceptance of pharmacotherapy in adults with PSUD, no systematic research has evaluated the efficacy and safety of psychotropic medications in the treatment of adolescents with PSUD.

Pharmacotherapy in this population may be viewed as a new subset of pediatric psychopharmacology and has met with similar difficulties in developing and achieving recognition. Most of the dissimilarities between pharmacotherapy of adolescents with PSUD (with or without psychiatric comorbidity) and pediatric psychopharmacology stem from the adult-targeted, disease model–oriented treatment approach. This has dominated the addiction field for almost 60 years and lacks age-appropriate developmental perspective to meet the needs of adolescents.

Several factors contribute to the present limited scope of pediatric psychopharmacology clinical research and treatment. Biderman[7] noted the problematical controversy over the use of psychotropic agents in the treatment of individuals who have not completed their development. Furthermore, most parents face the dilemma of whether their offspring's potential to outgrow early-onset disorder without pharmacological intervention is a realistic expectation or merely a form of denial and rationalization that may permit the disorder to take a chronic and debilitating course across age groups. Unfavorable public perceptions of pediatric psychopharmacology are related to concerns about the inappropriate use of medications, especially with institutional patients.[7] Psychiatry bashing by the media or Scientology, which promotes the myth that psychopharmacological treatment is an experimental approach or at best a means of last resort (e.g., stimulants treatment for attention deficit hyperactivity disorder [ADHD]), has created a significant public image problem.

Lack of clarity about parents' and childrens' understanding of the efficacy and risks of pharmacotherapy has led to the emergence of ethical issues, which include the rights of minors to refuse treatment entirely or certain treatment modalities (e.g., medications) and the use of inactive placebos in adolescents in need of pharmacotherapy while participating in research trials.

Knowledge of pediatric pharmacokinetics is still relatively incomplete, and clear approvals or guidelines by the Food and Drug Administration (FDA) for the use of most psychotropics with minors are lacking.[7] A continuing decrease in the number of adolescents hospitalized and a shortened length of stay leading to closure of inpatient units, combined with reduction in research support, have had a neg-

ative impact on efforts to provide precise monitoring based on lengthy delivery of psychopharmacological treatment. Finally, the number of pediatric psychopharmacologists is too small to meet the needs of the field and to continuously advocate for its national recognition.

As noted earlier in this section, the unique factors of pharmacological treatment of adolescents with PSUD that differentiate this subset from pediatric psychopharmacology at large are embedded in philosophical, conceptual, and economical aspects that create a special environment and "politics" of treatment.[8] Hoffmann and colleagues[8] referred to the hesitancy of self-help groups such as Alcoholics Anonymous (AA) to recognize and accept the importance of accurate medical and psychiatric differential diagnoses and the need for pharmacotherapy that may accompany PSUD (with or without psychiatric comorbidity). Sponsors of dually diagnosed adolescents in self-help groups may have a strong objection to any medication, even those without known abuse potential (i.e., lithium, neuroleptics), thus exposing adolescents to increased risk for relapse of both disorders.[5]

Pharmacotherapy and Treatment Outcome

A study on treatment outcome of adolescents with PSUD was conducted in a unit for dually diagnosed patients.[6] Staff, treatment completers', and noncompleters' perceptions of the value of treatment variables for the recovery process were examined. Kaminer and colleagues[6] hypothesized that the smaller the discrepancy between the staff and a patient's perception of the value of treatment variables, the higher the likelihood that a patient would complete treatment. Ten therapeutic modalities including pharmacotherapy were used in the program. Psychotropic medications were administered to patients as necessary based on strict medical criteria and usually only after a medication-free evaluation phase. Comparison was made using a standard rank-ordering system. The data were analyzed using the binomial theorem to investigate group differences.

Staff ranked psychotropic medications and substance addiction education equally as the most important therapeutic components.[6] In contrast, the two groups of patients ranked medications at the bottom of the list. The sharp disagreement in perceptions of the value of medications for treatment outcome, particularly between staff and treatment completers, is intriguing because even inactive treatment effect (i.e., placebo effect) is accepted as a beneficial intervention, especially in short-term treatment, when recommended by a trusted therapist. Also, treatment experiences and a patient's perception of the treatment environment are strong predictors of outcome.[9] Conversely, patients' misconception of treatment (i.e., the level of discrepancy in treatment expectations) is negatively correlated with treatment retention.[10]

Thus, regardless of the disagreement about the role of medications in the therapeutic process, other therapeutic interventions in the treatment program contributed to create a beyond-threshold treatment dosage effect (a descriptive term encompassing frequency, quality, quantity, type, and specificity of intervention). This effect is responsible for achieving patient-treatment matching and the necessary change for completion of planned treatment. In this study, a contract-based individual treatment plan, therapeutic group meeting (modified psychotherapeutic process focusing on the "here and now"), and educational counseling were perceived to be significant (clinically and statistically) for completion of the treatment program by staff and completers.

Kaminer and colleagues[11] reported another study that prospectively assessed attrition from treatment by the same cohort of patients previously assessed. The researchers found that DSM-III-R mood and adjustment disorders were more prevalent among completers, whereas noncompleters were more likely to be assigned a conduct disorder diagnosis.[1] A higher percentage of treatment completers than noncompleters received psychotropic medications (28% vs. 7%). Kaminer and associates[11] suggested that it may be a mood or an adjustment disorder that protects an adolescent with or without a comorbid conduct disorder from terminating treatment either because of the nature of the disorder or the patient's perception of symptoms of these disorders. Also, results from studies of psychotropic medications for the treatment of these disorders in adolescents may support findings that medications improved the likelihood of treatment completion in adult alcoholics.[12, 13]

Drug-Specific Pharmacotherapy

To consider pharmacological intervention of drug-specific pathopsychophysiological symptoms, it is imperative to comprehend what is known about the specific origin of these symptoms, including body organs, brain structures, and the behavioral mechanisms involved. It is also of great importance to define the goals of treatment (i.e., complete abstinence only, psychosocial adaptation) and to recognize the fact that polysubstance addiction is common and may hamper any treatment process focusing only on the drug addiction of choice.

Detoxification from opioids, alcohol, barbiturates, benzodiazepines, and other psychoactive agents needs to follow rigorous procedures in a timely fashion. No empirical studies have investigated detoxification of adolescents with PSUD; however, clinical experience suggests that there is no reason to assume that this therapeutic process should be any different from that of adults with PSUD as long as legal consent is obtained.[5] Therefore, detoxification procedures are not reviewed here.

Four drug-specific pharmacological strategies are commonly used for the treatment of PSUD[6]: (1) Make psychoactive substance administration aversive (e.g., disulfiram for alcohol dependence), (2) substitute for the psychoactive substance (e.g., methadone for heroin dependence), (3) block the reinforcing effects of the psychoactive substance (e.g., naltrexone for opioids addiction), (4) relieve craving/withdrawal (e.g., clonidine for heroin dependence; desipramine for cocaine dependence). To use any one of these approaches, it is necessary not only to identify an appropriate agent but also to increase its appeal by promoting a feeling of well-being that encourages a patient to comply with the assigned treatment.

Pharmacotherapy for the addiction of and dependence on nicotine, alcohol, cocaine, and opioids is reviewed next, with special emphasis on adolescents' needs.

CIGARETTE SMOKING (NICOTINE)

The Annual National High School Senior Survey[14] provides epidemiological data on psychoactive substance use. No clinical implications can be directly drawn from this study. However, based on the relative stability of 30-day prevalence, daily use of half a pack or more of cigarettes in the past 5 years, and the high addictive potential of nicotine, it appears that nicotine dependence among adolescents is common.

Pharmacotherapy of nicotine dependence uses the strategy of finding a substitute for the psychoactive substance. The invention of nicotine gum and its successor the nicotine transdermal patch as self-administering agents was a breakthrough in the treatment of cigarette dependence. The efficacy of these agents doubled the success rates of treatment programs from about 15% (validated long-term abstinence) to about 30%.[15] Furthermore, their success in reducing nicotine craving improved even more when behavioral or cognitive therapy sessions were also part of a comprehensive treatment plan.[16]

Only one study of 612 subjects who had received a prescription for nicotine gum included adolescents.[17] No special reference was made to the characteristics and treatment outcome of these adolescents in the outpatient clinic sample studied.

Side effects of nicotine gum include bad taste and sore mouth and jaws because it is hard to chew. The patch may increase nicotine toxicity, particularly if the person continues to smoke. It can irritate the user's skin and disrupt sleep if left on for 24 hours. Also, some people find it difficult to wean themselves off it.[16] Neither the gum nor the patch should be used by an active smoker. Unfortunately, advertisements by pharmaceutical companies recommend these agents for decreasing smoking as well as for smoking cessation, and these agents thus may induce nicotine intoxication.

No specific contraindications for the use of the nicotine gum or patch by adolescents with nicotine dependence are known. It appears that any therapeutic trial should start as a carefully designed case study on an individual basis for consenting adolescents with severe dependence.

New developments in the nicotine substitute field include nicotine inhalers and nicotine sprays.[18] These devices offer a person the choice of when and where to use them (similar to cigarette smoking). A potential concern is that it could be difficult to quit using such a device.

ALCOHOL

Alcohol dependence has been characterized as a set of disorders named the *alcoholisms*,[19] a term that reflects its phenomenological and etiological heterogeneity.[20] The presumed heterogeneity of patients' typologies led to the development of research attempting to subtype alcoholics. This effort generated Cloninger's type 1 and, more importantly for adolescents, type 2 (male-limited) alcoholism.[21] Type 2 alcoholism may first be diagnosed in adolescence. It is characterized by an early onset of spontaneous alcohol-seeking behavior, fighting, and arrests when drinking. Also, three personality traits characterize these patients: high novelty seeking, low harm avoidance, and low reward dependence. Buydens-Branchey and colleagues[22] reported that patients with early-onset alcoholism were incarcerated more frequently for violent crimes, were three times more likely to be depressed, and were four times more likely to have attempted suicide than patients with late-onset alcoholism (type 1—milieu limited) according to Cloninger.[21] The typological distinction drawn by these investigators resembles the alcoholism type A and B typology of Babor and colleagues[23] in the areas of familial alcoholism and early onset of drinking, antisocial behavior, and comorbid psychiatric disorders. Furthermore, Buydens-Branchey and associates[24] reported among the early-onset group an inverse relationship between a measure of central serotonergic activity and measures of depression and aggression. Based on the dichotomous typology of alcoholism supported by these data, treatment planning and objectives need to take into consideration the heterogeneity of patient populations.

The most common unidimensional pharmacotherapy to prevent alcohol consumption is aversive therapy with disulfiram. This antidipsotropic agent produces a reaction with ethanol by inhibiting the liver enzyme aldehyde dehydrogenase, which catalyzes the oxidation of aldehyde (the major metabolic product of ethanol to acetate). The resulting accumulation of acetaldehyde is responsible for the aversive symptoms. These symptoms are expected to be cognitively paired with ethanol consumption and to create negative reinforcement for alcohol-drinking behavior. The success of this controversial pharmacotherapy has been mediocre at best.[25]

Aversive therapy in children and adolescents has always been controversial and was used only in extreme cases of violent behavior or severe self-injurious behavior among mentally retarded individuals.[26] It appears unlikely that aversive pharmacotherapy will be introduced to adolescents with alcohol dependence owing to ethical and legal reasons. A study of two adolescent males who had alcohol dependence and who were introduced to disulfiram failed to show successful treatment outcome.[27]

Studies of the pharmacotherapy of alcoholism generated interest in the impact of alcohol consumption on opioid receptors and the potential utility of an opioid antagonist such as naltrexone to block the reinforcing properties of alcohol.[28] Also, the serotonergic system appears to have a role in the pathophysiology of alcohol dependence. Fluoxetine, a selective antagonist, was found to reduce alcohol consumption significantly.[29] According to the results of the study by Buydens-Branchey and colleagues,[24] it could be of heuristic value to test a hypothesis that adolescent males with type 2 or type B active alcoholism would benefit from pharmacotherapy with serotonin uptake antagonists because serotonin is the neuromodulator affecting behavioral inhibition.[21]

COCAINE

Despite encouraging reports implying that adolescents continue for the sixth consecutive year to move away from the use of cocaine,[14] a need remains for efficacious interventions to address psychophysiological changes secondary to cocaine dependence and withdrawal symptoms resulting from cessation after chronic use.

The neurotransmitter dopamine emerged as the leading catecholamine responsible for the specific reinforcing effects of cocaine and the suggested mechanisms for craving/withdrawal.[30] Neuroleptics were hypothesized to block the cocaine-induced euphoria initiated by mesolimbic and mesocortical neuranatomical reward pathways, leading to attenuation of cocaine self-administration by animals.[31] However, in humans, neuroleptics are known to produce anhedonia and extrapyramidal side effects, and compliance has been problematical. Flupenthixol decanoate is a neuroleptic agent that was reported in an open trial to rapidly decrease cocaine craving and use and to increase the average time retained in treatment.[31] It has been postulated that compliance with this medication would be satisfactory because of the lack of anhedonic effect.

Sporadic case reports about the capacity of lithium to block cocaine-induced euphoria were not confirmed even in cocaine addicts with bipolar spectrum disorders.[32] The pharmacological treatment strategy for cocaine abuse has mainly been focused on the reduction/elimination of cocaine abstinence-related craving. This is essential to improve relapse prevention rates by reducing attrition from treatment and to enable the introduction of additional therapeutic interventions.

Based on the theory that chronic stimulant use results in depletion of dopamine and reduction in dopaminergic activity, it was hypothesized that craving for cocaine would be reduced by increasing dopaminergic stimulation. Evidence to support the depletion therapy is sparse. However, the following direct and indirect dopamimetic agents have shown some efficacy in open trials: L-dopa, carbidopa, bromocriptine, amantadine, methylphenidate, and mazindol.[33] Another theory that appears to have superior neurobiological support suggests that craving is mediated by supersensitivity of presynaptic inhibiting dopaminergic autoreceptors. The tricyclic antidepressant desipramine was found to desensitize these receptors and facilitate cocaine abstinence by attenuating craving for 7 to 14 days from the onset of therapy. Gawin and colleagues[34] reported a 6-week double-blind random assignment study of desipramine treatment for cocaine craving. The treated outpatient cocaine addicts were more frequently abstinent, were abstinent for longer periods, and had less craving for cocaine than did lithium- and placebo-treated patients. Kosten and colleagues[35] presented 6-month follow-up data on 43 of the 72 patients originally reported by Gawin's group.[34] It was found that self-reported cocaine abstinence during the 6-month period was significantly greater in patients treated with desipramine (44%) than in those treated with lithium (19%) or placebo (27%).

Only one case of facilitation of cocaine abstinence in an adolescent by desipramine has been reported.[36] A 6-month follow-up using the teen addiction severity index[37] confirmed continued abstinence and progress in other life domains. In this case, desipramine treatment was instituted for the treatment of three psychiatric disorders simultaneously: cocaine dependence, major depressive disorder (MDD), and ADHD, thus preventing polypharmacy. The intensity of cocaine craving was reported to be independent of depression during the first week in newly abstinent chronic cocaine addicts.[38] This finding suggests that withdrawal-related dysphoria during the first week of abstinence does not respond to the antidepressant properties of desipramine and may be alleviated earlier than the depressive symptoms of a patient diagnosed as cocaine dependent with MDD. This may also differentiate a cocaine-dependent adolescent from a dually diagnosed one. It is recommended that the conclusions drawn from a single case study be generalized with caution. I recently treated two cocaine-dependent adolescents.[39] One patient's clinical symptoms responded favorably to desipramine for about 30 days at which time the patient dropped out of treatment. The second patient developed postural hypotension, and the medication was discontinued. Additional side effects of desipramine are reviewed later in this chapter.

This case study did not confirm the three-phase model of cocaine abstinence (i.e., crash, withdrawal, extinction) suggested by Gawin and Kleber.[40] A two-stage process of cocaine craving response to treatment by desipramine characterized this case. Weddington and colleagues[41] describe findings similar to these in a study of 12 adult cocaine addicts.

A development in the pharmacological treatment of cocaine dependence is the use of carbamazepine in open trial.[42] The theoretical rationale for this intervention is that the agent blocks cocaine-induced kindling and increases dopamine concentration. The pattern of continued cocaine use despite decreased craving and dysphoria may suggest inherent limitations of the dopamine agonist approach to cocaine pharmacotherapy. Furthermore, dopamine system dysregulation is probably not the only mechanism underlying cocaine addiction. Many cocaine abusers are polysubstance addicts (heroin and methadone included). Buprenorphine is an opioid used for the treatment of cocaine and opioid addiction[43] and is discussed in the section on opioids.

Stimulants have proved to be useful for the treatment of children and adolescents found to have ADHD. The pharmacokinetic similarities between an illegal stimulant such as cocaine and therapeutic stimulants such as methylphenidate, magnesium pemoline, and dextroamphetamine led to the assumption that they might be useful for the treatment of cocaine abuse. Also, it was suggested that adult abuse of cocaine could be attributed to a residual type of attention deficit disorder.[44] Neither assumption was confirmed.[42] The abuse potential of therapeutic stimulants deserves comment. Regardless of the common perception that these agents may be abused by children and adolescents, only two cases of methylphenidate abuse by patients diagnosed with ADHD were reported.[45]

It is noteworthy that cocaine addicts show more conditioned responses than do any other drug addicts. It is hypothesized that many repetitions cause release of the neurotransmitter dopamine, which is suggested to be responsible for both the reinforcing effects of cocaine and for craving and withdrawal phenomenology. The memory of the experience alone, even with no cocaine present, may initiate dopamine release equaling cocaine effect and may lead to subsequent craving and withdrawal (C. O'Brien: Personal communication). A combination of pharmacological intervention and behavioral and cognitive therapy should be further explored for the treatment of cocaine addiction in adolescents.

Finally, as an alternative to therapeutic approaches that are based on the pharmacology of the cocaine receptor, the delivery process of cocaine could be interrupted. Antibodies that may catalyze degradation of cocaine to an inactive form followed by release of the inactive products and continued ability for further binding could provide a treatment for cocaine dependence by blunting reinforcement.[46] This form of passive immunization by an artificial enzyme could provide a new avenue for treatment.

OPIOIDS

Methadone maintenance (MM) is a common form of opioid substitution therapy and is usually reserved for the treatment of adult heroin addicts. The desired response from MM is threefold: (1) prevention of the onset of opioid abstinence syndrome, (2) elimination of drug hunger or craving, and (3) blockade of the euphoric effects of any illicitly self-administered opioids. As a general rule, patients who have not been dependent on opioids for at least 1 year or who have not previously made any attempt at withdrawal are not appropriate candidates for prolonged opioid maintenance.[47]

MM should not rely on methadone administration alone, even in adequate daily dose, to be a "magic bullet" for heroin addiction. McLellan and colleagues[48] reported that patients who were in an MM program and who also received a psychosocial services package fared better than two other groups of patients who received counseling in addition to MM or MM only.

MM and not opioid detoxification is the treatment of choice for pregnant adolescents who are addicted to heroin. This pharmacotherapy given every day eliminates the danger of contracting acquired immunodeficiency syndrome from a contaminated needle. It also ensures a relatively stable plasma level of methadone, which reduces a fetus's risk of developing intrauterine distress, as compared with heroin, which has a short half-life and causes abrupt changes in plasma level.[49]

No person younger than 18 years may be admitted to an MM treatment program unless an authorized adult signs an official consent form (FDA-2635 consent for MM treatment). Treatment programs for patients younger than 18 years need to consider the following: According to FDA regulations, patients younger than 18 years are required to have two documented attempts at short-term detoxification or drug-free treatment to be eligible for MM. A 1-week waiting period is required after a detoxification attempt. However, before an attempt is repeated, the program physician has to document in the minor's record that the patient continues to be or is again physiologically dependent on narcotic drugs.[50]

Two additional oral pharmacotherapies are examined in therapeutic trials and are expected to expand the arsenal of opioids available for maintenance treatment, L-acetyl-methadol (LAAM) and buprenorphine.

LAAM is an opioid that is similar to methadone in its pharmacological actions. It is converted into active metabolites that have longer biological half-lives than methadone. Opioid withdrawal symptoms are not experienced for 72 to 96 hours after the last oral dose; therefore, LAAM can be given only three times per week as compared with daily administration of methadone. LAAM has been shown to have equivalent effects to methadone in terms of suppressing illicit opioid addiction and encouraging a more productive lifestyle.[47]

Buprenorphine is a partial opioid agonist-antagonist available also as an analgesic because of its ability to produce morphine-like effects at low doses. This agent relieves opioid withdrawal, diminishes craving, and does not produce euphoria. It is more difficult to overdose on buprenorphine than on methadone because of its antagonist effects in high doses.[51]

Many heroin addicts also abuse cocaine, which speeds the rush from heroin injected alone (i.e., a speed ball). MM treatment does not reduce cocaine addiction for many patients. Based on preliminary data, buprenorphine may reduce cocaine use in opioid addicts.[43] The mechanism of action in combination with cocaine remains to be clarified.

Pharmacology of Comorbid Psychiatric Disorders

Psychiatric comorbidity in the form of dual and triple diagnosis has been found to be common among adolescents with PSUD.[4, 52] The most common psychiatric diagnoses are mood disorders and conduct disorder. Other diagnoses reported include anxiety disorders, eating disorders, ADHD, and schizophrenia. Also, personality disorders, especially cluster B of DSM-III-R,[1] which includes antisocial, borderline, histrionic, and narcissistic personality disorders, have been identified among these ado-

lescents, with or without additional comorbid psychiatric disorders.[5]

It is often unclear whether a patient's symptoms are a sequence of substance addiction per se or are indicative of a comorbid psychiatric disorder. Moreover, in such patients, the sequelae of psychoactive substance intoxication or withdrawal are often difficult to distinguish from the signs and symptoms of concurrent psychiatric disorder. It is important to reemphasize that dual diagnosis is a term limited to the relationship between disorders only and does not apply to symptoms associated with PSUD. These symptoms may serve as indications of the severity of PSUD.

The diagnostic process of comorbid psychiatric disorders and the reliability and stability of dual diagnosis are of great significance from a treatment perspective. A diagnosis of artificial comorbidity and a precocious introduction of medications may lead to errors in treatment. A washout period of at least 2 weeks and sometimes longer is recommended before initiating pharmacotherapy. This is especially true for antidepressants because even in children and adolescents with MDD without a comorbid PSUD, approximately 25% of those initially diagnosed as depressed have a spontaneous syndromatic recovery within 2 weeks.[53] The researchers noted that treatments initiated in this period could produce inflated recovery rates. Both biological and depressive severity differences are found between those who recover and those who remain syndromatically ill after a 2-week follow-up phase.

Major Depressive Disorder

Conceptual difficulties regarding the validity of depression as a distinct diagnostic entity in children and adolescents are still debated. Substantial lack of clarity still exists about what is being rated in depressed children and adolescents (individual symptoms, regularly occurring syndromes, or constitutionally based disorders). It is also unclear which mental status variables should be examined in depressed youth when evaluating treatment effects.[54] Empirical data do not support antidepressants efficacy in child and adolescent MDD, although they have been proved for the treatment of MDD in adults. Geller and coworkers[55] and Ryan and colleagues[56] tried to replicate studies with adult MDD that found that tricyclic antidepressant steady-state plasma levels of more than 125 μg/L predict response.[57] No relation was found between plasma levels of impramine or desipramine and clinical response in adolescents with MDD.

Lithium augmentation in refractory adolescent MDD and monoamine oxidase inhibitor (MAOI) treatment of adolescent atypical depression were reported in open design studies.[58–60] These reports suggest the potential use of these agents in the management of refractory MDD in adolescents. Further confirmation by controlled studies is awaited.

Clinical experience suggests that many patients with PSUD are diagnosed as depressed, especially on admission to inpatient treatment programs. This could be attributed to various factors other than primary depression such as the mood-altering effects of the drug or to withdrawal symptoms; loss of the availability of psychoactive substances and related lifestyle; or a reaction to the loss of freedom, friends, and family after the admission. Most of the patients experience a gradual and spontaneous lifting of the depressive symptoms within 2 weeks. Clinical experience suggests that regardless of the results of empirical studies, adolescents who are diagnosed with MDD are commonly being treated either with tricyclic antidepressants such as imipramine or amitriptyline or by the new selective serotonin reuptake inhibitors (SSRIs) such as fluoxetine (Prozac), sertraline (Zoloft), and paroxetine (Paxil). Clinical improvement following tricyclic medications is usually expected after 3 to 4 weeks of pharmacotherapy, as reported by Kaminer and colleagues,[54] who used an observational measurement of symptoms, the emotional disorders rating scale (EDRS), which has been found to be responsive to treatment of MDD. This result confirmed findings in the adult literature.[57] Clinical response to SSRIs occurs after a shorter period of treatment.

Ambrosini and colleagues[53] reviewed treatment studies of children and adolescents that have focused on tricyclic antidepressants. The researchers concluded that their superiority to placebo has not been proved. However, they pointed out that this finding does not preclude their routine clinical use in MDD because on the average, more than half of the subjects treated openly will respond. Ambrosini and coworkers[53] suggested that maximal benefits with antidepressants most likely emerge after 8 to 10 weeks of treatment while maintaining plasma levels of tricyclics in the 200 ng/ml range. Maintenance treatment should be continued for 5 to 6 months after remission of depressive symptoms.

In summary, it is of enormous importance to elucidate future conceptual and clinical implications of the response of MDD symptoms to antidepressants across age groups. The Maudsley study carried out by Harrington and colleagues[61] indicated that indeed, depression in children and adolescents shows substantial specific continuity into adulthood, although the majority of adults with MDD had not experienced a depressive disorder in their pre-adulthood years. However, the implications of the Maudsley data are that the 30% to 35% of adults who do not respond to antidepressants have a history of child and adolescent MDD.[53]

It appears that this group may represent a distinct biological subpopulation characterized by age of onset of MDD as a possible biological marker with specificity to different pharmacotherapeutic response patterns. This pattern has significant similarities to Cloninger's[21] alcohol typologies and to findings regarding the pharmacotherapy of alcoholism reviewed earlier in this chapter.

SIDE EFFECTS

Antidepressants generate side effects similar to those reported in adults. The tricyclics may be lethal in overdose situations, primarily because of cardiovascular toxicity.[62] Four cases of sudden death related to the specific use of Norpramin (desipramine) by children ages 8 to 12 years old were reported.[63] The speculated pathophysiological mechanism is that desipramine may increase noradrenergic neurotransmission, leading to increased cardiac sympathetic tone, and could predispose vulnerable persons to ventricular tachyarrhythmias, syncope, and sudden death.

Neurotoxicity of antidepressants includes seizures, behavioral changes, and delirium. Data on adolescents' exposure to tricyclic neurotoxicity are limited to sporadic case reports. Anticholinergic effects are usually correlated with plasma tricyclic levels and most commonly include dry mouth, drowsiness, nausea, constipation, urinary retention, tremor, flushed face, and excessive sweating. Tricyclic antidepressants can induce behavioral toxicity, primarily precipitation, induction, or rapid cycling of manic symptoms.[64] Also, one study investigated mania associated with treatment of five adolescents for depression with the SSRI fluoxetine.[65]

Abrupt discontinuation of tricyclics may produce withdrawal symptoms. The most common symptoms are cholinergic effects. Coadministration of SSRIs with tricyclic antidepressants or administration even a few weeks later is contraindicated because it may raise the plasma level of these agents to a toxic level, most likely because of interference with their hepatic oxidative metabolism. Side effects of SSRIs in adolescents have been reported in case studies and in preliminary studies. Ambrosini and colleagues[62] reviewed and classified these into gastrointestinal, neuropsychiatric, and behavioral.

It is noteworthy that abuse of amitriptyline for its sedative effects was reported by an adolescent and adults with PSUD.[66]

The risk of suicide among adolescents with PSUD is high.[67] SSRIs are less cardiotoxic in overdoses, and they lack sedative potentiation with alcohol as compared with tricyclic antidepressants; therefore, their use is preferable for MDD in impulsive or suicidal adolescents.

Current experience suggests that before initiating treatment of any psychopathology in adolescents with tricyclic medication, a baseline electrocardiogram needs to be performed. Also, the medical examination and medical history should emphasize the cardiovascular system of the patient and family members in order to detect any cardiac vulnerability. Resting pulse should not exceed 130 beats per minute, and blood pressure should not exceed 140/90 mm Hg. Prolongation of the PR interval on the electrocardiogram should not exceed 0.21 seconds, the QRS complex should not be prolonged by more than 30% over baseline, and the QTc interval in particular should be within normal limits.*

Bipolar Disorders

The core phenomenology of bipolar disorder is similar regardless of age; however, as in the treatment of MDD and alcoholism type 1 versus type 2, it is not clear whether age of onset influences treatment response.

Lithium is the pharmacotherapy of choice, although no large-scale systematic studies have observed children and adolescents.[68] Also, anticonvulsants such as carbamazepine and valproic acid serve as a second tier. It is noteworthy that combinations of these medications were reported to have a synergistic effect in adult patients resistant to lithium monotherapy. The following indications for the initiation of lithium treatment for adolescents were noted by Carlson[68]: presence or history of dis-

abling episodes of mania and depression; episode(s) of severe depression with a possible history of hypomania; presence of an acute severe depression characterized by psychomotor retardation, hypersomnia, and psychosis; positive family history of a bipolar disorder (these adolescents are at risk for developing a manic episode when treated with antidepressants and may develop a rapid cycling course); an acute psychotic disorder with affective features; and behavior disorders characterized by severe emotional lability and aggression in patients with a positive family history of major mood or bipolar disorder or lithium responsiveness. Indeed, children misdiagnosed with ADHD have been shown actually to suffer from bipolar mood disorder.[69, 70] Also, the effectiveness of lithium for acute symptoms and for long-term management of bipolar disorder has been well established in the adult literature; however, the failure rate for lithium in prevention of bipolar disorder is approximately 33%.[71]

Lithium side effects in adolescents are similar to the symptoms manifested in adults. Tremor, urinary frequency, nausea, and diarrhea are the most common ones. Relative contraindications for the use of lithium include heart and kidney disease, diuretic use, chronic diarrhea, and electrolyte imbalance. Basic laboratory studies include blood electrolytes, urea, and nitrogen levels; blood count with differential; thyroid function tests; and a pregnancy test owing to the potential teratogenic effects of lithium.

The recommended therapeutic blood level is within the therapeutic range of 0.7 to 1.2 mEq/L. A level of more than 1.4 mEq/L should not be exceeded because of a risk of toxicity. Signs of toxicity include severe neurobehavioral and gastrointestinal symptoms.

Anticonvulsants' recommended blood levels, contraindications, and side effects are similar among age groups. Compared with lithium, monitoring of fluid and electrolyte intake is not required and the risk of toxicity is lower should serum levels exceed the recommended therapeutic range. In some cases, bipolar disorder may be refractory to all of these agents. One alternative, verapamil (a calcium channel antagonist), has been used without consistently proving clear effectiveness in the treatment of adults with a bipolar disorder. In addition, verapamil is associated with depression.[72] However, successful use of verapamil and valproic acid in the treatment of prolonged mania in an adolescent was reported.[73] Another alternative based on a single case report of an adolescent with a rapid cycling bipolar disorder was de-

---

*QT interval represents the time required for ventricular electrical systole. It varies with heart rate, and one can estimate QTc (corrected QT) interval, normally less than 0.42 second in males and 0.43 second in females, by the following formula: QTc = QT/RR interval.

scribed by Berman and Wolpert.[74] The investigators noted that the disorder, which was precipitated by a tricyclic antidepressant, responded to electrocurrent therapy.

Adolescents with PSUD and a comorbid bipolar disorder are at very high risk for suicide and aggressive behavior and should be observed carefully. The need for blood level monitoring of lithium is a special challenge, particularly for outpatients.

Anxiety Disorder

Panic and obsessive-compulsive disorders (OCD) in youth share phenomenological similarities with the adult patterns; however, avoidant disorder, overanxious disorder, separation anxiety, and school phobia are unique to children and adolescents as delineated in DSM-III-R.[1] The use of medications with addictive properties for the pharmacotherapy of anxiety disorders in adolescents with PSUD is not recommended. Furthermore, benzodiazepines such as alprazolam (Xanax), which are commonly used among adults with anxiety disorders, have not unequivocally been proved to be more efficacious than tricyclic antidepressants.

Panic disorder and OCD among adolescents with PSUD are rare. However, the median age for the onset of anxiety disorders is 15 years.[75] No studies have investigated the pharmacological treatment of panic disorder in adolescents. A study of adults with panic disorder showed that both the benzodiazepine alprazolam and the antidepressant imipramine demonstrated efficacy during acute treatment of panic disorder on most measures of panic and nonpanic anxiety, as well as measures of phobic avoidance and panic-related social disability.[76] These clinical benefits were achieved without any concomitant behavioral therapy or psychotherapy, and they were sustained throughout an 8-month course of maintenance therapy without any dose escalation. The same research group studied short- and long-term outcome after drug taper.[77] The researchers concluded that "over the long term, patients originally treated with imipramine or placebo did as well at follow-up as patients treated with alprazolam, without the problems of physical dependence and discontinuation that any long-term alprazolam therapy entails."[77]

The psychopharmacological treatment of OCD has been studied and reviewed extensively.[78] Antianxiety agents appear to be ineffective, and the tricyclic antidepressant clomipramine was reported to have significant superiority over placebo in lessening OCD symptoms in children and adolescents.[79] Clomipramine appears to have better results than desipramine; however, this conclusion remains to be tested in future studies. Open studies with SSRIs such as fluoxetine, as reviewed by Ambrosini and colleagues,[62] suggest it may be effective in adolescent OCD with or without clomipramine.

Separation anxiety and school phobia have been studied for more than 20 years. In contrast to the early report regarding a positive response to imipramine compared with placebo,[80] more recent studies have failed to show superiority of tricyclic antidepressants (e.g., imipramine, clomipramine) over placebo.[81, 82] It is noteworthy that these disorders were found to be associated with adult forms of panic and depressive disorders.[83, 84]

A study on the effects of alprazolam on children and adolescents with overanxious and avoidant disorders was reported.[85] The findings failed to show efficacy of the medication in comparison with placebo. This result stands in marked contrast to the favorable effects reported in studies with adults. Simeon and colleagues[85] intend to increase the dose of alprazolam and the length of pharmacotherapy in a future study. The researchers have not discussed the implications of the addictive potential of alprazolam in this study. It is important to note that these DSM-III-R diagnoses have been dropped from the DSM-IV section called "Anxiety Disorders of Childhood or Adolescence."[86] Avoidant disorder has been included in the modified social phobia diagnosis, and overanxious disorder has been subsumed by generalized anxiety disorder.

Buspirone hydrochloride (Buspar) is a relatively new anxiolytic drug, pharmacologically different from the benzodiazepines. This agent has been marketed as a less-sedative anxiolytic that does not potentiate alcohol effects and has a low, if any, addiction potential. Buspar has been successfully used to treat an adolescent with overanxious disorder who did not tolerate treatment with desipramine.[87] Buspirone may be particularly useful for clinical trials with teens with PSUD and anxiety symptoms.

The studies reviewed in this section have significant importance for the treatment of adolescents with PSUD and anxiety disorders. Moreover, they have unequivocal implications for the treatment and detoxification of benzodiazepine addiction and dependence. Tricyclic antidepressants are useful substitutes for these medications, which are used addictively for their sedative properties.

Eating Disorders

Anorexia and bulimia nervosa are psychiatric disorders predominantly diagnosed in females. Striking similarities are noted between these disorders and PSUD. Biopsychosocial factors are responsible for shaping an individual's anorexic or bulimic behavior and neurophysiological adaptation. Strober and Katz[88] questioned the traditional linkage between anorexia and bulimia, which has been based on the common denominator of eating disorders.

One of the criteria for bulimia nervosa according to DSM-III-R[1] has included the use of laxatives or diuretics to prevent weight gain. The misuse of medications without an addictive potential and in the service of the disorder does not meet the criteria for PSUD. However, females in general and bulimic patients in particular tend to use diet pills. Indeed, Johnston and colleagues[14] reported that stimulants use among female high-school seniors equals males' rate of use, and use of diet pills was higher among females. The use of medications with addictive potential (e.g., stimulants sold over the counter) and the fashionable use of cocaine to lose weight create a nosological dilemma regarding whether a patient qualifies for the diagnosis of PSUD, particularly when the person is bulimic. The discussion of this issue is beyond the scope of this chapter and deserves a thorough discussion elsewhere.

Since the mid-1980s, pharmacological trials among adult patients have demonstrated the short-term efficacy of several antidepressants in diminishing bingeing frequencies in bulimic patients. These include imipramine, desipramine, phenelzine (MAOI), as well as several new-generation antidepressants including trazodone, bupropion, and fluoxetine.[89] The bulimic symptoms improved even in the absence of coexistent depression and were not correlated with pretreatment severity or plasma medication levels. These findings do not support early studies linking the cause of mood disorders and eating disorder based on epidemiological and family studies.[90] Lithium carbonate was reported to reduce bulimic episodes in open trial studies.[91]

Anorexia nervosa and PSUD is a rare dual diagnosis. No effective pharmacotherapy for anorexia nervosa has been reported in a double-blind placebo-controlled trial. Only a limited number of open trials with fluoxetine noted some short-term improvement.

Schizophrenia

No studies on the comorbidity of PSUD and schizophrenia have been reported yet among adolescents. However, no data even among adult patients suggest that there should be any difference between the pharmacotherapy of schizophrenic patients with or without accompanying PSUD. Therefore, neuroleptics remain the category of medications of choice.

Disruptive Behavior Disorders

Conduct disorder (CD), ADHD, and oppositional defiant disorder (ODD) represent the largest group of psychiatric referrals. Comorbidity among these disorders is very common, and ODD is most probably a mild variant or precursor of CD and not a discrete disorder.[92]

Attention Deficit Hyperactivity Disorder

The effectiveness of stimulant therapy for ADHD in childhood has been extensively documented.[93] Methylphenidate (Ritalin), dextroamphetamine (Dexedrine), and magnesium pemoline (Cylert) are the three most commonly used stimulants. Antidepressants, particularly imipramine, desipramine, and nortriptyline, have also been found to be effective in the treatment of the aggression, inattention, and hyperactivity that characterize the heterogeneous population of children found to have the disorder.[62, 94] Tricyclics and MAOI should remain a second alternative to stimulants, which have less severe side effects and produce a more consistent response from patients.[95] However, these antidepressants should be used when a patient with ADHD is manifesting a comorbid anxiety or depressive disorder. Side effects of stimulants include weight loss, decreased appetite, possible mood lability, and a potentially reversible growth suppression once the medication is discontinued. This issue still generates debate.

Abuse of therapeutic stimulants by patients with ADHD is rare; however, peers and relatives may become addicted to the medication either because of its availability or because they have PSUD.[11]

Neuroleptics, carbamazepine, and clonidine (including a patch form) have been tested as treatments for childhood ADHD. However, only equivocal reports about a certain level of efficacy were noted in uncontrolled studies of neuroleptics and carbamazepine and in controlled studies of clonidine, especially in patients with comorbid tic disorders.[96] Serious side effects that characterize these medications limit their use in this group.

Stimulant therapy for adolescents with ADHD has also been found to be effective.[97] Methylphenidate and dextroamphetamine appear to be more effective than pemoline. I have treated adolescents with PSUD and comorbid ADHD with methylphenidate, producing a positive response. Adults with the disorder also respond to this treatment.[98]

Conduct Disorder

Aggression in child and adolescent psychiatry is most commonly thought to occur with the diagnosis of CD. Pharmacological treatment of aggression in CD is part of a comprehensive treatment plan that also includes psychosocial and behavioral interventions.[99] Neuroleptics have been used for aggressive behavior with and without CD in adolescents since the 1960s.[100, 101] Campbell and colleagues[101] reported that lithium was superior to placebo for the treatment of aggression in subjects with CD.

Stimulants and anticonvulsants were also used in early studies, but the results were ambiguous mostly because of lack of differentiation between aggressive subjects with or without ADHD.[102, 103] Beta blockers have showed some usefulness in a small group of subjects with aggressive behavior and additional disruptive or organic disorders.[104] Treatment of violent children and adolescents ages 5 to 15 years with clonidine was reported in an open trial study.[105] Aggression decreased with minimal side effects in most children, and plasma gamma-aminobutyric levels increased in 5 of the 17 cases.

A high percentage of adolescents diagnosed with CD are found to have antisocial personality disorder, which is highly correlated with PSUD. No specific pharmacological treatment for personality disorders has yet been developed. However, symptomatic relief of depressive or anxiety disorders that may accompany CD or a personality disorder could be achieved by selective pharmacotherapy.[11]

The Legal Angle

It is of significant importance to assess the legal aspects of an adolescent's and a family's consent for treatment of PSUD including psychopharmacotherapy. Facilities that treat minors must follow some basic common rules and protect confidentiality. Consent for admission to an inpatient unit needs to be provided by the caretaker and adolescent (unless the adolescent has been committed). Any patient who is younger than 18 years and who is married, a parent, or emancipated has the right to consent on his or her behalf. Before rendering any care without parental consent, the facility must obtain a written acknowledgment from the minor stating that he or she was (1) advised of the purpose and nature of such treatment services; (2) told that he or she may withdraw the signed acknowledgment at any time; (3) aware that the facility will make attempts to convince the child of the need for involvement of other family members in treatment and the facility's preference for parental consent for the rendering of treatment services; and (4) advised that a medical/clinical record of his or her treatment services will be made and maintained by the facility. The provisions of various laws and regulations establish that parental consent is usually but not always required to deliver PSUD treatment for minors. Also, patients with PSUD must be notified of the protection afforded by the federal rules on admission.[5, 66]

The Future of Pharmacotherapy for Adolescents with PSUD and Comorbid Disorders

Eichelman[106] described four important principles for the pharmacological treatment of adults: Treat the primary illness, use the most benign interventions when treating empirically, have some quantifiable means of assessing efficacy, and institute drug trials systematically. These principles are even more important with younger subjects.

Ethical principles must govern research and treatment in adolescent PSUD and comorbid psychiatric disorders.[107] Improved communication with and education of the public, especially the parents of patients, about the nature of PSUD and the efficacy of pharmacotherapy is necessary. Promotion of the concept of treatment dosage as a summation of the effects of comprehensive treatment modalities based on patient treatment matching will improve the perceptions of treatment programs.

Patients who would like to maintain their motivation to comply with the medication regimen should join or develop chapters of "double-trouble" self-help groups (i.e., PSUD and comorbid psychiatric disorders) or MM anonymous for patients from MM programs. Parents and therapists in the treatment facility may be instrumental in helping them succeed in this effort.

Biderman[7] suggested a careful and systematic study of new therapeutic agents. Case reports and case series should be followed by open studies, which will lead to controlled double-blind studies. Collaboration between centers will increase the number of subjects studied and will improve the significance of the results.

McLellan and colleagues'[45] study, reviewed in the section on opioids, confirms empirically that the cumulative effect of more treatment modalities is better than just a single pharmacological intervention. Pharmacotherapy alone cannot deal with polysubstance addiction and the various domains that an adult or adolescent with PSUD struggles with in the recovery process. However, no single strategy appears to be superior to others in dealing with adolescents with PSUD. It would be helpful to have a measurement of units of treatment dosage regardless of the modality of treatment intervention used (i.e., net effect of change). The Treatment Services Review[108] is such an assessment instrument designed to quantify different treatment modalities in adults with PSUD as delineated in the addiction severity index.[109] A modification of this instrument for adolescents could prove to be beneficial, by using a similar approach according to the teen addiction severity index.[37]

Finally, the age of onset of a disorder (i.e., mood disorder, PSUD) and the age-specific response to medications may represent a biological marker. This marker may facilitate and improve identification of heterogeneous clinical subpopulations, the course of disorders, and long-term morbidity and may potentiate future research for specific treatments tailored to the identified groups.

REFERENCES

1. American Psychiatric Association: Diagnostic and Statistical Manual of Mental Disorders, 3rd ed, revised. Washington, DC, American Psychiatric Association, 1987.
2. Anderson JC, Williams S, McGee R, Silva PA: DSM-III disorders in preadolescent children. Arch Gen Psychiatry 44:69–76, 1987.
3. Bukstein OG, Glancy LJ, Kaminer Y: Patterns of affective comorbidity in a clinical population of dually diagnosed substance-abusing adolescents. J Am Acad Child Adolesc Psychiatry 31:1041–1046, 1992.
4. Kaminer Y: The magnitude of concurrent psychiatric disorders in hospitalized substance abusing adolescents. Child Psychiatry Hum Dev 22:89–95, 1991.
5. Kaminer Y: Adolescent Substance Abuse: A Comprehensive Guide to Theory and Practice. New York, Plenum, 1994.
6. Kaminer Y: Desipramine facilitation of cocaine abstinence in an adolescent. J Am Acad Child Adolesc Psychiatry 31:312–317, 1992.
7. Biderman J: New developments in pediatric psychopharmacology. J Am Acad Child Adolesc Psychiatry 31:14–15, 1992.
8. Hoffmann NG, Sonis WA, Halikas JA: Issues in the evaluation of chemical dependency treatment programs for adolescents. Pediatr Clin North Am 34:449–459, 1987.
9. Miller WR: Motivation for treatment: A review with special emphasis on alcoholism. Psychol Bull 98:84–107, 1985.
10. Zweben A, Li S: The efficacy of role induction in preventing early dropout from outpatient treatment of drug dependency. Am J Drug Alcohol Abuse 8:171–183, 1981.
11. Kaminer Y, Tarter RE, Bukstein OG, Kabene M: Comparison between treatment completers and noncompleters among dually diagnosed substance-abusing adolescents. J Am Acad Child Adolesc Psychiatry 31:1046–1049, 1992.
12. Gerard DL, Saenger G: Outpatient Treatment of Alcoholism. Toronto, University of Toronto Press, 1966.
13. Smart RG, Gray G: Multiple predictors of dropout from alcoholism treatment. Arch Gen Psychiatry 35:363–367, 1978.
14. Johnston L, Bachman JG, O'Malley RM: Details of Annual Drug Survey. Ann Arbor, University of Michigan News and Information Services, 1992.
15. West R: The "nicotine replacement paradox" in smoking cessation: How does nicotine gum really work? Br J Addict 87:165–167, 1992.
16. Lichtenstein E, Glasgow RE: Smoking cessation: What have we learned over the past decade? J Consult Clin Psychol 60:518–527, 1992.
17. Johnson RE, Stevens VJ, Hollis JF, Woodson GT: Nicotine chewing gum use in the outpatient care setting. J Fam Pract 34:61–65, 1992.
18. Tonnesen P, Norregaard J, Mikkelsen K, et al: A double-blind trial of a nicotine inhaler for smoking cessation. JAMA 269:1268–1271, 1993.
19. Jacobson GR: The Alcoholisms: Detection, Diagnosis, and Assessment. New York, Human Sciences Press, 1976.
20. Gilligan S, Reich T, Cloninger CR: Etiologic heterogeneity in alcoholism. Genet Epidemiol 4:395–414, 1987.
21. Cloninger CR: Neurogenetic adaptive mechanisms in alcoholism. Science 236:410–416, 1987.
22. Buydens-Branchey L, Branchey MH, Noumair D: Age of alcoholism onset: I. Relationship to psychopathology. Arch Gen Psychiatry 46:225–230, 1989.
23. Babor TF, Hofmann M, DelBoca FK, et al: Types of alcoholics: I. Evidence for an empirically-derived typology based on indicators of vulnerability and severity. Arch Gen Psychiatry 49:599–608, 1992.
24. Buydens-Branchey L, Branchey MH, Noumair D, Lieber CS: Age of alcoholism onset: II. Relationship

to susceptibility to serotonin precursor availability. Arch Gen Psychiatry 46:231–236, 1989.

25. Alterman AI, O'Brien CP, McLellan AT: Differential therapeutics for substance abuse. In Frances RJ, Miller SI (eds): Clinical Textbook of Addictive Disorders. New York: Guilford Press, 1991, pp 369–390.

26. Council on Scientific Affairs: Aversion therapy. JAMA 258:2562–2566, 1987.

27. Myers WC, Donahue JE, Goldstein MR: Disulfiram for alcohol use disorders in adolescents. J Am Acad Child Adolesc Psychiatry 33:484–489, 1994.

28. O'Malley SS, Jaffe AJ, Chang G, et al: Naltrexone and coping skills therapy for alcohol dependence. Arch Gen Psychiatry 49:881–887, 1992.

29. Naranjo CA, Kadlec KE, Sanhueza P, et al: Fluoxetine differentially alters alcohol intake and other consummatory behaviors in problem drinkers. Clin Pharmacol Ther 47:490–498, 1990.

30. Kosten TR: Neurobiology of abused drugs: Opioids and stimulants. J Nerv Ment Dis 178:217–227, 1990.

31. Gawin FH, Allen D, Humblestone B: Outpatient treatment of crack cocaine smoking with flupenthixol decanoate. Arch Gen Psychiatry 46:322–325, 1989.

32. Nunes EV, McGrath PJ, Steven W, Quitkin FM: Lithium treatment for cocaine abusers with bipolar spectrum disorders. Am J Psychiatry 147:655–657, 1990.

33. Meyer RE: New pharmacotherapies for cocaine dependence revisited. Arch Gen Psychiatry 49:900–904, 1992.

34. Gawin FH, Kleber HD, Byck R, et al: Desipramine facilitation of initial cocaine abstinence. Arch Gen Psychiatry 46:117–121, 1989.

35. Kosten TR, Gawin FH, Kosten TA, et al: Six month follow-up of short-term pharmacotherapy for cocaine dependence. Am J Addict 1:40–49, 1992.

36. Kaminer Y, Tarter RE, Bukstein OG, Kabene M: Staff, treatment completers', and noncompleters' perceptions of the value of treatment variables. Am J Addict 1:115–120, 1992.

37. Kaminer Y, Bukstein OG, Tarter RE. The Teen Addiction Severity Index (T-ASI): Rationale and reliability. Int J Addict 26:219–226, 1991.

38. Ho A, Cambor R, Bodner G: Intensity of craving is independent of depression in newly abstinent chronic cocaine abusers. Presented at the 53rd Annual Scientific Meeting of the Committee on Problems of Drug Dependence, Palm Beach, FL, 1991.

39. Kaminer Y (in press).

40. Gawin FH, Kleber HD: Abstinence symptomatology and psychiatric diagnosis in cocaine abusers. Arch Gen Psychiatry 43:107–113, 1986.

41. Weddington WW, Brown BS, Haertzen CA, et al: Changes in mood, craving and sleep during short-term abstinence reported by male cocaine addicts: A controlled residential study. Arch Gen Psychiatry 47:861–868, 1990.

42. Halikas JA, Kuhn KL, Madduz TL: Reduction of cocaine use among methadone maintenance patients using concurrent carbamazepine maintenance. Am Clin Psychiatry 2:3–6, 1990.

43. Kosten TR, Kleber HD, Morgan C: Treatment of cocaine abuse with buprenorphine. Biol Psychiatry 26:637–639, 1989.

44. Weiss RD, Pope HG, Mirin SM: Treatment of chronic cocaine abuse and attention deficit disorder residual type, with magnesium pemoline. Drug Alcohol Depend 15:69–72, 1985.

45. Kaminer Y: Clinical implications of the relationship between attention-deficit hyperactivity disorder and psychoactive substance use disorders. Am J Addict 1:257–264, 1992.

46. Landry DW, Zhao K, Yang XQ, et al: Antibody-catalyzed degradation of cocaine. Science 259:1899–1901, 1993.

47. Jaffe JH: Opioids. In Frances AI, Hales RE (eds): Annual Review, vol 5. Washington, DC, American Psychiatric Association, 1986, pp 137–159.

48. McLellan AT, Arndt IO, Metzger DS, et al: The effects of psychosocial services in substance abuse treatment. JAMA 269:1953–1959, 1993.

49. Finnegan LP, Kandall SR: Maternal and neonatal effects of alcohol and drugs. In Lowinson JH, Ruiz P, Millman RB, Langrod JG (eds): Substance Abuse, A Comprehensive Textbook. Baltimore, Williams & Wilkins, 1992, pp 628–656.

50. Parrino MW: State Methadone Maintenance Treatment Guidelines. Rockville, MD, US Dept of Health and Human Services, 1992.

51. Rosen MI, Kosten TR: Buprenorphine: Beyond methadone. Hosp Community Psychiatry 42:347–349, 1991.

52. Bukstein OG, Brent D, Kaminer Y: Comorbidity of substance abuse and other psychiatric disorders in adolescents. Am J Psychiatry 146:1131–1141, 1989.

53. Ambrosini PJ, Bianchi MD, Rabinovich H, Elia J: Antidepressant treatments in children and adolescents: I. Affective disorders. J Am Acad Child Adolesc Psychiatry 32:1–6, 1993.

54. Kaminer Y, Seifer R, Mastrian A: Observational measurement of symptoms responsive to treatment of major depressive disorder in children and adolescents. J Nerv Ment Dis 180:639–643, 1992.

55. Geller B, Cooper TB, Graham DL, et al: Double-blind placebo controlled study of nortriptyline in depressed adolescents using a "fixed plasma level" design. Psychopharmacol Bull 26:85–90, 1990.

56. Ryan N, Puig-Antich J, Cooper T, et al: Imipramine in adolescent major depression: Plasma level and clinical response. Acta Psychiatr Scand 73:275–288, 1986.

57. Nelson C, Mazure C, Quinlan PM, Jatlow PI: Drug responsive symptoms in melancholia. Arch Gen Psychiatry 41:663–668, 1984.

58. Ryan N, Meyer V, Dachille S, et al: Lithium antidepressant augmentation in TCA-refractory depression in adolescents. J Am Acad Child Adolesc Psychiatry 27:371–376, 1988.

59. Ryan N, Puig-Antich J, Rabinovich H, et al: MAOI in adolescent major depression unresponsive to tricyclic antidepressants. J Am Acad Child Adolesc Psychiatry 27:755–758, 1988.

60. Strober M, Freedman R, Rigali J, et al: The pharmacotherapy of depressive illness in adolescence: II. Effects of lithium augmentation in nonresponders to imipramine. J Am Acad Child Adolesc Psychiatry 31:16–20, 1992.

61. Harrington R, Fudge H, Rutter M, et al: Adult outcomes of childhood and adolescent depression. Arch Gen Psychiatry 47:465–473, 1990.

62. Ambrosini PJ, Bianchi MD, Rabinovich H, Elia J: Antidepressant treatments in children and adolescents: II. Anxiety, physical, and behavioral disorders. J Am Acad Child Adolesc Psychiatry 32:483–492, 1993.

63. Riddle MA, Geller B, Ryan N: Another sudden death in a child treated with desipramine. J Am Acad Child Adolesc Psychiatry 32:792–797, 1993.

64. Strober M, Carlson G: Bipolar illness in adolescents with major depression, clinical, genetic, and psychopharmacologic predictions in a three-to-four perspective follow-up investigation. Arch Gen Psychiatry 39:549–555, 1982.

65. Venkataraman S, Naylor MW, King CA: Mania associated with fluoxetine treatment in adolescents. J Am Acad Child Adolesc Psychiatry 31:276–281, 1992.

66. Kaminer Y: Tricyclic antidepressants: Therapeutic use for cocaine craving and potential for abuse. J Am Acad Child Adolesc Psychiatry 33:592, 1994.

67. Kaminer Y: Psychoactive substance abuse and dependence as a risk factor in adolescent attempted and completed suicide. Am J Addict 1:21–29, 1992.

68. Carlson GA: Bipolar disorders in children and adolescents. In Garfinkel BD, Carlson GA, Weller EB (eds): Psychiatric Disorders in Children and Adolescents. Philadelphia, WB Saunders, 1990, pp 21–36.

69. DeLong GR, Aldershof AL: Long-term experience with lithium treatment in childhood: Correlation with clinical diagnoses. J Am Acad Child Adolesc Psychiatry 26:389–394, 1987.

70. Isaac G: Bipolar disorder in prepubertal children in a special education setting: Is it rare? J Clin Psychiatry 52:165–168, 1991.

71. Prien RE, Gelenberg AJ: Alternative to lithium for preventive treatment of bipolar disorder. Am J Psychiatry 146:840–848, 1989.

72. Barton B, Gitlin MJ: Verapamil in treatment-resistant mania: An open trial. J Clin Psychopharmacol 7:101–103, 1987.

73. Kastner T, Friedman DL: Verapamil and valproic acid treatment of prolonged mania. J Am Acad Child Adolesc Psychiatry 31:271–275, 1992.

74. Berman E, Wolpert EA: Intractable manic-depressive psychosis with rapid cycling in an 18-year-depressive adolescent successfully treated with electroconvulsive therapy. J Nerv Ment Dis 175:236–239, 1987.

75. Christie KA, Burke JD, Regier DA, et al: Epidemiologic evidence for early onset of mental disorders and higher risk of drug abuse in young adults. Am J Psychiatry 145:971–975, 1988.

76. Schweizer E, Rickels K, Weiss S, Zavodnick S: Maintenance drug treatment of panic disorder. I. Results of a prospective, placebo controlled comparison of alprazolam and imipramine. Arch Gen Psychiatry 50:51–60, 1993.

77. Rickels K, Schweizer E, Weiss S, Zavondnick S: Maintenance drug treatment for panic disorder. II. Short- and long-term outcome after drug taper. Arch Gen Psychiatry 50:61–68, 1993.

78. Rapoport JL: Pediatric psychopharmacology: The last decade. In Meltzer HY (ed): Psychopharmacology: The Third Generation of Progress. New York, Raven Press, 1987, pp 1211–1214.

79. DeVeaugh-Geiss J, Moroz G, Biederman J, et al: Clomipramine hydrochloride in childhood and adolescent obsessive-compulsive disorder—a multicenter trial. J Am Acad Child Adolesc Psychiatry 31:45–49, 1992.

80. Gittelman-Klein R, Klein DF: Controlled imipramine treatment of school phobia. Arch Gen Psychiatry 25:204–207, 1971.

81. Bernstein GA: Anxiety disorders. In Garfinkel BD, Carlson GA, Weller EB (eds): Psychiatric Disorders in Children and Adolescents. Philadelphia, WB Saunders, 1990, pp 64–83.

82. Klein RG, Koplewicz HS, Kanner A: Imipramine treatment of children with separation anxiety disorder. J Am Acad Child Adolesc Psychiatry, 31:21–28, 1992.

83. Gittelman R, Klein DF: Relationship between separation anxiety and panic and agoraphobic disorders. Psychopathology 17(Suppl 1):56–65, 1984.

84. Weissman MM, Leckman JF, Merikangas KR, et al: Depression and anxiety disorders in parents and children. Results from the Yale family study. Arch Gen Psychiatry 41:845–852, 1984.

85. Simeon JG, Ferguson HB, Knott V, et al: Clinical, cognitive, and neurophysiological effects of alprazolam in children and adolescents with overanxious and avoidant disorders. J Am Acad Child Adolesc Psychiatry 31:29–33, 1992.

86. American Psychiatric Association: Diagnostic and Statistical Manual of Mental Disorders, 4th ed. Washington, DC, American Psychiatric Association, 1994.

87. Kranzler HR: Use of buspirone in an adolescent with overanxious disorder. J Am Acad Child Adolesc Psychiatry 27:789–790, 1988.

88. Strober M, Katz JL. Do eating disorders and affective disorders share a common etiology? A dissenting opinion. Int J Eat Disord 6:171–180, 1987.

89. Kennedy SH, Garfinkel P: Advances in diagnosis and treatment of anorexia nervosa and bulimia nervosa. Can J Psychiatry 37:309–315, 1992.

90. Hudson JI, Pope HG, Jonas JM, Yurgelum-Todd D: Phenomenologic relationship of eating disorders to major affective disorder. Psychol Res 9:345–354, 1983.

91. Hsu LKG: Treatment of bulimia with lithium. Am J Psychiatry 141:1260–1262, 1984.

92. Abikoff H, Klein RG: Attention-deficit hyperactivity and conduct disorder: Comorbidity and implications for treatment. J Consult Clin Psychol 60:881–892, 1992.

93. Greenhill LL: Attention deficit hyperactivity disorder in children. In Garfinkel BD, Carlson GA, Weller EB (eds): Psychiatric Disorders in Children and Adolescents. Philadelphia, WB Saunders, 1990, pp 149–182.

94. Biderman J, Gastfriend DR, Jellinek MS: Desipramine in the treatment of children with attention deficit disorder. J Clin Psychopharmacol 6:359–363, 1986.

95. Pliszka SR: Tricyclic antidepressants in the treatment of children with attention deficit disorder. J Am Acad Child Adolesc Psychiatry 26:127–132, 1987.

96. Steingard R, Biderman J, Spencer T, et al: Comparison of clonidine response in the treatment of attention-deficit hyperactivity disorder with and without comorbid tic disorders. J Am Acad Child Adolesc Psychiatry 32:350–353, 1993.

97. Klorman R, Brumaghin JT, Fitzpatrick PA, Borgstedt AD: Clinical effects of a controlled trial of methylphenidate on adolescents with attention deficit disorder. J Am Acad Child Adolesc Psychiatry 29:702–709, 1990.

98. Wender PH, Wood DR, Reimherr FW: Pharmacological treatment of attention deficit disorder, residual type (ADD, RT, minimal brain dysfunction, hyperactivity) in adults. Psychopharmacol Bull 21:222–231, 1985.

99. Stewart JT, Myers WC, Burket RC, Lyle WB: A review of the pharmacotherapy of aggression in children and adolescents. J Am Acad Child Adolesc Psychiatry 29:269–277, 1990.

100. Werry JS, Aman MG: Methylphenidate and haloperidol in children. Arch Gen Psychiatry 32:790–795, 1975.

101. Campbell M, Small AM, Green WH, et al: A comparison of haloperidol and lithium in hospitalized aggressive conduct disordered children. Arch Gen Psychiatry 41:650–656, 1984.

102. Conners CK, Kramer R, Rothchild GH, et al: Treatment of young delinquent boys with diphenylhydantoin sodium and methylphenidate. Arch Gen Psychiatry 24:156–160, 1971.

103. Hechtman L: Adolescent outcome of hyperactive children treated with stimulants in childhood: A review. Psychopharmacol Bull 21:178–191, 1985.

104. Kuperman S, Stewart MA: Use of propranolol to decrease aggressive outbursts in younger patients. Psychosomatics 28:315–319, 1987.

105. Kemph JP, DeVane CL, Levin GM, et al: Treatment of aggressive children with clonidine: Results of an open pilot study. J Am Acad Child Adolesc Psychiatry 32:577–581, 1993.

106. Eichelman B: Toward a rational pharmacotherapy for

aggressive and violent behavior. Hosp Community Psychiatry 39:31–39, 1988.

107. Munir K, Earls F: Ethical principles governing research in child and adolescent psychiatry. J Am Acad Child Adolesc Psychiatry 31:408–414, 1992.

108. McLellan AT, Alterman AI, Cacciola JS, et al: A new measure of substance abuse treatment: Initial studies of the Treatment Survey Review. J Nerv Ment Dis 180:101–110, 1992.

109. McLellan AT, Luborsky L, Woody GE, O'Brien CP: An improved diagnostic evaluation instrument for substance abuse patients: The Addiction Severity Index. J Nerv Ment Disease 168:26–33, 1980.

110. Strober M, Mozzell W, Burroughs J, et al: A family study of bipolar I disorder in adolescence: Early onset of symptoms linked to increased familial loading and lithium resistance. J Affect Disord 15:255–268, 1988.

Psychopharmacotherapy for the Dually Diagnosed: Novel Approaches

Bradley M. Pechter, MD •
Philip G. Janicak, MD • John M. Davis, MD

Information from rigorously controlled studies on medications used to treat patients with both a mental disorder and addictive illness is scarce. In general, clinicians tend to use drugs for the primary psychiatric disorder while integrating a concurrent treatment strategy for the addiction problem.[1, 2] Simultaneous treatment of both the mental and the addictive disorders constitutes an integrated model and appears to be the best approach for treatment of dual diagnoses.[3, 4] For the addiction, an abstinence-based model that typically uses a 12-step–based group therapy is most often used.[5] Physicians' medication-prescribing practices for addicted patients currently are anecdotally based, and attitudes toward this group may have a significant role in determining the treatment strategy.[2]

Despite the lack of controlled data and the inevitable complications associated with treating two different disorders, some optimism about the therapy of patients with a dual diagnosis may be appropriate.[6] For instance, evidence suggests that some drug dependence among dually diagnosed patients is less severe than in patients who have psychoactive substance-induced organic mental disorders or drug use disorders alone.[7] In this context, a study of patients receiving clozapine found that levels of overall psychopathology were lower in psychotic addicts than their nonaddicted counterparts.[8]

As Miller and Gold report, studies have supported a neurochemical origin for the addictive use of alcohol and other drugs, with reinforcement centers in the limbic system most often implicated. Thus, the ventral tegmental area in the midbrain, as well as its projections to the nucleus accumbens septi in the forebrain, are primary areas of interest. The connection between these two areas is the mesolimbic pathway, and dopamine is the principal neurotransmitter involved. Other neurotransmitters such as serotonin, gamma-aminobutyric acid (GABA), and norepinephrine may also contribute significantly.[4, 9, 10] Interestingly, these same neuroanatomical areas and their relevant neurotransmitters have also been implicated in the pathogenesis of several mental disorders. Thus, medications that impact on these systems may have effects not only on the addiction problem but the concurrent psychiatric disorder as well.

Proper diagnosis, important with any illness, is even more crucial in treatment planning for patients with a dual diagnosis. Because psychoactive substance use can obfuscate the diagnosis, special care must be taken to preclude organically based syndromes. Thus, adequate periods of abstinence must first be achieved, and then the patient reexamined for residual symptoms compatible with a nonaddictive, non–substance-induced psychiatric disorder.

Furthermore, important demographical information relevant to the pharmacotherapy of patients with a dual diagnosis can be gleaned from several studies. For example, Drake and Wallach,[11] in their study of chronic mentally ill patients, with or without addictions, found that the dually diagnosed were

- Generally younger
- Usually male
- More frequently hostile, suicidal, and disordered in their speech
- Less compliant with medication
- Less able to manage their lives in the community in terms of maintaining regular meals, adequate finances, stable housing, and regular activities

Smith and Hucker[12] note the following characteristics in the population of schizophrenic addicts included in their review of the literature:

- More violence
- More suicide
- More noncompliance
- Earlier psychotic breakdown
- Exacerbations of psychosis
- Relative antipsychotic refractoriness
- Increased rates of hospitalization
- Increased tardive dyskinesia
- Poor prognosis overall

Additionally, Noordsy and colleagues contribute data indicating that a family history of alcoholism in alcoholic schizophrenics is associated with a more severe course of illness, greater resistance to treatment, and more frequent abuse of other drugs.[13]

Psychopharmacotherapy for Specific Disorders

The use of psychotropic medication without simultaneous attention to the addictive disorder is not likely to produce the desired results for the addiction or the concurrent psychiatric condition. There are also some relative contraindications to using certain psychotropics in patients with a dual diagnosis. For example, benzodiazepines, despite their frequent benefit, are also subject to addictive use. In addition, antidepressants and antipsychotics with high anticholinergic properties should be used conservatively because of their potential for misuse.

PSYCHOTIC DISORDERS

Although it is unclear why schizophrenic patients misuse substances, Decker and Ries[14] summarize various theories of substance use by schizophrenics as

- Dampening of positive symptoms
- Overcoming negative symptoms
- Coping with unpleasant side effects

Aside from the self-medication hypotheses, Smith and Hucker[12] present other theories centering on

- Psychosocial factors that create opportunity, interaction, and acceptance
- Premorbid addictive use precipitating schizophrenia

Minimal evidence supports these theories, however, and drug addiction in schizophrenic patients may simply represent two concurrent diseases. It is interesting that in their assessment of the literature, Decker and Ries, as well as Smith and Hucker, found that no particular substance seems to be preferentially used by schizophrenic patients with addictions. Although they write that "there is little evidence that opiates contribute to increased psychosis," other substances are known to have some psychotogenic qualities such as paranoia or hallucinations, which can be associated with use of alcohol, cocaine or amphetamines, cannabis, and LSD or hallucinogens.[15]

In the area of therapy, Bowers and colleagues reported the results from a study using fixed doses of haloperidol or perphenazine to treat psychotic patients with and without concurrent addiction.[16] They found that psychotic males with prior use of addictive substances had a poorer early response (first 10 days) to antipsychotics than their counterparts who had no addictive use of substances. They hypothesized that such earlier drug use had contributed to increased psychosis and to relative antipsychotic refractoriness, perhaps mediated by dopaminergic mechanisms. Although this study had several methodological disadvantages (e.g., not blinded, no random assignment, no significant drug washout period, possibly suboptimal plasma levels, and short duration), it nonetheless suggests a diminished responsiveness to antipsychotics in the population with a dual diagnosis. This initial drug refractoriness may have important clinical and theoretical significance that clearly needs further investigation and may discourage a cautious optimism in treatment of such patients.

As noted earlier, patients with or without a history of substance addiction attained similar improvements on clozapine.[8] In light of this study, as well as other observations, it is hypothesized that clozapine may have a unique ability to decrease drug craving in schizophrenic patients with a dual diagnosis.

A third study reported that schizophrenic patients with a dual diagnosis show predominantly negative symptoms early in the course of their illness, which then progresses to a mixed (i.e., positive and negative symptoms) presentation.[17] This, it is noted, is in marked contrast to the usual course in schizophrenia, in which positive symptoms occur early in the course of illness and then recede as negative symptoms gain prominence. This observation may also have relevance for drug treatment strategies of dually diagnosed psychotic disorders.

Finally, desipramine was studied in a 12-week open-label design in 27 outpatient schizophrenic cocaine addicts who were also treated with appropriate antipsychotic regimens, relapse prevention, and social skills training programs.[18] The group receiving desipramine (100 to 150 mg/day) was more likely to complete the study, had fewer cocaine-positive urine samples, and had improved psychiatric symptoms during the study. Although these results are consistent with the outcome in some studies using desipramine for cocaine addiction without psychiatric comorbidity, we note that there is disagreement in the literature about desipramine's effectiveness in reducing cocaine dependence.[19–22] To our knowledge, this is the only study using antidepressants in the literature on psychotic patients with a dual diagnosis.

Opiate Antagonists

Naltrexone, naloxone, and other related compounds are opiate antagonists that have been used as adjunctive treatments in primary heroin dependence. Two well-controlled studies have produced evidence that naltrexone reduces drinking in alcoholic patients.[23, 24] Such data led to this agent's approval by the Food and Drug Administration for this labeled indication. Furthermore, earlier studies indicated that psychotic patients with comorbid alcohol disorders are also benefited by this drug. The pertinent literature for these two issues is reviewed next.

Alcohol Disorders. Volpicelli and colleagues studied naltrexone in a double-blind placebo-controlled trial of 70 male alcoholics during a 12-week period.[23] Naltrexone (50 mg/day) was compared with placebo in patients receiving a "standard rehabilitation" treatment program after alcohol detoxification. Eight of 35 (23%) naltrexone-treated subjects met criteria for relapse, in comparison with 19 of 35 (54%) on placebo. Of the 20 subjects who sampled alcohol in the placebo group, all but one suffered relapse, whereas only half of those who sampled alcohol in the naltrexone group suffered relapse (i.e., 8 of 16). Most notably, naltrexone reduced the monthly relapse rate by 56%.

In a second double-blind placebo-controlled study, O'Malley and associates randomly assigned 97 alcoholic subjects to a 12-week trial using naltrexone (50 mg/day) or placebo in addition to either coping skills/relapse prevention therapy or supportive therapy.[24] Sixty-one percent of the patients in the naltrexone/supportive therapy group abstained continuously for 12 weeks, in comparison with 28% of the naltrexone/coping skills subjects, 21% of placebo/coping skills subjects, and 19% of placebo/supportive subjects. For the total sample of patients in the coping skills or supportive therapy groups who received naltrexone, 13 and 15 drinks, respectively, were consumed during their time in the study. This compared favorably with the placebo control group, who consumed 47 and 29 drinks, respectively, during the study period. Thus, naltrexone clearly reduced relapse rates, craving, frequency of drinking, and quantity consumed. As noted earlier, such results have justified the labeled use of naltrexone as an adjunct to the psychosocial treatment of alcoholism.

Psychiatric Disorders with Comorbid Alcohol Problems. No naltrexone studies have yet focused on schizophrenic or bipolar alcoholic patients. The promising findings of the trials already mentioned, as well as the possible benefits of opiate antagonists in treating symptoms of schizophrenia or bipolar disorder without alcohol dependence, however, warrant studies in these difficult-to-treat populations.[25, 26]

Several studies, most of them single or double blind, have investigated the effects of naloxone or naltrexone on hallucinations in schizophrenic patients. Although about one third found that these drugs decreased hallucinations, two thirds failed to find such an effect. Of the two studies that examined the effects of naltrexone in mania, one found an attenuation of symptoms and the other did not.[27, 28]

Most of this literature studied the effects of one injection of naltrexone versus one injection of placebo to determine whether hallucinations and delusions decreased. Although one open naltrexone study that continued for several weeks reported benefit in many schizophrenic patients, several others have not.[29–34] Because these studies generally investigated naltrexone alone, its role as an adjunctive therapy with antipsychotics has not been adequately addressed. Given that no evidence suggests that naltrexone is deleterious in the treatment of psychiatric disorders, we believe it is important to determine if it might improve hallucinations and delusions when used to augment standard antipsychotic drug therapy.

In summary, we believe that naltrexone is an especially promising agent in the pharmacotherapy of coexisting psychiatric and addictive disorders. To this end, we are conducting a double-blind placebo-controlled study examining its effectiveness in alcoholics also diagnosed with major psychotic or mood disorders, especially when combined with effective psychosocial interventions.

Disulfiram

Disulfiram is sometimes quite helpful as an adjunct to nonpharmacological treatments for alcoholism. Although it has the potential to worsen psychosis, Kofoed cautions that these findings are based on untreated chronically affected patients given high doses.[35, 36] Kofoed and colleagues used disulfiram with a small number of dually diagnosed psychotic and alcohol-dependent patients after they were stabilized on appropriate antipsychotic medications. They found that compliance with disulfiram therapy in their dual-diagnosis group was as good as in primary alcoholic outpatients. They also reported no particular problems, concluding that disulfiram seemed less of a risk than continued alcohol misuse.[37, 38]

Methadone

We are aware of no evidence demonstrating that methadone interferes with antipsychotic function. It is the opinion of one group, based on a small trial, that methadone may have some inherent antipsychotic properties when used as an adjunct to standard antipsychotics.[39] For these reasons, we believe that psychosis itself is not a contraindication for otherwise eligible patients to receive this drug for maintenance therapy of their narcotic dependence. Furthermore, this agent may help stabilize patients sufficiently to enable them to participate in appropriate treatments for their dual-diagnosis problem.

MOOD DISORDERS
Unipolar Depression

Although depression in patients with a dual diagnosis is a frequently studied problem, con-

siderable difficulty is encountered in diagnosing a true, independent major depressive episode in the presence of concurrent addiction.[40] A period of abstinence is often necessary, but the minimum time necessary before attempting to finalize the diagnosis is unclear. For example, DSM-IV requires that depressive symptoms "persist for a substantial period of time (e.g., about a month)" after acute withdrawal or intoxication to be called substance-induced mood disorder.[15] Some transitory depressive symptoms are common in the first few weeks of abstinence after a prolonged period of substance use. This may be a part of the withdrawal or a reaction to the patient's "hitting bottom." Ample evidence shows that although alcoholism and depression are often associated, they may also present as distinct entities and not different presentations of identical processes.[41] As a result, common symptoms often overlap, making proper diagnosis much more difficult.

Clinical studies of depressed alcoholics give some suggestions of the course of treatments. Brown and coworkers demonstrated that those male patients in their sample who were dually diagnosed with alcohol dependence and a mood disorder did not demonstrate more severe depressive symptoms or a slower recovery than their counterparts with either diagnosis alone.[42] Evidence from another study shows that depression in schizophrenic alcoholics on acute inpatient admission resolves within the same time frame as does depression in non–dually diagnosed alcoholics.[43] If supported and broadened by further investigation, this finding would simplify treatment strategies by including patients with a dual diagnosis in established trends for mainstream addiction treatment.

Tricyclic Antidepressants

The role of tricyclics for depressed alcoholics has usually been limited to the period of acute withdrawal and not for longer-term maintenance. Other methodological problems with studies in this area include[44]

- Relative inattention to different subtypes of depression
- Inadequate use of therapeutic drug monitoring
- Failure to monitor both mood and drinking behavior in response to treatment

Despite these design flaws, many of the studies support the beneficial effects of tricyclic antidepressants in the treatment of depression associated with alcohol withdrawal. These benefits, however, do not exceed those of placebo after 3 weeks and thus may have only limited application in actual clinical practice.

Of the antidepressants now available, imipramine is the most extensively studied. A trial[45] assessing this agent's effectiveness for alcoholism with comorbid depression had certain advantages over its predecessors, including

- Lifetime histories to establish diagnoses of depression (thus avoiding transient depressive effects of alcohol)
- A double-blind design during the second phase of the study
- Adequacy of dosing as monitored by plasma levels

Unfortunately, the criteria for response are incomplete, but the researchers report that of 60 alcoholics who had major depression and who completed an initial 12-week open-label trial of imipramine, 27 (45%) responded, showing improvement in both mood (posttreatment Hamilton Depression Rating Scale score = 3; SD = 3) and drinking behavior (30% achieving abstinence and another 15% at a "much reduced level"). These response rates were further enhanced after dose increases or treatment with disulfiram. Patients who improved with imipramine in the initial open trial were then randomized into a subsequent 6-month double-blind maintenance phase. During this phase, 7 of 10 (70%) suffered a relapse on placebo, in contrast to only 4 of 13 (31%) on imipramine. Although the sample sizes were small, the investigators believed that this represented a significant improvement for those on medication in a common dual-diagnosis scenario.

Support for the efficacy of imipramine in treating depression in dual diagnosis was also found in one open-label trial of depressed patients in a methadone maintenance program.[46] The results of this preliminary evaluation suggested that both mood and illicit drug use improved.

Desipramine versus placebo was studied in a 12-week double-blind design comparing depressed with nondepressed cocaine-dependent patients receiving methadone maintenance.[20] Here, desipramine led to less overall cocaine use, and by week 10, the medicated depressed patients still in treatment had a 68% reduction in cocaine craving and a 96% reduction in cocaine use compared with their counterparts in the placebo group. By the final 2 weeks of the trial, 0% of urine toxicology screens were cocaine free for depressed patients in the placebo group, compared with 33% for the depressed patients receiving desipramine. The percentage of cocaine-free screens was 50%

during the same period when only study completers were included. Despite the small sample size, this study supports the efficacy of desipramine as an adjunctive therapy for cocaine addiction.

The Selective Serotonin Reuptake Inhibitors. New possibilities exist with the emergence of the selective serotonin reuptake inhibitors (SSRIs). Basic studies that used these agents in animals have substantiated a decrease in alcohol preference and consumption, whereas nonspecific monoamine uptake blockers (e.g., amitriptyline, doxepin) have not.[47] Using animal models of spontaneous alcohol consumption, Gorelick reported evidence that increased brain serotonin activity tended to decrease alcohol preference and consumption. Extrapolating these results from the laboratory to the clinical arena, Gorelick and Paredes then studied the effect of fluoxetine on alcohol consumption in 20 males with chronic dependence.[48] After a 28-day double-blind placebo-controlled period, they found that the fluoxetine group had a 14% lower alcohol intake, primarily during the first week. The beneficial effect was associated with a lower proportion of requests as well as less craving for alcohol. Unfortunately, as in the imipramine outcomes, these investigators did not find a significant effect in later weeks (i.e., virtually no differences in scores on the Hamilton Depression and Anxiety Scales or the abridged Hopkins Symptom Checklist).

Although the SSRIs' mechanism of action in treating alcohol dependence remains unclear, Gorelick and Paredes postulate that it is not due to motor inhibition or general sedation. Rather, they believe it may be "related to decreased appetite and food intake or a conditioned taste aversion mediated by increased brain serotonin activity."[48] Other competing theories have been summarized by Thomas,[49] including

- Antidepressant and anxiolytic effects
- Decrease in impulsivity
- Extinction of reward contingencies

Several outpatient studies of SSRIs used in early-stage problem drinkers and chronic alcoholics have also supported this trend by demonstrating reductions in various parameters used to measure drinking during variable time frames.[50–52]

We are currently aware of no studies using the SSRIs to address treatment specifically in patients with a dual diagnosis. In fact, the avoidance of significant depressive symptoms in subjects involved in these early studies was important to their design to avoid contaminating the outcome because of the specific antidepressant action of these agents. Thus, the need for trials with this class of antidepressants in the dually diagnosed population is an important next step, particularly in light of the positive findings with imipramine. Analogous to the treatment of depression, the SSRIs may offer similar benefits with considerably less risk than the tricyclic antidepressants.

BIPOLAR DISORDER

A high incidence of comorbid addiction is noted in bipolar disorder. The Epidemiological Catchment Area Study found that more than half of all patients with bipolar disorder abused alcohol or other drugs, and other investigators reported slightly lower but still substantial numbers.[53] Although the possible genetic links between alcoholism and bipolar illness are still debated, the comorbidity remains significant. Data on the population with bipolar disorder shows that concurrent substance users

- Had an earlier age of onset
- Were hospitalized twice as often for mood problems
- Were four times more likely to have other axis I disorders
- Were twice as likely to have dysphoric mania than their non–substance-abusing counterparts[54]

Diagnosis and treatment of this population is further complicated by the fact that many addictive substances produce maniclike symptoms. Indeed, even relatively benign drugs frequently used in the general population, such as caffeine and ephedrine, may induce or exacerbate manic episodes in those who are predisposed.

In general, all mood-stabilizing agents used for the dually diagnosed population can at least facilitate treatment of the psychiatric and the addictive disorder by stabilizing patients, thus promoting more appropriate participation in treatment. Lithium, still considered by many the treatment of choice for bipolar disorder, has not fulfilled its initial promise for the treatment of primary alcoholism with and without a concurrent affective disorder. Dorus and colleagues studied 457 male alcoholics in a Veterans Administration collaborative study and found that lithium did not alter the use of alcohol in either depressed or nondepressed alcoholics.[55] Specifically, they reported abstinence in 38% of lithium-treated nondepressed alcoholics (compared with 28% of placebo controls) and 32% of lithium-treated depressed al-

coholics (compared with 37% of their placebo controls). Fawcett and colleagues, who studied 104 alcoholics in a double-blind placebo-controlled design, report beneficial effects of lithium in this population, but they found that 19 of 51 (37%) patients given lithium and 22 of 53 (42%) patients on placebo were abstinent at the 6-month follow-up. The numbers become even more similar at 12-month follow-up.[56]

Although lithium no longer appears promising to treat alcohol dependence itself, it may yet have a place in pharmacotherapy of the overall syndrome. A small pilot study (n = 12) by Nagel and coworkers assessed lithium in a double-blind placebo-controlled design focusing on recently (3 to 7 days before entry into study) detoxified alcoholics who manifested a syndrome resembling hypomania.[57] Symptoms consisted of elevated psychomotor activity, grandiosity, irritability, a heightened desire for social contact, loquaciousness, and sexual preoccupation. The severity of symptoms was significantly decreased by treatment with low-dose lithium carbonate (serum levels 0.3 to 0.5 mEq/L) but was not affected by placebo treatment.

Anticonvulsants such as divalproex sodium and carbamazepine are effective mood-stabilizing agents and may be useful in withdrawal states secondary to alcohol, benzodiazepines, and cocaine.[58, 59] Because lithium may show some utility in certain patients dually diagnosed with bipolar disorder, and the anticonvulsants attenuate several types of withdrawal syndromes, the latter agents may possibly emerge as effective and safe treatments for alcoholic patients with bipolar disorder.

ANXIETY-RELATED DISORDERS

Anxiety is a common complaint that invariably complicates addictive illnesses. Decker and Ries cite estimates of comorbid anxiety and alcohol disorders ranging from 20% to 50%, with men more likely to self-medicate anxiety than women.[14, 60–62] Some investigators have also found increased rates of alcoholism in family members of patients with anxiety disorders.[63, 64] Patients with alcohol or drug dependence show a tendency to develop panic disorder earlier, and it has been suggested that repeated alcohol withdrawal may be the trigger for panic attacks in susceptible individuals.[65, 66] Finally, benzodiazepines, the primary pharmacological treatment for these disorders, are themselves addictive and sometimes associated with anxiety syndromes, especially on their discontinuation.[67]

Few studies have evaluated pharmacotherapy for coexisting anxiety and addictive disorders, but future investigations should consider buspirone, a nonbenzodiazepine partial serotonin agonist with anxiolytic properties. This agent may be particularly valuable in treating patients with a dual diagnosis because it is nonaddicting. In this light, Kranzler and colleagues'[68] placebo-controlled trial of buspirone in anxious alcoholics indicated that this agent led to

- A greater likelihood of completing treatment
- Reduction of anxiety symptoms
- A slower rate of heavy alcohol relapse
- More days of abstinence during the follow-up period

Conclusion

Miller and Gold argue that "pharmacological treatments for addictive disorders that suppress the appetitive, instinctual, or motivational drive states in the limbic system will likely have the most specific action on addictive disorders. The substrate for reinforcement of drug use uses the mesolimbic pathways, where neurotransmitter systems such as serotonin, GABA, and norepinephrine interact. The development of medications could be aimed at these target structures as primary generators of addictive drug and alcohol use."[69]

Indeed, abundant research efforts are focusing on these systems. Myers, in a review of these efforts in animal models of alcoholism, concurs that opioid, dopaminergic, and serotonergic systems are the most crucial ones modulating experimental alcoholism.[70] He reports that experimental medications such as amperozide modulate dopaminergic and serotonergic pathways while demonstrating some antipsychotic, antidepressant, anxiolytic, and "alcoholytic" actions. These experimental explorations meld with newer and established treatments for psychosis, depression, and anxi-

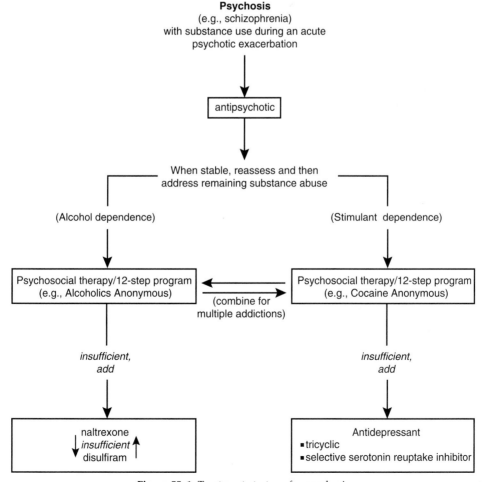

Figure 55–1. Treatment strategy for psychosis.

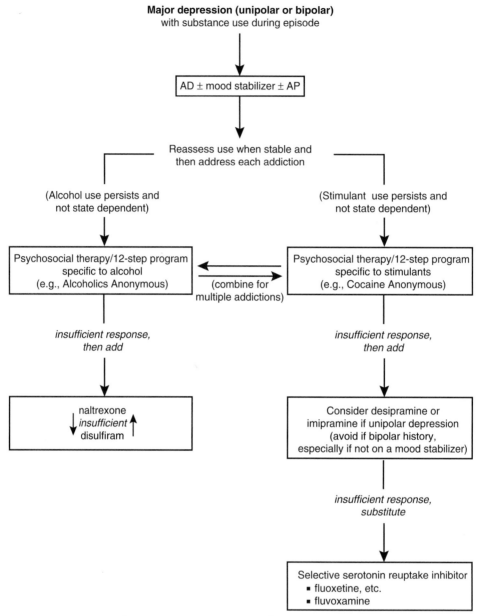

Figure 55–2. Treatment strategy for major depression.

ety, perhaps also establishing the foundation for treatment of patients with a dual diagnosis. Conceivably, future drug therapies may effectively and efficiently treat both conditions simultaneously.

Despite the complexities inherent in treating patients with a dual diagnosis, research and clinical practice must move forward to meet other challenges. Even as we begin to answer important questions in the area of dual diagnosis, questions about the treatment of triple diagnosis and beyond are emerging. For example, those with addiction, human immunode-

ficiency virus infection or acquired immunodeficiency syndrome, and a concurrent mental disorder are a natural extension of the simple dual-diagnosis paradigm.[71] Other scenarios might include mental retardation complicated by a psychiatric plus addictive illness and should also be the focus of future clinical research. Further controlled studies of medications to treat the dually diagnosed population are clearly needed.

Given our present state of knowledge, we have developed reasonable treatment strategies as outlined in Figures 55–1 to 55–3. These

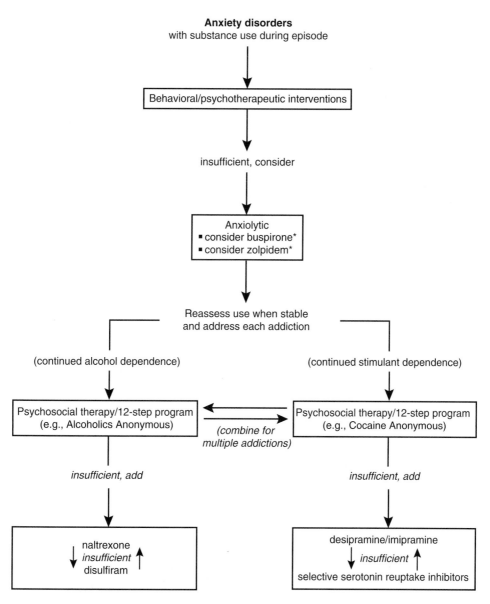

Anxiety disorders
with substance use during episode

Behavioral/psychotherapeutic interventions

insufficient, consider

Anxiolytic
▪ consider buspirone*
▪ consider zolpidem*

Reassess use when stable
and address each addiction

(continued alcohol dependence)

(continued stimulant dependence)

Psychosocial therapy/12-step program
(e.g., Alcoholics Anonymous)

*(combine for
multiple addictions)*

Psychosocial therapy/12-step program
(e.g., Cocaine Anonymous)

insufficient, add

insufficient, add

naltrexone
↓ *insufficient* ↑
disulfiram

desipramine/imipramine
↓ *insufficient* ↑
selective serotonin reuptake inhibitors

* These are nonaddictive, nonbenzodiazepine agents. Zolpidem may be especially effective with insomnia.

Figure 55–3. Treatment strategy for anxiety disorders.

figures address the treatment of psychotic, affective, and severe anxiety disorders complicated by alcohol or stimulant dependence (or the combination). We have chosen these substances, in part, to represent the most commonly encountered dual-diagnosis scenarios.

REFERENCES

1. Adelman SA, Fletcher KE, Bahnassi A, et al: The scale for treatment integration of the dually diagnosed (STIDD): An instrument for assessing intervention strategies in the pharmacotherapy of mentally ill substance abusers. Drug Alcohol Depend 27:35–42, 1991.
2. Adelman SA, Fletcher KE, Bahnassi A: Pharmacotherapeutic management strategies for mentally ill substance abusers. J Subst Abuse Treat 10:353–358, 1993.
3. Minkoff K: An integrated treatment model for dual diagnosis of psychosis and addiction. Hosp Community Psychiatry 40:1031–1036, 1989.
4. Miller NS: Issues in the diagnosis and treatment of comorbid addictive and other psychiatric disorders. Directions in Psychiatry 14(25):1–8, 1994.
5. Roman PM: Inpatient alcohol and drug treatment: A national study of treatment centers. Executive Report. Supported by National Institute of Alcohol Abuse and Addiction. Athens, GA, Institute for Behavioral Research, University of Georgia, 1989, pp 1–22.
6. Drake RE, Bartels SJ, Teague GB, et al: Treatment of substance abuse in severely mentally ill patients. J Nerv Ment Dis 181(10):606–611, 1993.
7. Lehman AF, Myers CP, Cortey E, et al: Severity of substance use disorders among psychiatric inpatients. J Nerv Ment Dis 182(3):164–167, 1994.
8. Buckley P, Thompson P, Way L, et al: Substance abuse among patients with treatment-resistant schizophrenia: Characteristics and implications for clozapine therapy. Am J Psychiatry 151(3):385–389, 1994.
9. Gold MS, Miller NS: Seeking drugs/alcohol and avoiding withdrawal. Psychiatr Ann 22(8):430–435, 1922.
10. Miller NS, Gold MS: A neurochemical model for alcohol and drug addiction. J Psychoactive Drugs 25(2):121–128, 1993.
11. Drake RE, Wallach MA: Substance abuse among the chronic mentally ill. Hosp Community Psychiatry 40(10):1041–1045, 1989.
12. Smith J, Hucker S: Schizophrenia and substance abuse. Br J Psychiatry 165:13–21, 1994.
13. Noordsy DL, Drake RE, Biesanz JC, et al: Family history of alcoholism in schizophrenia. J Nerv Ment Dis 182:651–655, 1994.
14. Decker KP, Ries RK: differential diagnosis and psychopharmacology of dual disorders. Psychiatr Clin North Am 16(4):703–719, 1993.
15. American Psychiatric Association: Diagnostic and Statistical Manual of Mental Disorders, 4th ed. Washington, DC, American Psychiatric Association, 1994.
16. Bowers MB, Mazure CM, Nelson JC, et al: Psychotogenic drug use and neuroleptic response. Schizophr Bull 16(1):81–85, 1990.
17. Rosenthal RN, Hellerstein DJ, Miner CR: Positive and negative syndrome typology in schizophrenic patients with psychoactive substance use disorders. Compr Psychiatry 35(2):91–98, 1994.
18. Ziedonis D, Richardson T, Lee E, et al: Adjunctive desipramine in the treatment of cocaine abusing schizophrenics. Psychopharmacol Bull 28(3):309–314, 1992.
19. Gawin FH, Kleber HD, Byck R, et al: Desipramine facilitation in initial cocaine abstinence. Arch Gen Psychiatry 46:117–121, 1989.
20. Ziedonis DM, Kosten TR: Depression as prognostic factor for pharmacological treatment of cocaine dependence. Psychopharmacol Bull 27:337–343, 1991.
21. Weddington WW, Brown BS, Haertzen CA, et al: Comparison of amantadine and desipramine combined with psychotherapy for treatment of cocaine dependence. Am J Drug Alcohol Abuse 17(2):137–152, 1991.
22. Arndt IO, McLellan AT, Dorozynsky L, et al: Desipramine treatment for cocaine dependence. J Nerv Ment Dis 182(3):151–156, 1994.
23. Volpicelli JR, Alterman AI, Hayashida M, et al: Naltrexone in the treatment of alcohol dependence. Arch Gen Psychiatry 49:876–880, 1992.
24. O'Malley SS, Jaffe AJ, Chang G, et al: Naltrexone and coping skills therapy for alcohol dependence. Arch Gen Psychiatry 49:881–887, 1992.
25. Berger P, Watson S, Akil H, et al: The effects of naloxone in chronic schizophrenia. Am J Psychiatry 138:913–915, 1981.
26. Watson SJ, Berger PA, Akil H, et al: Effects of naloxone in schizophrenia: Reduction in hallucinations in a subpopulation of subjects. Science 201:73–76, 1978.
27. Janowsky DS, Judd L, Huey L, et al: Naloxone effects on manic symptoms and growth-hormone levels. Lancet i:320, 1978.
28. Verhoeven WMA, van Praag HM, de Jong JTVM: Use of naloxone in schizophrenic psychoses and manic syndromes. Neuropsychobiology 7:159–168, 1981.
29. Emrich HM, Cording C, Piree S, et al: Indication of an antipsychotic action of the opiate antagonist naloxone. Pharmacopsychiatry 10:265–270, 1977.
30. Ragheb M, Berney S, Ban T: Naltrexone in chronic schizophrenia. Int Pharmacopsychiatry 15:1–5, 1980.
31. Simpson GM, Branchey MH, Lee JH: A trial of naltrexone in chronic schizophrenia. Curr Ther Res 22(6):909–913, 1977.
32. Mielke DH, Gaillant DM: An oral opiate antagonist in chronic schizophrenia: A pilot study. Am J Psychiatry 134:1430–1431, 1977.
33. Gitlin M, Rosenblatt M: Possible withdrawal from endogenous opiates in schizophrenics. Am J Psychiatry 135(3):377–378, 1978.
34. Dysken MW, Davis JM: Naloxone in amylobarbitone responsive catatonia (letter). Br J Psychiatry 133:476–480, 1978.
35. Major LF, Lerner P, Ballenger JC, et al: Dopamine beta-hydroxylase in the cerebrospinal fluid: Relationship to disulfiram-induced psychosis. Biol Psychiatry 14:337–344, 1979.
36. Kofoed L: Outpatient vs. inpatient treatment for the chronically mentally ill with substance use disorders. J Addict Dis 12(3):123–137, 1993.
37. Kofoed L, Kania J, Walsh T, et al: Outpatient treatment of patients with substance abuse and coexisting psychiatric disorders. Am J Psychiatry 143:867–872, 1986.
38. Kofoed LL: Chemical monitoring of disulfiram compliance: A study of alcoholic outpatients. Alcohol Clin Exp Res 11:481–485, 1987.
39. Britzer DA, Hartman N, Sweeney J, et al: Effect of methadone plus neuroleptics on treatment-resistant chronic paranoid schizophrenia. Am J Psychiatry 142:1106–1107, 1985.
40. Dackis CA, Gold MS, Pottash ALC, et al: Evaluating depression in alcoholics. Psychiatry Res 17:105–109, 1986.
41. Merikangas KR, Leckman JF, Prusoff BA, et al: Familial transmission of depression and alcoholism. Arch Gen Psychiatry 42(4):367–372, 1985.

42. Brown SA, Inaba RK, Gillin JC, et al: Alcoholism and affective disorder: Clinical course of depressive symptoms. Am J Psychiatry 152:45–52, 1995.
43. Brady KT, Killeen T, Jarrell P: Depression in alcoholic schizophrenic patients. Am J Psychiatry 150:1255–1256, 1993.
44. Ciraulo DA, Jaffe JH: Tricyclic antidepressants in the treatment of depression associated with alcoholism. J Clin Psychopharamacol 1:146–150, 1981.
45. Nunes EV, McGrath PJ, Quitkin FM, et al: Imipramine treatment of alcoholism with comorbid depression. Am J Psychiatry 150(6):963–965, 1993.
46. Nunes EV, Quitkin FM, Brady R, et al: Imipramine treatment of methadone maintenance patients with affective disorder and illicit drug use. Am J Psychiatry 148(5):667–669, 1991.
47. Gorelick DA: Serotonin uptake blockers and the treatment of alcoholism. Recent Dev Alcohol 7:267–281, 1989.
48. Gorelick DA, Paredes A: Effect of fluoxetine on alcohol consumption in male alcoholics. Alcohol Clin Exp Res 16(2):261–265, 1992.
49. Thomas R: Fluvoxamine and alcoholism. Int Clin Psychopharmacol 6(3):84–92, 1991.
50. Amit Z, Brown Z, Sutherland Z, et al: Reduction in alcohol intake in humans as a function of treatment with zimeldine: Implications for treatment. In Naranjo CA, Sellers EM (eds): Research Advances in New Psychopharmacological Treatments for Alcoholism. Amsterdam, Excerpta Medica, 1985, pp 189–198.
51. Naranjo CA, Sellers EM, Jullivan JT, et al: The serotonin uptake inhibitor citalopram attenuates ethanol intake. Clin Pharmacol Ther 41:266–274, 1987.
52. Naranjo CA, Sellers EM, Roach CA, et al: Zimeldine-induced variations in alcohol intake by non-depressed heavy drinkers. Clin Pharmacol Ther 35:374–381, 1984.
53. Winokur G, Cook B, Liskow B, et al: Alcoholism in manic depressive (bipolar) patients. J Stud Alcohol 54:574–576, 1993.
54. Sonne SC, Brady KT, Morton WA: Substance abuse and bipolar affective disorder. J Nerv Ment Dis 182(6):349–352, 1994.
55. Dorus W, Ostrow DG, Anton R, et al: Lithium treatment of depressed and nondepressed alcoholics. JAMA 262:1646–1652, 1989.
56. Fawcett J, Clark DC, Gibbons RD, et al: Evaluation of lithium therapy for alcoholism. J Clin Psychiatry 45:494–499, 1984.
57. Nagel K, Adler LE, Bell J, et al: Lithium carbonate and mood disorder in recently detoxified alcoholics: A double-blind, placebo-controlled pilot study. Alcohol Clin Exp Res 15(6):978–981, 1991.
58. Halikas J, Kuhn K, Carlsan G: The effect of carbamazepine on cocaine use. Am J Addict 1(1):30–39, 1992.
59. Kosten TR, Gawin FH, Kosten TA, et al: Six month follow-up of short-term pharmacotherapy for cocaine dependence. Am J Addict 1(1):40–49, 1992.
60. Bowen RC, Cipywnyk D, D'Arcy C, et al: Alcoholism, anxiety disorders, and agoraphobia. Alcohol Clin Exp Res 8:48–50, 1984.
61. Smail P, Stockwell T, Canter S, et al: Alcohol dependence and phobic anxiety states I. A prevalence study. Br J Psychiatry 144:53–57, 1984.
62. Reich J, Chaudhry D: Personality of panic disorder alcohol abusers. J Nerv Ment Dis 175:224–228, 1987.
63. Cloninger CR, et al: Follow-up and family study of anxiety neurosis. In Klein DF, Rabkin J (eds): Anxiety: New Research and Changing Concepts. New York, Raven Press, 1981.
64. Crowe RR, Crowe RC, Pauls DL, et al: A family study of anxiety neurosis: Morbidity risk in families of patients with and without mitral valve prolapse. Arch Gen Psychiatry 37:77–79, 1980.
65. Starcevic V, Uhlenhuth EH, Kellner R, et al: Comorbidity in panic disorder: II. Chronology of appearance and pathogenic comorbidity. Psychiatry Res 46:285–293, 1993.
66. George DT, Nutt DJ, Dwyer BA, et al: Alcoholism and panic disorder: Is the comorbidity more than coincidence? Acta Psychiatr Scand 81:97–107, 1990.
67. Janicak PG, Davis JM, Preskorn SH, Ayd FJ Jr: Principles and Practice of Psychopharmacotherapy. Baltimore, Williams & Wilkins, 1993.
68. Kranzler HR, Burleson JA, Del Boca FK, et al: Buspirone treatment of anxious alcoholics: A placebo-controlled trial. Arch Gen Psychiatry 51:720–731, 1994.
69. Miller NS, Gold MS: The psychiatrist's role in integrating pharmacological and nonpharmacological treatments for addictive disorders. Psychiatr Ann 22(8):436–440, 1992.
70. Myers RD: New drugs for the treatment of experimental alcoholism. Alcohol 11(6):439–451, 1994.
71. Batki SL: Drug abuse, psychiatric disorders, and AIDS. Dual and triple diagnosis. West J Med 152(5):547–552, 1990.

Experimental Pharmacological Agents to Reduce Alcohol, Cocaine, and Opiate Use*

Raye Z. Litten, Ph.D. • John P. Allen, Ph.D. •
David A. Gorelick, M.D., Ph.D. •
Kenzie Preston, Ph.D.

The past decade has witnessed significant advances in understanding the neurobiological bases of substance use and abuse and in identifying psychoactive agents that may influence these systems. Perhaps the most tangible evidence of this is that long-acting orally administered opiate agonists (methadone, L-acetylmethadol [LAAM]) and antagonists (naltrexone) have been approved by the Food and Drug Administration (FDA) and have achieved widespread clinical application.

Four basic pharmacological approaches have guided development of new pharmacotherapies for substance addiction.[1, 2]

1. Maintenance substitution treatment with a long-acting, cross-tolerant medication. The feasibility of this strategy is contingent on existence of a cross-tolerant medication that is not liable to produce significant medical or psychiatric complications with long-term use. This approach is typified by agents to treat opiate dependence.

2. Maintenance treatment with medication that blocks the effects of the abused drug.

This approach is useful when the abused drug exerts its clinically significant psychoactive effects predominantly at a single binding site that can be blocked by an antagonist. As with maintenance substitution, this strategy is currently available only for opiate dependence.

3. Medications that blunt the reinforcing effects of the abused drug or the craving for it other than by a direct action of the medication at the drug's receptor or binding site. This approach is attracting considerable attention for experimental pharmacotherapy of alcohol and cocaine addiction.

4. Alteration of drug metabolism to either enhance elimination of the drug from the body, thereby reducing its effects, or make its use aversive rather than reinforcing. The latter approach is currently exemplified only by disulfiram treatment for alcoholism.

Medications may facilitate clinical management of substance addiction at various stages from alleviating acute intoxication or withdrawal to remediating physical and psychological sequelae resulting from abuse and comorbid psychiatric disorders. This chapter

---

*All material in this chapter is in the public domain, with the exception of any borrowed figures or tables.

addresses psychopharmacological agents whose intended action is primarily to reduce use of abused substances. The primary focus is on pharmacotherapies that have demonstrated promise in clinical trials with human subjects but that are considered experimental in that they have not yet received either FDA approval for marketing in the United States or widespread clinical acceptance based on replicated controlled clinical trials.

Pharmacotherapies to Reduce Problematical Drinking

The primary focus of experimental pharmacotherapy for alcoholism has been on reducing the reinforcing effects of and craving for alcohol by influencing the neurotransmitter pathways that underlie these effects. A large body of research with animal models dealing with spontaneous alcohol intake has identified several classes of neuropharmacological agents that markedly influence alcohol intake.[3] Several of these agents also seem to attenuate drinking in humans. These include opioid antagonists; serotonergic agents including selective serotonin reuptake inhibitors (SSRIs), $5HT_{1A}$ agonists, $5HT_2$ antagonists, and $5HT_3$ antagonists; gamma-aminobutyric acid (GABA) agonists; and dopamine agonists and antagonists.[4, 5]

OPIOID ANTAGONISTS

Brain opioid systems profoundly influence patterns of alcohol consumption,[3, 5] and current preclinical research has explored the role of specific opioid receptor subtypes.[6] The opioid antagonists naltrexone, naloxone, and nalmefene all reduce alcohol consumption in rats and monkeys.[5, 7] Trials of naltrexone with human subjects suggest similar effects. The efficacy of naltrexone has been demonstrated by independent randomized, double-blind, placebo-controlled outpatient clinical trials by Volpicelli and colleagues[8] and O'Malley and associates.[9] Both studies found that daily administration of naltrexone (50 mg orally) reduced drinking episodes and diminished total level of consumption in alcohol-dependent subjects. Further, naltrexone significantly curbed propensity, duration, and severity of relapse to heavy drinking. For example, in the Volpicelli study,[8] 54% of placebo subjects had severe relapses, compared with only 23% for the naltrexone-treated subjects. Secondary data analysis suggested that the effectiveness of naltrexone may be based on reduction in the reinforcement properties of alcohol. Although subjects taking naltrexone often "sampled" alcohol during treatment, they tended to moderate subsequent consumption spontaneously and to cease drinking far more readily than did the placebo-treated subjects. Neither study reported any clinically significant side effects of naltrexone.

The O'Malley study[9] also evaluated the interaction of naltrexone with two types of psychosocial treatment, supportive therapy to encourage abstinence and structured coping skills/relapse prevention therapy. The naltrexone/supportive therapy group maintained abstinence longer. Among subjects who did initiate drinking, however, those receiving naltrexone in conjunction with coping skills/relapse prevention therapy were less likely to suffer major relapse.

In a later study with a more heterogeneous population of alcohol-dependent patients, Volpicelli and his colleagues[10] found that individuals highly compliant with naltrexone therapy and attending scheduled follow-up evaluations drank on fewer days and suffered lower rates of relapse than did subjects less compliant with naltrexone therapy or those assigned to the compliant or less compliant placebo group. The magnitude of drinking reduction was similar to that in their first study. Patients less compliant with naltrexone demonstrated minimal changes in drinking behavior.

An open-label trial with nondependent heavy drinkers also found that naltrexone treatment combined with brief counseling decreased self-reported desire to drink, drinking frequency, and amount of alcohol consumed.[11] A double-blind placebo-controlled trial is currently under way to corroborate these findings.

Several investigators are exploring the neurophysiological mechanisms for naltrexone's effect in reducing drinking. A clue to this may be that patients taking naltrexone report experiencing less euphoria from alcohol during their first "slip."[12] In a placebo-controlled laboratory study with nondependent social drinkers, those receiving 50 mg of naltrexone an hour earlier reported less reinforcement but greater sedative effect from a standard dose of alcohol.[13]

The opioid antagonist nalmefene is also under investigation as a potential treatment for alcoholism. A 12-week pilot study found that subjects on 40 mg of nalmefene daily experienced fewer drinking days and lower relapse rates than did those on 10 mg of nalmefene daily or on placebo.[14] Both nalmefene groups reported lower alcohol consumption per drinking day than did placebo-treated patients. Nalmefene was well tolerated and elicited few side effects. A large-scale trial of nalmefene is currently under way to confirm these early findings.

SEROTONERGIC AGENTS

Selective Serotonin Reuptake Inhibitors

SSRIs have consistently been shown to reduce intake of and preference for alcohol in rodents, an effect not produced by other classes of antidepressant medications.[15, 16] Several clinical studies have reported favorably on their potential in reducing alcohol consumption.[15, 17] Naranjo and coworkers[18–22] conducted a series of short-duration (1 to 4 weeks) double-blind outpatient trials with several SSRIs, including zimeldine, citalopram, viqualine, and fluoxetine. Subjects were early problem drinkers consuming at least 28 drinks per week, not clinically depressed, and receiving no treatment other than medication. Modest (10% to 20%) reductions in alcohol intake were observed. The nature of the effects was somewhat medication specific.[20–22] Fluoxetine and viqualine primarily diminished level of consumption per drinking occasion. Zimeldine and citalopram decreased frequency of drinking episodes. A long-term open-label study also found beneficial effects of zimeldine in alcohol-dependent men treated for 6 months.[23]

On the other hand, five other human studies with SSRIs have reported less promising results. A 12-week placebo-controlled trial of fluoxetine in subjects with mild to moderate alcohol dependence found that both groups fared equally well, a result attributed to the therapeutic effects of the concurrent relapse prevention therapy given to all subjects.[24] A shorter, 1-month study found that fluoxetine reduced alcohol consumption only in subjects with a positive family history of alcoholism.[25] A trial of fluvoxamine found its use limited by side effects.[26] It is interesting that Balldin and colleagues[27] found that citalopram was effective in reducing drinking in moderate but not heavy drinkers. Finally, Naranjo and associates[28] found that citalopram was more effective than placebo in reducing alcohol intake in mild to moderate drinkers during the first week of treatment, an effect that disappeared in the remaining 11 weeks of treatment. Subjects may have quickly developed tolerance to the medication.

In the single published inpatient trial of an SSRI, fluoxetine produced a statistically significant 14% decrease in consumption in severely alcohol-dependent nondepressed men during the first week of treatment, with no significant side effects.[29] However, despite continued medication, alcohol consumption returned to baseline levels during the next 3 weeks, again suggesting possible rapid tolerance to SSRIs.

As antidepressants, SSRIs might well prove more effective in alcoholics with comorbid depression. In an open-label 8-week trial with depressed alcoholics, those treated with fluoxetine demonstrated a decrease in depressive symptoms and in amount of alcohol consumed.[30] Early results from a double-blind placebo-controlled study with fluoxetine in similar subjects also revealed a 75% decrease in alcohol intake and a trend toward decrease in depression.[31] It would be of interest to determine if the effect of fluoxetine on drinking was direct or if, by diminishing depression, fluoxetine indirectly reduced alcohol intake.

In summary, SSRIs have shown some potential to reduce drinking behavior in nondepressed drinkers, especially with individuals who are nondependent or who are from families in which alcoholism is prevalent. They may show particular promise for alcoholics with comorbid depression. Most SSRIs are well tolerated even by drinking patients. Nevertheless, a few, such as zimeldine and fluvoxamine, have produced clinically significant adverse effects.[5, 26] Future research needs to more fully specify optimal dosage and duration of treatment with these medications, the kinds of patients who may profit most from them, and the basis for their pharmacological effect.

5HT$_{1A}$ Agonists

Animal studies suggest that 5HT$_{1A}$ receptors also influence alcohol consumption, perhaps owing to their modulation of brain dopamine activity.[32] Several 5HT$_{1A}$ agonists, including gepirone, ipsapirone, 1-[3-(trifluoromethyl)-phenyl]-piperazine (TFMPP), 8-hydroxy-2-(di-N-propylamino) tetralin (8-OH DPAT), and FG 5893, reduce alcohol intake in rodents.[33–36] Buspirone, a partial 5HT$_{1A}$ agonist clinically used as an antianxiety medication, is the only pharmacological agent of this class that has been evaluated in clinical trials. If ultimately proved effective, it could be a useful therapeutic agent, because it is not itself a sedative, does not impair psychomotor or driving performance, has no abuse liability, and does not interact with alcohol.[37–39]

Five trials of buspirone have been conducted in alcoholics with comorbid anxiety disorders; four of these yielded favorable results. Bruno's project[40] revealed that buspirone reduced craving and anxiety and improved retention in treatment. In an open trial, Kranzler and Meyer[41] also found that buspirone significantly reduced both anxiety and craving for alcohol. In a subsequent placebo-controlled trial, Kranzler and colleagues[42] found that buspirone reduced drinking days and improved treatment retention. In another trial enrolling alcoholics who had been abstinent for 30 to 90 days, buspirone reduced both drinking and anxiety and increased treatment retention.[43] The one negative study found no change from placebo in drinking behavior during 6 months of buspirone treatment in male alcoholics who had been abstinent at least 14 days at the start of treatment.[44] The lack of efficacy in this study may have been related to a greater degree of alcohol dependence in the subjects and the absence of any psychosocial treatment.

5HT$_2$ and 5HT$_3$ Antagonists

5HT$_2$ and 5HT$_3$ receptors modulate brain dopamine activity, with receptor stimulation enhancing dopamine release and receptor antagonists inhibiting dopamine release.[32] Agents that selectively block 5HT$_2$ and 5HT$_3$ receptors have also shown promise in animal studies, although human studies remain in early stages. Several studies have suggested that 5HT$_2$ antagonists, including the antidepressant ritanserin, amperozide, and risperidone (a mixed 5HT$_2$ and dopamine D2 antagonist antipsychotic medication), reduce alcohol intake in rats.[45–48] Preliminary results of a single-blind study of chronic alcoholics revealed that ritanserin diminished depression, anxiety, and desire to drink.[49] A multisite clinical trial of ritanserin in alcohol-dependent outpatients is now in progress.

Blockers of 5HT$_3$ receptors, including the antiemetic ondansetron, zacopride, MDL 72222, GR38932F, and ICS 205–930, also decrease alcohol intake in animals.[50–52] These agents are believed to block alcohol-induced release of dopamine in the mesocorticolimbic system, thereby decreasing reinforcing effects of alcohol.[52] Only ondansetron has been evaluated in clinical studies. It has been shown to decrease desire to drink in social drinkers.[52] In a 6-week trial, patients taking a low dose of ondansetron

(0.25 mg) consumed less alcohol than did those taking a higher dose (2.0 mg) or placebo.[53]

GABA Agonists

Studies have also implicated the GABAergic system in mediating drinking behavior.[5] Acamprosate, a GABAergic derivative of taurine, increased length of abstinence in chronic alcoholics during 3 months of treatment.[54] In a subsequent 3-month multisite study with alcohol-dependent patients, use of acamprosate was associated with lower plasma levels of gamma-glutamyl transpeptidase (GGT), further evidencing reduction in drinking.[55] Acamprosate has also been effective in attenuating drinking in alcoholic patients without a family history of alcoholism but not in those with such a history.[25]

Gamma-hydroxybutyric acid (GHB), a metabolite of GABA thought to enhance the GABAergic system, is also being investigated. Gallimberti and colleagues[56] found that GHB-treated alcohol-dependent subjects reported reduced craving for alcohol, drank on fewer days (26% vs. 8%), and consumed fewer drinks per day (4.7 vs. 9.9) than did subjects on placebo.

Dopamine Agonists and Antagonists

Dopaminergic neurons in the brain, especially in the mesolimbocortical system, are believed to mediate many of the reinforcing actions of abused substances, including alcohol.[57] Both agonists and antagonists of dopamine reduce alcohol intake in animals. Interestingly, the effects on pattern of drinking vary, apparently reflecting agent-specific effects on underlying receptor types (D1 or D2), sites (presynaptic versus postsynaptic), and brain area primarily affected.[58–62]

Bromocriptine, a dopamine agonist primarily of D2 type, has produced mixed results, improving social functioning and mood level while reducing craving for alcohol in one study,[63] but it appeared no better than placebo in reducing drinking behavior in another.[64]

European studies have suggested that tiapride, a dopamine D2 antagonist, may prove helpful in treatment of alcoholism. A 6-month study with alcohol-dependent subjects suffering comorbid anxiety or depression found that tiapride led to a 79% increase in abstinence rates and a 43% decrease in daily intake.[65] It also relieved symptoms of depression and anxiety and improved self-esteem and overall life satisfaction. In a subsequent 3-month study, tiapride was found to reduce alcohol consumption and enhance abstinence rate, self-esteem, and satisfaction with life situations in recently detoxified alcoholics.[66] An 11-site trial with tiapride is currently under way in Germany.

Research Directions and Conclusions

Of the agents studied to date, the most promising appears to be naltrexone, which has been approved for marketing in the United States as an adjunctive treatment for alcoholism. Projects currently under way are investigating its mechanisms of action and evaluating its effectiveness in various patient populations. Several studies suggest that the SSRIs, buspirone, and tiapride may reduce alcohol consumption, especially in patients with comorbid psychiatric problems. Various medications may improve the outcome of alcoholism treatment yet may have very different effects on the parameters of drinking behavior. Some may assist in maintaining abstinence longer (i.e., delay the occurrence of relapse). Others may moderate duration and intensity of relapse. Still others may reduce average level and frequency of consumption. Preclinical research on the neuropharmacological mechanisms of alcohol's effects, such as the role of the N-methyl-D-aspartate (NMDA) glutamate receptor system,[67] may also lead to the development of clinically useful medications.

Pharmacotherapies to Reduce Cocaine Use

More than a dozen medications already approved in the United States for other indications are currently being used in the treatment of cocaine addiction.[68] These agents can be considered experimental in that none has been FDA approved for this indication and none has consistently demonstrated efficacy in controlled clinical trials.[2, 17] The typical pattern of findings has been a promising result in the initial small-scale open-label trial, followed by inconsistent or negative results in later controlled clinical trials.

Most medications considered to date have been selected on a theoretical basis because they are thought to act according to one or more of the first three mechanisms outlined earlier—that is, maintenance with a cross-tolerant stimulant (e.g., methylphenidate), maintenance with a cocaine antagonist (i.e., a medication blocking a cocaine binding site, e.g., mazindol), or reduction of the reinforcing ef-

fects of or craving for cocaine. Most attention has focused on the latter mechanism, especially on dopaminergic agents because of the evidence linking cocaine's reinforcing psychoactive properties to its action on the mesolimbic brain reward system.[57, 69] No clinical trials have yet been conducted with the expressed intent of modifying cocaine's metabolism, although this is a growing area of preclinical research.[2]

STIMULANTS

Treatment with a stimulant medication might reduce cocaine craving and use, analogous to the successful use of the opiate agonist methadone in the treatment of heroin addiction. However, limited experience with the schedule II stimulants methylphenidate and phenmetrazine has actually shown them detrimental, because patients reported increased cocaine craving and use.[70, 71] One exception is methylphenidate use in patients with definite or possible comorbid attention deficit disorder. In these patients, methylphenidate may decrease cocaine use by direct therapeutic effect on the attention deficit disorder.[72]

Two schedule IV stimulants, pemoline and diethylpropion, have shown promising results in small pilot studies.[73, 74] Because these medications have less abuse potential than cocaine or other schedule II agents, they offer a promising area for future controlled clinical trials. Mazindol, an unscheduled medication that can be considered a very mild stimulant, has shown mixed results in three small pilot studies.[71, 75, 76] Mazindol blocks cocaine binding to the presynaptic dopamine reuptake pump and so could be acting as a cocaine antagonist in the direct pharmacological sense.

COCAINE ANTAGONISTS

Because of cocaine's key role in inhibiting the presynaptic dopamine reuptake pump (transporter), most attention has focused on medications that block the binding of cocaine to the transporter without themselves affecting dopamine reuptake or binding to the transporter but exerting less effect on dopamine reuptake than does cocaine itself.[77] Mazindol and bupropion block cocaine binding to the dopamine transporter. They also themselves inhibit dopamine reuptake but less rapidly and intensely than does cocaine; thus, they appear liable to little or no abuse potential. Despite these actions, mazindol did not alter the acute subjective effects of intravenous cocaine use in the laboratory[78] nor reduce cocaine use in a short placebo-controlled crossover clinical trial.[76] Neither mazindol nor bupropion has demonstrated consistent efficacy in larger open-label clinical trials.[2] Research with more selective dopamine transporter ligands, which act more as full cocaine antagonists, is continuing at both preclinical and clinical levels (discussed later).

Another approach to cocaine antagonism is blockade of the postsynaptic dopamine receptors on which synaptic dopamine would act when its presynaptic reuptake is blocked. Available neuroleptics, used to treat schizophrenia and other psychotic conditions, are potent dopamine receptor antagonists (chiefly D2) but do not block the acute effects of injected cocaine in the laboratory setting[79] and do not appear to reduce cocaine use in cocaine-abusing schizophrenic patients receiving chronic neuroleptic treatment.[80] However, in both a small open-label trial and an ongoing double-blind controlled clinical trial,[81] the neuroleptic flupenthixol, not marketed in the United States, has been reported to reduce cocaine use in nonschizophrenic cocaine addicts. Flupenthixol's efficacy may be related to its possible preferential action on presynaptic, rather than postsynaptic, dopamine receptors at the low doses used in these studies. Limited evidence from both animal and human studies shows that neuroleptic treatment could be detrimental to cocaine users, who may be at greater risk of neuroleptic-induced movement disorders[82] and neuroleptic malignant syndrome.[83] Further, neuroleptics may exacerbate acute cardiovascular effects of cocaine.[84]

DOPAMINERGIC MANIPULATION

Various medications that increase brain dopamine activity have been used, under the rationale that they would alleviate the presumed dopamine hypoactivity caused by chronic cocaine use.[85] Results of open-label trials[2] have been inconsistent in showing benefit of increasing dopamine synthesis by administration of its amino acid precursors tyrosine or L-dopa, an effective strategy in the treatment of Parkinson's disease. A single published double-blind trial[86] failed to find this strategy effective in reducing cocaine craving.

The presynaptic dopamine releaser amantadine, an antiparkinsonism agent, seems beneficial for methadone-maintained cocaine addicts but not for non–opiate-dependent patients.[2, 17] Some evidence suggests that its effectiveness may dissipate if use continues beyond several weeks. Bromocriptine has been found effective in most open-label and double-blind outpatient studies.[2, 17] Nevertheless, this finding should be further elucidated because several of the open-label studies included patients suffering comorbid attention deficit disorder, a condition that may respond directly to bromocriptine. Also, several of the double-blind studies failed to include cocaine use as an outcome measure, thus allowing only indirect inferences about efficacy. Current studies are using more specific, potent, and long-acting D2 agonists, such as pergolide and lisuride. Results are still inconclusive. One factor limiting use of D2 agonists is poor compliance owing to uncomfortable side effects such as headache and gastrointestinal distress, which occur at higher doses or with too rapid dose escalation. Further, these agents should be avoided in postpartum women because of risk of stroke and seizure.[87]

One strategy for increasing brain dopamine activity is concurrent use of two medications that act by different mechanisms, with the goal of an additive if not synergistic effect and an interruption of normal compensatory mechanisms that might limit the intensity or duration of the increase in dopamine activity. Such a combined medication approach has been successfully used in the treatment of Parkinson's disease.[88] The combination of bromocriptine and bupropion has shown early promise in a small open-label trial for the treatment of cocaine dependence.[89]

Another strategy to increase brain dopamine activity is inhibition of monoamine oxidase (MAO) type B, the chief dopamine-metabolizing enzyme in the brain. Although it was not effective in a small open-label study,[71] selegiline, an MAO inhibitor approved as a treatment for parkinsonism, is currently undergoing clinical trials for cocaine addiction. At low doses, selegiline selectively inhibits only MAO-B while sparing MAO-A. Because inhibition of MAO-A in the gastrointestinal tract mediates the hypertensive crises associated with ingestion of amine-containing foods or catecholaminergic medications, selegiline may be a safer medication for use in cocaine addicts. Older MAO inhibitors, such as phenelzine, inhibit both MAO-A and MAO-B, thus possibly precipitating a hypertensive crisis. Phenelzine has been used effectively in one small open-label trial. Patients' fear of a severe reaction if they used cocaine while taking the medication was proposed as one possible mechanism of action.[90] This would make phenelzine's action analogous to that of disulfiram in the treatment of alcoholism.

Many heterocyclic antidepressant medications inhibit presynaptic reuptake of dopamine, thereby increasing brain activity. These have been the most widely used treatment medications during the past decade, perhaps reflecting the observation that depression is a frequent symptom among cocaine addicts seeking treatment. The tricyclic antidepressant desipramine is most commonly used and was the first agent reported effective in a double-blind controlled clinical trial.[91] The efficacy of desipramine at typical antidepressant doses (150 to 300 mg daily, about 2.5 mg/g) was replicated in some early trials[92] but was not confirmed in several later and larger controlled trials.[2, 17]

Several patient clinical characteristics and pharmacokinetic factors may account for some of the variability in outcome reported in clinical trials of desipramine. Retrospective analyses of completed trials suggest that patients with depression fare well on desipramine,[93] whereas those with antisocial personality disorder fare poorly.[94] Evidence from a few clinical trials suggests a possible therapeutic plasma concentration ceiling for desipramine's efficacy, with concentrations greater than 200 ng/ml associated with poorer outcome.[95] This effect may be related to anecdotal reports of some patients' taking higher desipramine doses and experiencing subjective effects similar to those of cocaine, thus resulting in stimulation of cocaine craving.[96] Methadone increases desipramine plasma concentrations by inhibiting desipramine metabolism.[97] Thus, patients on concurrent methadone maintenance may have higher than optimum desipramine plasma concentrations despite receiving standard doses.

Two other heterocyclic antidepressants, maprotiline and imipramine, have been effective in single small open-label trials,[98, 99] but neither study has been replicated.

SEROTONERGIC AGENTS

Animal studies and later clinical trials indicating a prominent role for brain serotonin systems in inhibiting appetitive behaviors, such as food and alcohol intake (discussed earlier[15, 100]) have fostered interest in serotonergic agents as treatment for cocaine addiction. This interest has been sustained by animal studies showing that inhibition of the presynaptic serotonin transporter with SSRIs reduced cocaine self-administration and drug discrimination.[101] As in the treatment of alcoholism, various approaches to manipulating brain serotonin activity have been applied to the treatment of cocaine addiction, although no agent has yet shown conclusive efficacy.

Selective Serotonin Reuptake Inhibitors

Antidepressant SSRIs, such as fluoxetine and sertraline, have been the most widely used serotonergic medications for treatment of cocaine addiction. Early studies with doses in the antidepressant range (20 to 45 mg daily) found that fluoxetine reduced acute subjective effects of intravenous cocaine in a laboratory setting[102] and reduced cocaine use and craving in two of three small open-label outpatient clinical trials.[2, 17] However, two double-blind controlled clinical trials with fluoxetine did not find the medication more effective than placebo, even at plasma levels therapeutic for depression.[103]

5HT$_{1A}$ Agonists

The 5HT$_{1A}$ agonists buspirone and gepirone, developed as anxiolytics, were not effective in a small open-label trial[71] or multisite double-blind controlled clinical trial,[104] respectively. This finding contrasts with replicated results on the effectiveness of buspirone in the treatment of alcoholism (discussed earlier).

A preliminary report that the partial 5HT agonist m-chlorophenylpiperazine reduced cocaine craving in hospitalized cocaine addicts[105] suggests a possible role for 5HT$_{1A}$ receptors in mediating cocaine craving.

5HT$_2$ and 5HT$_3$ Antagonists

Ritanserin, a 5HT$_2$ antagonist developed as an antidepressant, reduces cocaine self-administration in animals[106] and some acute subjective effects of intravenous cocaine in a human laboratory setting.[107] Based on these promising results, ritanserin is currently undergoing several clinical trials as a pharmacotherapy for cocaine addiction. Ondansetron, a 5HT$_3$ antagonist, does not alter cocaine self-administration in animals[100] but does reduce some acute subjective effects of intravenous cocaine use in a human laboratory setting.[108]

OPIOID AGENTS

Opioid receptor antagonists such as naltrexone and naloxone reduce self-administration of drugs, including alcohol (discussed earlier) and nicotine,[109] in animals and humans. However, the extent of this influence on cocaine self-administration has not yet been demonstrated. Opioid receptor antagonists do not reduce cocaine self-administration in animals,[110] do not alter the acute subjective effects of intravenous cocaine in human laboratory settings,[111] and do not reduce cocaine use in outpatients dually dependent on both cocaine and alcohol.[112] No clinical trials of opioid antagonists in patients dependent only on cocaine have yet been conducted.

The role of opioid agents may differ in patients dually dependent on cocaine and opioids. Buprenorphine, a mixed or partial opioid agonist, reduces cocaine self-administration in animals[113] and is currently being evaluated as a treatment for opioid dependence. When used as an open-label maintenance treatment for opioid dependence, buprenorphine was reported to decrease concurrent cocaine use.[114] This effect, however, was not evident in double-blind clinical trials at doses up to 8 mg daily, levels that have been found to reduce opioid use significantly.[115, 116] Clinical experience suggests that higher buprenorphine doses of 12 to 16 mg daily might reduce cocaine use,[117] but this has not yet been confirmed by controlled clinical trials.

OTHER AGENTS

Various other medications have been tried for the treatment of cocaine dependence, often with little or no clinical evidence of efficacy.[68] Lithium has been tried because of reports that it could reduce the acute subjective effects of other stimulants. However, several studies suggest it is effective only in patients with comorbid bipolar disorder or cyclothymia.[118] The anticonvulsant carbamazepine, which blocks the development of cocaine-induced kindling in rodents, has been tried because of the hypothesis that kindling mediates cocaine craving in human cocaine users. Although several early open-label studies showed efficacy, this has not been confirmed by three double-blind controlled clinical trials.[121]

Calcium channel blockers, several of which remediate cardiovascular difficulties, have revealed potential in some animal and human laboratory studies. Their use is based on the known role of calcium influx in mediating neurotransmitter release, including release of dopamine.[119] In animal studies, calcium channel blockers have blocked cocaine-induced increases in brain dopamine and blocked or reduced behavioral effects of cocaine in some but not all studies.[119] In human laboratory studies, nifedipine and nimodipine were found to

block the acute subjective effects of intravenous cocaine administration[120] and to reduce cocaine craving,[121] respectively. However, two studies in clinical settings found that neither nifedipine nor diltiazem reduced cocaine use among outpatients,[71] nor did nimodipine reduce cocaine craving among inpatients.[122] Further advances may come from the development and use of blockers that target the N-type calcium channels specific to neurons rather than to cardiovascular tissue.

Another therapeutic approach beginning to undergo clinical evaluation is concurrent use of two different medications, with the goal of enhancing efficacy while minimizing side effects.[2] In addition to targeting a single neurotransmitter system by two different mechanisms, as described earlier for dopaminergic manipulations, this approach is being used to manipulate two different neurotransmitter systems concurrently. One medication combination that has generated promising open-label case reports is fenfluramine, which enhances serotonin activity, and phentermine, which enhances catecholamine activity.[123]

RESEARCH DIRECTIONS AND CONCLUSIONS

Of the agents studied to date, the most promising appear to be those that alter brain dopamine function, including dopamine agonists such as bromocriptine and pergolide, presynaptic releasers such as amantadine, and stimulants with low abuse potential such as pemoline. Preclinical research on selective dopamine receptor antagonists and on potent selective inhibitors of the presynaptic dopamine transporter (which can block cocaine binding without substantially interfering with dopamine transport[124]) should result in additional clinically useful agents. Serotonergic agents such as $5HT_2$ and $5HT_3$ antagonists and calcium channel blockers also show some promise in early studies. Further in the future, preclinical studies on other neurotransmitter receptor systems, such as excitatory amino acids (e.g., NMDA glutamate) and sigma receptors,[125] may eventually lead to development of new classes of therapeutic agents. Finally, as suggested earlier, research on combinations of medications may also prove useful.

Pharmacotherapies for Treatment of Opiate Abuse

Opiates have two major aspects that lead to initiation and maintenance of their use: They are strongly reinforcing, and they can produce a high degree of physical dependence. Medications currently exist to treat both these phenomena effectively. The two major approaches to treatment are the use of other agents to maintain dependence and attenuate the effects of illicit opiates and use of medications to alleviate discomfort associated with opiate withdrawal.

MAINTENANCE TREATMENT

The most effective pharmacological regimen for treatment of opiate dependence is opiate agonist maintenance therapy in which patients receive constant doses of the agonist at regular intervals from daily to every other day for months or years. Methadone and LAAM are the only opiate agonists yet approved in the United States for maintenance treatment. Maintenance administration of these long-acting agents attenuates the acute subjective effects of heroin and other illicit opiates through cross-tolerance. In addition, these agents decrease the intoxication/withdrawal cycle that occurs several times daily in individuals who are physically dependent on heroin.[126-128] Treatment retention and physiological stability afforded by agonist maintenance facilitate use of concurrent psychosocial or behavioral therapy that can be directed at improving patients' functioning and decreasing high-risk behaviors associated with transmission of human immunodeficiency virus. Opiate agonist maintenance has been shown to be effective in decreasing opiate and other illicit drug use, crime, and needle sharing and in retaining patients in treatment.[129-132]

An alternative to opiate agonist therapy is maintenance treatment with the opiate antagonist naltrexone. Naltrexone antagonizes opiates without itself producing physical dependence.[133] It is, however, not very useful as a maintenance agent.[134] Initiation of naltrexone therapy can be difficult because patients should be opiate free for approximately 1 week before naltrexone can be used, because it produces significant withdrawal in opiate-dependent individuals. In addition, compliance with treatment is low, probably because naltrexone does not produce any morphinelike subjective effects that might help retain patients in treatment.

The most promising new medication for treatment of opiate dependence is buprenorphine. Widely used as an analgesic, it is now being developed as a pharmacotherapy for opiate dependence in a joint effort by its manufacturer, Reckitt and Colman Pharmaceuticals, and the National Institute on Drug Abuse.[135]

Buprenorphine has a unique pharmacological profile that makes it suitable for opioid dependence treatment. It binds with high affinity to mu and kappa opioid receptors and acts as a partial agonist at the mu receptor and as an antagonist at the kappa receptor.[136] Because it is a partial mu agonist, buprenorphine, even in high doses, does not produce respiratory depression in healthy individuals.[136a] In addition, it can also act as an antagonist and precipitate withdrawal in opioid-dependent individuals under some conditions.[137] When given acutely, buprenorphine produces morphinelike subjective effects, substitutes for heroin, and suppresses opiate withdrawal.[138-140] It is active by intravenous, subcutaneous, intramuscular, and sublingual routes[136a, 141-143] and is administered sublingually in maintenance treatment with a potency ratio of 1.5 sublingual to subcutaneous. Buprenorphine has a long duration of action and thus needs to be taken only once every day or two.[144, 145]

The efficacy of buprenorphine as a maintenance medication has been well established by a number of clinical trials. A buprenorphine maintenance dose of 8 mg can be established within 3 days safely and with minimal withdrawal symptoms.[140] Daily administration of buprenorphine produces cross-tolerance and dose-related blockade of the subjective and physiological effects of opioids,[139, 146, 147] along with a decrease in heroin self-administration.[148, 149] In outpatient clinical trials, 8 mg/day of buprenorphine has proved as effective as 50 to 60 mg/day doses of methadone and superior to a lower methadone dose of 20 mg/day in treatment retention and decreasing opiate use.[115, 150] At least one trial, however, has found buprenorphine at doses of 2 and 6 mg/day less effective than methadone in the range of 35 to 65 mg/day.[151] Buprenorphine has low liability for producing physical dependence,[136] and unlike withdrawal from methadone treatment, cessation of buprenorphine maintenance leads to only relatively mild withdrawal.[139, 144, 148] Thus, as a maintenance agent, buprenorphine is safe, suppresses opiate withdrawal, blocks the effects of opioid agonists, does not require frequent or parenteral administration, decreases heroin use, retains patients in treatment, and can be withdrawn with relative ease.

Buprenorphine produces morphinelike subjective effects and thus may be abused. In fact, misuse of the analgesic preparation has been reported in a number countries.[152] Efforts to decrease likelihood of diversion and abuse of buprenorphine have centered on the addition of an opioid antagonists to the pharmaceutical preparation. Introduction of a buprenorphine/naloxone combination product in New Zealand has decreased but not completely suppressed buprenorphine abuse.[152] The abuse potential of a combination product may be low because, when administered parenterally, naloxone at least partially blocks the agonist effects of buprenorphine in nondependent opioid abusers[153] and produces withdrawal in patients receiving methadone maintenance.[154] However, buprenorphine binds more tightly to mu opioid receptors than methadone or heroin, and small doses of opiate antagonists can be administered to patients maintained on buprenorphine without precipitation of withdrawal.[155] Thus, patients could be switched from maintenance on buprenorphine alone to maintenance on a combination product with minimal difficulty. Development of a combination product for use in maintenance is under way.[135]

DETOXIFICATION

The second approach to treatment of opiate dependence is detoxification. Opiate detoxification is usually palliative in nature and not effective in the long term. It is, however, indicated in some situations, such as some medical conditions and very early in opiate dependence. Opiate agonists, including methadone, suppress withdrawal signs and symptoms and are usually prescribed in tapered doses to minimize patients' discomfort.[156] Clonidine is the only nonopiate to decrease signs of abstinence in opiate withdrawal.[157–159] It has become a mainstay in the medical treatment of opiate detoxification and is widely used by opiate addicts to self-treat their withdrawal. Clonidine has been used in combination with opiate antagonist administration to expedite detoxification and facilitate initiation of maintenance on naltrexone.[160]

Buprenorphine has been evaluated as a potential medication for facilitating transition from opiate dependence to a drug-free state and appears safe and efficacious in suppressing withdrawal in opiate detoxification. Buprenorphine is as effective as methadone in outpatients gradually detoxified from heroin over 90 days, with no differences between buprenorphine- and methadone-treated groups in retention, self-reported withdrawal, and drug use.[146] Gradual tapering of the buprenorphine dose is superior to rapid taper in suppressing withdrawal symptoms and illicit opiate use

and maintaining treatment retention in outpatients.[161] In short inpatient detoxification from heroin, buprenorphine given in a 3-day, dose-tapering regimen produces greater suppression of withdrawal symptoms early in treatment and less hypotensive effects than a 5-day clonidine regimen.[162] Further research is under way to evaluate detoxification with buprenorphine in patients hospitalized for medical reasons and in developing procedures for initiating antagonist pharmacotherapy. Combination treatment with buprenorphine and the opioid antagonist naltrexone appears to increase the magnitude acutely but decrease the overall duration of withdrawal[163] and may facilitate transition to naltrexone maintenance.[164]

Finally, analogues of dynorphin, an endogenous peptide with kappa agonist activity, are being evaluated for treating detoxification. Dynorphin analogues have shown effectiveness in attenuating withdrawal in morphine-dependent rats and rhesus monkeys[165, 166] and in heroin addicts.[167]

RESEARCH DIRECTIONS AND CONCLUSIONS

Considerable progress has been made in developing pharmacotherapies for opiate dependence. Methadone and LAAM can substitute for illicit opiates, relieving drug craving, blocking effects of opiates of dependence, and enhancing participation in psychosocial treatment programs. Buprenorphine shares these properties and allows rather easy withdrawal. Future research should be conducted to develop other agents that require even less frequent administration and have no abuse potential. As in the use of agents to decrease drinking and use of cocaine, it is also important to identify more precisely the subtypes of opiate abusers who will respond most favorably to the substitute agents and what types of conjunct medication-psychosocial interventions are most effective. Finally, research on how drug-taking lifestyle and psychological variables contribute to the desire to engage in illicit opiate use may also lead to development of new types of medications that address these needs.

Conclusion

Several topics related to pharmacotherapy for substance addiction require further research attention. Most importantly, we need to specify how medications should be integrated with psychosocial interventions to optimize patient-treatment matching. Although some studies suggest that the potential therapeutic contribution of a medication may be overwhelmed by a particularly potent psychosocial treatment regimen,[24] others suggest that the effect of a psychotherapeutic may be modified by the type of behavioral intervention with which it is combined.[9] Further, some agents may enhance the psychosocial treatment by improving retention of patients, as may be the case for opiate agonist maintenance treatment for opiate dependence. Research on counseling and behavioral therapies for alcoholism clearly suggests that different subtypes of alcoholic patients respond differentially to alternative therapies.[168] Growing evidence demonstrates that medications may also display such patient-treatment matching effects—for example, that antidepressants are more effective in substance addicts suffering comorbid depression and less effective in those with antisocial personality disorder. Thus, it is important in future research to identify not only the main effect of the pharmacological intervention but also its differential effects on various subtypes of patients and its interaction with different types of psychosocial interventions.

Dose-response relationships, duration of administration, effects of medications on various outcome measures, and underlying pharmacodynamics for various agents must also be further delineated.

The field of pharmacotherapy for substance addiction is still in early stages. Nevertheless, the progress achieved suggests that future research will yield great benefits in enhancing treatment effectiveness.

REFERENCES

1. Gorelick DA: Overview of pharmacologic treatment approaches for alcohol and other drug addiction: Intoxication, withdrawal, and relapse prevention. Psychiatr Clin North Am 16(1):141–156, 1993.
2. Gorelick DA: Pharmacological therapies of cocaine addiction. In Miller NS, Gold MS (eds): Pharmacological Therapies for Drug and Alcohol Addictions, New York, Marcel Dekker, 1995, pp 143–157.
3. Myers RD: New drugs for the treatment of experimental alcoholism. Alcohol 11:439–451, 1994.
4. Gorelick DA: Pharmacological treatment. Recent Dev Alcohol 11:413–427, 1993.
5. Litten RZ, Allen JP: Reducing the desire to drink: Pharmacology and neurobiology. In Galanter M (ed): Recent Developments in Alcoholism, vol 11: Ten Years of Progress. New York, Plenum, 1993, pp 325–344.
6. Froehlich JC, Li TK: Opioid peptides. In Galanter M (ed): Recent Developments in Alcoholism, vol 11: Ten Years of Progress. New York, Plenum, 1993, pp 187–206.
7. Volpicelli JR, Clay KL, Watson NT, et al: Naltrexone and the treatment of alcohol dependence. Alcohol Health and Research World 18:272–278, 1994.
8. Volpicelli JR, Alterman AI, Hayashida M, et al: Naltrexone in the treatment of alcohol dependence. Arch Gen Psychiatry 49:876–880, 1992.
9. O'Malley SS, Jaffe AJ, Chang G, et al: Naltrexone and coping skills therapy for alcohol dependence. Arch Gen Psychiatry 49:881–887, 1992.
10. Volpicelli JR, O'Brien CP, Watson NT: Naltrexone therapy for alcoholism: Recent findings. Presented at American Psychiatric Association Annual Meeting, Philadelphia, PA, May 1994.
11. Bohn MJ, Kranzler HR, Beazoglou D, et al: Naltrexone and brief counseling to reduce heavy drinking. Am J Addict 3:91–99, 1994.
12. Volpicelli JR, Watson NT, King AC, et al: Effect of naltrexone on alcohol "high" in alcoholics. Am J Psychiatry 152:613–615, 1995.
13. Swift RM, Whelihan W, Kuznetsov O, et al: Naltrexone-induced alterations in human ethanol intoxication. Am J Psychiatry 151:1463–1467, 1994.
14. Mason BJ, Ritvo EC, Morgan RO, et al: A double-blind, placebo-controlled pilot study to evaluate the efficacy and safety of oral nalmefene HCl for alcohol dependence. Alcohol Clin Exp Res 18:1162–1167, 1994.
15. Gorelick DA: Serotonin uptake blockers in the treatment of alcoholism. Recent Dev Alcohol 7:267–281, 1989.
16. LeMarquand D, Pihl RO, Benkelfat C: Serotonin and alcohol intake abuse, and dependence: Clinical evidence. Biol Psychiatry 36:326–337, 1994.
17. Gorelick DA: Pharmacologic therapies for cocaine and other stimulant addiction. In Miller NS (ed): Principles of Addiction Medicine. Washington, DC, American Society of Addiction Medicine, 1994.
18. Naranjo CA, Sellers EM, Roach CA, et al: Zimelidine-induced variations in alcohol intake by nondepressed heavy drinkers. Clin Pharmacol Ther 35:374–381, 1984.
19. Naranjo CA, Sellers EM, Sullivan JT, et al: The serotonin uptake inhibitor citalopram attenuates ethanol intake. Clin Pharmacol Ther 41:266–274, 1987.
20. Naranjo CA, Sullivan JT, Kadlec KE, et al: Differential effects of viqualine on alcohol intake and other consummatory behaviors. Clin Pharmacol Ther 46:301–309, 1989.
21. Naranjo CA, Kadlec KE, Sanhueza P, et al: Fluoxetine differentially alters alcohol intake and other consummatory behaviors in problem drinkers. Clin Pharmacol Ther 47:490–498, 1990.
22. Naranjo CA, Poulos CX, Bremner KE, et al: Citalopram decreases desirability, liking, and consumption of alcohol in alcohol-dependent drinkers. Clin Pharmacol Ther 51:729–739, 1992.
23. Balldin J, Berggren U, Bokstrom K, et al: Six-month open trial with zimelidine in alcohol-dependent patients: Reduction in days of alcohol intake. Drug Alcohol Depend 35:245–248, 1994.
24. Kranzler HR, Burleson JA, Korner P, et al: Placebo-controlled trial of fluoxetine as an adjunct to relapse prevention in alcoholics. Am J Psychiatry 152:391–397, 1995.
25. Gerra G, Caccavari R, Delsignore R, et al: Effects of fluoxetine and Ca-acetyl-homotaurinate on alcohol intake in familial and nonfamilial alcoholic patients. Curr Ther Res 52:291–295, 1992.
26. Kranzler HR, Del Boca F, Korner P, et al: Adverse effects limit the usefulness of fluvoxamine for the

treatment of alcoholism. J Subst Abuse Treat 10:283–287, 1993.

27. Balldin J, Berggren U, Engel J, et al: Effect of citalopram on alcohol intake in heavy drinkers. Alcohol Clin Exp Res 18:1133–1136, 1994.
28. Naranjo CA, Bremner KE, Lanctot KL: Effects of citalopram and a brief psycho-social intervention on alcohol intake, dependence and problems. Addiction 90:87–99, 1995.
29. Gorelick DA, Paredes A: Effect of fluoxetine on alcohol consumption in male alcoholics. Alcohol Clin Exp Res 16:261–265, 1992.
30. Cornelius JR, Salloum IM, Cornelius MD, et al: Fluoxetine trial in suicidal depressed alcoholics. Psychopharmacol Bull 29:195–199, 1993.
31. Cornelius JR, Salloum IM, Cornelius MD, et al: Fluoxetine vs. placebo in depressed alcoholics. Presented at the meeting of New Clinical Drug Evaluation Unit (NCDEU), Marco Island, FL, June 1994.
32. Nissbrandt H, Waters N, Hjorth S: The influence of serotoninergic drugs on dopaminergic neurotransmission in rat substantia nigra, striatum and limbic forebrain in vivo. Naunyn Schmiedebergs Arch Pharmacol 346:12–19, 1992.
33. Knapp DJ, Benjamin D, Pohoreck LA: Effects of gepirone on ethanol consumption, exploratory behavior, and motor performance in rats. Drug Dev Res 26:319–341, 1992.
34. McBride WJ, Murphy JM, Lumeng L, et al: Serotonin, dopamine, and GABA involvement in alcohol drinking of selectively bred rats. Alcohol 7:199–205, 1990.
35. Singh GK, Kalmus GW, Bjork AK, et al: Alcohol drinking in rats is attenuated by the mixed 5-HT$_1$ agonist/5-HT$_2$ antagonist FG 5893. Alcohol 10:243–248, 1993.
36. Svensson L, Fahlke C, Hard E, et al: Involvement of the serotonergic system in ethanol intake in the rat. Alcohol 10:219–224, 1993.
37. Mattila MJ, Aranko K, Seppala T: Acute effects of buspirone and alcohol on psychomotor skills. J Clin Psychiatry 43(12):56–60, 1982.
38. Smiley A, Moskowitz H: Effects of long-term administration of buspirone and diazepam on driver steering control. Am J Med 80 (Suppl 3B):22–29, 1986.
39. Taylor DP, Eison MS, Riblet LA: Pharmacological and clinical effects of buspirone. Pharmacol Biochem Behav 23:687–694, 1985.
40. Bruno F: Buspirone in the treatment of alcoholic patients. Psychopathology 22 (Suppl 1):49–59, 1989.
41. Kranzler HR, Meyer RE: An open trial of buspirone in alcoholics. J Clin Psychopharmacol 9:379–380, 1989.
42. Kranzler HR, Burleson JA, Del Boca FK, et al: Buspirone treatment in anxious alcoholics: A placebo-controlled trial. Arch Gen Psychiatry 51:720–731, 1994.
43. Tollefson GD, Montague-Clouse J, Tollefson SL: Treatment of comorbid generalized anxiety in a recently detoxified alcoholic population with a selective serotonergic drug (buspirone). J Clin Psychopharmacol 12:19–26, 1992.
44. Malcolm R, Anton RF, Randall CL, et al: A placebo-controlled trial of buspirone in anxious inpatient alcoholics. Alcohol Clin Exp Res 16:1007–1013, 1992.
45. Panocka I, Pompei P, Massi M: Suppression of alcohol preference in rats induced by risperidone, a serotonin 5-HT$_2$ and dopamine D$_2$ receptor antagonist. Brain Res Bull 31:595–599, 1993.
46. Myers RD, Lankford MF, Bjork A: 5-HT$_2$ receptor blockage by amperozide suppresses ethanol drinking in genetically preferring rats. Pharmacol Biochem Behav 45:741–747, 1993.
47. Panocka I, Massi M: Long-lasting suppression of alcohol preference in rats following serotonin receptor blockade by ritanserin. Brain Res Bull 28:493–496, 1992.
48. Meert TF, Janssen PAJ: Ritanserin, a new therapeutic approach for drug abuse. Part 1: Effects on alcohol. Drug Dev Res 24:235–249, 1991.
49. Monti JM, Alterwain P: Ritanserin decreases alcohol intake in chronic alcoholics. Lancet 337:60, 1991.
50. Oakley NR, Jones BJ, Tyers MB, et al: The effect of GR38032 on alcohol consumption in the marmoset. Br J Pharmacol 95:870P, 1988.
51. Hodge CW, Samson HH, Lewis RS, et al: Specific decreases in ethanol- but not water-reinforced responding produced by the 5-HT$_3$ antagonist ICS 205-930. Alcohol 10:191–196, 1993.
52. Johnson BA, Cowen PJ: Alcohol-induced reinforcement: Dopamine and 5-HT$_3$ receptor interactions in animals and humans. Drug Dev Res 30:153–169, 1993.
53. Sellers EM, Toneatto T, Romach MK, et al: Clinical efficacy of the 5-HT$_3$ antagonist ondansetron in alcohol abuse and dependence. Alcohol Clin Exp Res 18:879–885, 1994.
54. Lhuintre JP, Daoust M, Moore ND, et al: Ability of calcium bis acetyl homotaurine, a GABA agonist, to prevent relapse in weaned alcoholics. Lancet 1:1014–1016, 1985.
55. Lhuintre JP, Moore N, Tran G, et al: Acamprosate appears to decrease alcohol intake in weaned alcoholics. Alcohol 25:613–622, 1990.
56. Gallimberti L, Ferri M, Davide S, et al: Gamma-hydroxybutyric acid in the treatment of alcohol dependence: A double-blind study. Alcohol Clin Exp Res 16:673–676, 1992.
57. Koob GF: Drugs of abuse: Anatomy, pharmacology and function of reward pathways. Trends Pharmacol Sci 13:177–184, 1992.
58. Ng GY, George SR: Dopamine receptor agonist reduces ethanol self-administration in the ethanol-preferring C57BL/6J inbred mouse. Eur J Pharmacol 269:365–374, 1994.
59. Pfeffer AO, Samson HH: Haloperidol and apomorphine effects on ethanol reinforcement in free feeding rats. Pharmacol Biochem Behav 29:343–350, 1988.
60. Dyr W, McBride WJ, Lumeng L, et al: Effects of D$_1$ and D$_2$ dopamine receptor agents on ethanol consumption in the high-alcohol-drinking (HAD) line of rats. Alcohol 10:207–212, 1993.
61. Rassnick S, Pulvirenti L, Koob GF: SDZ-205, 152, a novel dopamine receptor agonist, reduces oral ethanol self-administration in rats. Alcohol 10:127–132, 1993.
62. Rassnick S, Pulvirenti L, Koob GF: Oral ethanol self-administration in rats is reduced by the administration of dopamine and glutamate receptor antagonists into the nucleus accumbens. Psychopharmacology 109:92–98, 1992.
63. Borg V: Bromocriptine in the prevention of alcohol abuse. Acta Psychiatr Scand 68:100–110, 1983.
64. Dongier M, Vachon L, Schwartz G: Bromocriptine in the treatment of alcohol dependence. Alcohol Clin Exp Res 15:970–977, 1991.
65. Shaw GK, Majumdar SK, Waller S, et al: Tiapride in the long-term management of alcoholics of anxious or depressive temperament. Br J Psychiatry 150:164–168, 1987.
66. Shaw GK, Waller S, Majumdar SK, et al: Tiapride in the prevention of relapse in recently detoxified alcoholics. Br J Psychiatry 165:515–523, 1994.
67. Tsai G, Gastfriend DR, Coyle JT: The glutamatergic basis of human alcoholism. Am J Psychiatry 152:332–340, 1995.

68. Gorelick DA, Halikas JA, Crosby RD: Pharmacotherapy of cocaine dependence in the United States: Comparing scientific evidence and clinical practice. Substance Abuse 15:209–213, 1994.

69. Johanson CE, Fischman MW: The pharmacology of cocaine related to its abuse. Pharmacol Rev 41:3–52, 1989.

70. Gawin FH, Riordan CA, Kleber HD: Methylphenidate use in non-ADD cocaine abusers—a negative study. Am J Drug Alcohol Abuse 11:193–197, 1985.

71. Tennant F, Tarver A, Sagherian A, et al: A placebo-controlled elimination study to identify potential treatment agents for cocaine detoxification. Am J Addict 2:299–308, 1993.

72. Khantzian EJ, Gawin FH, Riordan C, et al: Methylphenidate treatment of cocaine dependence: A preliminary report. J Subst Abuse Treat 1:107–112, 1984.

73. Weiss RD, Pope HG, Mirin SM: Treatment of chronic cocaine abuse and attention deficit disorder, residual type, with magnesium pemoline. Drug Alcohol Depend 15:69–72, 1985.

74. Alim TN, Rosse RB, Vocci FJ Jr, et al: Diethylpropion pharmacotherapeutic adjuvant therapy for inpatient treatment of cocaine dependence: A test of the cocaine-agonist hypothesis. Clin Neuropharmacol 18:183–195, 1995.

75. Berger R, Fawin F, Kosten TR: Treatment of cocaine abuse with mazindol. Lancet 1:283, 1989.

76. Kosten TR, Steinberg M, Diakogiannis IA: Crossover trial of mazindol for cocaine dependence. Am J Addict 2:161, 1993.

77. Kosten TA, Kosten TR: Pharmacological blocking agents for treating substance abuse. J Nerv Ment Dis 179:583–592, 1991.

78. Preston KL, Sullivan JT, Berger P, et al: Effects of cocaine alone and in combination with mazindol in human cocaine abusers. J Pharmacol Exp Ther 207:296–307, 1993.

79. Sherer MA, Kumor KM, Jaffe JH: Effects of intravenous cocaine are partially attenuated by haloperidol. Psychiatr Res 27:117–125, 1989.

80. Gawin FH: Neuroleptic reduction of cocaine-induced paranoia but not euphoria? Psychopharmacology 90:142–143, 1986.

81. Gawin FH, Khalsa ME, Brown J, et al: Flupenthixol treatment of crack users: Initial double-blind results. NIDA Res Monogr 132:319, 1993.

82. Decker KP, Ries RK: Differential diagnosis and psychopharmacology of dual disorders. Psychiatr Clin North Am 16:703–718, 1993.

83. Kosten TR, Kleber HD: Rapid death during cocaine abuse: A variant of the neuroleptic malignant syndrome? Am J Drug Alcohol Abuse 12:335–346, 1988.

84. Goldfrank LR, Hoffman RS: The cardiovascular effects of cocaine. Ann Emerg Med 20:165–175, 1991.

85. Dackis CA, Gold MS: Pharmacological approaches to cocaine addiction. J Subst Abuse Treat 2:139–145, 1985.

86. Chadwick MJ, Gregory DL: A double-blind amino acids, L-tryptophan and L-tyrosine, and placebo study with cocaine-dependent subjects in an inpatient chemical dependency treatment center. Am J Drug Alcohol Abuse 16:275–286, 1990.

87. Bakht FR, Kirshon B, Baker T, et al: Postpartum cardiovascular complications after bromocriptine and cocaine use. Am J Obstet Gynecol 162:1065–1066, 1990.

88. Zimmerman T, Sage J: Comparison of combination pergolide and levodopa to levodopa alone after 63 months of treatment. Clin Neuropharmacol 14:165–169, 1991.

89. Montoya ID, Preston KL, Cone EJ, et al: Safety and efficacy of bupropion combined with bromocriptine for treatment of cocaine dependence. Am J Addict 5:69–75, 1996.

90. Brewer C: Treatment of cocaine abuse with monoamine oxidase inhibitors. Br J Psychiatry 163:815–816, 1993.

91. Gawin FH, Kleber HD, Byck R, et al: Desipramine facilitation of initial cocaine abstinence. Arch Gen Psychiatry 46:117–121, 1989.

92. Levin FR, Lehman AF: Meta analysis of desipramine as an adjunct in the treatment of cocaine addiction. J Clin Psychopharmacol 11:374–378, 1991.

93. Ziedonis DM, Kosten TR: Pharmacotherapy improves treatment outcome in depressed cocaine addicts. J Psychoactive Drugs 23:417–425, 1991.

94. Arndt IO, McLellan AT, Dorzynsky L, et al: Desipramine treatment for cocaine dependence. J Nerv Ment Dis 182(3):151–156, 1994.

95. Khalsa ME, Gawin FH, Rawson R, et al: A desipramine ceiling in cocaine abusers. NIDA Res Monogr 132:318, 1993.

96. Weiss RD, Mirin SM: Tricyclic antidepressants in the treatment of alcoholism and drug abuse. J Clin Psychiatry 50 (Suppl 7):4–9, 1989.

97. Kosten TR, Gawin FH, Morgan C, et al: Evidence for altered desipramine disposition in methadone-maintained patients treated for cocaine abuse. Am J Alcohol Drug Abuse 16:329–336, 1990.

98. Brotman AW, Witkie SM, Gelenberg AJ, et al: An open trial of maprotiline for the treatment of cocaine abuse. J Clin Psychopharmacology 8:125–127, 1988.

99. Rosecan JS: The treatment of cocaine abuse with imipramine, L-tyrosine and L-tryptophan. Presented at the Seventh World Congress of Psychiatry, Vienna, Austria, July 13–19, 1983.

100. Sellers EM, Higgins GA, Tomkins DM, et al: Opportunities for treatment of psychoactive substance use disorders with serotonergic medications. J Clin Psychiatry 52 (Suppl 12):49–54, 1991.

101. Spealman RD: Modification of behavioral effects of cocaine by selective serotonin and dopamine uptake inhibitors in squirrel monkeys. Psychopharmacology 112:93–99, 1993.

102. Walsh SL, Preston KL, Sullivan JT, et al: Fluoxetine alters the effects of intravenous cocaine in humans. J Clin Psychopharmacol 14:396–407, 1994.

103. Covi L, Hess JM, Kreiter NA, Haertzen CA: Effects of combined fluoxetine and counseling in the outpatient treatment of cocaine abusers. Am J Drug Alcohol Abuse 21:327–344, 1995.

104. Jenkins SW, Warfield NA, Blaine JD, et al: A pilot trial of gepirone vs. placebo in the treatment of cocaine dependency. Psychopharmacol Bull 28:21–26, 1992.

105. Branchey M, Buydens-Branchey L: Decrease in cocaine craving after administration of serotonin agonist M-CPP. Biol Psychiatry 33:152A, 1993.

106. McMillen BA, Jones EA, Hill LJ, et al: Amperozide, a 5-HT$_2$ antagonist, attenuates craving for cocaine by rats. Pharmacol Biochem Behav 46:125–129, 1993.

107. Sullivan JT, Testa MP, Preston KL, et al: Psychoactivity of ritanserin and its interaction with intravenous cocaine. NIDA Res Monogr 141:377, 1994.

108. Sullivan JT, Jasinski DR, Preston KL, et al: Cocaine blocking effects of ondansetron. NIDA Res Monogr 119:466, 1992.

109. Gorelick DA, Rose JE, Jarvik ME: Effect of naloxone on cigarette smoking. J Subst Abuse 1:153–159, 1989.

110. Stine SM, Freeman M, Burns B: Effect of methadone dose on cocaine abuse in a methadone program. Am J Addict 1:294–303, 1992.

111. Walsh SL, Sullivan JT, Preston KL, et al: Naltrexone

interactions with cocaine, hydromorphone, and a "speedball" combination in substance abuses. NIDA Res Monogr 141:26, 1994.

112. Carroll KM, Ziedonis D, O'Malley S, et al: Pharmacologic interventions for alcohol- and cocaine-abusing individuals. Am J Addict 2:77–79, 1993.

113. Mello NK, Mendelson JH, Lukas SE, et al: Buprenorphine treatment of opiate and cocaine abuse: Clinical and preclinical studies. Harvard Rev Psychiatry 1:168–183, 1993.

114. Gastfriend DR, Mendelson JH, Mello NK, et al: Buprenorphine pharmacotherapy for concurrent heroin and cocaine dependence. Am J Addict 2:269–278, 1993.

115. Johnson RE, Jaffe JH, Fudala PJ: A controlled trial of buprenorphine treatment for opioid dependence. JAMA 267:2750–2755, 1992.

116. Kosten TR, Rosen MI, Schottenfeld R, et al: Buprenorphine for cocaine and opiate dependence. Psychopharmacol Bull 28:15–19, 1992.

117. Schottenfeld R, Pakes J, Ziedonis D, et al: Buprenorphine: Dose-related effects on cocaine and opioid use in cocaine-abusing opioid-dependent humans. Biol Psychiatry 34:66–74, 1993.

118. Nunes EV, McGrath PJ, Wager S, et al: Lithium treatment for cocaine abusers with bipolar spectrum disorders. Am J Psychiatry 147:655–657, 1990.

119. Schindler CW, Tella SR, Prada J, et al: Calcium channel blockers antagonize some of cocaine's cardiovascular effects, but fail to alter cocaine's behavioral effects. J Pharmacol Exp Ther 272:791–798, 1995.

120. Muntaner C, Kumor KM, Nagoshi C, et al: Effects of nifedipine pretreatment on subjective and cardiovascular responses to intravenous cocaine in humans. Psychopharmacology 105:37–41, 1991.

121. Montoya ID, Levin FR, Fudala PJ, et al: Double-blind comparison of carbamazepine and placebo for treatment of cocaine dependence. Drug Alcohol Depend 38:213–219, 1995.

122. Rosse RB, Alim TN, Fay-McCarthy M, et al: Nimodipine pharmacotherapeutic adjuvant therapy for inpatient treatment of cocaine dependence. Clin Neuropharmacol 17:348–358, 1994.

123. Rothman RB, Gendron T, Hitzig P: Combined use of fenfluramine and phentermine in the treatment of cocaine addiction. J Subst Abuse Treat 11:273–275, 1994.

124. Baumann MH, Char GU, De Costa BR, et al: GBR12909 attenuates cocaine-induced activation of mesolimbic dopamine neurons in the rat. J Pharmacol Exp Ther 271:1216–1222, 1994.

125. Witkin JM: Pharmacotherapy of cocaine abuse: Preclinical development. Neurosci Biobehav Rev 18:121–142, 1994.

126. Dole VP, Nyswander ME, Kreek MJ: Narcotic blockade. Arch Intern Med 118:304–309, 1966.

127. Goldstein A: Heroin addiction and the role of methadone in its treatment. Arch Gen Psychiatry 26:291–297, 1972.

128. Martin WR, Jasinski DR, Haertzen CA: Methadone—a reevaluation. Arch Gen Psychiatry 28:286–295, 1973.

129. Ball J, Corty E, Bond H, et al: The reduction of intravenous heroin use, non-opiate abuse and crime during methadone maintenance treatment: Further findings. In Harris LS (ed): Problems of Drug Dependence, 1987: Proceedings of the 49th Annual Scientific Meeting, The Committee on Problems of Drug Dependence, Inc. NIDA Res Monogr 81:224–225, 1988.

130. Ball J, Lange WR, Myers CP, et al: Reducing the risk of AIDS through methadone maintenance. J Health Soc Behav 29:214–226, 1988.

131. Cooper JR: Methadone treatment and acquired immunodeficiency syndrome. JAMA 262:1664–1668, 1989.

132. Strain EC, Stitzer ML, Liebson IA, et al: Dose-response effects of methadone in the treatment of opioid dependence. Ann Intern Med 119:23–27, 1993.

133. Martin WR, Jasinski DR, Mansky PA: Naltrexone, an antagonist for the treatment of heroin dependence. Arch Gen Psychiatry 28:784–791, 1973.

134. Gonzalez JP, Brogden RN: Naltrexone: A review of its pharmacodynamic and pharmacokinetic properties and therapeutic efficacy in the management of opioid dependence. Drugs 35:192–213, 1988.

135. Segal DL, Schuster CR: Buprenorphine: What interests the National Institute on Drug Abuse? In Cowan A, Lewis JW (eds): Buprenorphine: Combating Drug Abuse with a Unique Opioid. New York: Wiley-Liss, 1995, pp 309–320.

136. Cowan A: Update on the general pharmacology of buprenorphine. In Cowan A, Lewis JW (eds): Buprenorphine: Combating Drug Abuse with a Unique Opioid. New York, Wiley-Liss, 1995, pp 309–320.

136a. Walsh SL, Preston KL, Stitzer ML, et al: Clinical pharmacology of buprenorphine: Ceiling effects at high doses. Clin Pharmacol Ther 55:569–580, 1994.

137. Strain EC, Preston KL, Liebson IA, et al: Buprenorphine effects in methadone-maintained volunteers: Effects at two hours after methadone. J Pharmacol Exp Ther 272:628–638, 1995.

138. Banys P, Clark HW, Tusel DJ, et al: An open trial of low dose buprenorphine in treating methadone withdrawal. J Subst Abuse Treat 11:9–15, 1994.

139. Jasinski DR, Pevnick JS, Griffith JD: Human pharmacology and abuse potential of the analgesic buprenorphine. Arch Gen Psychiatry 35:501–516, 1978.

140. Johnson RE, Cone EJ, Henningfield JE, et al: Use of buprenorphine in the treatment of opioid addiction. I. Physiologic and behavioral effects during a rapid dose induction. Clin Pharmacol Ther 46:335–343, 1989.

141. Pickworth WB, Johnson RE, Holicky BA, et al: Subjective and physiologic effects of intravenous buprenorphine in humans. Clin Pharmacol Ther 53:570–576, 1993.

142. Jasinski DR, Fudala PJ, Johnson RE: Sublingual versus subcutaneous buprenorphine in opiate abusers. Clin Pharmacol Ther 45:513–519, 1989.

143. Preston KL, Bigelow GE, Bickel WK, et al: Drug discrimination in human postaddicts: Agonist-antagonist opioids. J Pharmacol Exp Ther 250:184–196, 1989.

144. Fudala PJ, Jaffe JH, Dax EM, et al: Use of buprenorphine in the treatment of opioid addiction. II. Physiological and behavioral effects of daily and alternate-day administration and abrupt withdrawal. Clin Pharmacol Ther 47:525–534, 1990.

145. Amass L, Bickel WK, Higgins ST, et al: Alternate-day dosing during buprenorphine treatment of opioid dependence. Life Sci 54:1215–1228, 1994.

146. Bickel WK, Stitzer ML, Bigelow GE, et al: A clinical trial of buprenorphine: Comparison with methadone in the detoxification of heroin addicts. Clin Pharmacol Ther 43:72–78, 1988.

147. Bickel WK, Stitzer ML, Bigelow GE, et al: Buprenorphine: Dose-related blockade of opioid challenge effects in opioid dependent humans. J Pharmacol Exp Ther 247:47–53, 1988.

148. Mello NK, Mendelson JH: Buprenorphine suppresses heroin use by heroin addicts. Science 207:657–659, 1980.

149. Mello NK, Mendelson JH, Huehnle JC: Buprenorphine effects on human heroin self-administration. J Pharmacol Exp Ther 223:30–39, 1982.

150. Strain EC, Stitzer ML, Liebson IA, et al: Comparison of buprenorphine and methadone in the treatment of opioid dependence. Am J Psychiatry 151:1025–1030, 1994.
151. Kosten TR, Schottenfeld R, Ziedonis D, et al: Buprenorphine versus methadone maintenance for opioid dependence. J Nerv Ment Dis 181:358–364, 1993.
152. Robinson GM, Dukes PD, Robinson BJ, et al: The misuse of buprenorphine and a buprenorphine-naloxone combination in Wellington, New Zealand. Drug Alcohol Depend 33:81–86, 1993.
153. Weinhold LL, Preston KL, Farre M, et al: Buprenorphine alone and in combination with naloxone in non-dependent humans. Drug Alcohol Depend 30:263–274, 1992.
154. Preston KL, Bigelow GE, Liebson IA: Buprenorphine and naloxone alone and in combination in opioid-dependent humans. Psychopharmacology 94:484–490, 1988.
155. Kosten TR, Krystal JH, Charney DS, et al: Opioid antagonist challenges in buprenorphine maintained patients. Drug Alcohol Depend 25:73–78, 1990.
156. Fishbain DA, Rosomoff HL, Cutler R, Rosomoff RS: Opiate detoxification protocols: A clinical manual. Ann Clin Psychiatry 5:53–65, 1993.
157. Charney DS, Sternberg DE, Kleber HD, et al: The clinical use of clonidine in abrupt withdrawal from methadone. Arch Gen Psychiatry 38:1273–1277, 1981.
158. Gold MS, Pottash AM, Sweeney DR, et al: Opiate withdrawal using clonidine: A safe, effective, and rapid nonopiate treatment. JAMA 243:343–346, 1980.
159. Jasinski DR, Johnson RE, Kocher TR: Clonidine in morphine withdrawal: Differential effects on signs and symptoms. Arch Gen Psychiatry 42:1063–1066, 1985.
160. Charney DS, Heninger GR, Kleber HD: The combined use of clonidine and naltrexone as a rapid, safe, and effective treatment of abrupt withdrawal from methadone. Am J Psychiatry 143:831–837, 1986.
161. Amass L, Bickel WK, Higgins ST, et al: A preliminary investigation of outcome following gradual or rapid buprenorphine detoxification. In Magura S, Rosenblum A (eds): Experimental Therapeutics in Addiction Medicine. Binghamton, NY, Haworth Press, 1994, pp 33–45.
162. Cheskin LJ, Fudala PF, Johnson RE: A controlled comparison of buprenorphine and clonidine for acute detoxification from opioids. Drug Alcohol Depend 36:115–121, 1994.
163. Montoya ID, Mann DJ, Ellison PA, et al: Inpatient medically supervised opioid withdrawal with buprenorphine alone and in combination with naltrexone. Clin Pharmacol Ther 55:131, 1994.
164. Rosen M, Kosten TR: Detoxification and induction onto naltrexone. In Cowan A, Lewis JW (eds): Buprenorphine: Combating Drug Abuse with a Unique Opioid. New York, Wiley-Liss, 1995, pp 289–305.
165. Green PG, Lee NM: Dynorphin A- (1–13) attenuates withdrawal in morphine-dependent rats: Effect of route of administration. Eur J Pharmacol 145:267–272, 1988.
166. Bowman ER, Aceto MD: Dynorphine- (2–17) suppressed withdrawal in morphine-dependent rhesus monkeys. In Harris LS (ed): Problems of Drug Dependence, 1993: Proceedings of the 55th Annual Scientific Meeting, The Committee on Problems of Drug Dependence, Inc. NIDA Res Monogr 141:108, 1994.
167. Wen HL, Ho WKK: Suppression of withdrawal symptoms by dynorphin in heroin addicts. Eur J Pharmacol 82:183–186, 1982.
168. Mattson ME, Allen JP, Longabaugh R: A chronological review of empirical studies matching alcoholic clients to treatment. J Stud Alcohol 12 (Suppl):16–29, 1994.

INDEX

Note: Page numbers in *italics* indicate figures; those with a t indicate tables.

ISBN 0-7216-5211-5